Workbook
EMERGENCY
CARE

14th Edition

Workbook
EMERGENCY CARE

14th Edition

BOB ELLING

DANIEL LIMMER | MICHAEL F. O'KEEFE

MEDICAL EDITOR
EDWARD T. DICKINSON, MD, FACEP

LEGACY AUTHORS

Harvey D. Grant | Robert H. Murray, Jr. | J. David Bergeron

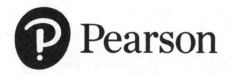

Pearson

Senior Vice President, Product Management: Adam Jaworski
Director, Product Management: Katrin Beacom
Content Manager: Kevin Wilson
Development Editor: Rachel Bedard
Vice President, Content Production and Digital Studio:
   Caroline Power
Managing Producer, Health Science: Melissa Bashe
Content Producer: Faye Gemmellaro
Operations Specialist: Maura Zaldivar-Garcia
Director, Digital Production: Amy Peltier
Digital Studio Producer: William Johnson
Digital Content Team Lead: Brian Prybella
Product Marketing Coordinator: Brian Hoehl

Full-Service Project Management and Composition:
   SPi Global
Inventory Manager: Vatche Demirdjian
Manager, Rights & Permissions: Gina Cheselka
Interior and Cover Design: Studio Montage
Cover Art: Pearson photo by Michal Heron
Managing Photography Editor: Michal Heron
Photographers: Michal Heron, Kevin Link, Maria Lyle,
   Isaac Turner
Back Cover Photo: © Daniel Limmer
Printer/Binder: LSC Communications, Inc.
Cover Printer: Phoenix Color/Hagerstown

Notice on Care Procedures

It is the intent of the authors and publisher that this text be used as part of a formal Emergency Medical Technician (EMT) education program taught by qualified instructors and supervised by a licensed physician. The procedures described in this textbook are based on consultation with EMT and medical authorities. The authors and publisher have taken care to make certain that these procedures reflect currently accepted clinical practice; however, they cannot be considered absolute recommendations.

The material in this text contains the most current information available at the time of publication. However, federal, state, and local guidelines concerning clinical practices, including (without limitation) those governing infection control and universal precautions, change rapidly. The reader should note, therefore, that the new regulations may require changes in some procedures.

It is the reader's responsibility to familiarize himself or herself with the policies and procedures set by federal, state, and local agencies as well as the institution or agency where the reader is employed. The authors and the publisher of this text and the supplements written to accompany it disclaim any liability, loss, or risk resulting directly or indirectly from the suggested procedures and theory, from any undetected errors, or from the reader's misunderstanding of the text. It is the reader's responsibility to stay informed of any new changes or recommendations made by any federal, state, or local agency as well as by his or her employing institution or agency.

Notice on Gender Usage

The English language has historically given preference to the male gender. Among many words, the pronouns *he* and *his* are commonly used to describe both genders. Society evolves faster than language, and the male pronouns still predominate in our speech. The authors have made great effort to treat the two genders equally, recognizing that a significant percentage of EMTs are women. However, in some instances, male pronouns may be used to describe both males and females solely for the purpose of brevity. This is not intended to offend any women readers.

Notice regarding "Case Studies"

The names used and situations depicted in the Case Studies throughout this text are fictitious.

Notice on Medications

The authors and the publisher of this text have taken care to make certain that the equipment, doses of drugs, and schedules of treatment are correct and compatible with the standards generally accepted at the time of publication. Nevertheless, as new information becomes available, changes in treatment and in the use of equipment and drugs become necessary. The reader is advised to carefully consult the instruction and information material included in the page insert of each drug or therapeutic agent, piece of equipment, or device before administration. This advice is especially important when using new or infrequently used drugs. Prehospital care providers are warned that use of any drugs or techniques must be authorized by their Medical Director, in accordance with local laws and regulations. The publisher disclaims any liability, loss, injury, or damage incurred as a consequence, directly or indirectly, of the use and application of any of the contents of this text.

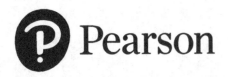

ISBN 10:   0-13-537907-5
ISBN 13: 978-0-13-537907-3

24 2023

Dedicated to my beautiful daughters: Laura, Caitlin and Destinee, and to my lovely wife, Kirsten. May you always maintain humility as your accomplishments meet the stars!

B.E.

Contents

SECTION 4 MEDICAL EMERGENCIES

SECTION 5 TRAUMA

SECTION 6 SPECIAL POPULATIONS

SECTION 7 OPERATIONS

APPENDIX

©2021 Pearson Education, Inc.
Emergency Care, 14th Ed.

Introduction

Overview

This workbook is designed to accompany the textbook *Emergency Care,* 14th Edition. The workbook covers the course knowledge and National Highway Traffic Safety Administration (NHTSA) Education Standards to which all standardized testing instruments will be referenced. In all areas where the textbook goes beyond the national core standards to present current trends in medical care, this workbook also follows along very closely. It is neither meant to replace the text nor to be a substitute for a well-designed course in emergency care.

This is a self-instructional workbook. It has been designed to allow you to work at your own pace and evaluate your own progress. To benefit from this workbook, follow the procedures in this introduction. Thousands of EMT students before you have used prior editions of this workbook as part of their emergency medical training. The system works, having helped them to learn and excel on state and national certification and registration examinations. By doing your best on each chapter, you and the patients to whom you deliver emergency care will benefit.

This edition continues the emphasis of the Education Standards on patient assessment. In addition, there are several updated sections and the new chapters as found in the text. There are Case Studies as well as a "Gray Zone" discussion that addresses areas of prehospital care that simply are not "black and white" but rather involve shades of gray. There are three Interim Exams as well as a full-length comprehensive final EMT exam in Appendix B.

Features

The chapters in this workbook contain most of these elements:

- **Match Terminology and Definitions:** In this section, you are asked to match chapter terminology with appropriate definitions, which appear in the chapter's running text or in the chapter glossary or both.

- **Multiple-Choice Review:** This section provides, on average, 20 to 40 questions. Emphasis is placed on multiple-choice questions because this is the format of state and national examinations used for certification or registration. Practice in answering multiple-choice questions can help to improve your understanding of the material as well as your course grades. These multiple-choice questions generally appear in the same order in which the topics appear in the textbook, enabling you to build on prior knowledge.

- **Complete the Following:** This section focuses on your recalling and listing specific information on chapter objectives, such as the signs and symptoms of shock or the five stages of grief.

- **Label the Diagram/Photograph and Complete the Chart:** In a few chapters, you are asked to study a visual and to identify its content or to complete a partially filled-in chart. These diagrams, photographs, and charts correspond to those in the textbook.

- **Pathophysiology:** Many chapters have questions that are based on this feature found in the text. It specifically delves into the physiology of trauma or diseases so that the reader can reflect on what is happening "inside" the body and "outside" the body.

- **Case Study:** The case study is designed to require you to synthesize information that you have learned up to that point in the course and to apply this knowledge to a real-life situation. As each step of the case is presented, you are asked a series of questions that build on the facts of the case. There are some "Gray Zone" questions that are designed not to have a "black or white" answer. The answers often lie in the shades of gray and incorporate your using good clinical judgment to make a decision as you would in the field. They are proceeded by the abbreviation, *GZQ*.

- **Answer Key:** The Answer Key is found at the back of the workbook. It provides answers for all the workbook elements. For the Multiple-Choice Review questions, rationales are provided where appropriate, along with the textbook page reference(s) where each topic is discussed.

Steps for Success

To get the most out of this workbook, you should complete the following seven steps:

Step 1: Learn the Course Objectives/Outcomes

Each chapter of the textbook begins with objectives or outcomes that were developed as part of the NHTSA's National Education Standard Instructional Guidelines. Most state and national certifying examinations are based on these objectives. To score well on those exams, you must learn the outcomes of the course. Use the outcomes in the textbook in the following way:

1. Read them over.
2. Read the text.
3. Reread the outcomes in the form of a question.
4. Write down your answer to each question on a blank piece of paper.
5. Perform a self-assessment or ask your instructor to assess how well you understand the material in the chapter.

Step 2: Learn the EMT's Language

Emergency Medical Services (EMS) is clearly a medical field. Therefore, it is necessary for the EMT to learn and understand the language of medicine. This will help you to communicate with the other members of the health care team in a clear, concise, and accurate manner. In addition, learning the language of medicine will facilitate your understanding of medical and trade journal articles as you work to keep current in the constantly changing EMS field.

First, review the medical terminology in the text and then put aside the text. Next, test your understanding of the terminology by completing the Match Terminology and Definitions exercises in each workbook chapter. Complete the entire set of matching exercises before checking your answers against the Answer Key. If there were terms that you were unable to match, write the word on one side of an index card and write the definition on the other side of the card.

Carry these cards in your pocket and refer to them frequently to help you learn the terms.

Step 3: Learn the Body's Structure

The language of medicine also includes learning the names and locations of the structures of the human body. Imagine being unable to take a peripheral pulse because you could not find the radial artery in the wrist! To help you learn the structures of the body, anatomical drawings and diagrams are provided in workbook chapters in which they are appropriate. For example, the drawing of the respiratory system in the workbook has blank numbered lines that point to each of the system's different structures. Label each structure as requested and check your answers in the answer key at the back of the workbook. If you miss any body structures, go to the textbook page suggested and study the body structure again.

Step 4: Answer the Multiple-Choice Questions

For each Multiple-Choice Review, complete the entire exercise at one sitting. Read each question and all the answer choices before you mark your answer. If you jump to a conclusion without fully reading the question, you could answer incorrectly. Also, watch out for questions with negative expressions or the word *except*. Once you have completed the exercise, refer to the Answer Key to check your performance. A textbook page reference has been provided for the theory or principle tested in each question. Many answers have an author comment whenever it is appropriate to clarify the answer to a question.

You will need to practice reading, and not reading into, multiple-choice questions. If it has been many years since you took a standardized test, leave extra time to review this section of each workbook chapter. If you notice any trends in your performance on these questions, you may wish to consult your instructor for test-taking assistance.

Step 5: Use the Pathophysiology

This feature is written to enrich your understanding of the content of the chapter.

Step 6: Take the Interim and Final Exams

Once you have completed each individual workbook chapter, move on to the next chapter and repeat steps 1 to 5. Three full-length Interim Exams are included in the workbook and are similar to the interim exams your instructor may use in the EMT course. Each exam covers material in the chapters that precede it. Therefore, when you have completed all the material in the chapters preceding

©2021 Pearson Education, Inc.
Emergency Care, 14th Ed.

an exam, it's time to take the Interim Exam. The comprehensive final exam is in Appendix B.

Step 7: Pay Close Attention Case Studies

The case studies integrated in the workbook help you to synthesize your knowledge and apply it to real-life situations. They put you at a scene and require you to think quickly and accurately. Answers at the back of the workbook will help you sort out any problems you confront. The Gray Zone areas are discussed in the answer key.

So that's it: seven simple steps. It will take time and commitment to work through each of the steps. This is a self-instructional workbook, so it will be up to you to reward yourself for doing well on chapters. At the same time, you need to be honest with yourself. If you are having difficulty with a chapter, let your instructor know immediately so that he or she can offer additional assistance.

It is the hope of the *Emergency Care* authors and development team that using this workbook as an integral part of your EMT training package will help you to improve your understanding of the material and enhance your performance in the field. After all, isn't high-quality patient care what EMS is all about? See you in the streets!

Acknowledgments

The author of the *Emergency Care Workbook*, 14th Edition, extends appreciation to Dan Limmer and Mike O'Keefe for their friendship, confidence, and the opportunity to partake in this important project. Special thanks, too, to a dear friend and mentor, J. David Bergeron.

About the Author

Bob Elling, MPA, EMT-P, has been passionately involved in EMS for more than four decades. He is currently a paramedic with the Times Union Center, Whiteface Mountain Medical Services, and an Adjunct Faculty at Hudson Valley Community College and North Country Community College. He retired after 34 years of service to the Town of Colonie and 23 years with Albany Medical Center. He is a dedicated advocate for the American Heart Association, having served in many leadership roles, most notably as the Chairman of Advocacy for NYS as well as the Guidelines 2005 Editor. He is also Regional Faculty for the NYS Bureau of EMS. Bob has served as a paramedic and lieutenant for the NYC EMS, Program Director for the HVCC Paramedic Program, Associate Director of NYS EMS, and Education Coordinator for PULSE: Emergency Medical Update. Bob enjoys writing and is the author, coauthor, or editor of more than fifty EMS publications. Bob lives in Lake Placid, New York, where he enjoys distance running (he has completed thirty marathons), skiing, cycling, hiking, photography, and spending time with his family. You can reach him at his e-mail address: bobelling@me.com.

1

Introduction to Emergency Medical Services

Core Concepts

- The chain of human resources that forms the EMS system
- How the public activates the EMS system
- Your roles and responsibilities as an EMT
- The process of EMS quality improvement

Outcomes

After reading this chapter, you should be able to:

1.1 Describe the components of the EMS system. (pp. 3–8)
- Describe the connections between EMS history and EMS today.
- Recognize components that make up EMS systems.
- Diagram the chain of human resources in EMS systems.
- Describe the communications system by which the public can access EMS.
- Explain the different levels of EMS training.

1.2 Summarize the roles and responsibilities of EMTs. (pp. 9–15)
- Describe the tasks within the roles and responsibilities of an EMT.
- Explain the traits of an EMT that convey professionalism.
- Explain the EMT's role in quality improvement.
- Explain the role of an EMS system physician Medical Director.

1.3 Describe the connection between public health and EMS systems. (pp. 16–17)
- List ways that EMS systems can support public health.

1.4 Summarize the role of evidence-based research in EMS. (pp. 17–19)
- Identify ways research impacts EMS.
- Explain the evidence-based process for EMTs.
- Compare the different methods of medical research.
- Explain how to evaluate medical research.

Match Key Terms

A. A system for telephone access to report emergencies

B. A process of continuous self-review with the purpose of identifying and correcting aspects of the system that require improvement

C. Oversight of the patient-care aspects of an EMS system by the Medical Director

D. A physician who assumes ultimate responsibility for the patient-care aspects of the EMS system

E. Standing orders issued by the Medical Director that allow EMTs to give certain medications or perform certain procedures without speaking to the Medical Director or another physician at that moment

F. Lists of steps, such as assessments and interventions, to be taken in different situations

G. Policies or protocols issued by a Medical Director that authorize EMTs and others to perform particular skills in certain situations

H. Orders from the on-duty physician given directly to an EMT in the field by radio or telephone

I. Submitted to a professional journal and reviewed by several of the researcher's peers

J. The long-term survival of patients

K. Techniques or practices that are supported by scientific evidence of their safety and efficacy, rather than merely supposition and tradition

_____ **1.** Evidence-based techniques

_____ **2.** Off-line medical direction

_____ **3.** On-line medical direction

_____ **4.** 911 system

_____ **5.** Medical direction

_____ **6.** Medical Director

_____ **7.** Quality improvement

_____ **8.** Protocols

_____ **9.** Standing orders

_____ **10.** Patient outcomes

_____ **11.** Peer reviewed

Multiple-Choice Review

_____ **1.** The earliest documented Emergency Medical Service was in:
   A. England in the 1890s.
   B. France in the 1790s.
   C. Seattle in the 1970s.
   D. Miami in the 1960s.

_____ **2.** In 1966, the _____ charged the United States _____ with developing EMS standards and helping the states to upgrade the quality of their prehospital emergency care.
   A. Uniform Traffic Act; Department of Transportation
   B. President; Fire Academy
   C. National Highway Safety Act; Department of Transportation
   D. American Medical Association; Department of Health and Human Services

_____ **3.** Which of the following is *not* a major component of the National Highway Traffic Safety Administration's EMS system assessment standards?
   A. Transportation
   B. Computerization
   C. Communications
   D. Evaluation

_____ **4.** An example of a specialty hospital in the EMS system is a(n):
   A. emergency department.
   B. correctional facility.
   C. trauma center.
   D. primary care center.

_____ **5.** The National Registry of Emergency Medical Technicians (NREMT) provides certification, based on successful completion of examinations for EMS training in all of the following *except*:
  A. advanced first aid.
  B. emergency medical responder.
  C. advanced EMT.
  D. paramedic.

_____ **6.** The major emphasis of EMT education deals with _____ of the ill or injured patient in the prehospital setting.
  A. treatment but non-transport
  B. interpretation of electrocardiograms
  C. basic-level assessment and care
  D. techniques of advanced airway care

_____ **7.** Patient care provided by the EMT should be:
  A. delayed until transportation.
  B. based on assessment findings.
  C. guided by the service's attorney.
  D. based on the patient's diagnosis.

_____ **8.** An example of ensuring continuity during the transfer of care of the patient would be:
  A. providing pertinent patient information to the hospital staff.
  B. performing more hospital procedures in the field.
  C. giving a report only directly to a physician.
  D. staying to assist the hospital staff in their management.

_____ **9.** Patient advocacy is:
  A. assessing your patient.
  B. abandoning your patient.
  C. executing your primary responsibility as an EMT.
  D. speaking up for your patient.

_____ **10.** Good personality traits are very important to the EMT. You should be:
  A. cooperative and resourceful.
  B. respectful and condescending.
  C. cunning and inventive.
  D. emotionally stable and shy.

_____ **11.** An EMT who is *not* in control of personal habits might:
  A. be disrespectful or condescending.
  B. make inappropriate decisions.
  C. render improper care.
  D. do all of the above.

_____ **12.** To prevent violating patient confidentiality, the EMT should:
  A. communicate with medical direction.
  B. perform an accurate interview.
  C. avoid inappropriate conversation about the patient.
  D. develop the ability to listen to others.

_____ **13.** An EMT may maintain up-to-date knowledge and skills through continuing education such as:
  A. rereading the EMT textbook.
  B. repeating the EMT course.
  C. attending EMS conferences.
  D. riding many shifts each week.

_____ **14.** A process of continuous self-review of all aspects of an EMS system for the purpose of identifying and correcting aspects of the system that require change is called:
  A. off-line medical direction.
  B. patient advocacy.
  C. quality improvement.
  D. continuing education.

_____ **15.** In some states, the role of EMTs has been expanded to assist local Public Health Departments with:
  A. cancer screening exams.
  B. seasonal flu vaccinations.
  C. water quality testing.
  D. rodent control.

_____ **16.** Participation in continuing education and keeping carefully written documentation are examples of the EMT's role in:
  A. patient advocacy.
  B. medical direction.
  C. quality improvement.
  D. transfer of care.

_____ **17.** Every EMS service or agency will have a:
   A. minimum of three EMTs on each vehicle.
   B. call review on a monthly basis.
   C. contract with the local hospital.
   D. Medical Director.

_____ **18.** It is important that each EMT know his or her Medical Director. An EMT is operating as the Medical Director's:
   A. employee.   **C.** eyes and ears in the field.
   B. replacement.   **D.** peer.

_____ **19.** The difference between on-line and off-line medical direction is that:
   A. off-line medical direction does not need protocols.
   B. off-line orders are given by the on-duty physician, usually over the radio or phone.
   C. on-line medical direction uses standing orders.
   D. on-line orders are given by the on-duty physician, usually over the radio or phone.

_____ **20.** An example of a pharmaceutical carried by EMTs that may require a physician consultation to administer is:
   A. lidocaine.   **C.** oxygen.
   B. pain relievers.   **D.** aspirin.

_____ **21.** As a new EMT, you will witness many changes in the EMS system and patient care, moving from practices that have been based on _____ to those that are based on _____.
   A. in-hospital care; prehospital care   **C.** instinct; traditions
   B. tradition; research   **D.** research; tradition

_____ **22.** The EMT has many jobs to do. It is the responsibility of the EMT to treat patients:
   A. as quickly as possible.
   B. in their community or district.
   C. in a nonjudgmental and fair manner.
   D. if they are insured or injured at work.

_____ **23.** Your Medical Director has stated that EMS is moving closer to science-based guidelines. A general procedure involved in making evidence-based patient care decisions is:
   A. reviewing the literature.   **C.** forming a hypothesis.
   B. evaluation of evidence.   **D.** all of these.

_____ **24.** Your service has been seeing an increase in injuries to the aging population, and your leadership is planning a program to do something about it. Injury prevention for geriatric patients and campaigns are examples of:
   A. hospital responsibilities.   **C.** the nursing domain.
   B. an EMT's role in public health.   **D.** off-line medical direction.

_____ **25.** In a process developed by Galileo almost 400 years ago, called _____, general observations are turned into a _____.
   A. guidelines development; set of protocols
   B. the scientific method; hypothesis
   C. predicting the outcome; theory
   D. the big bang theory; story tale

_____ **26.** Which of the following is *not* a challenge when EMTs conduct research in the field?
   A. an unstable work environment   **C.** lengthy patient encounters
   B. obtaining consent from patients   **D.** disjointed data collection

Complete the Following

1. List at least six of the categories and standards of an EMS system established by the National Highway Traffic Safety Administration.

   A. _____

   B. _____

   C. _____

   D. _____

   E. _____

   F. _____

2. List five types of specialty hospitals.

   A. _____

   B. _____

   C. _____

   D. _____

   E. _____

3. List the four levels of EMS certification.

   A. _____

   B. _____

   C. _____

   D. _____

4. List at least six of the responsibilities of an EMT.

   A. _____

   B. _____

   C. _____

   D. _____

   E. _____

   F. _____

Case Study: Introduction to the "Gray-Zone"

In most of the chapters of this EC14 Workbook there will be a feature called the Case Study. Since there is a limited amount of content that has been covered so far, in Chapter 1: Introduction to Emergency Medical Services, this first Case Study will be used to familiarize you with the format and discuss the concept of the "Gray-Zone." In this sample case you may come across some terms or concepts you have not yet learned in your EMT course. Don't worry. They are here to illustrate how these cases will evolve.

- Typically you will be given some dispatch information such as: "Your unit and the police are dispatched to the scene of an attempted suicide with shots fired."

- Often on the way to the call you may be given some updates from the dispatcher such as: "The police have arrived and advise that the scene is secure (safe) and that you should respond directly to the scene."

- You may also be given some descriptive information about the scene that you would observe on arrival such as: "The home is a private residence in a suburban community."

- As you first encounter the patient you would be given information that makes up your general impression such as: "You find a 48-year-old male lying with his face covered with blood. He is moaning, and his chest and abdomen appear to be moving as he breathes."

- Next, information will be provided that would be found during your primary assessment of the patient such as: "After donning protective gloves, mask, and goggles, both you and your partners carefully provide manual stabilization of the neck and consider moving the patient with the scoop stretcher."

- The case will proceed to provide primary assessment findings such as: "The mandible and tongue are severely lacerated. The mouth and nose are bubbling with blood as the patient attempts to breathe and you can hear gurgling."

- At this point in the case you will be asked a couple of questions on how you should proceed such as: "How should you open the airway of this trauma patient?" or "Does this patient need to be suctioned?" There may also be follow-up questions like, "How long should you suction and with what device?"

- Next, the case will proceed with some additional pertinent information being presented such as: "Once the patient's airway is opened and cleared, you consider applying oxygen to this patient. He has no other obvious injuries, yet you are treating him for a possible spinal injury due to the impact of the bullet and his backward fall from his desk chair during the incident. The police think that the bullet struck the front of his chin and face rather than travelling into his head as originally intended. You will be given baseline vital signs at an appropriate time in the case development. Following are a few examples of such information: "You evaluate the patient's breathing rate as 28, shallow, and labored; pulse as 120, weak, and regular; and SP0$_2$ as 94%."

- At this point you may again be asked more questions relevant to the case and your management of the patient, such as: "What device should be used to administer oxygen to this patient?" and "What is the proper liter flow to set the regulator for the device you chose to use?"

- Finally, you will be given some additional information about the secondary assessment, patient condition update, and effect of your treatment, or you may be asked about your decision to call for a paramedic unit and where and when you will be transporting the patient. For example, "The patient has a blood pressure of 100/70 mmHg and his oxygen saturation is 95%, so you decide his priority is (A) [high, low]. The major problem with this patient is his (B) [spinal injury, facial injury]. He should be transported (C) [right away, in a few minutes] to the (D) [local hospital, trauma center]." "From your knowledge of your EMS system, what ALS (advanced life support) treatment(s) might be helpful to this patient if you can arrange for an ALS intercept?" and "What should you do if you hear hissing or bubbling around the mask as you ventilate?"

Some of the answers to the questions asked during the cases are simple ones where there is a clear right answer and a clear wrong answer that can be found in the chapter in your book.

©2021 Pearson Education, Inc.
Emergency Care, 14th Ed.

Occasionally you will be asked questions that do not have a clear yes/no or black/white answer. That is because they require your best clinical judgment to answer. This is the "gray zone," and many of your decisions are made in this area. As you learn more about Emergency Medical Services you will see that many times the best clinical judgment on how to treat a patient could be found in the gray zone. There are also some procedures and interventions that you will learn to do that are being studied and evaluated. As the latest research updates becomes available, your Medical Director or the State or Regional EMS System may update what you have learned. These research results could mean updates to the protocols you use to treat patients. Some of these controversial topics are also discussed in the Gray Zone of this workbook. Hopefully you will find this to be an enlightening and stimulating discussion! Throughout the workbook Gray Zone Questions will be identified with *GZQ*, as you can see below.

Here are a couple of questions, covered in this chapter, that relate to this case discussion:

GZQ **1.** What is the role of a Paramedic?

_____

GZQ **2.** What is the role of a Medical Director?

_____

GZQ **3.** What are treatment protocols?

_____

Well-Being of the EMT

2

Core Concepts

- Standard Precautions, or how to protect yourself from transmitted diseases
- The kinds of stress caused by involvement in EMS and how they can affect you, your fellow EMTs, and your family and friends
- The impact that dying patients can have on you and others
- How to identify potential hazards and maintain scene safety

Outcomes

After reading this chapter, you should be able to:

2.1 Describe how specific healthy habits can affect the EMT's well-being. (pp. 24–38)
- Identify the role of a support system in maintaining well-being.
- Recognize the health benefits of an exercise program.
- Relate the importance of sleep to performance as an EMT.
- Identify the health benefits of eating right.
- List the negative impacts of excess consumption of alcohol and caffeine.
- Recognize the importance of regular visits to your physician, including keeping current on vaccines.
- Explain the concepts of personal protection from communicable diseases.

2.2 Explain why EMS can be a particularly stressful job. (pp. 38–45)
- Describe what happens in each stage of stress.
- Contrast acute, delayed, and cumulative stress reactions.
- Give examples of types of situations in EMS that have a higher probability than routine circumstances of causing a stress reaction in EMS providers.
- Recognize when an EMT is exhibiting signs and symptoms of stress.
- Identify the components of an employer's comprehensive system for stress management.
- Interpret the statements and behaviors of a dying patient or that patient's family members in terms of emotional stages of grief.
- Given a scenario, translate generic approaches for dealing with death and dying patients into actions specific to the situation.

2.3 Summarize concepts of scene safety in EMS. (pp. 46–51)
- State the rationale for the priority given to scene safety in EMS.
- List the most common causes of EMS line-of-duty deaths (LODD).
- State the primary actions expected of EMTs upon encountering a potential hazardous materials situation.
- State actions EMTs can take in advance to plan for encountering violence on an EMS call.
- Explain specific observations EMTs should make on every call to detect potential indications of violence.
- Given a scenario, translate the generic approach to reacting to danger to situation-specific actions.

Match Key Terms

A. A strict form of infection control that is based on the assumption that all blood and other body fluids are infectious; also known as body substance isolation (BSI).

B. A comprehensive system that includes education and resources to both prevent stress and deal with stress appropriately when it occurs.

C. The introduction of dangerous chemicals, disease, or infectious materials.

D. Equipment that protects the EMS worker from infection and/or exposure to the dangers of rescue operations.

E. The organisms that cause infection, for example, viruses and bacteria.

F. An emergency involving multiple patients.

G. The removal or cleansing of dangerous chemicals and other dangerous or infectious materials.

H. The release of a harmful substance into the environment.

I. Toughness; an ability to recover quickly from difficult situations.

J. A state of physical and/or psychological arousal to a stimulus.

_____ **1.** Contamination

_____ **2.** Pathogens

_____ **3.** Multiple-casualty incident (MCI)

_____ **4.** Standard Precautions

_____ **5.** Critical incident stress management (CISM)

_____ **6.** Decontamination

_____ **7.** Hazardous material incident

_____ **8.** Stress

_____ **9.** Personal protective equipment (PPE)

_____ **10.** Resilience

Multiple-Choice Review

_____ **1.** While providing care for a 45-year-old female who has a fever of unknown origin, you may have been exposed to an organism that causes infection. Such an organism is referred to as a(n):
  A. airborne organism.   **C.** allergen.
  B. bloodborne micro-organism.   **D.** pathogen.

_____ **2.** Procedures that protect you from the blood and body fluids of the patient and protect the patient from your blood and body fluids are referred to as:
  A. universal precautions.   **C.** Standard Precautions.
  B. general isolation.   **D.** quarantine isolation.

_____ **3.** To provide the appropriate level of precautions to protect from infectious disease in the field, the EMT may need to use:
  A. hand washing and SCBA.   **C.** disposable gloves and eye protection.
  B. a HEPA mask and shoe covers. **D.** a paper gown and leather gloves.

4. When an EMT covers a patient's mouth and nose with a mask to prevent the spread of an airborne disease, the EMT should:
A. monitor the patient's respirations and airway closely.
B. write "TB alert" on the patient's prehospital care report.
C. wear a surgical mask to reduce the spread of TB.
D. notify his or her supervisor before transporting the patient.

5. The EMT can plan safety precautions in advance of the call in all of the following ways *except* by:
A. keeping his or her tetanus immunization current.
B. maintaining a list of communicable patients in your district.
C. obtaining a flu shot.
D. obtaining the hepatitis B vaccine.

6. All EMTs who work or volunteer for an ambulance service or first responder agency should be immunized with all of the following vaccines *except*:
A. tetanus.
B. hepatitis B.
C. tuberculin skin test (TST).
D. influenza.

7. A federal organization responsible for issuing guidelines for employee safety around bloodborne pathogens is (the):
A. Food and Drug Administration (FDA).
B. Federal Communications Commission (FCC).
C. Occupational Safety and Health Administration (OSHA).
D. Public Health Service (PHS).

8. Every employer of EMTs must provide all employees, free of charge, a:
A. yearly physical examination.
B. life insurance policy.
C. hepatitis B vaccination.
D. universal health insurance policy.

9. The federal act that establishes procedures by which emergency response workers can find out whether they have been exposed to life-threatening infectious diseases is:
A. OSHA 1910.1030.
B. the Ryan White CARE Act.
C. NFPA 1207.
D. OSHA 1910.1200.

10. After contact with the blood or body fluids of a patient, an EMT should submit a request for a determination of exposure to his or her:
A. employer.
B. Medical Director.
C. designated officer.
D. local hospital.

11. Sometimes the EMT does not have the complete SAMPLE history for every patient when deciding which level of Standard Precautions to utilize. Always assume that any person with _____ has _____.
A. a cold; a bloodborne disease
B. a productive cough; TB
C. a fever; typhus
D. dehydration and sores; AIDS

12. From an EMT's perspective, what do the diseases chickenpox, German measles, and whooping cough have in common?
A. They are all caused by bloodborne pathogens.
B. They are all spread by exposure to oral secretions during suctioning.
C. They are all spread by airborne droplets.
D. They all can be prevented by eating the right foods.

13. The EMT can safeguard his or her well-being by:
A. understanding and dealing with job stress.
B. ensuring scene safety.
C. practicing Standard Precautions.
D. all of these.

_____ 14. All of the following are examples of calls that have a high potential for causing acute stress reactions in the EMT *except*:
  A. trauma to multiple children.
  B. an adult with femur fracture.
  C. a plane crash with many victims.
  D. death or serious injury of a coworker.

_____ 15. You should be aware of the signs that you, your crew, or your patients may be affected by stress. Some warning signs that an EMT is being affected by stress include:
  A. overeating and ringing in the ears.
  B. frequent urination and sweating.
  C. indecisiveness and guilt.
  D. increased sexual activity and sleep.

_____ 16. All of the following are lifestyle changes that may benefit an EMT in preventing and dealing with EMS job stress *except*:
  A. developing more healthful and positive dietary habits.
  B. devoting time to relaxing.
  C. exercising.
  D. avoiding discussion about feelings.

_____ 17. After the crash of a van in which six children were severely injured, the EMS Director conferred with the Medical Director. and they decided to set up a meeting of all the providers who were involved in the call. A meeting held by a team of peer counselors and mental health professionals within 24 to 72 hours after an incident like this is called a(n):
  A. incident critique.
  B. MCI critique.
  C. critical incident stress debriefing.
  D. quality circle.

_____ 18. A smaller meeting conducted within a few hours with the rescuers who were directly involved in the most stressful aspects of a call is called a:
  A. defusing session.
  B. CISD.
  C. Code Green.
  D. eSCAPe.

_____ 19. Most medical professionals and EMS leaders agree that the best course of action for an EMT who is experiencing significant stress from a serious call that involved multiple deaths is to:
  A. seek help from a mental health professional who is experienced in these issues.
  B. take a week off from work.
  C. exercise vigorously.
  D. talk with other EMTs.

_____ 20. A patient who finds out that he or she is dying may go through which of the following emotional stages?
  A. Anger and laughter
  B. Denial and empathy
  C. Depression and acceptance
  D. Bargaining and elation

_____ 21. As an EMT, you have been assigned to take a terminally ill patient back and forth to radiation therapy on multiple trips for the past few weeks. You have come to know the patient and realize that he has been going through emotional stages that fall roughly in the following order:
  A. Acceptance, rage, depression, acceptance, bargaining
  B. Denial, anger, bargaining, depression, acceptance
  C. Bargaining, acceptance, denial, anger, depression
  D. Depression, bargaining, denial, acceptance, anger

_____ 22. An EMT will occasionally need to assist the patient who has a terminal illness. Experts suggest all of the following *except*:
  A. listening empathetically to the patient.
  B. telling the patient that everything will be fine.
  C. being tolerant of angry reactions from the patient or family members.
  D. trying to recognize the patient's needs.

_____ **23.** You are on a call that suddenly becomes violent to you and your crew. All of the following words sum up actions required to respond to danger *except*:
  A. plan.   **C.** run.
  B. observe.   **D.** react.

_____ **24.** The body's response to stress was studied by a Canadian physician named Dr. Hans Selye. He found that there is a(n):
  A. resistance syndrome.   **C.** general adaptation syndrome.
  B. excess of the chemical cortisone. **D.** exhaustion syndrome.

_____ **25.** The phases of adaptation to stress include alarm, exhaustion, and:
  A. reaction.   **C.** resistance.
  B. distress.   **D.** rest.

_____ **26.** A stress reaction that involves either physical or psychological behavior manifested days or weeks after an incident is called a(n):
  A. acute stress reaction.   **C.** cumulative stress reaction.
  B. posttraumatic stress disorder. **D.** burnout.

_____ **27.** If you suspect your patient may have active tuberculosis, when transporting it is appropriate for the EMT to:
  A. wear disposable gloves.   **C.** wear N-95 or HEPA mask.
  B. wear an eye shield.   **D.** all of the above.

_____ **28.** The normal mode of transmission of the disease chickenpox (varicella) is thought to be through:
  A. blood or stool.   **C.** airborne droplets.
  B. accidental needlesticks.   **D.** ventilation systems.

_____ **29.** Each of the following diseases is thought to be spread by respiratory secretions or oral or nasal secretions *except*:
  A. hepatitis.   **C.** pneumonia.
  B. bacterial meningitis.   **D.** influenza.

_____ **30.** A disease that mothers are thought to be able to pass to their unborn children is:
  A. chickenpox (varicella).   **C.** tuberculosis.
  B. AIDS.   **D.** mumps.

_____ **31.** The patient that you are assessing has a respiratory complaint and is running a fever. He also complains of the chills and just got back from a region of Africa where Ebola is prevalent. What is the incubation period for this disease?
  A. One week   **C.** 2 days after symptoms develop
  B. 2 to 21 days   **D.** 42 days

_____ **32.** On closer examination of the patient described in the previous question, after taking the appropriate level of PPE, you note that the patient has signs that would be considered "late signs" such as:
  A. photophobia.   **C.** extensive bruising.
  B. flushed skin.   **D.** unequal pupils.

_____ **33.** You responded to a motor vehicle crash involving an overturned propane truck. Which of the following is an excellent resource to assist you with determining a safe distance to park your ambulance?
  A. The State EMS Code   **C.** The NFPA handbook
  B. Emergency Response Guidebook   **D.** The Regional EMT Protocols

_____ **34.** When arriving at the scene of a call where you suspect danger, the best policy would be to:
  A. instruct bystanders to wait across the street.
  B. call for a police backup to secure the scene.
  C. assume the perpetrator has left the scene.
  D. tell emotional family members they must calm down or leave.

_____ **35.** The eSCAPe curriculum is designed to help patients and EMS providers deal
with posttraumatic stress. What does the "A" stand for?
  A. Always (provide a debriefing)   **C.** Airway (open and clear always)
  B. Ambulate (get moving right away)   **D.** Anticipate (what happens next)

Complete the Following

1. List five types of calls with a high potential of stress for EMS personnel.

   A. _____

   B. _____

   C. _____

   D. _____

   E. _____

2. List five signs or symptoms of stress.

   A. _____

   B. _____

   C. _____

   D. _____

   E. _____

3. List five of the eight critical elements of the standard Title 29 Code of Federal
   Regulation 1910.1030.

   A. _____

   B. _____

   C. _____

   D. _____

   E. _____

4. List four factors to address in planning for a potentially violent call.

   A. _____

   B. _____

   C. _____

   D. _____

Case Study: Just a Fall in the Kitchen

Your unit is responding to a call for an elderly patient who fell in her kitchen and cannot get up. On your arrival, you are met by her 30-year-old son, who states that he always checks in on his 70-year-old mother every day or so. He goes on to state that he has been away for the past week in the Bahamas and called his mother a couple of times, but she never answered the phone. On his return, he came right over to the house to find her lying on the floor in the kitchen. She may have fallen four or five days ago.

You put on PPE per protocol and introduce yourself to the patient and find that she is verbally responsive only, cold, and confused. She has apparently not had anything to eat or drink since she fell. She has the look of a patient who has a broken hip. She is lying in a pool of urine and feces. As you complete the primary assessment, your partner quickly gets the stretcher and a long backboard as well as some additional PPE to make it possible to move the patient.

1. What Standard Precautions would be appropriate in this situation?

   _____

2. Would it be appropriate to remove the patient's clothing and clean her up in the house?

   _____

3. Once you determine that the patient is breathing, has an open airway, and has a pulse, what exam should you conduct on her?

   _____

The patient has no complaints of neck pain or head pain, but her back is very uncomfortable from lying on the floor, and she has an obviously deformed right hip. You carefully move her to the stretcher, using the backboard and a pillow and straps. Before moving her to the ambulance, you decide to get a full set of baseline vital signs and note the following: respirations of 24, pulse of 90 and regular, blood pressure of 110/70 mmHg, and SpO_2 of 97%.

4. What medical history would be appropriate to obtain from the patient's son?

   _____

5. Based on the potential for exposure to body fluids, how should you handle this patient?

   _____

6. If you noticed that your glove was ripped, what should you do to maintain your own personal protection?

   _____

After transporting the patient to the hospital ED, you give a complete report of the assessment and management you provided as well as what you found on the patient's history. The nurse in the ED checks the patient's hospital record and informs you that the patient has a history of prior falls and hepatitis B as well as the open sores on her legs, which may be shingles.

7. Does the updated information that you were given in the ED change how you should have managed the hazards in this situation for your own protection?

   _____

©2021 Pearson Education, Inc.
Emergency Care, 14th Ed.

3

Lifting and
Moving Patients

Core Concepts

- How using body mechanics to lift and move patients can help prevent injury
- When it is proper to move a patient and how to do so safely
- The various devices used to immobilize, move, and carry patients

Outcomes

After reading this chapter, you should be able to:

3.1 Describe the considerations in preventing injury to the EMS crew when lifting and moving patients. (pp. 56–58)
- Given descriptions of situations, estimate whether it is safe to attempt to lift the patient.
- Distinguish between proper use of body mechanics and improper lifting and moving technique.

3.2 Summarize the considerations in moving patients. (pp. 58–76)
- Given a selection of descriptions, categorize the need to move the patients as emergent, urgent, or nonurgent.
- Recognize the specific techniques used for each method of moving a patient.
- Identify patient-carrying devices.
- Given a description of a situation, select the most appropriate patient-carrying device.
- Contrast the general considerations for moving a patient with a suspected spine injury and one with no suspected spine injury.
- Distinguish between techniques for moving a patient without suspected spine injury onto a carrying device.
- Match descriptions of patient problems with considerations for positioning the patient.

Match Key Terms

A. Having to do with patients who are significantly overweight or obese.

B. A method of lifting and carrying a patient from ground level to a stretcher in which two or more rescuers kneel, curl the patient to their chests, stand, then reverse the process to lower the patient to the stretcher.

C. Gripping with as much hand surface as possible in contact with the object being lifted, all fingers bent at the same angle and hands at least 10 inches apart.

D. A method of transferring a patient from bed to stretcher, in which two or more rescuers curl the patient to their chests, then reverse the process to lower the patient to the stretcher.

E. The proper use of the body to facilitate lifting and moving and prevent injury.

F. A method of lifting and carrying a patient during which one rescuer slips hands under the patient's armpits and grasps the wrists, while another rescuer grasps the patient's knees.

G. A lift from a squatting position with weight to be lifted close to the body, feet apart and flat on the ground, body weight on or just behind balls of feet, and the back locked in. The upper body is raised before the hips.

H. A method of transferring a patient from bed to stretcher by grasping and pulling the loosened bottom sheet of the bed.

_____ 1. Power grip

_____ 2. Body mechanics

_____ 3. Direct carry

_____ 4. Direct ground lift

_____ 5. Draw-sheet method

_____ 6. Bariatric

_____ 7. Extremity lift

_____ 8. Power lift

Multiple-Choice Review

_____ 1. To ensure your personal safety when lifting an adult patient, it is important to:
   A. always wear a back brace.
   B. keep the weight as far away from your body as possible.
   C. use your legs, not your back, to lift.
   D. avoid lifting a patient who weighs more than you do.

_____ 2. When lifting a patient, you should do all of the following *except*:
   A. communicate your plan clearly with your partner.
   B. twist while you and your partner lift the patient.
   C. know your partner's physical ability and limitations.
   D. communicate frequently with your partner.

_____ 3. EMTs lift the cot or stretcher on most calls. When lifting this device, you should:
   A. use four rescuers if on rough or uneven terrain.
   B. keep both of your feet together and flat on the ground.
   C. use a third person positioned on the heaviest side.
   D. compensate by using your back if you are using only one hand.

_____ 4. When you place all fingers and the palm in contact with the stretcher as you prepare to lift, you are using the hand technique known as the:
   A. power grip.   C. lock grip.
   B. power lift.   D. grip lift.

_____ **5.** You are in a situation in which the only way to move a heavy object is to pull it. When you must pull an object, you should:
   A. keep the line of pull through the center of your body by bending your knees.
   B. pull from an overhead position, keeping your knees locked.
   C. keep the weight you are pulling at least 20 inches away from your body.
   D. keep your elbows straight with arms close to your sides.

_____ **6.** You must decide whether to move a patient using an emergency move. The situations in which an emergency move would be used include all of the following *except*:
   A. the scene is hazardous because of an immediate danger of fire.
   B. explosives or other hazardous chemicals are present.
   C. care of life-threatening conditions requires repositioning the patient.
   D. the dispatcher is holding another EMS call.

_____ **7.** You and your partner are assigned to quickly move as many patients as possible from the hallway of a nursing facility because of a fire in another wing of the building. The next patient you come to is on the floor, and you have decided to use an emergency move. How should the EMT move this patient to safety?:
   A. rolling the patient like a log.
   B. using a spine board and strapping the patient down.
   C. pulling on the patient's clothing in the neck and shoulder area.
   D. using one rescuer on each extremity.

_____ **8.** If your 55-year-old male patient has an altered mental status, you should consider a(n) _____ move.
   A. emergency   **C.** nonurgent
   B. urgent   **D.** immediate

_____ **9.** You and your crew have decided to use a log roll to get your patient onto a long backboard. When doing a log roll, you should lean from your hips and:
   A. keep your back curved only while leaning over the patient.
   B. position yourself at least 10 inches from the patient.
   C. use your shoulder muscles to help with the roll.
   D. roll the patient as fast as possible.

_____ **10.** The final step in packaging a patient for transport to the hospital on a wheeled stretcher involves:
   A. securing the stretcher to the ambulance.
   B. placing a towel under the patient's head.
   C. covering the patient with a top sheet.
   D. adjusting the position of the back rest.

_____ **11.** Your 65-year-old female patient is in a bedroom that is on the second floor of her residence. If you and your partner are going to be carrying her down the stairway, you should:
   A. flex at the waist with bent knees.
   B. keep your lower back muscles loose.
   C. place one hand on the railing for balance.
   D. use a stair chair instead of a stretcher.

_____ **12.** Your 55-year-old male patient, who is approximately 650 pounds, has a chief complaint of "chest pain and difficulty breathing." While you are conducting the primary assessment and care, it would be helpful to have your partner call for:
   A. powered loading equipment.   **C.** additional crew members.
   B. a bariatric stretcher.   **D.** all of these.

_____ **13.** You have a 28-year-old male patient who was injured while working on the rooftop of a three-story structure. The fire department will be using the ladder bed to lower the patient to the ground. Which device should the patient be placed in first?
   A. basket stretcher.
   B. Reeves stretcher.
   C. short spine board.
   D. scoop stretcher.

_____ **14.** A 52-year-old male has injured his spine in a motor vehicle crash. The trauma center is 35 minutes away. Which of the following patient carrying devices would be best suited to protecting the patient's spine during transport?
   A. The padded ambulance cot
   B. A long spine board
   C. A vest-type extrication device
   D. A Stokes basket

_____ **15.** The pack strap carry is an example of a(n) _____ move for a patient who has no spine injury.
   A. emergency
   B. urgent
   C. immediate
   D. nonurgent

_____ **16.** Another name for the squat-lift used by EMTs is the:
   A. leg lift.
   B. power lift.
   C. thigh thrust.
   D. power grip.

_____ **17.** How should the EMT's feet be positioned when lifting?
   A. Comfortable distance apart.
   B. Weight on balls of feet.
   C. Flat on the ground.
   D. All of these.

_____ **18.** The EMT who has to lift with one hand, as in a litter carry, must be careful *not* to:
   A. lift with the legs.
   B. compensate by leaning.
   C. lift with the weight close to the body.
   D. take breaks if they are needed.

_____ **19.** A more comfortable device that can be used to transport a patient in the supine position who has sustained a spinal injury is a:
   A. scoop stretcher.
   B. stair chair with tracks.
   C. vacuum mattress.
   D. KED.

_____ **20.** When a vacuum mattress is used, the patient is placed on the device and the air is _____ by a pump. Then the mattress will form a _____ and conforming surface around the patient.
   A. inflated; rigid
   B. withdrawn; rigid
   C. inflated; soft
   D. withdrawn; soft

Complete the Following

1. List five patient-carrying devices.

   A. _____

   B. _____

   C. _____

   D. _____

   E. _____

2. List four general principles that will help you prevent injury when reaching for a patient.

A. _____

B. _____

C. _____

D. _____

3. List five general principles that will help you prevent injury when pushing or pulling a patient.

A. _____

B. _____

C. _____

D. _____

E. _____

4. List three situations that may require an emergency move.

A. _____

B. _____

C. _____

Label the Photographs

Fill in the name of each emergency move on the line provided.

1. _____   2. _____

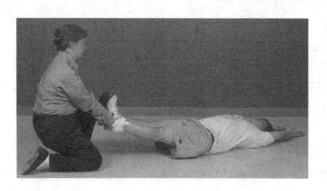

3. _____

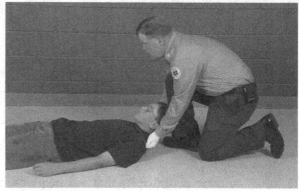

4. _____

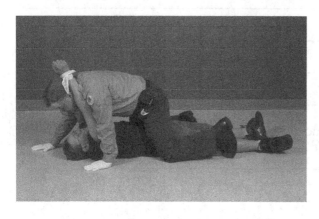

5. _____

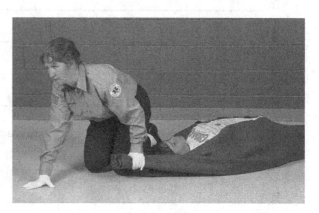

6. _____

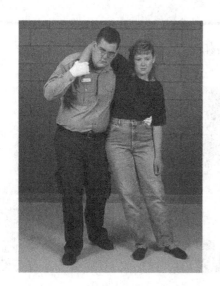

7. _____

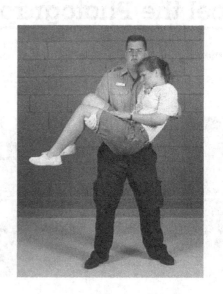

8. _____

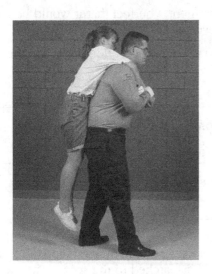

9. _____

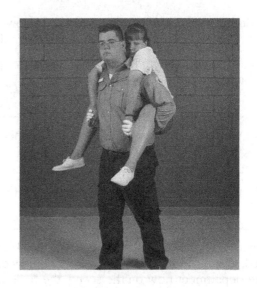

10. _____

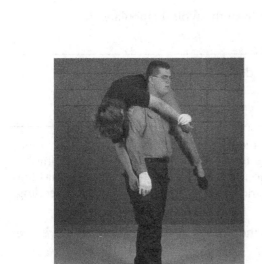

11. _____

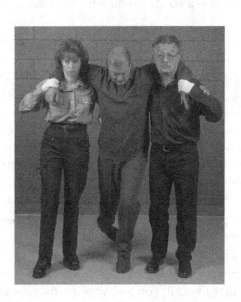

12. _____

Case Study: More Than the Average Patient

Your unit is on the scene of a patient whose daughter called EMS because her father cannot get out of bed. According to the daughter, who identified herself as Mary Ann, her dad, Mr. Joe Thomas, has continued to gain weight over the past few years. He has gotten so obese that he can barely get himself out of bed. She states that she has been giving him a bedpan and/or a urinal to relieve himself for the past couple of weeks. Today he is complaining of back pain and has chills and a fever.

After donning protective gloves, mask, eye shield, and a disposable gown because the patient has feces on him, you decide to call the dispatcher to have the fire department dispatched to the scene for assistance. You conduct a primary assessment and find a 50-year-old male who you estimate to weigh about 500 pounds. He states that his back hurts and he cannot roll on his side anymore. He is lying on a mattress that is directly on the floor, as the bed frame could no longer handle his weight. He has a long history of urinary tract infections and kidney stones, but it is difficult to tell whether he may have a kidney stone or urinary tract infection now. After your assessment, you feel that it would be most appropriate for him to go to the emergency department for evaluation.

1. Normally, a stair chair is used to remove patients who are on the second floor. Would it be appropriate in this case?

_____

2. Would a direct ground lift or a draw-sheet method be more appropriate for this patient?

_____

3. Why would you decide to call the fire department in this situation?

_____

Once the fire department arrives, you work together to devise a plan to get the patient out of the bed, down the stairs, and into the ambulance. With your supervisor and an engine company from the fire department now on the scene, the regional bariatric unit is dispatched to the scene. The patient is visibly embarrassed but does appropriately answer all of your questions about his medical history. He has not seen his physician for quite some time.

4. What is a bariatric unit, and how might that be different from the typical ambulance?

_____

GZQ **5.** The EMTs choose the Reeves stretcher to get the patient down the stairs. Would the scoop stretcher have been a safer or equally safe choice?

_____

It takes five EMTs and rescue workers to carefully roll the patient onto the Reeves stretcher and then to drag the patient and stretcher down the steps and exit the house. Fortunately, the bariatric unit has a special stretcher that is rated for obese patients and a lift to make it possible to get Mr. Thomas into the ambulance. On the way to the hospital, you call ahead and alert the ED that you will be needing extra assistance on arrival.

6. If you were unable to get the patient down the stairs in the Reeves stretcher, what may have been another useful device to consider?

_____

GZQ **7.** After the call, you and your partner discuss it and decide that a lot of rescuers were involved but every one was absolutely necessary. What is the highest priority in these calls and why?

_____

4

Medical, Legal, and Ethical Issues

Core Concepts

- The scope of practice of an EMT
- How a patient may consent to or refuse emergency care
- The legal concepts of torts, negligence, and abandonment
- What it means to have a duty to act
- The responsibilities of an EMT at a crime scene

Outcomes

After reading this chapter, you should be able to:

4.1 Summarize the relationship between scope of practice and standard of care. (pp. 81–82)
- Classify tasks and procedures as either within or outside of an EMT's scope of practice.
- Give examples of ways an EMT can maintain the expected standard of care.

4.2 Give a synopsis of concepts of patient consent to and refusal of care and ethical challenges that arise in the EMT's work. (pp. 82–90)
- Describe when each of the types of consent applies.
- Recognize the criteria that must be met when a patient refuses emergency medical care.
- Given scenarios, derive specific actions from the general steps for interacting with a patient who refuses emergency medical care.
- Describe the EMT's obligations when confronted with different types of Physician's Orders for Life-Sustaining Treatment (POLST).
- Recognize the presence of an ethical challenge.
- Explain various actions that could be taken to address an ethical challenge.
- Predict how various decisions about ethical challenges might play out.

4.3 Outline concepts associated with legal issues that affect EMTs. (pp. 90–99)
- Given a scenario in which a patient makes a claim of negligence against an EMT, determine whether the elements required to prove negligence are present.
- Differentiate between a tort and a criminal act.
- Summarize what Good Samaritan laws are.
- Identify ways in which EMTs may inadvertently violate a patient's confidentiality.
- Describe how the Health Insurance Portability and Accountability Act (HIPAA) impacts the legality of what patient information can be shared by EMTs.

- Identify situations with potential for slander or libel.
- State how medical identification devices and organ donor status identification can guide the decisions of a EMTs.
- Describe the purpose of "safe haven" laws.
- Give examples of observations EMTs should make and document at crime scenes.
- Given scenarios, translate the general list of actions EMTs should take at crime scenes into specific actions.

Match Key Terms

Part A

A. The consent that it is presumed a patient or patient's parent or guardian would give if they could, such as for an unconscious patient or a child whose parents cannot be contacted when care is needed.

B. Physician orders that state not only the patient's wishes regarding resuscitation attempts but also the patient's wishes regarding artificial feeding, antibiotics, and other life-sustaining care if the person is unable to state the person's desires later.

C. Being held legally responsible.

D. An obligation to provide care to a patient.

E. Consent given by adults who are of legal age and mentally competent to make a rational decision with regard to their medical well-being.

F. Permission from the patient for care or other action by the EMT.

G. A series of laws, varying by state, designed to provide limited legal protection for citizens and some health care personnel when they are administering emergency care.

H. A set of regulations that define the scope, or extent and limits, of the EMT's job.

I. A law that permits a person to drop off an infant or child off at a police, fire, or EMS station or to deliver the infant or child to any available public safety personnel.

J. A finding that there was failure to act properly in a situation in which there was a duty to act that needed care as would reasonably be expected of the EMT was not provided, and that harm was caused to the patient as a result.

K. A legal document, usually signed by the patient and physician, which states that the patient has a terminal illness and does not wish to prolong life through resuscitative efforts.

L. The obligation not to reveal information obtained about a patient except to other health care professionals involved in the patient's care, or under subpoena, or in a court of law, or when the patient has signed a release of confidentiality.

M. Leaving a patient after care has been initiated and before the patient has been transferred to someone with equal or greater medical training.

_____ **1.** Abandonment

_____ **2.** Slander

_____ **3.** Confidentiality

_____ **4.** Consent

_____ **5.** "Safe haven" law

_____ **6.** Do not resuscitate (DNR) order

_____ **7.** Duty to act

_____ **8.** Expressed consent

_____ **9.** Good Samaritan laws

_____ **10.** HIPAA

_____ **11.** Implied consent

_____ **12.** Liability

_____ **13.** Negligence

_____ **14.** Organ donor

_____ **15.** Scope of practice

_____ **16.** Physician's Orders for Life-Sustaining Treatment (POLST)

©2021 Pearson Education, Inc.
Emergency Care, 14th Ed.

N. A person who has completed a legal document that allows for donation of organs and tissues in the event of death.

O. The Health Insurance Portability and Accountability Act, a federal law protecting the privacy of patient-specific health care information and providing the patient with control over how this information is used and distributed.

P. False, injurious information stated verbally.

Part B

A. A civil, not a criminal, offense; an action or injury caused by negligence from which a lawsuit may arise.

B. Regarding, personal standards or principles of right and wrong.

C. False, injurious information in written form.

D. For an EMT providing care for a specific patient in a specific situation, the care that would be expected to be provided by an EMT with similar training when caring for a patient in a similar situation.

E. Placing a person in fear of bodily harm.

F. Literally "in place of a parent," indicating a person who may give consent for care of a child when the parents are not present or able to give consent.

G. Causing bodily harm or restraining a person.

H. A Latin term meaning "the thing speaks for itself."

I. Regarding a social system or social or professional expectations for applying principles of right and wrong.

J. The location where a crime has been committed or any place where evidence relating to a crime may be found.

K. A DNR order; instructions written in advance of an event.

_____ **1.** *In loco parentis*

_____ **2.** Assault

_____ **3.** Battery

_____ **4.** Tort

_____ **5.** *Res ipsa loquitur*

_____ **6.** Moral

_____ **7.** Ethical

_____ **8.** Libel

_____ **9.** Advance directive

_____ **10.** Crime scene

_____ **11.** Standard of care

Multiple-Choice Review

_____ **1.** The collective set of regulations governing the EMT is called the EMT's:
  A. duty to act.   **C.** advance directives.
  B. scope of practice.   **D.** Good Samaritan laws.

_____ **2.** Laws that govern the skills and treatments that an EMT may perform are:
  A. standardized (uniform) throughout the country.
  B. different from state to state.
  C. standardized (uniform) for regions within a state.
  D. governed by the U.S. DOT.

_____ **3.** When the EMT advocates for the physical/emotional needs of the patient, this is considered a(n) _____ for the EMT.
  A. advance directive   **C.** ethical responsibility
  B. protocol   **D.** legal responsibility

_____ 4. Which one of the following is *not* a type of consent required for any treatment or action by an EMT?
A. Child and mentally incompetent adult
B. Implied
C. Applied
D. Expressed

_____ 5. When you inform the adult patient of a procedure you are about to perform and its associated risks, you are asking for the patient's:
A. expressed consent.   C. implied consent.
B. in loco parentis.   D. applied consent.

_____ 6. You are assessing a 28-year-old male patient who was found unconscious at the bottom of a stairwell. Consent that is based on the assumption that this patient would approve your life-saving care is called:
A. expressed.   C. implied.
B. involuntary.   D. applied.

_____ 7. You are treating a 22-year-old female who decides that she does not want a cervical collar and definitely does not want to be transported to the hospital. The record of her refusal of medical care and/or transport should include all of the following *except*:
A. informing the patient of the risks and consequences of refusal.
B. documenting the steps you took.
C. signing of the form by the Medical Director.
D. obtaining a release form with the patient's witnessed signature.

_____ 8. It is clear that your 24-year-old competent male patient does not want to go to the hospital. Forcing him to go to the hospital against his will may result in _____ charges against the EMT.
A. abandonment   C. implied consent
B. assault   D. negligence

_____ 9. Which of the following is an action the EMT should *not* take if a 36-year-old female refuses care?
A. Leave phone stickers with emergency number should she change her mind.
B. Recommend that a relative call the family physician to report the incident.
C. Tell the patient to call her family physician if the problem recurs.
D. Call a relative or neighbor who can stay with her.

_____ 10. You are at the home of a very sick patient who has a terminal illness. Her daughter states that she has DNR paperwork. Another name for a DNR order is a(n):
A. delayed nervous response.   C. refusal of treatment.
B. duty not to react.   D. advance directive.

_____ 11. There may be varying degrees of DNR orders in your state, which may be expressed through a variety of detailed instructions that may be part of the order, such as:
A. allowing CPR only if cardiac or respiratory arrest was observed.
B. allowing comfort-care measures such as endotracheal intubation.
C. disallowing the use of long-term life-support measures.
D. specifying that only 5 minutes of artificial respiration will be attempted.

_____ 12. In a hospital, long-term life-support and comfort-care measures would consist of intravenous feeding and:
A. routine inoculations.
B. the use of a respirator.
C. infection control by the health care providers.
D. hourly patient documentation.

13. If an EMT with a duty to act fails to provide the standard of care and if this failure causes harm or injury to the patient, the EMT may be accused of:
A. *res ipsa loquitur*.   C. battery.
B. negligence.   D. assault.

14. Leaving your 82-year-old male patient on a hallway stretcher in a busy ED and leaving without giving a report to a health care professional is an example of:
A. liability infraction.   C. abandonment.
B. battery.   D. breach of duty.

15. The EMT should not discuss information about a patient except to relay pertinent information to the physician at the ED. Information that is considered confidential includes:
A. patient history gained through interview.
B. assessment findings.
C. treatment rendered.
D. all of these.

16. The EMT should not release confidential patient information. The exception to this rule would be to:
A. inform other health care professionals who need to know information to continue care.
B. report incidents the police asked you about.
C. comply with a patient's family request.
D. share with the other victims of the motor vehicle collision.

17. A medical identification device worn to indicate serious medical conditions is available in each of the following formats *except*:
A. bracelets.   C. cards.
B. necklaces.   D. patches.

18. You responded to a high-speed collision involving a motorcycle and an automobile. The 26-year-old female cyclist has a severe head injury and is not likely to live until morning. When treating this woman, who happens to have an organ donor card, you should:
A. transport without delay and document a DNR.
B. treat the patient the same as any other patient and inform the ED physician.
C. withhold oxygen therapy from the patient to keep the organ hypoxic.
D. all of these.

19. You are at the scene of a home invasion where the 55-year-old male homeowner was shot in the head multiple times by the perpetrators. The police have called you to determine whether there are any signs of life. At this crime scene, you should:
A. avoid disturbing any evidence at the scene unless emergency care requires.
B. immediately remove the patient from the scene.
C. move all obstacles from around the patient to make more room to work.
D. search the house for clues to the cause of the crime.

20. You mention to your partner, out of view of the patient, that once you get to the ED and turn over the patient, there will be some reports to file. Commonly required reporting situations in most states include all of the following *except*:
A. child and elder abuse.   C. sexual assault.
B. crimes in public places.   D. suspected human trafficking.

21. The extent of limits of an EMT's occupation is referred to as the:
A. ethical dilemma.   C. scope of practice.
B. national curriculum.   D. regional protocol.

_____ **22.** You were called to a bar fight where a 28-year-old male was knocked unconscious. On your arrival, he is awake and has a broken nose but no life threats. He admits to drinking "half a dozen beers" in the last 90 minutes. He wants to refuse medical attention. Why should you discourage the patient from refusing care and transport?
   A. He is not legally old enough to consent.
   B. He may not be mentally competent at this time.
   C. Patients die from broken noses all the time.
   D. He is unable to actually sign the release.

_____ **23.** The federal law designed to protect the patient's private medical information is called:
   A. NHTSA.   **C.** HIPAA.
   B. ANSI.   **D.** OSHA.

_____ **24.** You are on the scene where a 40-year-old male barricaded himself and his wife in their home and threatened to do harm. After 2 hours, the wife escaped through the bathroom window, and the police rushed in and restrained the husband. It is your responsibility to transport him to the local ED. What should be your highest priority?
   A. Monitoring the patient's mental status and vital signs.
   B. Making sure your documentation shows that you did not apply handcuffs.
   C. Restraining the patient further so that he is not able to move.
   D. Explaining to the patient that he no longer has any rights to refuse care.

_____ **25.** The police are concerned about the presence of microscopic evidence at the scene of a violent assault. Your crew was asked to be careful and limit their involvement in the scene to essential patient care. What are examples of microscopic evidence?
   A. The position in which the patient was initially found
   B. Any dirt and carpet fibers
   C. Fingerprints that were found at the scene
   D. The condition of the scene

_____ **26.** You are on the scene where a 46-year-old female who is refusing to go to the hospital. After arguing for 20 minutes you decide to just restrain her and remove to the ED as her family wishes so they can get a break from her complaining. If the patient is of sound mind you could be charged with:
   A. assault.   **C.** liability.
   B. battery.   **D.** obstruction of justice.

_____ **27.** The concept used in _____ law is _res ipsa loquitur_ which is a Latin term for:
   A. criminal: "the situation is fluid."
   B. tort: "in the presence of a parent."
   C. tort: "the thing speaks for itself."
   D. criminal: "the case smells of negligence."

_____ **28.** When conducting a physical exam of an unconscious adult patient with a suspected medical problem, you remember that there was a "Vial of Life" sticker on the front door of the residence. This is important because it may:
   A. reveal the patient's name.
   B. give clues to the patient's home address.
   C. reveal that additional medical identification is in the refrigerator.
   D. be the cause of the emergency.

©2021 Pearson Education, Inc.
Emergency Care, 14th Ed.

Complete the Following

1. List four conditions that must be fulfilled for a patient to refuse care or transport.

   A. _____

   B. _____

   C. _____

   D. _____

2. A finding of negligence, or failure to act properly, requires that all of the following circumstances be proven.

   A. _____

   B. _____

   C. _____

3. Four medical conditions that may be listed on a medical identification device (such as a necklace, bracelet, or card) are:

   A. _____

   B. _____

   C. _____

   D. _____

4. Describe the purpose of the typical state "safe haven" law and how it may affect your EMS agency.

   _____

   _____

Case Study: A Witnessed Collision: First on the Scene

It's a summer morning, and you are traveling on an interstate highway with your family, heading to the lake. Although the speed is posted at 55 mph, traffic has been moving at least 10 mph faster. All of a sudden, you observe, a few cars in front of yours, an SUV going from the center lane to the passing lane, cutting off another car, and then veering off the center of the road down into a ravine. The SUV rolls over numerous times before coming to rest on its roof.

1. If you are an off-duty EMT, are you legally required to stop and offer assistance?

   _____

2. Are you protected from a lawsuit? Explain your answer.

_____

3. Are you protected from a liability suit provided that your treatment is appropriate?

_____

As you secure your vehicle safely off the shoulder and assign another motorist to carefully set out some flares, your spouse uses a mobile phone to call for emergency assistance.

4. In most communities, what is the universal emergency phone number?

_____

5. What types of questions would you expect the dispatcher to ask about the collision?

_____

_____

6. Which emergency response agencies would you expect to dispatch personnel to the scene?

_____

As you carefully climb down through the brush to the car, you notice two patients who were ejected from the vehicle. Another citizen arrives, and she identifies herself as an EMT in the state. You ask her to check the two ejected patients while you check the car for additional patients. After a few minutes, she reports back to you that one ejected patient is dead and the other is unconscious with an obvious head injury.

7. As additional helpers arrive, how can they help with the head injured patient?

_____

8. What types of injuries could the patient have?

_____

9. Do you need permission to treat the patient? Explain.

_____

Inside the car is a conscious 40-year-old male who appears to have been injured by the steering wheel in the left upper quadrant of his abdomen. He also has an obviously fractured left femur. After obtaining some additional help, you decide to carefully move this patient out of the car.

10. What additional potential injuries might this patient have?

_____

11. How can you help to minimize further injury to the leg?

_____

12. Do you need permission to treat this patient? Explain.

_____

Once the patient is out of the car, two ambulances arrive, as does the fire department with a paramedic engine and a heavy rescue truck. Meanwhile, the police have arrived and are dealing with the traffic congestion that has developed.

13. Because plenty of help is now on the scene, can you leave?

_____

14. What would be the problem if you left before the help arrived on the scene?

_____

5. Medical Terminology

Core Concepts

- Medical terminology and how terms are constructed
- Directional terms
- Positional terms

Outcomes

After reading this chapter, you should be able to:

5.1 Demonstrate communication in the language of medicine. (pp. 104–107)
- Analyze the meanings of medical terminology components.
- Recognize the meanings of common acronyms, mnemonics, and abbreviations used in the language of medicine.
- Distinguish between circumstances in which an EMT should use medical terminology, abbreviations, and acronyms; and situations in which plain language is a better choice.

5.2 Apply terms of position and direction to describe a location on the human body. (pp. 107–112)
- Identify the anatomic regions of the body.
- Match anatomic terms of position and direction to their definitions.

Match Key Terms

Part A

A. A word root with an added vowel that can be joined with other words, roots, or suffixes to form a new word.

B. The study of body structure.

C. A word part added to the end of a root or word to complete its meaning.

D. A word part added to the beginning of a root or word to modify or qualify its meaning.

E. A word formed from two or more whole words.

_____ **1.** Compound

_____ **2.** Root

_____ **3.** Combining form

_____ **4.** Prefix

_____ **5.** Suffix

_____ **6.** Anatomy

©2021 Pearson Education, Inc.
Emergency Care, 14th Ed.

F. Foundation of a word that is not a word that can stand on its own.

G. The study of body function.

H. Toward the midline of the body.

I. An imaginary line drawn down the center of the body, dividing it into right and left halves.

J. A flat surface formed when slicing through a solid object.

K. To the side, away from the midline of the body.

L. The back of the body or body part.

M. A line drawn vertically from the middle of the armpit to the ankle.

N. The front of the body or body part.

O. Limited to one side.

P. On both sides.

Q. The standard reference position for the body in the study of anatomy.

_____ **7.** Physiology

_____ **8.** Anatomic position

_____ **9.** Plane

_____ **10.** Midline

_____ **11.** Medial

_____ **12.** Lateral

_____ **13.** Bilateral

_____ **14.** Unilateral

_____ **15.** Midaxillary line

_____ **16.** Anterior

_____ **17.** Posterior

Part B

A. Away from the head.

B. Toward the head.

C. Referring to the front of the body.

D. Closer to the torso.

E. Referring to the back of the body or the back of the hand or foot.

F. Referring to the sole of the foot.

G. Referring to the palm of the hand.

H. The trunk of the body; without the head and extremities.

I. The line through the center of each clavicle.

J. Farther away from the torso.

K. Lying on the back.

L. divisions of the abdomen used to describe the location of a pain or injury:

M. A sitting position.

N. Lying facedown.

O. Lying on the side.

_____ **1.** Ventral

_____ **2.** Dorsal

_____ **3.** Superior

_____ **4.** Inferior

_____ **5.** Proximal

_____ **6.** Distal

_____ **7.** Torso

_____ **8.** Palmar

_____ **9.** Plantar

_____ **10.** Midclavicular line

_____ **11.** Abdominal quadrants

_____ **12.** Supine

_____ **13.** Prone

_____ **14.** Recovery position

_____ **15.** Fowler position

Multiple-Choice Review

_____ **1.** The word *electrocardiogram* is actually a combination of:
   A. three roots.
   B. two suffixes.
   C. a prefix and a suffix.
   D. two prefixes.

_____ **2.** If a patient is lying on his or her side, the patient is said to be in the
   _____ position.
   A. Fowler's
   B. recovery
   C. left supine
   D. left prone

_____ **3.** When a patient who has been having difficulty breathing is placed in a sitting-up
   position on a stretcher, this position is called:
   A. prone.
   B. supine.
   C. Fowler.
   D. lateral recumbent.

_____ **4.** A patient lying flat on his back would be in the _____ position.
   A. prone
   B. supine
   C. Fowler
   D. Semi-Fowler

_____ **5.** Your patient is being treated for heart disease and was referred to a specialist
   for further treatment. The type of physician she is going to see is most likely
   a(n):
   A. cardiologist.
   B. internist.
   C. asthmatologist
   D. pulmonologist.

_____ **6.** When you see the suffix "itis" in a patient's chart, it means:
   A. a person afflicted with.
   B. a patient suffering from.
   C. inflammation.
   D. a hole or opening.

_____ **7.** Your service encourages the use of abbreviations and acronyms on the
   prehospital care report to save time. What is the downside of using them?
   A. They are not understood by the patient.
   B. They can lead to communication errors.
   C. They take time to learn.
   D. Not all EMT courses teach what acronyms are.

_____ **8.** The reference position of the body used when discussing human anatomy is
   called the:
   A. universal position.
   B. unilateral position.
   C. erect position.
   D. anatomic position.

_____ **9.** A patient who has absent lung sounds in both the right and left upper lobes is
   said to have _____ findings.
   A. superior
   B. unilateral
   C. bilateral
   D. inferior

_____ **10.** Your patient was stabbed in the front of the chest on the left side, and you
   suspect that his heart may have been injured. Which of the following is the best
   description of this location using the terminology you learned in this chapter?
   A. The wound is at the left anterior axillary line.
   B. The wound is at the left nipple level in the mid-clavicular line.
   C. The wound is at the left posterior border of the fourth rib.
   D. The wound is at the left lateral border of the thorax.

©2021 Pearson Education, Inc.
Emergency Care, 14th Ed.

Complete the Following

1. Describe each of the following planes or directional terms:

   A. Midline _____

   B. Medial _____

   C. Lateral _____

   D. Midaxillary line _____

   E. Anterior _____

   F. Posterior _____

   G. Superior _____

   H. Inferior _____

   I. Midclavicular line _____

2. Name the organ(s) or body system that is the specialty of each of the following doctors:

   A. Pulmonologist _____

   B. Gastroenterologist _____

   C. Cardiologist _____

   D. Neurologist _____

3. Define the following medical prefixes:

   A. Ante _____

   B. Brady _____

   C. Contra _____

   D. Dys _____

   E. Hyper _____

   F. Inter _____

   G. Peri _____

   H. Poly _____

   I. Super/Supra _____

   J. Uni _____

Pathophysiology: Dissecting a Compound Word

Your 52-year-old female patient is complaining of abdominal pain. She tells you that this happens every time she eats greasy fried food. She also says that she loves to eat fried fish on Fridays and often suffers the consequences. Her husband states that she has been treated previously for similar symptoms and the diagnosis was cholecystitis.

1. If you break this medical term down into three parts, they are _____, _____, and _____.

2. What does each part mean? _____, _____, _____.

3. The gallbladder is an organ that secretes a substance called bile, which helps in the digestive process to break down fats. Why would it be a good idea for your patient to find something else to eat on Fridays?

Label the Diagrams

Anatomic Postures

Fill in the name of each anatomical position on the line provided.

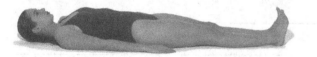

1. _____

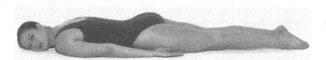

2. _____

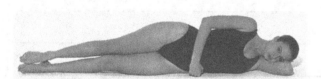

3. _____

Anatomical Positions

Fill in the appropriate directional terms and landmarks on the numbered lines provided following Diagrams 1 and 2.

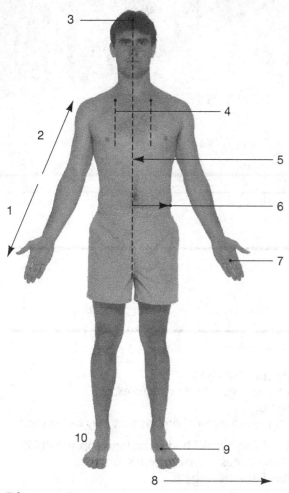

Diagram 1

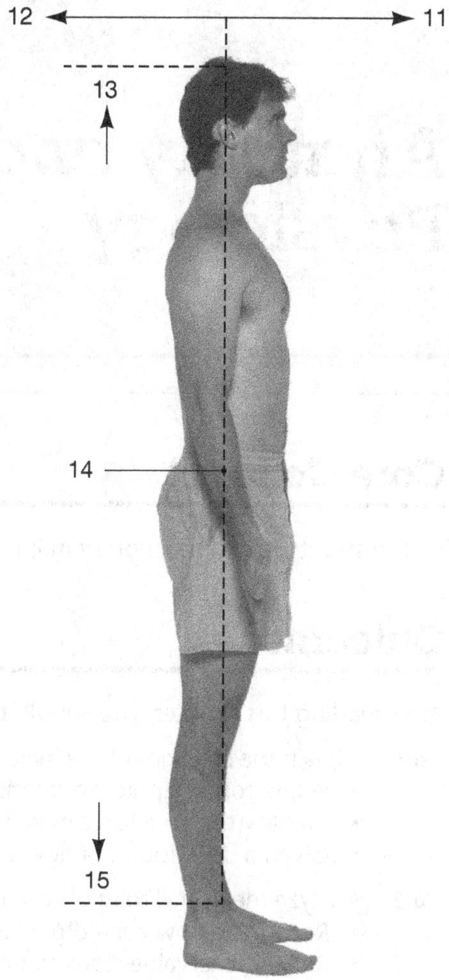

Diagram 2

1. _____
2. _____
3. _____
4. _____
5. _____
6. _____
7. _____
8. _____
9. _____
10. _____

11. _____
12. _____
13. _____
14. _____
15. _____

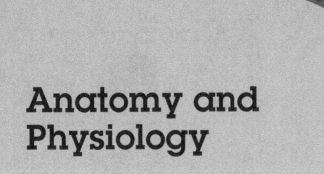

Anatomy and Physiology

Core Concept

• The structure and function of major body systems

Outcomes

After reading this chapter, you should be able to:

6.1 Explain the locations of the major systems in the body. (pp. 118–149)
   • Relate topographic landmarks to the locations of underlying body structures.
   • Identify the structures in various diagrams of organs.
   • Given a description of how a patient was injured, predict internal organs that may be harmed.

6.2 Analyze the overall roles of each organ system in maintaining normal body functions. (pp. 118–149)
   • Recognize how each organ system in the body contributes to that system's function.
   • Relate observable signs to potential dysfunctions of internal organs.

Match Key Terms

Part A

A. The bony structure of the head.

B. The lower jaw.

C. Bones that comprise the nasal cavity.

D. Bones that form the structure of the cheeks.

E. Tissue that connects bone to bone.

F. The bones of the body.

G. The wing-shaped plate of cartilage that sits anterior to the larynx and forms the Adam's apple.

H. The study of body structure.

I. Tissue that connects muscle to bone.

J. The top, back, and sides of the skull.

_____ **1.** Anatomy

_____ **2.** Physiology

_____ **3.** Thyroid cartilage

_____ **4.** Musculoskeletal system

_____ **5.** Skeleton

_____ **6.** Muscle

_____ **7.** Ligament

_____ **8.** Tendon

_____ **9.** Skull

©2021 Pearson Education, Inc.
Emergency Care, 14th Ed.

K. The two fused bones forming the upper jaw.

L. A system that helps manage the pH of the blood.

M. The bones of the spinal column.

N. Tissue that can contract to allow movement of a body part.

O. The system of bones and skeletal muscles that support and protect the body and permit movement.

P. The study of body function.

Q. The bony structures around the eyes.

_____ **10.** Cranium

_____ **11.** Mandible

_____ **12.** Maxillae

_____ **13.** Nasal bones

_____ **14.** Orbits

_____ **15.** Zygomatic arches

_____ **16.** Vertebrae

_____ **17.** Buffer system

Part B

A. The pelvic socket into which the ball at the proximal end of the femur fits to form the hip joint.

B. The kneecap.

C. The lateral and smaller bone of the lower leg.

D. The ankle bones.

E. The lower, posterior portions of the pelvis.

F. The basin-shaped bony structure that supports the spine and is the point of attachment for the lower extremities.

G. The superior portion of the sternum.

H. The chest.

I. The medial anterior portion of the pelvis.

J. The large bone of the thigh.

K. The medial and larger bone of the lower leg.

L. Bony protrusions seen on either side of the ankle joint.

M. Composed of organs, tissues, and vessels these help to maintain the fluid balance of the body and contributes to the body's immune system.

N. The superior and widest portion of the pelvis.

O. The inferior portion of the sternum.

P. The breastbone.

Q. The foot bones.

_____ **1.** Thorax

_____ **2.** Sternum

_____ **3.** Manubrium

_____ **4.** Xiphoid process

_____ **5.** Pelvis

_____ **6.** Ilium

_____ **7.** Ischium

_____ **8.** Pubis

_____ **9.** Acetabulum

_____ **10.** Femur

_____ **11.** Patella

_____ **12.** Tibia

_____ **13.** Fibula

_____ **14.** Malleolus

_____ **15.** Tarsals

_____ **16.** Metatarsals

_____ **17.** Lymphatic system

Part C

A. The medial bone of the forearm.

B. The hand bones.

C. Muscle that can be consciously controlled.

D. Specialized involuntary muscle found only in the heart.

_____ **1.** Calcaneus

_____ **2.** Phalanges

_____ **3.** Clavicle

_____ **4.** Scapula

E. The bone of the upper arm, between the shoulder and the elbow.

F. The highest portion of the shoulder.

G. The collarbone.

H. The heel bone.

I. The lateral bone of the forearm.

J. Artery of the lower arm; the artery felt when taking the pulse at the thumb side of the wrist.

K. The point where two bones come together.

L. Muscle that responds automatically to brain signals but cannot be consciously controlled.

M. The ability of the heart to generate and conduct electrical impulses on its own.

N. The joint where the acromion and the clavicle meet.

O. The shoulder blade.

P. The bones of the fingers and toes.

Q. The wrist bones.

_____ 5. Acromion process

_____ 6. Acromioclavicular joint

_____ 7. Humerus

_____ 8. Radius

_____ 9. Ulna

_____ 10. Carpals

_____ 11. Metacarpals

_____ 12. Joint

_____ 13. Voluntary muscle

_____ 14. Involuntary muscle

_____ 15. Cardiac muscle

_____ 16. Automaticity

_____ 17. Radial artery

Part D

A. The organs where the exchange of atmospheric oxygen and waste carbon dioxide takes place.

B. The microscopic sacs of the lungs where gas exchange with the bloodstream takes place.

C. A leaf-shaped structure that prevents food and foreign matter from entering the trachea.

D. The mechanical process of moving gases to and from the alveoli.

E. The ring-shaped structure that forms the lower portion of the larynx.

F. An active process in which the intercostal (rib) muscles and the diaphragm contract, increasing the size of the chest cavity and causing air to flow into the lungs.

G. The area directly posterior to the nose.

H. The muscular structure that divides the chest cavity from the abdominal cavity; a major muscle of respiration.

I. The process of moving oxygen and carbon dioxide between circulating blood and the cells.

J. The two large sets of branches that come off the trachea and enter the lungs. There are right and left bronchi.

K. The system of nose, mouth, throat, lungs, and muscles that brings oxygen into the body and expels carbon dioxide.

L. A passive process in which the intercostal (rib) muscles and the diaphragm relax, causing the chest cavity to decrease in size and air to flow out of the lungs.

_____ 1. Respiratory system

_____ 2. Oropharynx

_____ 3. Nasopharynx

_____ 4. Pharynx

_____ 5. Epiglottis

_____ 6. Larynx

_____ 7. Cricoid cartilage

_____ 8. Trachea

_____ 9. Lungs

_____ 10. Mainstem bronchi

_____ 11. Alveoli

_____ 12. Diaphragm

_____ 13. Inhalation

_____ 14. Exhalation

_____ 15. Ventilation

_____ 16. Respiration

M. The "windpipe"; the structure that connects the pharynx to the lungs.

N. The area directly posterior to the mouth and nose; made up of the oropharynx and the nasopharynx.

O. The voice box.

P. The area directly posterior to the mouth.

Part E

A. The largest artery in the body. It transports blood from the left ventricle to begin systemic circulation.

B. The large neck arteries, one on each side of the neck, that carry blood from the heart to the head.

C. A structure that opens and closes to permit the flow of a fluid in only one direction.

D. Artery supplying the foot, lateral to the large tendon of the big toe.

E. Any blood vessel carrying blood away from the heart.

F. Major artery of the upper.

G. The two lower chambers of the heart.

H. The major artery supplying the leg.

I. The smallest kind of artery.

J. The vessels that carry deoxygenated blood from the right ventricle of the heart to the lungs.

K. The system made up of the heart and the blood vessels.

L. Artery supplying the foot, behind the medial ankle.

M. The blood vessels that supply the muscle of the heart (myocardium).

N. This is the major venous structure that returns blood from the body to the right atrium.

O. A system of specialized muscle tissues that conducts electrical impulses that stimulate the heart to beat.

P. The two upper chambers of the heart.

_____ **1.** Cardiovascular system

_____ **2.** Atria

_____ **3.** Ventricles

_____ **4.** Venae cava

_____ **5.** Valve

_____ **6.** Cardiac conduction system

_____ **7.** Artery

_____ **8.** Coronary arteries

_____ **9.** Aorta

_____ **10.** Pulmonary arteries

_____ **11.** Carotid arteries

_____ **12.** Femoral artery

_____ **13.** Brachial artery

_____ **14.** Posterior tibial artery

_____ **15.** Dorsalis pedis artery

_____ **16.** Arteriole

Part F

A. The rhythmic beats caused as waves of blood move through and expand arteries.

B. The carotid and femoral pulses, which are examples of these.

C. The fluid portion of the blood.

D. The supply of oxygen to and removal of wastes from, the cells and tissue of the body as a result of the flow of blood through the capillaries.

_____ **1.** Capillary

_____ **2.** Venule

_____ **3.** Vein

_____ **4.** Pulmonary veins

_____ **5.** Plasma

_____ **6.** Red blood cells

E. Components of the blood. They help the body fight infection.

F. The pressure created in the arteries when the left ventricle contracts and forces blood into circulation.

G. Any blood vessel returning blood to the heart.

H. The pressure caused by blood exerting force against the walls of blood vessels.

I. Inability of the body to adequately circulate blood to the body's cells to supply them with oxygen and nutrients.

J. The radial, brachial, posterior tibial, and dorsalis pedis pulses are all examples of these.

K. A thin-walled, microscopic blood vessel where the oxygen/carbon dioxide and nutrient/waste exchange with the body's cells takes place.

L. The pressure remaining in the arteries when the left ventricle is refilling.

M. Components of the blood. These participate in the clotting of blood.

N. The vessels that carry oxygenated blood from the lungs to the left atrium of the heart.

O. Components of the blood. They transport oxygen and carbon dioxide.

P. The smallest kind of vein.

_____ **7.** White blood cells

_____ **8.** Platelets

_____ **9.** Pulse

_____ **10.** Peripheral pulses

_____ **11.** Central pulses

_____ **12.** Blood pressure

_____ **13.** Systolic blood pressure

_____ **14.** Diastolic blood pressure

_____ **15.** Perfusion

_____ **16.** Hypoperfusion

Part G

A. The outer layer of the skin.

B. A gland located behind the stomach that produces insulin and juices that assist in digestion of food in the duodenum of the small intestine.

C. The brain and spinal cord.

D. The largest internal organ of the body, which produces bile to assist in breakdown of fats and assists in the metabolism of various substances in the body.

E. The layer of tissue between the body and the external environment.

F. A small tube located near the junction of the small and large intestines in the right lower quadrant of the abdomen.

G. The nerves that enter and leave the spinal cord and travel between the brain and organs without passing through the spinal cord.

H. An organ located in the left upper quadrant of the abdomen that acts as a blood filtration system and a reservoir for blood.

_____ **1.** Nervous system

_____ **2.** Central nervous system

_____ **3.** Peripheral nervous system

_____ **4.** Autonomic nervous system

_____ **5.** Digestive system

_____ **6.** Stomach

_____ **7.** Small intestine

_____ **8.** Large intestine

_____ **9.** Liver

_____ **10.** Gallbladder

_____ **11.** Pancreas

©2021 Pearson Education, Inc.
Emergency Care, 14th Ed.

I. The inner (second) layer of the skin, rich in blood vessels and nerves, found beneath the epidermis.

J. The system of brain, spinal cord, and nerves that governs sensation, movement, and thought.

K. A sac on the underside of the liver that stores bile produced by the liver.

L. The muscular tube between the stomach and the large intestine, divided into the duodenum, the jejunum, and the ileum, which receives partially digested food from the stomach and continues digestion. Nutrients are absorbed by the body through its walls.

M. The muscular tube that removes water from waste products received from the small intestine and moves anything not absorbed by the body toward excretion from the body.

N. The division of the peripheral nervous system that controls involuntary motor functions.

O. The muscular sac between the esophagus and the small intestine where digestion of food begins.

P. The system by which food travels through the body and is digested, or broken down into absorbable forms.

_____ **12.** Spleen

_____ **13.** Appendix

_____ **14.** Skin

_____ **15.** Epidermis

_____ **16.** Dermis

Part H

A. The female organ of reproduction used for both sexual intercourse and as an exit from the uterus for the fetus.

B. The male organs of reproduction used for the production of sperm.

C. A system of glands that produce chemicals called hormones that help to regulate many body activities and functions.

D. The tube connecting the bladder to the vagina or penis for excretion of urine.

E. The female organ of reproduction that is used to house the developing fetus.

F. Egg-producing organs within the female reproductive system.

G. A hormone produced by the pancreas to help with glucose transport into cells.

H. The organ of male reproduction responsible for sexual intercourse and the transfer of sperm.

I. The body system that regulates fluid balance and the filtration of blood.

J. The layers of fat and soft tissues found below the dermis.

K. The body system that is responsible for human reproduction.

L. The round saclike organ of the renal system used as a reservoir for urine.

_____ **1.** Subcutaneous layers

_____ **2.** Endocrine system

_____ **3.** Insulin

_____ **4.** Epinephrine

_____ **5.** Renal system

_____ **6.** Kidneys

_____ **7.** Bladder

_____ **8.** Ureters

_____ **9.** Urethra

_____ **10.** Reproductive system

_____ **11.** Testes

_____ **12.** Penis

_____ **13.** Ovaries

_____ **14.** Uterus

_____ **15.** Vagina

M. The tubes connecting the kidneys to the bladder.

N. A hormone produced by the body. As a medication, dilates respiratory passages and is used to relieve severe allergic reactions.

O. Organs of the renal system that filter blood and regulate fluid levels in the body.

Multiple-Choice Review

_____ **1.** All the following are body systems _except_:
    A. respiratory.   **C.** abdominal.
    B. cardiovascular.   **D.** musculoskeletal.

_____ **2.** The musculoskeletal system has four functions. It supports and protects the body, provides for movement, and:
    A. gives the body sensation.
    B. forms blood cells and stores minerals.
    C. provides for the body's outer covering.
    D. allows transport of oxygen into the cells.

_____ **3.** Your patient was involved in a fight in a bar. You suspect that he has broken his upper jaw. What is the name of the bone involved?
    A. Mandible   **C.** Maxillae
    B. Orbit   **D.** Nasal bone

_____ **4.** The spinal column includes the _____ vertebrae.
    A. thoracic and coccyx   **C.** lumbar and sternal
    B. cervical and orbit   **D.** sacrum and pelvic

_____ **5.** An injury to the spinal cord at the _____ level may be fatal because control of the muscles of breathing arise from the spinal cord at this level.
    A. lumbar   **C.** cervical
    B. sacral   **D.** thoracic

_____ **6.** Your patient was standing on the street corner when a truck cut the corner too close, knocked him down, and ran over his legs. The bones in the lower extremities that he may have broken include the:
    A. femur, calcaneus, and phalanges.   **C.** orbit, lumbar, and shin.
    B. ischium, tibia, and ulna.   **D.** radius, fibula, and metatarsals.

_____ **7.** The bones in the upper extremities include the:
    A. humerus and radius.   **C.** phalanges and tibia.
    B. humerus and calcaneus.   **D.** ulna and cervical.

_____ **8.** The types of muscle tissue include:
    A. voluntary.   **C.** cardiac.
    B. involuntary.   **D.** all of these.

_____ **9.** A patient who is walking is using:
    A. voluntary muscle.   **C.** cardiac muscle.
    B. involuntary muscle.   **D.** smooth muscle.

_____ **10.** Involuntary (smooth) muscle is found in the:
    A. thyroid.   **C.** heart.
    B. blood vessels.   **D.** quadriceps and biceps.

_____ **11.** The structure in the throat that is described as the voice box is called the:
    A. pharynx.   **C.** trachea.
    B. larynx.   **D.** sternum.

©2021 Pearson Education, Inc.
Emergency Care, 14th Ed.

_____ **12.** A leaf-shaped valve that prevents food and foreign objects from entering the trachea during swallowing is called the:
    A. pharynx.   **C.** larynx.
    B. epiglottis.   **D.** bronchi.

_____ **13.** Oxygen passes from the environment to the lungs in what order?
    A. Nose, bronchi, larynx, trachea, lung
    B. Larynx, esophagus, trachea, bronchi, alveoli
    C. Mouth, pharynx, trachea, bronchi, alveoli
    D. Epiglottis, trachea, pharynx, bronchi, alveoli

_____ **14.** When the diaphragm and intercostal muscles relax, the size of the chest cavity:
    A. increases, causing inhalation.   **C.** decreases, causing exhalation.
    B. increases, causing exhalation.   **D.** decreases, causing inhalation.

_____ **15.** The difference between the adult airway and the pediatric airway is that:
    A. the adult's tongue takes up proportionally more space in the mouth than the child's.
    B. the trachea is softer and more flexible in an adult.
    C. the cricoid cartilage is softer in an adult.
    D. all structures are smaller and more easily obstructed in a child.

_____ **16.** The body system that is responsible for the breakdown of food into absorbable forms is called the _____ system.
    A. nervous   **C.** endocrine
    B. digestive   **D.** integumentary

_____ **17.** A hollow organ containing acidic gastric juices that begin the breakdown of food into components that the body will be able to convert to energy is the:
    A. large intestine.   **C.** stomach.
    B. small intestine.   **D.** liver.

_____ **18.** The major artery in the thigh is called the:
    A. carotid.   **C.** radial.
    B. femoral.   **D.** brachial.

_____ **19.** The vessel that carries oxygen-poor blood from the portions of the body below the heart and back to the right atrium is called the:
    A. posterior tibial.   **C.** inferior vena cava.
    B. internal jugular.   **D.** aorta.

_____ **20.** The heart has a right and left side as well as upper and lower chambers. The left atrium:
    A. receives blood from the veins of the body.
    B. receives blood from the pulmonary veins.
    C. pumps blood to the lungs.
    D. pumps blood to the body.

_____ **21.** The fluid that carries the blood cells and nutrients is called:
    A. platelets.   **C.** plasma.
    B. urine.   **D.** none of these.

_____ **22.** The formed blood component that is essential to the formation of blood clots is called:
    A. plasma.   **C.** white blood cells.
    B. platelets.   **D.** red blood cells.

_____ **23.** The components of the blood involved in destroying microorganisms (germs) and producing antibodies are the:
    A. platelets   **C.** red blood cells
    B. leukocytes   **D.** erythrocytes

_____ **24.** The two main divisions of the nervous system are:
- **A.** central and peripheral.
- **B.** bones and muscles.
- **C.** brain and skin.
- **D.** spinal cord and brain.

_____ **25.** The nerves that carry information from throughout the body to the spinal cord and brain are _____ nerves.
- **A.** motor
- **B.** cardiac
- **C.** spinal
- **D.** sensory

_____ **26.** One of the functions of the integumentary system is to:
- **A.** eliminate excess oxygen into the atmosphere.
- **B.** regulate the diameter of the blood vessels in the circulation.
- **C.** aid in temperature regulation.
- **D.** allow environmental water to carefully enter the body.

_____ **27.** The system that secretes hormones, such as insulin and epinephrine and that is responsible for regulating many body activities is called the _____ system.
- **A.** integumentary
- **B.** nervous
- **C.** endocrine
- **D.** gastrointestinal

_____ **28.** The kidneys and ureters are structures of the _____ system.
- **A.** endocrine
- **B.** digestive
- **C.** renal/urinary
- **D.** integumentary

_____ **29.** Fluid balance of the body and a contribution to the body's immune system are functions of the _____ system.
- **A.** blood
- **B.** nervous
- **C.** endocrine
- **D.** lymphatic

_____ **30.** The organs which are part of the lymphatic system include the thymus, adenoids, and the:
- **A.** gall bladder.
- **B.** spleen.
- **C.** pancreas.
- **D.** liver.

_____ **31.** As food is digested, water is removed from waste products prior to their elimination from the body by the:
- **A.** small intestine.
- **B.** stomach.
- **C.** ureters.
- **D.** large intestine.

_____ **32.** When epinephrine and norepinephrine are released by the adrenal gland they can cause:
- **A.** increased cardiac force of contraction.
- **B.** increased heart rate.
- **C.** bronchiole dilation.
- **D.** all of the above.

Complete the Following

1. List the names of nine arteries in the body. (pp. 133–134)

A. _____

B. _____

C. _____

D. _____

E. _____

F. _____

G. _____

H. _____

I. _____

2. List four structures found in the integumentary system. (p. 121)

A. _____

B. _____

C. _____

D. _____

3. List five structures in the heart's conduction system. (p. 132)

A. _____

B. _____

C. _____

D. _____

E. _____

Pathophysiology: Recognizing Sympathetic Nervous System Response

The 72-year-old female patient discussed in the chapter of the textbook (p. 142) is having a silent MI, which is an MI that is painless. A significant number of these patients do not present with the "classic" symptoms of "crushing substernal chest pain" radiating down the left arm, so it is important always to consider the possibility of a heart attack in a patient who is not feeling well and has shortness of breath (dyspnea).

1. Elderly patients, females, and what other group of patients have silent MIs? _____

2. When the brain signals to the adrenal glands that the body is undergoing severe stress, such as that which occurs during an MI, the adrenal glands secrete two chemicals: epinephrine and norepinephrine. What do these two chemicals cause the body to do? _____

3. Of what body system is the adrenal gland a component? _____

4. Of what body system is the heart a component? _____

Label the Diagrams

Fill in the name of the structures for each of the following anatomical body system illustrations.

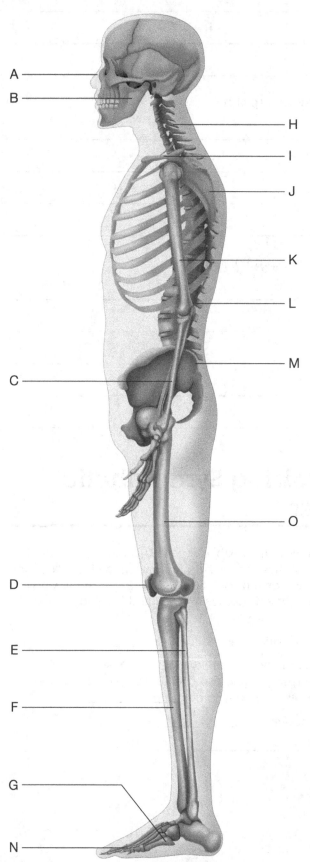

1. Skeletal system

A. _____

B. _____

C. _____

D. _____

E. _____

F. _____

G. _____

H. _____

I. _____

J. _____

K. _____

L. _____

M. _____

N. _____

O. _____

©2021 Pearson Education, Inc.
Emergency Care, 14th Ed.

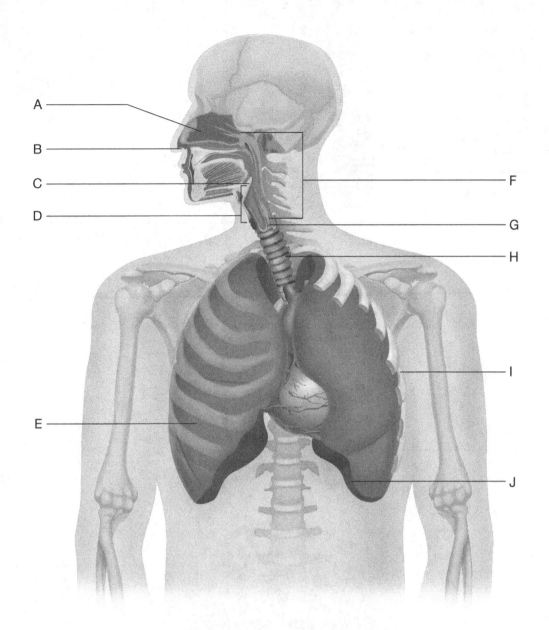

2. Respiratory system

A. _____   F. _____

B. _____   G. _____

C. _____   H. _____

D. _____   I. _____

E. _____   J. _____

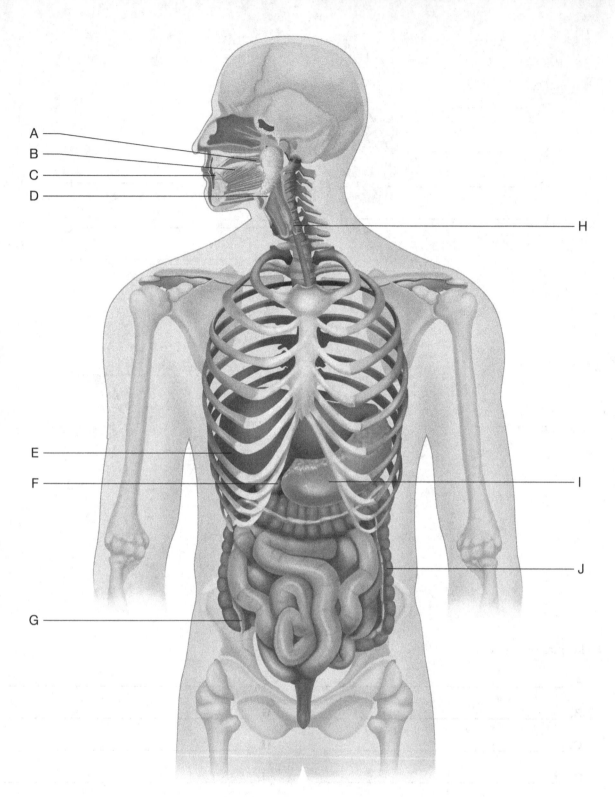

3. Digestive system

A. _____   F. _____

B. _____   G. _____

C. _____   H. _____

D. _____   I. _____

E. _____   J. _____

Principles of Pathophysiology

Core Concepts

- The cell, cellular metabolism, and results of the alteration of cellular metabolism
- The cardiopulmonary system and its combined respiratory and cardiovascular functions
- The respiratory system and the importance of oxygenation and ventilation
- The cardiovascular system and the movement of blood
- The principles of perfusion, hypoperfusion, and shock
- Disrupted physiology of major body systems

Outcomes

After reading this chapter, you should be able to:

7.1 Summarize the structures and functions of body cells. (pp. 157–159)
- Describe the influence of water on cells.
- Describe the role of glucose in cells.

7.2 Summarize the coordinated processes required of the cardiopulmonary system to maintain perfusion. (pp. 159–174)
- Contrast the processes of aerobic and anaerobic metabolism in cells.
- Relate the composition of air with the demands of the cardiopulmonary system.
- Distinguish between the processes of ventilation, respiration, and perfusion.
- Identify the structures of the airway.
- Explain the impact on the body of changes in the tidal volume, minute volume, and dead air space.
- Explain circumstances that lead to respiratory dysfunction.
- Describe the mechanism by which the body attempts to compensate for disruptions of respiration.
- Describe the functions of the various components of blood.
- Describe the consequences of reduction of blood volume, red blood cells, and water-retaining proteins.
- Distinguish the functions of arteries, veins, and capillaries.
- Outline the process of gas (oxygen and carbon dioxide) exchange in the body.
- Explain how the nervous system can correct low and high blood pressure.
- Analyze how loss of blood vessel tone, increased permeability, and increased systemic vascular resistance affect blood pressure.

- Illustrate the interaction of stroke volume, cardiac preload, cardiac contractility, and cardiac output.
- Given a change in the balance of sympathetic and parasympathetic components of the nervous system, predict the impact on heart function.
- Predict the consequences of mechanical and electrical dysfunctions of the heart.
- Explain the concept of V/Q (ventilation-perfusion) match.

7.3 Summarize the pathophysiology of shock. (pp. 174–176)
- Describe the mechanism which underlies all forms of shock.
- Contrast hypovolemic, distributive, cardiogenic, and obstructive shock.
- Given descriptions of patient presentations, categorize them as being in either compensated or decompensated shock.

7.4 Summarize fluid balance in the body. (pp. 176–178)
- Recall the distribution of water throughout the spaces of the body.
- Explain the distribution of water throughout the spaces of the body.
- Identify the structures that regulate fluid distribution throughout the spaces of the body.
- Describe disruptions of fluid balance.

7.5 Give a synopsis of general concepts of nervous system dysfunction. (p. 179)
- Explain how trauma can result in nervous system dysfunction.
- Explain how medical problems can result in nervous system dysfunction.
- Given a scenario, predict whether a patient has nervous system dysfunction.

7.6 Describe the mechanism by which the endocrine system contributes to control of body functions. (p. 180)
- Recall the structures primarily at the root of endocrine dysfunction.
- Explain the general categories of endocrine disorders.

7.7 Describe the relationship between perfusion and the gastrointestinal system. (p. 180)
- Describe the anatomy that can contribute to the severity of gastrointestinal bleeding.
- Recall potential causes of nausea and vomiting.
- Describe the consequences of ongoing loss of blood or fluid through the gastrointestinal tract.

7.8 Summarize the mechanism by which a response by the immune system can lead to shock. (p. 181)
- Give examples of types of substances that may provoke a hypersensitivity reaction.
- Compare normal immune response to foreign substances with allergic reactions.
- Describe the impact on body tissues of excess release of histamine.

Match Key Terms

A. The amount of blood ejected from the heart in one contraction.

B. The amount of blood ejected from the heart in one minute (HR × SV).

C. A substance that, when dissolved in water, separates into charged particles.

D. Fraction of inspired oxygen; the concentration of oxygen in the air we breathe.

E. The amount of air breathed in during each respiration multiplied by the number of breaths per minute.

F. Swelling associated with the movement of water into the interstitial space.

G. An abnormally low amount of water in the body.

H. An exaggerated response by the immune system to a particular substance.

_____ **1.** Pathophysiology

_____ **2.** Electrolyte

_____ **3.** Metabolism

_____ **4.** Aerobic metabolism

_____ **5.** Anaerobic metabolism

_____ **6.** Patent

_____ **7.** Tidal volume

_____ **8.** Dead air space

©2021 Pearson Education, Inc.
Emergency Care, 14th Ed.

I. The supply of oxygen to and removal of wastes from the cells and tissues of the body as a result of the flow of blood through the capillaries.

J. The study of how disease processes affect the function of the body.

K. The pressure within a blood vessel that tends to push water out of the vessel.

L. Sensors in the blood vessels designed to identify internal pressure.

M. The pressure in the peripheral blood vessels that the heart must overcome to pump blood in the system.

N. The volume of air moved in one cycle of breathing.

O. Open and clear; free from obstruction.

P. The cellular process in which oxygen is used to metabolize glucose.

Q. Air that occupies the space between the mouth and alveoli but does not actually reach the area of gas exchange.

R. The cellular function of converting nutrients into energy.

S. Chemical sensors in the brain and blood vessels that identify changing levels of oxygen and carbon dioxide.

T. The cellular process in which glucose is metabolized into energy without oxygen.

U. The pull exerted by large proteins in the plasma portion of blood that tends to pull water from the tissues into the bloodstream.

V. This implies that the alveoli are supplied with enough air and that the air in the alveoli is matched with sufficient blood in the pulmonary capillaries to permit optimum exchange of oxygen and carbon dioxide.

W. Sweating: condition of cool, pale, and moist/sweaty skin. sweating.

X. The non-medical term referring to hypoperfusion.

Y. The inability of the body to adequately circulate blood to the body's cells to supply them with oxygen and nutrients.

_____ 9. Chemoreceptors

_____ 10. Plasma oncotic pressure

_____ 11. Hydrostatic pressure

_____ 12. Cardiac output

_____ 13. Systemic vascular resistance (SVR)

_____ 14. V/Q match

_____ 15. Perfusion

_____ 16. Dehydration

_____ 17. Edema

_____ 18. Hypersensitivity

_____ 19. Stretch receptors

_____ 20. FiO_2

_____ 21. Minute volume

_____ 22. Stroke volume

_____ 23. Hypoperfusion

_____ 24. Shock

_____ 25. Diaphoresis

Multiple-Choice Review

_____ 1. The study of how disease processes affect the function of the body is called:
  A. anatomy.
  B. physiology.
  C. pathophysiology.
  D. kinetics.

_____ 2. The cell structure that contains the DNA is called the:
  A. endoplasmic reticulum.
  B. nucleus.
  C. mitochondria.
  D. Golgi apparatus.

_____ 3. Water management by the cells of the body is important because:
   A. it influences the concentrations of electrolytes.
   B. too much water interrupts basic cellular functions.
   C. too little water causes cells to dehydrate and die.
   D. all of these are true.

_____ 4. When the legs are crushed under a slab of concrete, the blood supply is diminished to the cells in the legs. This condition may result in:
   A. carbon monoxide being produced.   C. aerobic metabolism.
   B. lactic acid being produced.   D. all of these.

_____ 5. Movement of air into and out of the chest requires:
   A. a patent airway.
   B. an alert mental status.
   C. a large tidal volume to overcome the dead space.
   D. all of these.

_____ 6. You are assessing the ventilations of a 35-year-old female who appears to be having an asthma attack. The best assessment of the amount of air that gets into and out of the lungs each minute is the:
   A. end-tidal CO_2.   C. minute volume.
   B. tidal volume.   D. SPO_2.

_____ 7. An example of a patient whose minute volume is likely to have diminished considerably would be:
   A. a 35-year-old female experiencing an asthma attack.
   B. a 22-year-old male who has overdosed on a narcotic.
   C. a 16-year-old who just broke multiple ribs.
   D. all of these.

_____ 8. The respiratory control center of the brain is the:
   A. medulla oblongata.   C. cerebellum.
   B. foramen magnum.   D. cerebrum.

_____ 9. Respiration is activated by changing pressure within the thorax.
   _____ is a(n) _____ process, and _____ is a(n) _____ process.
   A. Exhalation; active; inhalation; passive
   B. Inhalation; active; exhalation; passive
   C. Exhalation; active; inhalation; voluntary
   D. Inhalation; passive; exhalation; involuntary

_____ 10. Your patient is beginning to have respiratory difficulties because his chest was crushed in a car crash. The sensory information provided to the respiratory system to increase the rate and/or tidal volume originates with the:
   A. ribs and chest vault.
   B. nervous system and spinal cord.
   C. chemoreceptors in the brain and vascular system.
   D. pressure sensors located in the aortic arch and carotids.

_____ 11. Energy for the cell is produced largely by the _____, which are responsible for conversion of glucose and nutrients into:
   A. lysosome: ATP.   C. endoplasmic reticulum: DNA.
   B. mitochondria: ATP.   D. mitochondria: RNA.

_____ 12. Your patient is dehydrated yet also has massive edema. This can be due to any of the following, *except*:
   A. changes in cell wall permeability.
   B. kidney function.
   C. the size and volume of proteins in blood plasma.
   D. hyperventilating under stress.

_____ **13.** When a patient's blood vessels constrict because of external blood loss, this process was originated by the brain because of messages received from the:
   A. chemoreceptors in the aortic arch.   C. marrow in the long bones.
   B. stretch receptors in certain blood   D. pulmonary system.
   vessels.

_____ **14.** Anaerobic metabolism is inefficient because it causes:
   A. acids to leak out of the cells.
   B. the body to expend more energy to eliminate CO_2.
   C. breakdown of fats.
   D. all of these.

_____ **15.** Patients who develop sepsis are prone to problems that affect:
   A. glucose production.   C. blood vessel constriction.
   B. level of insulin.   D. control of respirations.

_____ **16.** The average person ejects approximately 70 mL of blood per contraction of the heart. This is known as:
   A. afterload.   C. preload.
   B. vascular resistance.   D. stroke volume.

_____ **17.** The more forceful the squeezing of the heart, the greater the stroke volume. This concept refers to the _____ of the heart.
   A. resistance   C. preload
   B. contractility   D. afterload

_____ **18.** The patient's stroke volume depends on:
   A. afterload.   C. preload.
   B. contractility.   D. all of these.

_____ **19.** A 60-year-old female patient is experiencing a fight-or-flight situation, and her body is attempting to compensate by increasing her cardiac output by:
   A. decreasing her pulse rate.   C. increasing the heart rate.
   B. decreasing the stroke volume. D. decreasing the respiratory rate.

_____ **20.** When a cardiac patient has a repeat heart attack and cardiac output drops, this is often due to:
   A. ventricular irritability.
   B. a decrease in the tidal volume.
   C. a decrease in the strength of contractions.
   D. an increase in the heart rate.

_____ **21.** Fluid distribution is determined by:
   A. the brain and kidneys regulating thirst and eliminating excess fluid.
   B. the large proteins in blood plasma pulling fluid into the bloodstream.
   C. the permeability of both cell membranes and the walls of the capillaries helping to determine how much water can be held in and pushed out of cells and blood vessels.
   D. all of these.

_____ **22.** You are treating a 50-year-old male patient who has had severe vomiting and diarrhea for the past day. You suspect that he may have:
   A. an excess of body fluids.   C. edema in the extremities.
   B. a condition called dehydration. D. all of these.

_____ **23.** You are assessing a patient who you suspect may be having a stroke. He has signs of neurologic impairment, including:
   A. inability to speak or difficulty speaking.
   B. visual or hearing disturbance.
   C. weakness (sometimes limited to one side).
   D. all of these.

_____ **24.** An example of a condition in which glands of the body are producing too much of a hormone is:
- **A.** Graves' disease.
- **B.** diabetes.
- **C.** meningitis.
- **D.** a stroke.

_____ **25.** The most common disorders of the digestive system are diarrhea and:
- **A.** dizziness.
- **B.** nausea and vomiting.
- **C.** severe thirst.
- **D.** chills and fever.

_____ **26.** When the brain cells are significantly deprived of glucose a patient will develop signs and symptoms that mimic the signs and symptoms of:
- **A.** heart attack.
- **B.** stroke.
- **C.** shock.
- **D.** allergic reaction.

_____ **27.** A 42-year-old female with a history of blood clots in her left leg suddenly developed difficulty breathing as a result of a clot moving to the:
- **A.** heart.
- **B.** brain.
- **C.** spinal cord.
- **D.** lung.

_____ **28.** When a patient develops an infection that reaches the brain and spinal cord, the body system most affected is the:
- **A.** nervous system.
- **B.** respiratory system.
- **C.** cardiovascular system.
- **D.** endocrine system.

_____ **29.** A patient with severe nausea and vomiting due to a digestive problem can quickly become:
- **A.** unresponsive.
- **B.** dehydrated.
- **C.** constipated.
- **D.** hypertensive.

_____ **30.** Endocrine disorders most commonly occur due to:
- **A.** traumatic events.
- **B.** stroke.
- **C.** illness.
- **D.** pregnancy.

_____ **31.** A patient who is experiencing a new stroke might exhibit which sign?
- **A.** Malnutrition
- **B.** Electrolyte imbalance
- **C.** Rectal bleeding
- **D.** Visual disturbance

_____ **32.** When a pediatric patient experiences vasoconstriction, it is a very powerful response. It can be sustained through massive volume loss and therefore the EMT should:
- **A.** have the patient drink plenty of fluids.
- **B.** disregard the vital sign changes.
- **C.** not wait for hypotension to recognize shock.
- **D.** encourage the patient to sit up.

_____ **33.** Infants and young children rely a great deal on heart rate to compensate for poor perfusion. This is because:
- **A.** their vessels rarely constrict.
- **B.** they have very little fluid volume.
- **C.** they have so little fat.
- **D.** they have less contractile heart muscle cells than an adult.

_____ **34.** A clinical finding that EMTs can use to indicate poor perfusion, considered helpful in children but less reliable in adults, is:
- **A.** central pulses.
- **B.** capillary refill time.
- **C.** blood sugar test.
- **D.** heart rate.

_____ **35.** When assessing a pediatric patient who has fallen off a skateboard, the EMT should be especially concerned in finding _____, which may be the earliest indicator of compensation in a young child.
- **A.** an increased heart rate
- **B.** an increased blood pressure
- **C.** pallor and sweating
- **D.** nervousness and anxiety

©2021 Pearson Education, Inc.
Emergency Care, 14th Ed.

Complete the Following

1. For the "air to go in and air to go out and blood to go round and round," the system must be working. List what needs to be functioning properly.

   A. In the respiratory system: _____

   B. In the cardiovascular system: _____

2. A ventilation/perfusion (V/Q) match involves:

   A. _____

   B. _____

3. Shock is commonly defined as:

   _____

4. Four groupings of shock are:

   A. _____

   B. _____

   C. _____

   D. _____

5. Water comprises approximately 60 percent of the body's weight. What percent of water is in each of these three spaces?

   A. Intracellular fluid - _____

   B. Intravascular fluid - _____

   C. Interstitial fluid - _____

Pathophysiology: Recognizing Compensation

On the basis of the discussion of recognizing compensation in the text, list five things that happen to the body during a fight-or-flight situation.

   1. _____

   2. _____

   3. _____

   4. _____

   5. _____

Case Study: Major Life-Threatening Bleeding Injury

On a fall evening, you respond to a car that crashed into a utility pole at a high rate of speed. The vehicle is a small car, and most of the front end is displaced, literally wrapped around the pole. Both the police and rescue are responding to the call. There will definitely be a need to remove the roof and doors of the vehicle because the driver, a 22-year-old male, is pinned behind the steering column. The patient has left upper abdominal pain and an open left femur fracture. Your first set of vital signs reveals a pulse of 110 and thready, respirations of 22, blood pressure of 100/70 mmHg, and SpO_2 of 94%.

1. What do you suspect is the problem with the abdomen?

_____

2. If the patient is in shock, what type of shock would you suspect?

_____

GZQ **3.** What oxygen therapy should be used for this patient?

_____

As the rescue company pops the door of the car and removes the roof, it becomes easier to visualize how to get the patient out of the vehicle. Because of the severity of the damage to the vehicle, you have decided to use a spine board and collar and take the patient out through the top of the vehicle.

4. How much time do you have on the scene, as a goal, with this patient? Why?

_____

5. As the patient's body attempts to compensate for the blood loss, what signs would you expect to see for compensated shock?

_____

As you move the patient into the ambulance, the medic unit is on the scene, and a paramedic jumps into your unit to ride along to the hospital. You take another set of vital signs, and they are pulse 120, respiratory rate of 22, BP of 98/68, and SPO_2 of 93%. The patient's mental status is still verbal, although he is very anxious. The paramedic states, "I'll get an IV started on the way to the trauma center." You recheck the injured leg, which is now splinted, and the bleeding has slowed down.

GZQ **6.** What can you do to shorten the time the patient will spend in the ED?

_____

7. What sign is leading you to believe that the patient is moving towards decompensated shock?

_____

©2021 Pearson Education, Inc.
Emergency Care, 14th Ed.

8

Life Span Development

Core Concepts

- The physiologic (physical) characteristics of different age groups from infancy through late adulthood
- The psychosocial (mental and social) characteristics of different age groups from infancy through late adulthood

Outcomes

After reading this chapter, you should be able to:

8.1 Distinguish between the physiologic characteristics of people of different age groups. (pp. 186–196)
- Recall the physiologic characteristics of infants.
- Categorize infants' vital signs as normal or abnormal.
- Given descriptions of physical stimulation of an infant, explain the reflexes that should occur.
- Match infant age ranges with cognitive (mental) developmental milestones.
- Categorize toddlers' vital signs as normal or abnormal.
- Explain the increased susceptibility of toddlers to infectious diseases.
- Categorize a preschooler's vital signs as normal or abnormal.
- Categorize a school-age child's vital signs as normal or abnormal.
- Describe the physiologic changes that characterize adolescence.
- Differentiate between normal and abnormal adolescent vital signs.
- Compare the physiologic characteristics of early, middle, and late adulthood.
- Differentiate between normal and abnormal adult vital signs.

8.2 Compare the psychosocial characteristics of people. (pp. 186–196)
- Describe the cognitive (mental) and emotional characteristics expected in normally developing infants.
- Match toddler age ranges with cognitive (mental) developmental milestones.
- List the benefits to preschoolers of social interaction.
- Describe the psychosocial characteristics of school-age children.
- Describe the psychosocial characteristics of adolescents.
- Compare the psychosocial characteristics of early, middle, and late adulthood.

Match Key Terms

A. A reflex in which stroking a hungry infant's lips causes the infant to start sucking.

B. A reflex response in which a hungry infant automatically turns toward the stimulus when the cheek or one side of the mouth is touched.

C. The infant's reaction to the infant's environment.

D. Stage of life from 12 to 36 months.

E. Stage of life from 13 to 18 years.

F. Stage of life from 19 to 40 years.

G. Stage of life from 61 years and older.

H. Stage of life from birth to 1 year of age.

I. A grasping reflex in which an infant grabs onto a finger placed in the infant's palm.

J. Concept developed from an orderly, predictable environment versus a disorderly, irregular environment.

K. Stage of life from 6 to 12 years.

L. Stage of life from 41 to 60 years.

M. Building on what one already knows.

N. Stage of life from 3 to 5 years.

O. The sense that needs will be met.

P. A response to being startled in which the infant throws out both arms, spreads the fingers, then grabs with the fingers and arms.

_____ **1.** Infancy

_____ **2.** Moro reflex

_____ **3.** Palmar reflex

_____ **4.** Rooting reflex

_____ **5.** Sucking reflex

_____ **6.** Bonding

_____ **7.** Trust versus mistrust

_____ **8.** Scaffolding

_____ **9.** Temperament

_____ **10.** Toddler phase

_____ **11.** Preschool age

_____ **12.** School age

_____ **13.** Adolescence

_____ **14.** Early adulthood

_____ **15.** Middle adulthood

_____ **16.** Late adulthood

Multiple-Choice Review

_____ **1.** Your patient is primarily a nose breather, and her head is equal to 25 percent of her total body weight. What age group is she in?
   A. Toddler
   B. Infancy
   C. School age
   D. Preschool age

_____ **2.** You are assessing an infant who is very congested. Why can nasal congestion be a major problem in the first few months of life?
   A. Because these children breathe with their diaphragm.
   B. Because the liver is so large in a patient of this age.
   C. Because children of this age are primarily nasal breathers.
   D. Because it is an indication of life-threatening airway compromise.

_____ **3.** Infants get their immunity and antibodies from:
   A. breastfeeding from their mother.
   B. the vaccinations they receive.
   C. producing their own antibodies from exposure to diseases.
   D. all of these.

©2021 Pearson Education, Inc.
Emergency Care, 14th Ed.

_____ **4.** You are evaluating an infant whose mother states that the infant "has been very sleepy all day." Which of the following nervous system reflexes is *not* normally found in an infant?
   A. The Cushing reflex   **C.** The rooting reflex
   B. The Moro reflex   **D.** The sucking reflex

_____ **5.** When the mother strokes the infant's lips and the baby starts sucking, this is a nervous system reflex known as the:
   A. Moro reflex.   **C.** palmar reflex.
   B. sucking reflex.   **D.** rooting reflex.

_____ **6.** A mother states that her baby daughter is developing her reactions to the environment. This is also known as the psychosocial characteristic of:
   A. trust versus mistrust.   **C.** bonding.
   B. temperament.   **D.** scaffolding.

_____ **7.** When an infant develops anxiety and insecurity, this is often due to the psychosocial characteristic of:
   A. trust versus mistrust.   **C.** bonding.
   B. temperament.   **D.** scaffolding.

_____ **8.** A toddler has continuing developments and changes from infancy. Examples include each of the following *except* that:
   A. the brain is now 90 percent of an adult's brain weight.
   B. the alveoli increase in numbers.
   C. the child is less susceptible to illness.
   D. all of the primary teeth should be in place.

_____ **9.** The adolescent years often include the beginning of:
   A. self-destructive behaviors.
   B. excellent decision-making skills.
   C. nasal breathing.
   D. the replacement of primary teeth.

_____ **10.** The peak physical condition occurs between the ages of _____ and _____.
   A. 12; 16   **C.** 30; 40
   B. 19; 26   **D.** 35; 45

_____ **11.** You have been called to the home of a woman who fell in the kitchen. When you get a medical history, you find that she is taking medicine for control of high cholesterol, and she states that she has been dieting this week and was a little dizzy. According to your understanding of typical activities of different age groups, what is her most likely age group?
   A. School age   **C.** Early adulthood
   B. Adolescent   **D.** Middle adulthood

_____ **12.** You are treating a patient in his late adulthood. Some examples of the psychosocial challenges that a person in late adulthood faces include:
   A. financial burdens.   **C.** living environment.
   B. self-worth.   **D.** all of these.

_____ **13.** EMTs may need to make some adjustments in how they conduct their assessment according to the patient's stage of life. How might the age of the patient affect your assessment?
   A. The parent or caregiver will need to help you when you assess an infant.
   B. The patient who is in late adulthood is likely to have cardiovascular disorders.
   C. The adolescent often experiments with alcohol and tobacco.
   D. All of these are challenges that you might come across.

_____ **14.** An EMT's ability to communicate with a school-aged patient can be compli-
cated by all of the following *except*:
 A. negative self-esteem.   **C.** separation anxiety.
 B. moral reasoning.   **D.** internal self-control of behavior.

_____ **15.** During the adolescent years of development, both males and females:
 A. begin to develop self-esteem.   **C.** replace their primary teeth.
 B. reach reproductive maturity.   **D.** All of these are correct.

_____ **16.** Girls are usually finished growing by the age of:
 A. 14.   **C.** 18.
 B. 16.   **D.** 20.

_____ **17.** Boys are usually finished growing by the age of:
 A. 14.   **C.** 18.
 B. 16.   **D.** 20.

_____ **18.** Serious family conflicts occur in some _____ as the child strives for
 _____ and the parents strive for _____.
 A. school-age children; freedom; control
 B. adolescents; independence; control
 C. early adults; control; independence
 D. preschoolers; independence; control

_____ **19.** The leading cause of death in the early adulthood age group is/are:
 A. overdose.   **C.** accidents.
 B. heart attack.   **D.** stroke.

_____ **20.** The highest levels of job stress occur in which age group?
 A. Adolescent   **C.** Middle adult
 B. School-age   **D.** Early adult

Complete the Following

1. List the eight life stages of life discussed in the textbook.

 A. _____

 B. _____

 C. _____

 D. _____

 E. _____

 F. _____

 G. _____

 H. _____

2. Many changes occur during the first months of life. List a developmental
characteristic for each of the following months in the child's first year:

 A. 2 months: _____

 B. 3 months: _____

C. 4 months: _____

D. 5 months: _____

E. 6 months: _____

F. 7 months: _____

G. 8 months: _____

H. 9 months: _____

I. 10 months: _____

J. 11 months: _____

K. 12 months: _____

3. You are assessing the vital signs of your patient. What would the normal pulse rate be for each of the following age groups?

A. Newborn: _____

B. Infant: _____

C. Toddler: _____

D. Preschooler: _____

E. School age: _____

F. Adolescence: _____

4. List four psychosocial changes in the early adulthood years:

A. _____

B. _____

C. _____

D. _____

Airway Management

Core Concepts

- Physiology of the airway
- Pathophysiology of the airway
- How to recognize an adequate or an inadequate airway
- How to open an airway
- How to use airway adjuncts
- Principles and techniques of suctioning

Outcomes

After reading this chapter, you should be able to:

9.1 Describe the structure and function of the normal airway. (pp. 203–206)
  - Differentiate the structures of the upper airway from those of the lower airway.
  - Match airway structures to their functions.

9.2 Explain concepts of airway pathophysiology. (pp. 206–210)
  - List causes of obstruction of the upper and lower airway.
  - List the steps to airway assessment in the primary assessment.
  - Distinguish between signs that indicate absent breathing, inadequate airway, and adequate airway.
  - List signs of inadequate airway that are more likely in children than in adults.
  - Explain how to determine whether a patient's airway status may worsen.

9.3 Describe the use of manual maneuvers to open the airway. (pp. 210–216)
  - Given a scenario, provide a rationale for selecting the type of manual maneuver that is best for the patient in the scenario.

9.4 Explain the use of adjunctive equipment to manage a patient's airway. (pp. 216–234)
  - State the importance of having a suction device immediately available during airway management procedures.
  - Given scenarios, identify adherence to general rules for using airway adjuncts.
  - Describe how the features of an oropharyngeal airway allow it to provide an air passage in patients who cannot maintain their own airways.
  - List the sequence of steps used in the insertion of oropharyngeal airway.

- Identify instances when a nasopharyngeal airway offers benefits over an oropharyngeal airway.
- List the sequence of steps used in the insertion of a nasopharyngeal airway.
- Describe the minimum features required of suction units.
- Match the components and attachments of suction devices with their designed purposes.
- Suggest responses to complications encountered when suctioning a patient's airway.
- Recall the general rules that apply to suctioning techniques.
- Describe decision-making considerations in choosing approaches to suctioning.

Match Key Terms

A. A means of correcting blockage of the airway by moving the jaw forward without tilting the head or neck. Used when trauma, or injury, is suspected to open the airway without causing further injury to the spinal cord in the neck.

B. A curved device inserted through the patient's mouth into the pharynx to help maintain an open airway.

C. An airway that is open and clear to the passage of air into and out of the body.

D. Vomiting or retching that results when something is placed in the back of the pharynx. This is tied to the swallow reflex.

E. The passageway by which air enters or leaves the body. The structures of the airway are the nose, mouth, pharynx, larynx, trachea, bronchi, and lungs.

F. A means of correcting blockage of the airway by the tongue by tilting the head back and lifting the chin. Used when no trauma, or injury, is suspected.

G. Use of a vacuum device to remove blood, vomitus, and other secretions or foreign materials from the airway.

H. A flexible device inserted through the patient's nostril into the pharynx to help maintain an open airway.

I. The space between the vocal cords that defines the boundary between the upper and lower airways.

J. A high-pitched inspiratory sound generated from partially obstructed airflow in the upper airway.

K. The contraction of smooth muscle that lines the bronchial passages that result in a decreased internal diameter of the airway and increased resistance to flow.

_____ **1.** Airway

_____ **2.** Patent airway

_____ **3.** Head-tilt, chin-lift maneuver

_____ **4.** Jaw-thrust maneuver

_____ **5.** Oropharyngeal airway

_____ **6.** Nasopharyngeal airway

_____ **7.** Gag reflex

_____ **8.** Suctioning

_____ **9.** Bronchoconstriction

_____ **10.** Stridor

_____ **11.** Glottic opening

Multiple-Choice Review

_____ **1.** The movement of air into and out of the lungs requires that:
- **A.** oxygen exits on the exhalation phase.
- **B.** carbon dioxide enters on the inhalation phase.
- **C.** airflow is unobstructed and moving freely.
- **D.** the mouth be open at all times that the patient is breathing.

_____ **2.** When a patient inhales, air enters the body and finally travels through the
_____ prior to entering the trachea.
  A. nasopharynx   **C.** laryngopharynx
  B. oropharynx   **D.** both B and C.

_____ **3.** The hypopharynx is also called the:
  A. nares.   **C.** trachea.
  B. laryngopharynx.   **D.** glottis.

_____ **4.** The large leaflike structure that protects the opening to the trachea is called the:
  A. oropharynx.   **C.** epiglottis.
  B. xiphoid process.   **D.** cricoid cartilage.

_____ **5.** When we say that a patient is experiencing lower airway obstruction, it is likely
that the:
  A. patient is choking on a foreign object.
  B. patient's bronchial passages or alveoli are congested.
  C. patient's tongue is swollen.
  D. epiglottis is inflamed.

_____ **6.** You believe that your patient is exhibiting signs of an inadequate airway. These
signs will include all of the following *except*:
  A. absent air movement.
  B. air that can be felt at the nose or mouth on expiration.
  C. unusual hoarse or raspy sound quality to the voice.
  D. abnormal noises such as wheezing, crowing, or stridor.

_____ **7.** When inserting an OPA into a pediatric patient:
  A. insert it straight in.
  B. do not rotate or flip over the tongue.
  C. consider using a tongue depressor.
  D. all of the above.

_____ **8.** If the choking infant becomes unconscious you should:
  A. initiate abdominal thrusts.
  B. continue with backslaps.
  C. begin CPR.
  D. place the infant in the prone position.

_____ **9.** If a conscious infant is choking severely, you must:
  A. encourage the child to cough.
  B. intervene with backslaps and chest thrusts.
  C. begin chest compressions at 100 per minute.
  D. reach into the mouth and feel for an obstruction.

_____ **10.** One indication that a child is experiencing labored breathing is that she:
  A. has a headache.
  B. complains of nausea.
  C. has nasal flaring when she breathes.
  D. is dizzy when standing.

_____ **11.** The optimal airway position in unresponsive infants and children can be achieved by:
  A. hyperextending the neck.
  B. keeping the neck in flexion.
  C. aligning the patient's ear to the level of the suprasternal notch.
  D. utilizing the modified-jaw thrust.

_____ **12.** You are about to manage the airway of a 22-year-old male who fell face first down a
flight of stairs. What is the importance of mechanism of injury to airway care?
  A. An injured patient will need more oxygen.
  B. Trauma victims may require the jaw-thrust maneuver to open the airway.
  C. Patients without a mechanism of injury will have an open airway.
  D. An injury can make airway care easier to manage than a medical emergency.

_____ **13.** Your patient has sustained a high-energy impact to the head and neck. To open the airway of a patient with a suspected head, neck, or spine injury, the EMT should use a _____ maneuver.
   A. jaw-thrust
   B. head-tilt, chin-lift
   C. head-tilt, neck-lift
   D. sniffing position

_____ **14.** You are deciding which airway adjunct to use to assist in keeping open the airway of a 30-year-old female who you suspect has sustained a basilar skull fracture. You note clear fluid running out of her ears. It is best to choose:
   A. no airway if she is unconscious.
   B. an OPA if she has no gag reflex.
   C. a NPA to allow the fluid to drain.
   D. a NPA in each of the nares.

_____ **15.** When performing the jaw-thrust maneuver, the EMT should do each one of the following *except*:
   A. kneeling at the top of the patient's head.
   B. gently place one hand on each side of patient's lower jaw.
   C. using the index fingers to push the angles of the patient's lower jaw forward.
   D. tilting the head by applying gentle pressure to the patient's forehead.

_____ **16.** The main purpose of the jaw-thrust maneuver is to:
   A. open the mouth with only one hand.
   B. open the airway without moving the head or neck.
   C. create an airway for the medical patient.
   D. create an airway when it is not possible to jut the jaw.

_____ **17.** An oral or nasal airway should be:
   A. cleaned for reuse after the call.
   B. inserted in all critically injured patients.
   C. used to help keep an airway open.
   D. used to prevent the need for suctioning.

_____ **18.** It is always important to be careful when inserting an OPA. If something is placed in the patient's throat, the gag reflex may cause the patient to:
   A. take deep breaths.
   B. pass out.
   C. vomit or retch.
   D. all of these.

_____ **19.** You will be inserting an OPA in your patient. First you will need to measure the correct size. An OPA of proper size extends from the:
   A. corner of the patient's mouth to the tip of the earlobe.
   B. lips to the larynx.
   C. nose to the angle of the jaw.
   D. none of these.

_____ **20.** In an adult patient an OPA should be inserted:
   A. upside down, with the tip toward the roof of the mouth, then flipped 180 degrees over the tongue.
   B. right side up, using a tongue depressor to press the tongue down and forward to keep it from obstructing the airway.
   C. either of these.
   D. neither of these.

_____ **21.** A nasopharyngeal airway should be:
   A. inserted with the bevel on the lateral side of the nostril.
   B. measured from the patient's nostril to the tip of the earlobe or angle of the jaw.
   C. inserted into the left nostril when possible.
   D. turned 180 degrees with the tip facing the roof of the mouth.

_____ **22.** To assist in airway maintenance, you have decided to use a nasopharyngeal airway (NPA). When inserting an NPA, lubricate the outside of the tube with:
   A. petroleum jelly.
   B. an oil-based lubricant.
   C. a silicone-based gel.
   D. a water-based lubricant.

_____ 23. Your service requires that you bring the suction unit on all priority calls where you might need to use it. The purposes of suctioning may include removal of:
   A. teeth and large pieces of solid material.
   B. excess oxygen from the patient.
   C. blood, vomitus, and other secretions.
   D. all of these.

_____ 24. When a patient begins to vomit or produce a gurgling sound, it is essential that you have a(n) _____ ready to go at the patient's side.
   A. suction unit   C. blood pressure cuff
   B. oxygen tank   D. pocket mask

_____ 25. You are treating a 29-year-old female who has major airway problems. She has thick secretions and blood in her upper airway that need to be suctioned with a Yankauer. Which of the following is *not* true of the Yankauer suction tip?
   A. It has a rigid tip.
   B. It allows for excellent control over the distal end of the device.
   C. It is used most successfully with responsive patients.
   D. It has a larger bore than flexible catheters.

_____ 26. Compared to an adult's airway structures, the pediatric patient's respiratory system includes:
   A. a narrower trachea.   C. a smaller mouth and nose.
   B. a softer and more flexible trachea.   D. all of the above.

_____ 27. Why is nasal obstruction a more urgent problem in an infant as opposed to an adult?
   A. the nose is proportionately larger than adults.
   B. infants and newborns typically breathe through their noses.
   C. the trachea is narrower.
   D. children depend more on their diaphragms for breathing.

_____ 28. It can be problematic to lay a small child flat who has altered mental status because:
   A. it makes it hard to breathe thru the nose.
   B. flexion of the neck can cause airway obstruction.
   C. the child will become anxious.
   D. all of the above.

_____ 29. Suctioning in pediatrics is not very different than suctioning in adults. Both rigid and flexible suction catheters have appropriate pediatric sizes. The difference is:
   A. time stimulating the hypopharynx should be minimized.
   B. infants are very sensitive to vagal stimulation.
   C. bulb syringes are used in the emergency childbirth setting.
   D. all of the above are true.

_____ 30. Some patients will benefit from a supraglottic airway. If these devices are included in your protocols, they should be considered when:
   A. proper positioning will not work.
   B. manual airway opening and adjuncts cannot keep the airway open.
   C. The patient does not have a gag reflex.
   D. all of the above.

_____ 31. In a supine patient an optimal airway position can be achieved by:
   A. using the jaw thrust maneuver.
   B. turning the patient on one side and inserting an OPA.
   C. creating a head elevated, sniffing position.
   D. flexing the neck with padding behind the head.

_____ **32.** You are suctioning a young child who sustained a broken nose after falling from a tricycle. You notice the pulse is slowing down. What could be going on?
   A. The child has internal bleeding leading to shock.
   B. Vagal stimulation caused by catheter contact when suctioning the hypopharynx.
   C. The bleeding is causing a gag reflex in the child.
   D. The child is calming down because of receiving care.

_____ **33.** Compared to an adult's airway physiology, the pediatric airway includes:
   A. More dependency on the diaphragm for breathing.
   B. A chest wall that is softer than an adult's.
   C. A tongue that takes up proportionately more space in the mouth.
   D. All of the above.

Pathophysiology: Sounds of a Partially Obstructed Airway

1. Of the abnormal sounds that patients make when the airway is partially obstructed, which sound is typically high-pitched?

   _____

2. What sound may be an early finding due to a developing respiratory burn?

   _____

3. Which sound is caused by the soft tissue of the upper airway causing partial obstruction to the flow of air?

   _____

4. Which sound is usually due to liquid in the airway?

   _____

Complete the Following

1. List eight signs of an inadequate airway in adults and/or pediatric patients.

   A. _____

   B. _____

   C. _____

   D. _____

   E. _____

   F. _____

   G. _____

   H. _____

2. List six general rules for the use of OPAs and NPAs.

A. _____

B. _____

C. _____

D. _____

E. _____

F. _____

3. Complete the missing information in this listing of the Airway in the Primary Assessment-ABC.

The Airway in the Primary Assessment-ABC

Is the airway open?
Is the patient able to speak?

Look

- _____

- _____

- _____

- _____

Listen

- _____

- _____

Feel

- _____

- _____

Will the airway stay open?

- _____

- _____

- _____

- _____

Are there potential threats that may develop later?

- _____
- _____
- _____
- _____

Case Study: Rapidly Changing Airway

Your BLS unit and the police are dispatched to the scene of a call for a woman who is having difficulty breathing. The call was made by a family member who came home and found his 45-year-old mother wheezing and struggling. The police arrive before you and advise that the scene is secure and that you should respond directly to the scene of a private home in a suburban community two minutes from your station. As you enter the house, you can hear a woman wheezing, and the sound gets louder as you go up the stairs. She is in the rear upper bedroom. After donning your protective gloves, mask, and eye shield, you begin to question the patient as your partner obtains a set of baseline vital signs. The patient talks in short, choppy sentences, and you can hear wheezing without the use of a stethoscope. It is clear to you that she is having a very severe asthma attack.

GZQ **1.** Do you suspect that this patient has an upper airway or lower airway obstruction?

_____

2. What is the significance of the patient being able to speak only in short, choppy sentences?

_____

3. If this patient becomes unconscious while you are providing care, what type of airway would be used first?

_____

4. When the patient is unconscious and placed on your stretcher, how would you manually open the airway?

_____

5. You are assisting the patient, who is now unconscious on your stretcher. ALS has been called for, and you are preparing to carry her out the front door to the ambulance. The patient starts to make a snoring noise. Her heart rate is 100, and her respiratory rate is 28 and labored with an SPO_2 of 92%. What is that noise, and what should you do about it?

_____

6. After dealing with the airway noise, you notice a gurgling sound. What causes this sound, and how do you take care of it?

_____

GZQ **7.** After dealing with the gurgling sound, you notice that there is hardly any wheezing sound either with or without a stethoscope. What is the significance of this finding at this point?

_____

Respiration and Artificial Ventilation

Core Concepts

- Physiology and pathophysiology of the respiratory system
- How to recognize adequate and inadequate breathing
- Principles and techniques of positive pressure ventilation
- Principles and techniques of oxygen administration

Outcomes

After reading this chapter, you should be able to:

10.1 Compare the physiology and pathophysiology of breathing. (pp. 239–241)
- Describe the mechanical process of breathing.
- Describe the physiology of respiration at the alveolar level.

10.2 Explain concepts of cardiopulmonary pathophysiology. (pp. 241–242)
- Explain how various conditions can interrupt the mechanical processes of breathing.
- Explain how various conditions can interrupt the process of gas exchange at the alveolar level.
- Explain how various impairments of circulation can interrupt the exchange of gases at the cellular level.

10.3 Summarize concepts of respiration. (pp. 243–248)
- List conditions necessary for adequate respiration.
- Recognize the consequences of inadequate breathing.
- Distinguish the pathophysiologies of respiratory distress and respiratory failure.

10.4 Describe the assessment of patients' breathing. (pp. 248–251)
- Describe the sequence of steps involved in assessing breathing.
- Evaluate breathing status based on assessment findings.
- Differentiate between patients who need only supplemental oxygen and those who need artificial ventilation with supplemental oxygen.

10.5 Summarize concepts of positive pressure ventilation. (pp. 251–264)
- Explain complications of positive pressure intervention.
- Describe the general approach to using artificial ventilation.
- Describe different techniques of artificial ventilation.
- Compare the approaches to artificial ventilation for patients with rapid breathing and those with slow breathing.
- Match the EMT's interventions with patients' respiratory statuses.

©2021 Pearson Education, Inc.
Emergency Care, 14th Ed.

- Identify the equipment used with each technique of artificial ventilation.
- List the sequence of steps for using each technique of artificial ventilation.
- List modifications of artificial ventilation for stoma breathers.
- Describe the indications for using an automatic transport ventilator (ATV).

10.6 Explain concepts related to administering supplemental oxygen. (pp. 264–281)
- Describe the major issues to consider when making a decision to provide patients with supplemental oxygen.
- Compare the features of various portable and fixed oxygen cylinders used in EMS system.
- Describe the EMT's obligations with respect to evaluating the supply of oxygen available.
- List the EMT's obligations with respect to safety related to oxygen use.
- Identify the equipment and supplies used in oxygen administration.
- Describe the purpose of each of the parts of an oxygen delivery system.
- List risks to patients who receive excessive amounts of supplemental oxygen.
- List the sequence of steps for preparing an oxygen delivery system for supplemental oxygen administration.
- Given a patient scenario, select the most appropriate approach to oxygen therapy.
- Describe considerations in responding to patients who have complications that can interfere with oxygen administration and artificial ventilation.
- Provide the rationales for modifying techniques of oxygenation and artificial ventilations in pediatric patients.

10.7 Explain the EMT's roles and responsibilities related to the use of advanced airway devices. (pp. 281–285)
- Recognize the types of devices used for advanced airway management.
- Identify what EMTs can do to assist in the advanced airway placement procedures.
- Describe considerations in ventilating a patient who has an advanced airway device in place.

Match Key Terms

Part A

A. A device, usually with a one-way valve, to aid in artificial ventilation. It also acts as a barrier to prevent contact with a patient's breath or body fluids.

B. A process by which molecules move from an area of high concentration to an area of low concentration.

C. The process of forcing air and/or oxygen into the lungs when breathing has stopped.

D. Increased work of breathing; a sensation of shortness of breath.

E. When breathing completely stops.

F. Forcing air or oxygen into the lungs when a patient has stopped breathing or has inadequate breathing.

G. The exchange of oxygen and carbon dioxide between cells and circulating blood.

H. A blue or gray color resulting from lack of oxygen in the body.

I. Breathing in and out (inhalation and exhalation).

J. The amount of air that reaches the alveoli during an inhalation.

_____ 1. Ventilation

_____ 2. Alveolar ventilation

_____ 3. Diffusion

_____ 4. Pulmonary respiration

_____ 5. Cellular respiration

_____ 6. Respiration

_____ 7. Hypoxia

_____ 8. Respiratory distress

_____ 9. Respiratory failure

_____ 10. Respiratory arrest

_____ 11. Cyanosis

_____ 12. Artificial ventilation

_____ 13. Positive pressure ventilation

_____ 14. Pocket face mask

K. The diffusion of oxygen and carbon dioxide between the alveoli and the blood and between the blood and the cells.

L. The reduction of breathing to the point at which oxygen intake is not sufficient to support life.

M. An insufficiency of oxygen in the body's tissues.

N. The exchange of oxygen and carbon dioxide between the alveoli and circulating blood in the pulmonary capillaries.

Part B

A. A device designed to be placed over a stoma or tracheostomy tube to provide supplemental oxygen.

B. A permanent surgical opening in the neck through which the patient breathes.

C. A face mask that delivers very specific concentrations of oxygen by mixing oxygen with inhaled air.

D. A valve that indicates the flow of oxygen in liters per minute.

E. A face mask and reservoir bag device that delivers high concentrations of oxygen. The patient's exhaled air escapes through a valve and is not rebreathed.

F. A face mask and reservoir oxygen bag with no flutter valves on the mask, allowing the patient to breath in atmospheric air along with oxygen.

G. A device that provides positive pressure ventilations. It includes settings designed to adjust ventilation rate and volume, is portable, and is easily carried on an ambulance.

H. A device that delivers low concentrations of oxygen through two prongs that rest in the patient's nostrils.

I. A handheld device with a face mask and self-refilling bag that can be squeezed to provide artificial ventilations to a patient.

J. A cylinder filled with oxygen under pressure.

K. A device connected to the flowmeter to add moisture to the dry oxygen coming from an oxygen cylinder.

L. A device connected to an oxygen cylinder to reduce cylinder pressure so that it is safe for delivery of oxygen to a patient.

_____ **1.** Bag-valve mask (BVM)

_____ **2.** Venturi mask

_____ **3.** Stoma

_____ **4.** Tracheostomy mask

_____ **5.** Automatic transport ventilator (ATV)

_____ **6.** Oxygen cylinder

_____ **7.** Pressure regulator

_____ **8.** Flowmeter

_____ **9.** Humidifier

_____ **10.** Nonrebreather (NRB) mask

_____ **11.** Nasal cannula

_____ **12.** Partial rebreather mask

Multiple-Choice Review

_____ **1.** During the process of ventilation:
   A. the intercostal muscles expand, causing the air to be forced out of the chest.
   B. carbon dioxide enters the body during each expiration.
   C. oxygen enters the body during each expiration.
   D. the diaphragm and chest muscles contract and relax to change the pressure in the chest.

©2021 Pearson Education, Inc.
Emergency Care, 14th Ed.

_____ **2.** Respiratory failure is:
   A. the complete cessation of inspiration.
   B. inadequacy of breathing with insufficient oxygen intake.
   C. another term for respiratory arrest.
   D. caused by electrocution in young children.

_____ **3.** You are assessing a 45-year-old female who called the ambulance because she was having difficulty breathing. Which of the following is a sign that she might not be breathing adequately?
   A. Air moving in and out of the chest.
   B. Equal expansion of both sides of the chest.
   C. Severely diminished breath sounds upon auscultation of the lungs.
   D. Skin color normal.

_____ **4.** You are assessing a 6-year-old male who is having difficulty breathing. Signs of inadequate breathing in a child this age may include:
   A. cyanotic skin, lips, tongue, or earlobes.
   B. retractions between and below the ribs.
   C. nasal flaring.
   D. all of these.

_____ **5.** Each of the following is a sign of labored breathing in an adult patient _except_:
   A. inspirations or expirations that are prolonged.
   B. breathing rate in an adult of 14 to 18 breaths per minute.
   C. breathing that is very shallow, is very deep, or appears labored.
   D. the patient is unable to speak in full sentences.

_____ **6.** You are treating a patient who has signs of inadequate breathing. These signs could include all of the following _except_:
   A. absent or minimal chest movement.
   B. air that can be felt at the nose or mouth on exhalation.
   C. diminished or absent breath sounds.
   D. noises such as wheezing, gurgling, stridor, or crowing.

_____ **7.** Your patient is a child who is approximately 4 years old and is in respiratory distress, which may be leading to respiratory failure. Inadequate breathing in a child this age is defined as:
   A. fewer than 12 breaths per minute.
   B. more than 36 breaths per minute.
   C. cyanosis of the lips and earlobes.
   D. any of these.

_____ **8.** Which of the following is a difference in signs between respiratory distress and respiratory failure?
   A. A patient with respiratory failure has cyanotic or gray skin color.
   B. A patient with respiratory failure shows an alert mental status.
   C. A patient with respiratory distress shows blue skin.
   D. A patient with respiratory distress results in a comatose patient.

_____ **9.** Your patient may be becoming cyanotic. You check for cyanosis by observing the patient's lips and:
   A. tongue.   **C.** nail beds.
   B. earlobes.   **D.** tongue, nail beds, earlobes.

_____ **10.** One indication that a patient is experiencing inadequate breathing is that she:
   A. has a headache.   **C.** talks in short, choppy sentences.
   B. complains of nausea.   **D.** is dizzy when standing.

_____ **11.** When the diffusion of oxygen and carbon dioxide takes place between the cells and circulating blood this accomplishes:
   A. pulmonary respiration.   **C.** passive diffusion.
   B. cellular respiration.   **D.** alveolar ventilation.

_____ **12.** Your patient has overdosed on a narcotic medication that was prescribed for pain after a surgical procedure. Apparently, she took four times the prescribed dose, thinking that she could completely eliminate the pain. This medicine has been known to depress respirations and lead to:

A. cyanosis.

B. hypoxia.

C. tachycardia.

D. delayed capillary refill.

_____ **13.** The normal, or adequate, breathing rate for a 50-year-old adult should be:

A. 6 to 10 breaths per minute.

B. 12 to 20 breaths per minute.

C. 15 to 30 breaths per minute.

D. 25 to 50 breaths per minute.

_____ **14.** When the EMT determines that the patient is not breathing or that breathing is inadequate, it is necessary to provide:

A. positive pressure ventilation.

B. artificial ventilation.

C. assistance with a BVM device.

D. any of these.

_____ **15.** The negative side effects of positive pressure ventilation include each of the following *except*:

A. hypothermia.

B. gastric distension.

C. decreasing cardiac output.

D. dropping blood pressure.

_____ **16.** You have been ventilating a patient with a BVM device. Your partner states that you should be careful not to hyperventilate the patient because it causes:

A. hypoxia in the heart tissue.

B. vasoconstriction and limited blood flow to the brain.

C. the blood pressure to increase excessively.

D. an excessive elevation of carbon dioxide in the blood stream.

_____ **17.** The EMT can use various techniques to provide artificial ventilation in the field. Given plenty of trained helpers, which would be the *least* effective?

A. One rescuer using a bag-valve mask

B. A flow-restricted, oxygen-powered ventilation device

C. Two rescuers using a bag-valve mask with high-concentration supplemental oxygen at 15 liters per minute

D. Mouth-to-mask with high-concentration supplemental oxygen at 15 liters per minute

_____ **18.** Which of the following indicates you are ventilating the patient adequately?

A. The patient's chest rises and falls with each ventilation.

B. The rate of ventilation is too slow or too fast.

C. The patient's color changes from cyanotic to ashen.

D. The patient's heart rate continues to slow with ventilations.

_____ **19.** If an adult has a tidal volume of 500 mL and is breathing at 12 times per minute, what would his/her alveolar ventilation volume be per minute?

A. 2,100

B. 3,000

C. 4,200

D. 6,000

_____ **20.** The adult sized bag-valve mask on your EMS unit should have a:

A. nonrefilling shell that is easily cleaned.

B. non-jam valve with an oxygen inlet.

C. standard 9/12-mm fitting.

D. manual disabling pop-off valve.

_____ **21.** The bag-valve mask should be capable of:

A. withstanding cold temperatures.

B. providing a high pressure in the chest and airway.

C. blowing off at pressures above 40 mm of water pressure.

D. receiving an oxygen inlet flow of 25 liters per minute.

_____ **22.** In ventilating a 35-year-old male head trauma patient with a bag-valve mask, it is most effective to do all of the following *except*:
  A. use a device with a volume of 1,000 to 1,600 mL.
  B. use two EMTs to perform the procedure.
  C. position the EMT who is maintaining the mask seal at the patient's head.
  D. maintain the head-tilt, chin-lift maneuver.

_____ **23.** In ventilating a 22-year-old unconscious female, a bag-valve mask should be used with:
  A. a reservoir bag.   **C.** an oxygen tank and liter flow regulator.
  B. an oral airway.   **D.** all of these.

_____ **24.** If the patient's chest does not rise and fall during ventilation using a bag-valve mask, the EMT should do all of the following *except*:
  A. reposition the head and reattempt ventilations.
  B. check for escape of air around the mask.
  C. use an alternative method of artificial ventilation.
  D. increase the rate at which the bag is squeezed.

_____ **25.** If the patient has a _____ and needs ventilatory assistance, the best device to use is a _____.
  A. stoma; oropharyngeal airway
  B. tracheotomy; positive pressure ventilator
  C. stoma; bag-valve mask
  D. tracheotomy; nasal airway

_____ **26.** When you question an elderly woman with a respiratory complaint, she speaks in short, two- or three-word sentences. Is this significant?
  A. No, she probably always speaks that way.
  B. Yes, she must have a completely blocked airway.
  C. No, elderly people always talk slowly.
  D. Yes, she is probably very short of breath.

_____ **27.** A prehospital modality of therapy for treating patients with inadequate breathing and respiratory distress that assists with ventilations of a breathing patient is:
  A. a nonrebreather mask.   **C.** CPAP.
  B. a BVM device.   **D.** a Venturi mask.

_____ **28.** When prolonged ventilations need to be done on a patient and there is only one EMT on the airway, you should consider using a/an:
  A. nonrebreather mask.
  B. automatic transport ventilator.
  C. pocket face mask.
  D. BVM device.

_____ **29.** A fully pressurized portable oxygen tank should have approximately _____ psi.
  A. 1,000   **C.** 2,000
  B. 1,500   **D.** 2,500

_____ **30.** Which portable oxygen cylinder, when full, lasts the longest when delivering oxygen?
  A. D   **C.** A
  B. E   **D.** M

_____ **31.** Before connecting a regulator to an oxygen supply cylinder, the EMT should:
  A. remove the protective seal and then open the valve.
  B. crack the main valve for one second.
  C. attach the nonrebreather mask to the flowmeter, then attach to the tank.
  D. do all of these.

_____ **32.** Humidified oxygen is:
   A. not possible in an ambulance.
   B. not used for patients on chronic oxygen therapy.
   C. not needed in adult patients who are being transported for short distances.
   D. habit forming.

_____ **33.** Concerns about the dangers of giving too much oxygen to patients with chronic COPD:
   A. are invalid in the out-of-hospital setting when clinically appropriate to administer.
   B. have been understated and proven to be a major problem.
   C. are invalid when the patient is over the age of 60.
   D. are dealt with by using a nonrebreather mask at low flow rates.

_____ **34.** Your patient may be having a heart attack. He is in moderate distress and his SpO_2 is 92%. The best method for you to use when giving a high concentration of oxygen to this breathing patient is a:
   A. nasal cannula.   **C.** simple face mask.
   B. Venturi mask.   **D.** nonrebreather mask.

_____ **35.** The oxygen concentration of a nonrebreather mask is between:
   A. 50% and 60%.   **C.** 70% and 80%.
   B. 60% and 70%.   **D.** 80% and 90%.

_____ **36.** You are treating a patient who is breathing on his own but is in respiratory distress, and his SpO_2 is 93%. The flow rate of a nonrebreather mask should be:
   A. adjusted so that when the patient inhales, the bag deflates by two-thirds.
   B. 12 to 15 liters per minute.
   C. adjusted to 6 liters per minute.
   D. all of these.

_____ **37.** The oxygen concentration of a nasal cannula is between:
   A. 4% and 6%.   **C.** 24% and 44%.
   B. 8% and 20%.   **D.** 50% and 6%.

_____ **38.** You are treating a 68-year-old female who fell and injured her ribs. She was found breathing at a rate of 44 and shallowly, yet she is starting to turn cyanotic. Why is this a serious threat to her life?
   A. She is inhaling too much oxygen.
   B. Her minute volume may be diminished.
   C. Her minute volume is excessive.
   D. She is exceeding her dead space.

_____ **39.** What is meant by anatomical dead space?
   A. The maximum amount of room for dying cells in the body
   B. The compartment where tissue swells like with edema
   C. Hollow chambers like the sinus
   D. The area in the lungs that does not participate in gas exchange.

_____ **40.** What is the most important consideration in assessing and managing the breathing of a child?
   A. The child's chest wall is more rigid and harder to ventilate.
   B. Children consume oxygen at a higher rate than adults do.
   C. The child's trachea is softer and less flexible.
   D. All of these are equally important.

Complete the Following

1. To determine the signs of adequate breathing, the EMT should:

   A. _____

   B. _____

   C. _____

   D. _____

   E. _____

2. The signs of inadequate breathing include the following:

   A. _____

   B. _____

   C. _____

   D. _____

   E. _____

   F. _____

   G. _____

   H. _____

   I. _____

   J. _____

   K. _____

3. List three mechanical failures of the cardiopulmonary system and two examples of each:

   A. _____

   • _____

   • _____

   B. _____

   • _____

   • _____

C. _____

   • _____

   • _____

Pathophysiology: Respiratory Distress to Respiratory Failure

1. When a patient is having an asthma attack and the respiratory system is trying to compensate, what happens to the respiratory rate?

   _____

2. When the fight-or-flight response is stimulated, what happens to the blood vessels in the arms and legs?

   _____

3. Why does the patient have wheezes when you listen with your stethoscope?

   _____

4. When the patient starts to get very anxious, what is the likely cause?

   _____

5. When the asthmatic patient starts to get tired, what is the potential result?

   _____

Case Study: Complicated Airway: The Self-Inflicted Shooting

Your unit and the police are dispatched to the scene of an attempted suicide at which shots were fired. The call was placed by a family member, who was called by the patient threatening to do harm to himself with a handgun. The police arrive before you and advise that the scene is secure and that you should respond directly to the scene, which is a private home in a suburban community. Upon arrival, you find a 48-year-old male lying with his face covered with blood. He is moaning, and his chest and abdomen appear to be moving as he breathes. After donning protective gloves, mask, and goggles, you and your partners carefully provide manual stabilization of the neck and place the patient onto a scoop stretcher. What is revealed is a mandible and tongue that are severely lacerated, and the mouth and nose are bubbling with blood as the patient attempts to breathe, and you can hear gurgling.

GZQ 1. How should you open the airway of this patient?

   _____

2. Does this patient need to be suctioned?

   _____

3. Should an airway adjunct be used on this patient?

   _____

Once the patient's airway is open and clear, you need to oxygenate him. He has no other obvious injuries, yet you are treating him for a possible spinal injury due to the impact of the bullet and his backward fall from his desk chair during the incident. The police think that the fall is why he shot his chin instead of his brain during the suicide attempt. You evaluate the patient's breathing rate as 28, shallow, and labored and his pulse as 120, weak, and regular. His SpO_2 is 94%.

GZQ **4.** What device should be used to administer oxygen to this patient?

_____

5. What is the proper liter flow to set the regulator for the device you chose in question number 4? If your unit has CPAP should you use it?

_____

Your portable D cylinder was full at the beginning of the shift, and this is your first call.

6. How many liters are in the tank? How much pressure is in the tank?

_____

7. How much time can you expect to get out of the tank, considering your service's policy is to refill tanks at 200 psi?

_____

8. As you prepare to transport the patient, you continue to suction him, making sure not to exceed _____ seconds per attempt because, as you suction, you are also removing _____. Which would be better to use: a rigid-tip or a flexible catheter?

_____

9. The patient has a blood pressure of 100/70 mmHg and his oxygen saturation is 95 percent, so you decide that his priority is _____ [high, low]. The major problem with this patient is his _____. He should be transported _____ [right away, in a few minutes] to the _____ [local hospital, trauma center].

10. From your knowledge of your EMS system, what ALS (advanced life support) treatment(s) might be helpful to this patient if you can arrange for an ALS intercept?

_____

11. What should you do if you hear hissing or bubbling around the mask as you ventilate?

_____

Interim Exam 1

Use the answer sheet provided to complete this exam. It is perforated, so it can be removed easily from this workbook.

1. Most EMT training programs are based on standards developed by the:
   A. American Red Cross (ARC).
   B. American Heart Association (AHA).
   C. National Highway Traffic Safety Administration (NHTSA).
   D. National Institutes of Health (NIH).

2. An EMT can inspire patient confidence and cooperation by:
   A. transporting the patient from the scene to a hospital.
   B. providing patient care without regard for the EMT's own personal safety.
   C. telling the patient that everything will be all right.
   D. being pleasant, cooperative, sincere, and a good listener.

3. If an on-duty EMT fails to provide the standard of care and this failure causes harm or injury to the patient, the EMT may be accused of:
   A. assault.   C. negligence.
   B. abandonment.   D. breach of promise.

4. You are treating a conscious and mentally competent adult patient who wants to refuse your care and transport to the hospital. This refusal must be _____ and documented.
   A. implied   C. involuntary
   B. actual   D. informed

5. The EMT is authorized to treat and transport an unconscious patient because of the legal consideration known as _____ consent.
   A. applied   C. triage
   B. implied   D. immunity

6. A child fell off the ladder of a sliding board at a park and twisted her ankle. The parents are not present, but the child agrees to care. The child's consent is:
   A. not needed.   C. implied.
   B. actual.   D. not sufficient.

7. In some states, _____ help to protect the off-duty EMT from lawsuits when the stop at the scene of a collision to offer assistance.
   A. professional associations
   B. blanket insurance policies
   C. Good Samaritan laws
   D. abandonment laws

8. The form of infection control that assumes that all body fluids should be considered potentially infectious is:
   A. infectious disease.
   B. Standard Precautions.
   C. immunity.
   D. universal precautions.

9. In planning to lift a patient using a nonurgent move the EMT should consider:
   A. utilizing a shoulder drag.
   B. lifting the patient with a firefighter's carry.
   C. whether the patient has an immediate life threat.
   D. how fast the patient can be moved into the ambulance.

10. When lifting an injured patient, the EMT should:
    A. keep the back loose and knees locked.
    B. twist or attempt to make the lift and other moves at the same time.
    C. use the leg muscles to do the lift.
    D. try not to talk to her or his partner.

11. All of the following are ways in which an EMT can avoid a potential back injury *except*:
    A. pushing, rather than pulling, a load.
    B. keeping the back locked in while lifting.
    C. keeping the arms straight when pulling.
    D. pushing or pulling from a kneeling position if the weight is below waist level.

12. The driver of an automobile was found unresponsive but breathing adequately. The EMT should use which patient carrying device to move the patient out of the vehicle?
    A. stair chair   C. scoop stretcher
    B. basket stretcher   D. long spine board

13. A method of lifting and carrying a patient in which one EMT slips both hands under the patient's armpits and grasps the wrists while another EMT grasps the patient's knees is called the:
    A. direct ground lift.
    B. extremity lift.
    C. draw-sheet method.
    D. direct carry method.

14. To achieve the optimal position for managing the airway of an infant, the EMT should place the patient on the back with:
    A. padding under the head.
    B. padding under the shoulders.
    C. head tilted back.
    D. head tilted down.

15. The venae cavae are two large veins that return blood to which part of the heart?
    A. right atrium.
    C. left atrium.
    B. right ventricle.
    D. left ventricle.

16. The heart receives its own blood supply from the:
    A. coronary arteries.
    B. pulmonary arteries.
    C. carotid arteries.
    D. aorta.

17. You are treating the driver of a vehicle that was involved in a collision. He is a 22-year-old male who requires immediate airway and bleeding control. You are unable to provide this treatment with him in the vehicle. You should:
    A. check the patient's vital signs.
    B. use an urgent move to extricate him.
    C. remove the patient on a short backboard.
    D. do all of these.

18. The component of the blood that carries oxygen and carbon dioxide are the:
    A. T cells
    B. red blood cells.
    C. white blood cells.
    D. platelets.

19. When a person sustains an injury that causes inadequate circulation of blood through the body, the EMT should recognize this condition is _____ and may lead to death.
    A. perfusion
    B. anaerobic metabolism
    C. hypoperfusion
    D. aerobic metabolism

20. The _____ system is composed of tissues, organs, and vessels that help maintain the body's immune system.
    A. nervous
    C. endocrine
    B. digestive
    D. lymphatic

21. The liver is located in which two abdominal quadrants?
    A. upper and lower right
    B. upper right and left
    C. upper and lower right
    D. lower left and right

22. If you are an EMT with a service that does not provide the appropriate personal protective equipment, why should you serve as an advocate for this equipment?
    A. Without the equipment, your crew members could be injured unnecessarily.
    B. Without the equipment, you could be seriously injured.
    C. An injured EMT is of little help to the patient, and the equipment would protect the EMT from injury.
    D. All of these are reasons to serve as an advocate.

23. During an EMS call, a lethal threat is made by a 24-year-old intoxicated male. The EMT should first:
    A. retreat to a safe area.
    B. radio for assistance.
    C. reevaluate the situation.
    D. remedy the situation.

24. Of the different types of stress, which is a positive form that helps the EMT work under pressure and respond effectively?
    A. Cumulative stress
    B. Eustress
    C. Distress
    D. Critical incident stress

25. In responding to a violent situation, observation begins when you:
    A. enter the scene.
    B. exit the ambulance.
    C. enter the neighborhood.
    D. arrive at the patient's side.

26. To ensure crew safety, members of the crew should always:
    A. remain in the ambulance.
    B. carry a portable radio.
    C. wear a bulletproof vest.
    D. carry a canister of pepper gas.

27. While you are treating a patient with a severely bleeding forearm, the patient's pet dog comes into the room. The patient states, "He won't hurt you. He's very friendly." Your best course of action, after or while quickly controlling the bleeding, would be to:
    A. have your partner observe the dog closely while you treat the patient.
    B. have the dog secured in another room.
    C. ignore the dog because the patient assures you that the dog is friendly and will not harm you.
    D. do all of these.

28. An advantage of the advance directive is that:
  A. the patient is not involved in making a decision about her treatment.
  B. the patient's expressed wishes may be followed.
  C. no matter what the family says, CPR is not given.
  D. it protects the EMT from charges of negligence.

29. Some EMTs participate in activities that attract legal actions, but most EMTs are rarely involved in legal entanglements. You can prevent most lawsuits if you:
  A. provide care within the scope of your practice.
  B. properly document your care.
  C. are courteous and respectful to all your patients.
  D. do all of these.

30. Which of the following is *not* a function of the musculoskeletal system?
  A. It gives the body shape.
  B. It protects the internal organs.
  C. It provides for body movement.
  D. It regulates body temperature.

31. The superior portion of the sternum is called the:
  A. xiphoid process.
  B. sternal body.
  C. manubrium.
  D. clavicle.

32. A young girl fell while ice skating and injured the protrusion on the inside of one of her ankles. The medical term for this location is the:
  A. acromion.
  B. medial malleolus.
  C. lateral malleolus.
  D. calcaneus.

33. The heart muscle has a property called _____. This means that the heart has the ability to generate and conduct electrical impulses on its own.
  A. contractility
  B. automaticity
  C. involuntary contraction
  D. conductibility

34. A division of the peripheral nervous system that controls involuntary motor functions is called the _____ nervous system.
  A. autonomic
  B. central
  C. sensory
  D. motor

35. When in the anatomic position, a person is facing:
  A. away from you. **C.** face down.
  B. the observer. **D.** face up.

36. An anatomic term that is occasionally used to refer to the sole of the foot is:
  A. calcaneus. **C.** dorsal.
  B. ventral. **D.** plantar.

37. The bones of the cheek are called the _____ bones.
  A. orbit **C.** zygomatic
  B. maxillae **D.** mandible

38. In comparing body structure positions, the knees are said to be _____ to the toes, and the toes are _____ to the knees.
  A. inferior; superior
  B. proximal; distal
  C. distal; dorsal
  D. anterior; posterior

39. A patient found lying on her back is in the _____ position.
  A. anatomical
  B. prone
  C. supine
  D. lateral recumbent

40. To assist in describing the location of abdominal organs, we divide the abdomen into _____ parts.
  A. two **C.** four
  B. three **D.** five

41. Your 18-year-old male patient has severe burns of the entire front (anterior) surface of the torso. The torso of the body is composed of the abdomen, pelvis, and:
  A. thorax.
  B. upper arms and legs.
  C. extremities.
  D. head.

42. The structure that divides the chest cavity from the abdominal cavity is the:
  A. meninges. **C.** diaphragm.
  B. duodenum. **D.** spinal column.

43. The anatomic name for the kneecap is the:
  A. ilium. **C.** patella.
  B. malleolus. **D.** phalange.

44. The cranium consists of the:
  A. facial bones.
  B. mandible and maxillae.
  C. top, back, and sides of the skull.
  D. zygomatic bones.

©2021 Pearson Education, Inc.
Emergency Care, 14th Ed.

45. The highest point in the shoulder is the:
  A. acromion process.
  B. humerus.
  C. metatarsal.
  D. clavicle.

46. When confronted with an unconscious minor without parents or a legal guardian present, the EMT should:
  A. seek a physician's approval before beginning care.
  B. consider consent for care to be implied and begin care.
  C. ask the child for consent and begin care.
  D. delay care until the parents are found.

47. The legal concept of negligence requires that three circumstances must be demonstrated. Which of the following is *not* one of the three circumstances?
  A. The EMT had a duty to act.
  B. The EMT committed a breach of duty.
  C. The EMT followed a local protocol.
  D. The breach of duty caused harm.

48. As an EMT, you have been assigned to take a terminally ill patient back and forth to chemotherapy multiple times a week for the next few weeks. You realize that the patient has been going through emotional stages of grief. These stages are often, if not always, experienced in the following order:
  A. depression, bargaining, denial, acceptance, anger.
  B. acceptance, rage, depression, acceptance, bargaining.
  C. denial, anger, bargaining, depression, acceptance.
  D. bargaining, acceptance, denial, anger, depression.

49. In 1970, the _____ was founded to establish professional standards.
  A. American Medical Association
  B. National Registry of Emergency Medical Technicians
  C. National Highway Traffic Safety Administration
  D. U.S. Department of Transportation

50. A continuous self-review with the purpose of identifying and correcting aspects of the EMS system that require improvement is called:
  A. standing orders.
  B. quality improvement.
  C. protocols.
  D. medical direction.

51. A physician who assumes the ultimate responsibility for the patient-care aspects of the EMS system is called the:
  A. Designated Agent.
  B. Medical Director.
  C. Off-line Director.
  D. Primary Care Physician.

52. There are high risks of a lawsuit against an EMS agency in cases of:
  A. patients who refuse care.
  B. on-scene deaths.
  C. cardiac arrest cases.
  D. pedestrians struck by cars.

53. The legal extent or limits of the EMT's skills are formally defined by the:
  A. patient.
  B. DOT curriculum.
  C. state.
  D. scope of practice.

54. Which is *not* generally considered a sign or symptom of stress?
  A. Decisiveness
  B. Guilt
  C. Loss of interest in work
  D. Difficulty sleeping

55. All the following are types of calls that have a high potential for causing excessive stress *except*:
  A. calls involving infants and children.
  B. patients with severe injuries.
  C. cases of abuse and neglect.
  D. motor vehicle collisions.

56. Lifestyle changes that can help the EMT deal with stress include all of the following *except*:
  A. exercise to burn off tension.
  B. increased consumption of fatty foods.
  C. decreased consumption of caffeine.
  D. decreased consumption of alcohol.

57. One of the functions of the integumentary system is to:
  A. regulate the diameter of the blood vessels in the circulation.
  B. eliminate excess oxygen into the atmosphere.
  C. allow environmental water to carefully enter the body.
  D. protect the body from the environment, bacteria, and other organisms.

58. Stress after a major EMS incident is:
  A. unusual and unexpected.
  B. a sign of weakness.
  C. normal and to be expected.
  D. part of the grieving process.

59. Retreating to a world of one's own after hearing one is going to die is a result of the stage of grief called:
  - **A.** bargaining.
  - **B.** depression.
  - **C.** denial.
  - **D.** anxiety.

60. A patient's lower extremities are trapped under a farm tractor, diminishing the blood supply, and thus oxygen, to the cells in the legs. This injury can result in:
  - **A.** no lactic acids being produced.
  - **B.** anaerobic metabolism.
  - **C.** no carbon dioxide being produced.
  - **D.** none of these.

61. A disease that is spread by exposure to an open wound or sore of an infected individual may be caused by a(n) _____ pathogen.
  - **A.** universal
  - **B.** airborne
  - **C.** bloodborne
  - **D.** intracellular

62. An infection that causes inflammation of the liver is called:
  - **A.** meningitis.
  - **B.** tuberculosis.
  - **C.** typhoid.
  - **D.** hepatitis.

63. A(n) _____ disease is one that is spread by inhaling or absorbing droplets from the air through the eyes, nose, or mouth.
  - **A.** bloodborne
  - **B.** noncommunicable
  - **C.** airborne
  - **D.** viral

64. The communicable disease that kills the most health workers every year in the United States is:
  - **A.** tuberculosis.
  - **B.** HIV/AIDS.
  - **C.** meningitis.
  - **D.** hepatitis B virus.

65. Always assume that any patient with a:
  - **A.** cold has a bloodborne disease.
  - **B.** productive cough has TB.
  - **C.** fever has typhoid.
  - **D.** rash has measles.

66. Which of the following is *not* true about the human immunodeficiency virus (HIV)?
  - **A.** It attacks the immune system.
  - **B.** It doesn't survive well outside the human body.
  - **C.** It can be introduced through puncture wounds.
  - **D.** It is an airborne pathogen.

67. Your patient has HIV. You are accidentally stuck with a needle that has some infected blood on it. Your chance of contracting the disease is less than:
  - **A.** 0.5%.
  - **B.** 5%.
  - **C.** 10%.
  - **D.** 15%.

68. If you think your patient has TB, you should wear the usual personal protective equipment plus a:
  - **A.** surgeon's mask.
  - **B.** gown.
  - **C.** HEPA or N-95 respirator.
  - **D.** Tyvek suit.

69. Instead of providing mouth-to-mouth ventilations to the nonbreathing patient, the EMT when acting alone should use:
  - **A.** a pocket mask with a one-way valve.
  - **B.** a one-way valve.
  - **C.** a bag-valve mask.
  - **D.** an endotracheal tube.

70. An act that establishes procedures through which emergency response workers can find out whether they have been exposed to life-threatening infectious diseases is called:
  - **A.** OSHA 1910.1030.
  - **B.** the Ryan White CARE Act.
  - **C.** the AIDS Protection Act.
  - **D.** OSHA 1910.120.

71. Each emergency response employer must develop a plan that identifies and documents job classifications and tasks in which there is the possibility of exposure to potentially infectious body fluids. This is required by:
  - **A.** OSHA 1910.1030.
  - **B.** the Ryan White CARE Act.
  - **C.** the AIDS Protection Act.
  - **D.** OSHA 1910.120.

72. Select the suffix that means "inflammation."
  - **A.** -itis
  - **B.** -algia
  - **C.** -ist
  - **D.** -plegia

73. The body's ability to maintain stability within cells and the body using nervous system feedback and messaging is called:
  - **A.** "fight or flight."
  - **B.** perfusion.
  - **C.** homeostasis.
  - **D.** metabolism.

74. An EMT is treating a conscious choking infant when suddenly the infant becomes unresponsive, the EMT should:
  - **A.** perform five back slaps.
  - **B.** begin CPR.
  - **C.** suction the airway.
  - **D.** insert a nasal pharyngeal airway.

75. Which of the following is *least likely* to be a high-risk area for TB?
  A. Correctional facilities
  B. Daycare centers
  C. Homeless shelters
  D. Nursing homes

76. If anyone at the scene is in possession of a weapon, the EMT should:
  A. notify the police immediately.
  B. ask the person to give it to you.
  C. ignore the person with the weapon.
  D. advise the person to leave the scene.

77. The reduction of breathing to the point at which oxygen intake is not sufficient to support life is called:
  A. respiratory failure.
  B. anoxic metabolism.
  C. respiratory arrest.
  D. respiratory support.

78. Signs of adequate breathing include all of the following *except*:
  A. equal expansion of both sides of the chest.
  B. air moving in and out of the nose.
  C. blue or gray skin coloration.
  D. present and equal breath sounds.

79. The widening of the nostrils of the nose with respirations is called:
  A. hyperventilating.
  B. nasal flaring.
  C. nasal gurgling.
  D. wheezing.

80. The condition in which a patient's skin or lips are blue or gray is called:
  A. stridor.
  C. pallor.
  B. cyanosis.
  D. anemia.

81. If a patient is unable to speak in full sentences, this could be a sign of:
  A. complete airway blockage.
  B. snoring.
  C. shortness of breath.
  D. respiratory arrest.

82. The procedures by which the EMT initially treats life-threatening respiratory problems include all of the following *except*:
  A. opening and securing the airway.
  B. inserting an endotracheal tube immediately.
  C. providing supplemental oxygen to the breathing patient.
  D. ensuring a clear airway with frequent suctioning.

83. You are assessing the airway of an unconscious male patient. You recall that most airway problems involve:
  A. the tongue.
  C. shock.
  B. asthma.
  D. the epiglottis.

84. You are treating a patient who fell down a flight of metal stairs. Which maneuver is most appropriate for an unconscious patient found lying at the bottom of a stairwell?
  A. Head-tilt, chin-lift
  B. Head-tilt, neck-lift
  C. Jaw-pull lift
  D. Jaw-thrust

85. Artificial ventilation may be inadequate if the:
  A. chest rises with each ventilation.
  B. heart rate returns to normal.
  C. rate of ventilation is too fast or too slow.
  D. skin becomes warm and dry.

86. The technique for inserting an oropharyngeal airway into a pediatric patient is:
  A. exactly the same as the technique for inserting one into an adult.
  B. to slide the device in from the corner of the mouth.
  C. to measure and lubricate the device prior to insertion.
  D. to insert the device straight in without any rotation.

87. A 6-year-old female is experiencing a seizure. She has snoring respirations and her teeth are clenched shut. What can the EMT do to manage the airway?
  A. Insert an oropharyngeal airway.
  B. Insert a nasopharyngeal airway.
  C. Suction the nostrils.
  D. Use a tongue depressor to open the mouth.

88. A proper oxygen flow rate in ventilating a patient with a bag-valve mask is _____ liters per minute.
  A. 5
  C. 15
  B. 10
  D. 20

89. According to American Heart Association guidelines, in ventilating a patient with a bag-valve mask that has supplemental oxygen, the volume administered should be:
  A. 400 milliliters.
  B. sufficient to achieve visible chest rise.
  C. 800 milliliters.
  D. as much as possible during the 1-second time frame.

90. The first step in providing artificial ventilation of a stoma breather is to:
- **A.** leave the head and neck in a neutral position.
- **B.** ventilate at the appropriate rate for the patient's age.
- **C.** clear any mucus or secretions obstructing the stoma.
- **D.** establish a seal using a pediatric-sized mask.

91. When suctioning the airway of an infant the EMT should be alert for _____ because the infant is very sensitive to vagal stimulation associated with suctioning.
- **A.** slowing heart rate
- **B.** increased heart rate
- **C.** increased vomiting
- **D.** decreased blood pressure

92. The two most common airway adjuncts are the oropharyngeal airway and the:
- **A.** nasal cannula.
- **B.** nasopharyngeal airway.
- **C.** endotracheal tube.
- **D.** Yankauer.

93. An oropharyngeal airway should be inserted in:
- **A.** all patients with inadequate breathing.
- **B.** trauma patients with a gag reflex.
- **C.** medical patients with a gag reflex.
- **D.** unconscious patients with no gag reflex.

94. When suctioning a 19-year-old patient who you suspect has bleeding into his throat, you should:
- **A.** suction on the way in and the way out.
- **B.** avoid using eyewear or a mask.
- **C.** try not to suction for longer than 10 seconds.
- **D.** hypoventilate before suctioning.

95. Which of the following statements about supraglottic airways is accurate?
- **A.** In some systems an EMT may use a supraglottic airway when a patient is in cardiac arrest.
- **B.** Inserting a supraglottic airway is a procedure only advanced providers may use.
- **C.** Supraglottic airways should never be used in pediatric patients.
- **D.** The supraglottic airway should only be used after an oropharyngeal airway was inserted first.

96. An insufficiency in the supply of oxygen to the body's tissues is called:
- **A.** anoxia.
- **B.** no-oxia.
- **C.** hypoxia.
- **D.** cyanosis.

97. Before the oxygen cylinder's pressure gauge reads a minimum of _____ psi, you must switch to a fresh cylinder.
- **A.** 200
- **B.** 400
- **C.** 800
- **D.** 1,000

98. When handling oxygen cylinders, the EMT should do all of the following *except*:
- **A.** have the cylinders hydrostatically tested every 5 years.
- **B.** ensure that valve seat inserts and gaskets are in good condition.
- **C.** store reserve cylinders in a warm, humid room.
- **D.** use medical-grade oxygen in all cylinders.

99. The best way to deliver high-concentration oxygen to a breathing patient is to use a:
- **A.** nonrebreather mask.
- **B.** partial rebreather mask.
- **C.** bag-valve mask.
- **D.** nasal cannula.

100. A nasal cannula provides between _____ percent and _____ percent oxygen concentrations.
- **A.** 10; 21
- **B.** 24; 44
- **C.** 36; 58
- **D.** 72; 96

101. You are assessing a 54-year-old woman who is unconscious and has a noisy upper airway. If she has dentures, during airway procedures you should:
- **A.** remove them right away.
- **B.** leave them in unless they are loose.
- **C.** remove the denture plates one at a time.
- **D.** hold them in place with a free hand.

102. When managing the airway of a child, you should remember that:
- **A.** the child's mouth and nose are smaller and more easily obstructed.
- **B.** the chest wall is firmer in a child.
- **C.** the child's trachea is wider and less easily obstructed.
- **D.** all of these are airway considerations in a child.

103. You are dealing with a patient who is in severe distress from a life-threatening asthma attack. If breathing stops completely, the patient is in:
- **A.** respiratory arrest.
- **B.** ventilatory reduction.
- **C.** artificial ventilation.
- **D.** respiratory failure.

©2021 Pearson Education, Inc.
Emergency Care, 14th Ed.

104. When using poor technique when providing positive pressure ventilation to on a patient with inadequate ventilation, one negative side effect can be:
  A. oxygen saturation will increase.
  B. an unresponsive patient may become responsive.
  C. the blood pressure will rise significantly.
  D. the stomach will fill with air.

105. A device that allows the control of oxygen in liters per minute is called a:
  A. flowmeter.
  B. G tank.
  C. humidifier.
  D. reservoir.

106. When the EMT ventilates a patient too quickly, too much carbon dioxide will leave the body resulting in:
  A. inadequate chest rise and fall.
  B. increased blood flow to the brain due to vasodilation of blood vessels.
  C. decreased blood flow to the brain due to vasoconstriction of blood vessels.
  D. a dangerous increase in blood pressure.

107. Why do some EMS systems use humidified oxygen?
  A. Lack of humidity can dry out the patient's mucous membranes.
  B. It provides a reservoir for the oxygen.
  C. It limits the risk of infection.
  D. It is helpful when transporting patients short distances.

108. The automatic transport ventilator is an alternative device to the bag-valve mask and includes:
  A. minimal mask seal.
  B. an alarm that detects low oxygen saturation.
  C. settings to adjust ventilation rate and volume.
  D. settings to adjust oxygen flow rates.

109. An important anatomic consideration in the airway management of a child is that:
  A. a child's metabolism consumes oxygen at a higher rate than an adult.
  B. a child's metabolism consumes oxygen at a slower rate than an adult.
  C. using an airway adjunct when ventilating a child is not as critical as it is with an adult.
  D. maintaining a patent airway in a child is much easier than an adult.

110. In using an air mattress, the patient is placed on the device and the air is _____ by a pump. The mattress will then form a _____ and conforming surface around the patient.

  A. inflated; rigid
  B. withdrawn; soft
  C. inflated; soft
  D. withdrawn; rigid

111. The body system that is responsible for the breakdown of food into absorbable forms is the _____ system.
  A. urinary
  B. nervous
  C. digestive
  D. integumentary

112. Providing positive pressure ventilations on an infant can cause gastric distention which:
  A. paralyzes the diaphragm.
  B. prevents the lungs from filling adequately.
  C. obstructs the upper airway.
  D. improves gas exchange.

113. When an adult patient is breathing at a respiratory rate of 12 times a minute, you would expect that the minute volume would be approximately _____ milliliters per minute.
  A. 3,000
  B. 4,500
  C. 5,000
  D. 6,000

114. Your patient is a 45-year-old female who has been vomiting and has had diarrhea for the past week. There is a danger that she may have:
  A. extremity edema.
  B. an excess of body fluid.
  C. dehydration.
  D. all of these.

115. You are questioning an older adult man who is sitting on a bench in the park. He has a respiratory complaint, and he speaks in short, two- or three-word sentences. Is this significant?
  A. Yes, he is probably very short of breath.
  B. No, older adults always talk slowly.
  C. No, he is probably always like that.
  D. Yes, he probably has a complete airway obstruction.

116. Why can nasal congestion be a major problem in the first few months of life?
  A. Because the liver is so large in patients in this age group.
  B. Because children in this age group are primarily nose breathers.
  C. Because it is an indication of life-threatening airway compromise.
  D. Because children in this age group breathe with their diaphragm.

117. When the mother strokes the infant's lips and the baby starts sucking, this is a nervous system reflex known as the _____ reflex.
A. Moro
C. palmar
B. sucking
D. rooting

118. The adolescent years are the beginning of:
A. better decision-making skills.
B. nasal breathing.
C. self-destructive behaviors.
D. all of these.

119. In a pediatric patient capillary refill is a reliable assessment finding to determine:
A. preload of the heart.
B. afterload of the heart.
C. mental status.
D. circulatory status.

120. Serious conflicts may occur in families as the issues of control and independence collide with children in which age group?
A. Toddler
C. School age
B. Preschool
D. Adolescent

121. Girls are usually finished growing by the age of:
A. 14.
C. 18.
B. 16.
D. 20.

122. You are examining an older woman sitting on a bench in front of the supermarket. She is sitting upright and leaning forward with her hands on her knees, to make it easier to breathe. What is this position called?
A. High Fowler position
B. Tripod position
C. Bench position
D. Trendelenburg position

123. You have been called to a restaurant for a female patient who collapsed at the table. According to a family member, she did not strike her head as she slid out of the chair when she lost consciousness. To open her airway, you should use a _____ maneuver.
A. modified jaw-thrust
B. head-tilt, chin-lift
C. head-tilt, neck-lift
D. modified chin-lift

124. A nasopharyngeal airway should be:
A. turned 180 degrees with the tip facing the roof of the mouth.
B. inserted with the bevel on the lateral side of the nostril.
C. measured from the patient's nostril to the earlobe.
D. inserted in the left nostril when possible.

125. You are treating a patient who initially had a chief complaint of severe difficulty breathing. You are concerned that this may be leading to respiratory failure, which is:
A. caused by excessive exercise in older adults.
B. another term used to describe respiratory arrest.
C. inadequate breathing and is a precursor to respiratory arrest.
D. the complete cessation of expiration.

©2021 Pearson Education, Inc.
Emergency Care, 14th Ed.

Interim Exam 1 Answer Sheet

Fill in the correct answer for each item. For scoring purposes, note that there are 125 questions valued at 0.8 point each.

1. [ ] A	[ ] B	[ ] C	[ ] D		**35.** [ ] A	[ ] B	[ ] C	[ ] D
2. [ ] A	[ ] B	[ ] C	[ ] D		**36.** [ ] A	[ ] B	[ ] C	[ ] D
3. [ ] A	[ ] B	[ ] C	[ ] D		**37.** [ ] A	[ ] B	[ ] C	[ ] D
4. [ ] A	[ ] B	[ ] C	[ ] D		**38.** [ ] A	[ ] B	[ ] C	[ ] D
5. [ ] A	[ ] B	[ ] C	[ ] D		**39.** [ ] A	[ ] B	[ ] C	[ ] D
6. [ ] A	[ ] B	[ ] C	[ ] D		**40.** [ ] A	[ ] B	[ ] C	[ ] D
7. [ ] A	[ ] B	[ ] C	[ ] D		**41.** [ ] A	[ ] B	[ ] C	[ ] D
8. [ ] A	[ ] B	[ ] C	[ ] D		**42.** [ ] A	[ ] B	[ ] C	[ ] D
9. [ ] A	[ ] B	[ ] C	[ ] D		**43.** [ ] A	[ ] B	[ ] C	[ ] D
10. [ ] A	[ ] B	[ ] C	[ ] D		**44.** [ ] A	[ ] B	[ ] C	[ ] D
11. [ ] A	[ ] B	[ ] C	[ ] D		**45.** [ ] A	[ ] B	[ ] C	[ ] D
12. [ ] A	[ ] B	[ ] C	[ ] D		**46.** [ ] A	[ ] B	[ ] C	[ ] D
13. [ ] A	[ ] B	[ ] C	[ ] D		**47.** [ ] A	[ ] B	[ ] C	[ ] D
14. [ ] A	[ ] B	[ ] C	[ ] D		**48.** [ ] A	[ ] B	[ ] C	[ ] D
15. [ ] A	[ ] B	[ ] C	[ ] D		**49.** [ ] A	[ ] B	[ ] C	[ ] D
16. [ ] A	[ ] B	[ ] C	[ ] D		**50.** [ ] A	[ ] B	[ ] C	[ ] D
17. [ ] A	[ ] B	[ ] C	[ ] D		**51.** [ ] A	[ ] B	[ ] C	[ ] D
18. [ ] A	[ ] B	[ ] C	[ ] D		**52.** [ ] A	[ ] B	[ ] C	[ ] D
19. [ ] A	[ ] B	[ ] C	[ ] D		**53.** [ ] A	[ ] B	[ ] C	[ ] D
20. [ ] A	[ ] B	[ ] C	[ ] D		**54.** [ ] A	[ ] B	[ ] C	[ ] D
21. [ ] A	[ ] B	[ ] C	[ ] D		**55.** [ ] A	[ ] B	[ ] C	[ ] D
22. [ ] A	[ ] B	[ ] C	[ ] D		**56.** [ ] A	[ ] B	[ ] C	[ ] D
23. [ ] A	[ ] B	[ ] C	[ ] D		**57.** [ ] A	[ ] B	[ ] C	[ ] D
24. [ ] A	[ ] B	[ ] C	[ ] D		**58.** [ ] A	[ ] B	[ ] C	[ ] D
25. [ ] A	[ ] B	[ ] C	[ ] D		**59.** [ ] A	[ ] B	[ ] C	[ ] D
26. [ ] A	[ ] B	[ ] C	[ ] D		**60.** [ ] A	[ ] B	[ ] C	[ ] D
27. [ ] A	[ ] B	[ ] C	[ ] D		**61.** [ ] A	[ ] B	[ ] C	[ ] D
28. [ ] A	[ ] B	[ ] C	[ ] D		**62.** [ ] A	[ ] B	[ ] C	[ ] D
29. [ ] A	[ ] B	[ ] C	[ ] D		**63.** [ ] A	[ ] B	[ ] C	[ ] D
30. [ ] A	[ ] B	[ ] C	[ ] D		**64.** [ ] A	[ ] B	[ ] C	[ ] D
31. [ ] A	[ ] B	[ ] C	[ ] D		**65.** [ ] A	[ ] B	[ ] C	[ ] D
32. [ ] A	[ ] B	[ ] C	[ ] D		**66.** [ ] A	[ ] B	[ ] C	[ ] D
33. [ ] A	[ ] B	[ ] C	[ ] D		**67.** [ ] A	[ ] B	[ ] C	[ ] D
34. [ ] A	[ ] B	[ ] C	[ ] D		**68.** [ ] A	[ ] B	[ ] C	[ ] D

69. [ ] A	[ ] B	[ ] C	[ ] D		98. [ ] A	[ ] B	[ ] C	[ ] D
70. [ ] A	[ ] B	[ ] C	[ ] D		99. [ ] A	[ ] B	[ ] C	[ ] D
71. [ ] A	[ ] B	[ ] C	[ ] D		100. [ ] A	[ ] B	[ ] C	[ ] D
72. [ ] A	[ ] B	[ ] C	[ ] D		101. [ ] A	[ ] B	[ ] C	[ ] D
73. [ ] A	[ ] B	[ ] C	[ ] D		102. [ ] A	[ ] B	[ ] C	[ ] D
74. [ ] A	[ ] B	[ ] C	[ ] D		103. [ ] A	[ ] B	[ ] C	[ ] D
75. [ ] A	[ ] B	[ ] C	[ ] D		104. [ ] A	[ ] B	[ ] C	[ ] D
76. [ ] A	[ ] B	[ ] C	[ ] D		105. [ ] A	[ ] B	[ ] C	[ ] D
77. [ ] A	[ ] B	[ ] C	[ ] D		106. [ ] A	[ ] B	[ ] C	[ ] D
78. [ ] A	[ ] B	[ ] C	[ ] D		107. [ ] A	[ ] B	[ ] C	[ ] D
79. [ ] A	[ ] B	[ ] C	[ ] D		108. [ ] A	[ ] B	[ ] C	[ ] D
80. [ ] A	[ ] B	[ ] C	[ ] D		109. [ ] A	[ ] B	[ ] C	[ ] D
81. [ ] A	[ ] B	[ ] C	[ ] D		110. [ ] A	[ ] B	[ ] C	[ ] D
82. [ ] A	[ ] B	[ ] C	[ ] D		111. [ ] A	[ ] B	[ ] C	[ ] D
83. [ ] A	[ ] B	[ ] C	[ ] D		112. [ ] A	[ ] B	[ ] C	[ ] D
84. [ ] A	[ ] B	[ ] C	[ ] D		113. [ ] A	[ ] B	[ ] C	[ ] D
85. [ ] A	[ ] B	[ ] C	[ ] D		114. [ ] A	[ ] B	[ ] C	[ ] D
86. [ ] A	[ ] B	[ ] C	[ ] D		115. [ ] A	[ ] B	[ ] C	[ ] D
87. [ ] A	[ ] B	[ ] C	[ ] D		116. [ ] A	[ ] B	[ ] C	[ ] D
88. [ ] A	[ ] B	[ ] C	[ ] D		117. [ ] A	[ ] B	[ ] C	[ ] D
89. [ ] A	[ ] B	[ ] C	[ ] D		118. [ ] A	[ ] B	[ ] C	[ ] D
90. [ ] A	[ ] B	[ ] C	[ ] D		119. [ ] A	[ ] B	[ ] C	[ ] D
91. [ ] A	[ ] B	[ ] C	[ ] D		120. [ ] A	[ ] B	[ ] C	[ ] D
92. [ ] A	[ ] B	[ ] C	[ ] D		121. [ ] A	[ ] B	[ ] C	[ ] D
93. [ ] A	[ ] B	[ ] C	[ ] D		122. [ ] A	[ ] B	[ ] C	[ ] D
94. [ ] A	[ ] B	[ ] C	[ ] D		123. [ ] A	[ ] B	[ ] C	[ ] D
95. [ ] A	[ ] B	[ ] C	[ ] D		124. [ ] A	[ ] B	[ ] C	[ ] D
96. [ ] A	[ ] B	[ ] C	[ ] D		125. [ ] A	[ ] B	[ ] C	[ ] D
97. [ ] A	[ ] B	[ ] C	[ ] D					

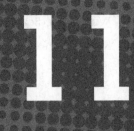

Scene Size-Up

Core Concepts

- Identifying hazards at a scene
- Determining whether a scene is safe to enter
- Mechanisms of injury and how they relate to patient condition
- Determining what additional assistance may be needed at a scene

Outcomes

After reading this chapter, you should be able to:

11.1 Analyze each of the components of scene size-up. (pp. 290–309)
- Recognize potential hazards at a scene.
- Explain the rationale for the priority of determining scene safety.
- Identify any modifications required to your personal protective equipment based on specific characteristics of a scene.
- Relate observations about the mechanism of injury to suspicions for patterns of patient injuries.
- Identify sources of information to advise you about the nature of a medical patient's illness.
- Given a scenario, determine the need for additional resources.

Match Key Terms

A. Injury caused by an object that passes into or through the skin.

B. Injury caused by a blow that does not penetrate the skin or other body tissues.

C. A force or forces that may have caused injury.

D. The area around the wreckage of a vehicle collision or other incident within which special safety precautions should be taken.

E. Awareness that there may be injuries based on mechanism of injury.

_____ **1.** Scene size-up

_____ **2.** Danger zone

_____ **3.** Mechanism of injury

_____ **4.** Penetrating trauma

_____ **5.** Blunt-force trauma

_____ **6.** Index of suspicion

_____ **7.** Nature of the illness

F. What is medically wrong with a patient.

G. Steps taken when approaching the scene of an emergency call.

Multiple-Choice Review

_____ **1.** The scene size-up is the first part of the patient assessment process. It begins as you approach the scene, surveying it to determine:
   A. whether there are any threats to your own safety.
   B. the number of injured patients at the scene.
   C. the personal safety of all those involved in the call.
   D. the mechanism of injury.

_____ **2.** Of the following situations, which is most likely to be too risky and involve the EMTs initially retreating from the location where the patient is located?
   A. A motor vehicle crash on a busy highway.
   B. A vehicle off the road which is in an unstable position.
   C. A fight at a party involving automatic weapons.
   D. A domestic disturbance with a lot of shouting going on.

_____ **3.** If you arrive at a multiple-vehicle collision scene where police, fire vehicles, and other ambulances are already present, you should:
   A. immediately begin patient care.
   B. conduct your own scene size-up.
   C. ensure that no bystanders are injured.
   D. all of these.

_____ **4.** Which of the following is _not_ an appropriate action when you near the scene of a traffic collision?
   A. Look and listen for other EMS units approaching from side streets.
   B. Look for signs of collision-related power outages.
   C. Observe traffic flow to anticipate blockage at the scene.
   D. Attempt to park your vehicle downhill from the scene.

_____ **5.** You have been dispatched to a multiple-car collision on the interstate. When you are in sight of the collision scene, you should watch for the signals of police officers because:
   A. they may have information about hazards or the location of injured persons.
   B. the first ones on the scene are considered to be in charge.
   C. federal law requires you to follow the command of other responders.
   D. they are considered the medical-care experts on the scene.

_____ **6.** When there are no apparent hazards, consider the danger zone to extend at least _____ feet in all directions from the wreckage.
   A. 25   **C.** 100
   B. 50   **D.** 200

_____ **7.** When a collision vehicle is on fire, consider the danger zone to extend at least _____ feet in all directions, even if the fire appears small and limited to the engine compartment.
   A. 25   **C.** 100
   B. 50   **D.** 200

_____ **8.** Your scene size-up should identify:
   A. the potential for a violent or dangerous situation.
   B. the exact name and quantity of a hazardous substance.
   C. the diagnosis of each of the patients on the scene.
   D. all of these.

_____ 9. The EMT's equipment/supplies for Standard Precautions during the scene size-up may include all of the following *except*:
   A. eye protection.
   B. disposable gloves.
   C. face mask or eye shield.
   D. nonrebreather mask.

_____ 10. Standard Precautions should be taken with all patients. The key element of Standard Precautions is to:
   A. always wear all the protective clothing.
   B. always have personal protective equipment readily available.
   C. place equipment on the patient as well as the rescuer.
   D. determine which body fluids pose a danger to the EMT.

_____ 11. Certain injuries are common to particular situations. Injuries to bones and joints are usually associated with:
   A. fights and drug usage.
   B. falls and vehicle collisions.
   C. fires and explosions.
   D. bullet wounds.

_____ 12. Some idea of potential forces involved in the mechanism of injury (MOI) assists the EMT in:
   A. immobilizing the patient's spine.
   B. determining which Standard Precautions to use.
   C. predicting various injury patterns.
   D. all of these.

_____ 13. The physical forces and energy that may be imparted on the patient are influenced by the laws of physics. One of those laws, the law of inertia, states that:
   A. the faster you enter a turn, the more your vehicle will be pulled straight.
   B. the slower the speed, the greater the energy loss.
   C. a body in motion will remain in motion unless acted upon by an outside force.
   D. the mass or weight of an object is the most important contributor to an injury.

_____ 14. You are treating a patient who was involved in a head-on collision. She was the unrestrained driver who took the "up-and-over" pathway. To which part of her body was she most likely to have sustained injuries?
   A. Skull
   B. Fibula
   C. Knees
   D. Femur

_____ 15. Which of the following is *least* likely to be considered a mechanism of injury (MOI) for an unrestrained patient who was in a head-on crash and followed the "up-and-over" pathway?
   A. Steering wheel
   B. Windshield
   C. Brake pedal
   D. Dashboard

_____ 16. You are on the scene of a car crash. Your patient has stable vital signs and is complaining of knee, leg, and hip pain. He also states that he was in the front passenger seat of the vehicle and was not wearing his seat belt. What type of collision did he most likely experience?
   A. Head-on, up-and-over
   B. Rear-end
   C. Head-on, down-and-under
   D. Rotational impact

_____ 17. Which type of collision is most serious when the occupant is not restrained because it has the potential for multiple impacts?
   A. Side impact
   B. Rear-end impact
   C. Head-on, up-and-over
   D. Rollover

_____ 18. You are walking around a vehicle that was involved in a collision. All of the following are indications of mechanisms of injury *except*:
   A. an 18-inch dent into the side door.
   B. a spiderweb crack in the windshield.
   C. a broken steering column.
   D. a flat rear tire.

_____ 19. You have just arrived at the scene of a severe fall involving an adult male patient. According the Centers for Disease Control and Prevention, a severe fall for an adult is:
   A. over 20 feet.
   B. often accompanied by an amputation.
   C. less than 10 feet.
   D. always fatal.

_____ 20. You are evaluating a patient who sustained a penetrating injury. In a _____ injury, the injury is usually limited to the penetrated area.
   A. low-velocity   **C.** high-velocity
   B. medium-velocity   **D.** super-velocity

_____ 21. The pressure wave around a bullet's track through the body is called:
   A. exsanguination.   **C.** cavitation.
   B. gas penetration.   **D.** hyperextension

_____ 22. You are evaluating a patient who sustained an injury caused by a blow that hit the body but did not penetrate the skin. This type of injury is called a(n):
   A. inertia trauma.   **C.** blunt-force trauma.
   B. cavitation.   **D.** rotational impact.

_____ 23. In which of the following situations would it be necessary for you and your partner to call for additional assistance?
   A. You are treating a patient who has flulike symptoms and also has a toddler with similar symptoms.
   B. Your patient is a 450-pound male who fell down the stairs and has a broken leg.
   C. You are treating a patient with a deep laceration in his right forearm.
   D. Your patient loses consciousness while you are carrying her to the ambulance.

_____ 24. You are in the living room of a private home, treating a patient for nausea, headache, and general body weakness when your eyes begin to tear. Three family members have the same symptoms. You should immediately:
   A. evacuate all people from the building.
   B. call for three additional ambulances.
   C. notify the police department.
   D. begin to flush out everyone's eyes.

_____ 25. If the number of patients is more than the responding units can effectively handle, the EMT should:
   A. involve bystanders in care of the injured.
   B. call for additional EMS resources immediately.
   C. advise medical direction that assistance is needed.
   D. do all of these.

_____ 26. When arriving at the scene of a collision, the EMT should:
   A. start placing flares across the road.
   B. don a reflective vest.
   C. immediately start additional units.
   D. contact medical direction on the radio.

_____ 27. A significant danger faced by the EMT is violence. On arriving at the scene of a private home, you hear screaming from inside. There are beer cans piled up on the front porch, and as you knock on the door, it suddenly gets very quiet inside. What should you do next?
   A. Enter the residence and search for weapons.
   B. Contact the dispatcher to inquire whether they have ever had violence at this location.
   C. Retreat to a safe location and ask for the police to respond to secure the scene.
   D. Yell into the house that you are EMS and not the police.

_____ **28.** You arrive on the scene of a large fire. If the personnel at the scene are using the incident command/management system, you should:
  A. follow the instructions of the Incident Commander.
  B. drive past the scene and park off the road.
  C. transport the first patient you come across.
  D. tag all of the patients.

_____ **29.** A fall over _____ feet for a 12-year-old child would be considered a severe fall by the CDC.
  A. 2   **C.** 10
  B. 5   **D.** 12

_____ **30.** Vehicles with airbags should still require the occupants to use passenger restraint systems properly because:
  A. they only deploy once during the collision.
  B. the airbag may cause injury itself.
  C. airbags may damage the windshield.
  D. all of the above are correct.

Complete the Following

1. List five signals that violence may be a danger on your call.

  A. _____

  B. _____

  C. _____

  D. _____

  E. _____

2. List the guidelines for establishing a danger zone around the wreckage of a vehicle collision.

  A. When there are no apparent hazards: _____

  B. When fuel has been spilled: _____

  C. When the vehicle is on fire: _____

  D. When electrical wires are down: _____

  E. When hazardous materials are involved: _____

3. List five types of motor vehicle collisions and the common injury patterns for each.

A. _____

B. _____

C. _____

D. _____

E. _____

4. When you are determining the nature of the illness this information can be obtained from:

A. _____

B. _____

C. _____

Label the Diagram

Add labels to the mechanism-of-injury diagram to identify the type of force (and direction, if appropriate) affecting the body parts listed or indicated by the arrows.

MECHANISM OF INJURY

The force that produced the injury, its intensity and direction.

TYPES OF FORCE

- Direct
- Twisting
- Forced Flexion or Hyperextension
- Indirect

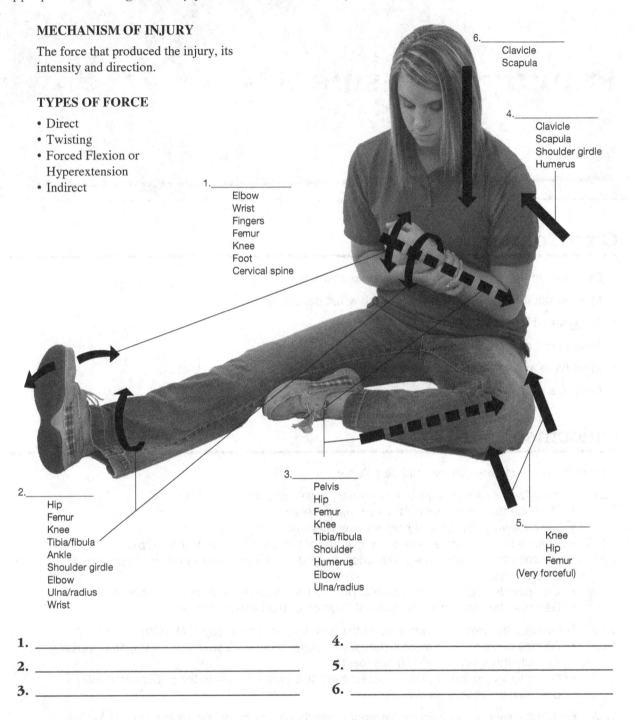

1._____
Elbow
Wrist
Fingers
Femur
Knee
Foot
Cervical spine

6._____
Clavicle
Scapula

4._____
Clavicle
Scapula
Shoulder girdle
Humerus

2._____
Hip
Femur
Knee
Tibia/fibula
Ankle
Shoulder girdle
Elbow
Ulna/radius
Wrist

3._____
Pelvis
Hip
Femur
Knee
Tibia/fibula
Shoulder
Humerus
Elbow
Ulna/radius

5._____
Knee
Hip
Femur
(Very forceful)

1. _____

2. _____

3. _____

4. _____

5. _____

6. _____

12

Primary Assessment

Core Concepts

- Deciding on the approach to the primary assessment
- Manual stabilization of the head and neck when necessary
- The general impression
- Assessment of mental status using the AVPU scale
- Identifying and treating problems with the airway, breathing, and circulation
- Making a priority decision

Outcomes

After reading this chapter, you should be able to:

12.1 Summarize the general approach to primary assessment. (pp. 314–321)
- Describe the components of the primary assessment.
- Describe why the steps of primary assessment are ongoing.
- Given a scenario, determine the sequence of the primary assessment steps.
- Describe the actions to be taken upon finding specific problems during the primary assessment.
- Compare the approaches to stable, potentially unstable, and unstable patients.
- Describe the concept of manual stabilization of the head and neck.

12.2 Summarize the specific components of the primary assessment. (pp. 321–329)
- Given a description of mental status, categorize a patient's status using the Alert/Verbal/Painful/Unresponsive (AVPU) approach.
- Given a description of primary assessment findings, categorize the patient as stable, potentially stable, or unstable.

12.3 Explain the concept of clinical judgement applied to the primary assessment. (pp. 330–334)
- Explain the evolution of clinical judgement from novice to expert EMTs.
- Explain how observations can modify the EMT's interpretation of the chief complaint.
- Analyze a primary assessment.

©2021 Pearson Education, Inc.
Emergency Care, 14th Ed.

Match Key Terms

A. Impression of the patient's condition that is formed on first approaching the patient, based on the patient's environment, chief complaint, and appearance.

B. Level of responsiveness.

C. Airway, breathing, and circulation.

D. In emergency medicine, the reason EMS was called, usually in the patient's own words.

E. The first element in a patient's assessment: steps taken for the purpose of discovering and dealing with any life-threatening problems.

F. A memory aid for classifying a patient's levels of responsiveness, or mental status. The letters stand for alert, verbal response, painful response, unresponsive.

G. Actions taken to correct or manage a patient's problem.

H. The decision regarding the need for immediate transport of the patient versus further assessment and care at the scene.

I. The use of specific procedures and equipment for limiting movement of the head, neck, and spine when spinal injury is possible or likely.

J. Using one's hands to prevent movement of a patient's head and neck until a cervical collar can be applied.

_____ 1. A-B-Cs

_____ 2. AVPU

_____ 3. Chief complaint

_____ 4. General impression

_____ 5. Interventions

_____ 6. Mental status

_____ 7. Primary assessment

_____ 8. Priority

_____ 9. Manual stabilization

_____ 10. Spinal motion restriction

Multiple-Choice Review

_____ 1. You are treating a 22-year-old male who is responsive and has a medical complaint. Which of the following steps is *not* part of the primary assessment for this patient?
   A. Assess the patient's mental status.
   B. Assess the adequacy of breathing.
   C. Determine the patient's priority.
   D. Obtain the patient's blood pressure.

_____ 2. The general impression is based on an evaluation of all of the following *except*:
   A. the patient's chief complaint.
   B. appearance.
   C. the environment.
   D. past medical history.

_____ 3. You are assessing a 27-year-old male and making observations about the scene. Finding drug-use paraphernalia at the scene of an emergency is an example of:
   A. an indication of the patient's chief complaint.
   B. the environment part of the general impression.
   C. an assessment of the scene safety.
   D. a medical history of drug addiction.

_____ 4. When a 45-year-old female tells you, in her own words, why she requested an ambulance, this is called the:
   A. general impression.
   B. chief complaint.
   C. primary assessment.
   D. secondary assessment.

_____ **5.** If your patient is not alert and breathing is inadequate due to an insufficient minute volume, you should:
  A. transport immediately.
  B. provide positive pressure ventilations.
  C. obtain a full set of vitals.
  D. all of the above.

_____ **6.** You are assessing a 25-year-old male cyclist who was racing and fell off his bike, landing on his right shoulder. First you determine his mental status using AVPU. What does the "A" in AVPU stand for?
  A. Action   **C.** Assess
  B. Airway   **D.** Alert

_____ **7.** You have determined that your patient is a "V" as far as mental status is concerned. What does the "V" in AVPU stand for?
  A. Violent reaction   **C.** Verbal response
  B. Very painful   **D.** Venous constriction

_____ **8.** One major decision outcome between the primary assessment of a responsive trauma patient and the primary assessment of an unresponsive trauma patient is:
  A. the assessment is done more quickly on the responsive patient.
  B. the unresponsive patient is a higher priority for immediate transport.
  C. there is no difference between the two assessments.
  D. a jaw-thrust maneuver should always be used on the responsive patient.

_____ **9.** You are assessing a 35-year-old female patient who was involved in a serious car crash. She is not alert, and her breathing rate is less than 8 per minute and shallow. As the EMT in charge, you should:
  A. give high-concentration oxygen via nonrebreather mask.
  B. quickly evaluate the patient's circulation and treat for shock.
  C. suction the patient and perform rescue breathing with a pocket mask.
  D. provide positive pressure ventilations with 100% oxygen.

_____ **10.** During your primary assessment of a 42-year-old female patient who is alert and has a breathing rate that is greater than 28 with signs of respiratory distress and SPO_2 of 93%, you should provide her with:
  A. positive pressure ventilations with 100% oxygen.
  B. high-concentration oxygen via nonrebreather mask.
  C. low-concentration oxygen via bag-valve mask.
  D. medium-concentration oxygen via nasal cannula.

_____ **11.** In the primary assessment of a 53-year-old male patient, the circulation assessment includes evaluating all of the following _except_:
  A. pulse.   **C.** severity of bleeding.
  B. skin characteristics.   **D.** blood pressure.

_____ **12.** You are evaluating a 29-year-old male patient. If his skin is warm, dry, and a normal color, it would indicate:
  A. a serious sunburn.   **C.** alcohol abuse.
  B. heat exposure.   **D.** good circulation.

_____ **13.** Your 38-year-old male patient has no life-threatening external hemorrhage, but his skin is cool, pale, and moist. This could indicate:
  A. increased perfusion.   **C.** poor circulation.
  B. high blood pressure.   **D.** cold exposure.

_____ **14.** To evaluate skin color in a dark-skinned patient, the EMT should also:
  A. evaluate the tissues of the lips or nail beds.
  B. evaluate the tissues of the heels of the feet.
  C. check the pupils of the eyes.
  D. do all of these.

©2021 Pearson Education, Inc.
Emergency Care, 14th Ed.

_____ **15.** When assessing the circulation during the primary assessment, the EMT should check for and control severe bleeding. This is important to do because:
   A. open wounds can become infected.
   B. bleeding may lead to long-term complications.
   C. a patient can bleed to death in minutes.
   D. the blood pressure may drop over time.

_____ **16.** When a life threat is observed in the primary assessment, the EMT should:
   A. complete the assessment, then treat.
   B. treat it immediately.
   C. determine the patient's priority, then treat.
   D. package the patient for transport.

_____ **17.** On completion of your primary assessment, you decide that your patient is a high priority. High-priority conditions include:
   A. poor general impression.   **C.** shock.
   B. unresponsive.   **D.** all of these.

_____ **18.** You are treating a patient who you have decided, after your primary assessment, should be a high-priority patient. All of the following would be considered high-priority conditions *except*:
   A. difficulty breathing.
   B. responsive but not following commands.
   C. an uncomplicated childbirth.
   D. chest pain consistent with cardiac problems.

_____ **19.** During the primary assessment of a 55-year-old female with a chief complaint of chest pain, you note that her breathing rate is 24 and SPO_2 is 89%. You should consider:
   A. providing oxygen to the patient.
   B. providing bag-valve mask ventilations.
   C. starting an IV.
   D. using a paper bag to slow down the rate.

_____ **20.** When doing an assessment on a patient who appears lifeless, the approach is adapted to include:
   A. the pulse check for at least 20 seconds.
   B. the C-A-B approach per AHA Guidelines.
   C. the routine A-B-C approach per AHA Guidelines.
   D. none of these are appropriate.

_____ **21.** For a patient to be considered stable he/she needs to:
   A. have only one life threat found during the primary assessment.
   B. have vital signs that are in the normal or just slightly abnormal range.
   C. be willing to sign the refusal form.
   D. have no history of today's problems.

_____ **22.** When assessing a child who is responsive and appears stable on general impression, it is helpful to take a moment to:
   A. kneel at her level.
   B. establish a rapport with the child.
   C. check the capillary refill.
   D. all of the above.

_____ **23.** In the early part of your patient assessment of a trauma patient, your primary concern is to treat the patient's _____ while providing:
   A. life threatening conditions: full spinal immobilization.
   B. medical complaints: oxygen.
   C. life threatening conditions: spinal motion restriction.
   D. obvious fractures: manual stabilization.

_____ **24.** If an infant is not initially alert you should _____ to stimulate
responsiveness or crying.
   A. shout a verbal stimulus
   B. squeeze the shoulder muscle
   C. gently provide a sternal rub
   D. ask the parent to wake the child

Complete the Following

1. The primary assessment is the first element in the total assessment of the
patient. List the six steps of the primary assessment.

   A. _____

   B. _____

   C. _____

   D. _____

   E. _____

   F. _____

2. State what the letters in AVPU stand for.

   A. _____

   V. _____

   P. _____

   U. _____

3. List five examples of patients who may be critical.

   A. _____

   B. _____

   C. _____

   D. _____

   E. _____

4. List the basic three possible results of a pulse-rate check during the
primary assessment.

   A. _____

   B. _____

   C. _____

5. List six high-priority conditions.

A. _____

B. _____

C. _____

D. _____

E. _____

F. _____

Case Study: Car-versus-Bike Crash

Your unit has been dispatched to a call for a car-versus-bike crash on Main Street on a Friday morning. The report from bystanders on the scene is that the male patient (the bike rider) is awake and in a lot of pain. The police have also been dispatched, and they arrive just as you are arriving at the scene.

1. With the police available to attend to the traffic control, what is your initial responsibility?

_____

As you turn to start attending to the patient, a bystander tells you that the cyclist was "tooling right along with the traffic when a guy in a parked car at the curb suddenly opened his driver's door." The bystander goes on to describe how the cyclist hit the door and flew off his bike into the air.

2. Following the scene size-up, what is the name for the the next phase of patient assessment?

_____

3. What is the term for how the injury occurred?

_____

4. How can information like this from a bystander be invaluable?

_____

You introduce yourself to the patient. He says that his name is Tony and he was in a big rush on his way to work, cycling at probably 20 miles per hour. He goes on to say, "That guy did not even look. He just opened his door right in front of me. I couldn't stop that fast." You notice that Tony was wearing a heavy coat and a bright reflective vest as well as a bike helmet. You also note that Tony seems to be protecting his right arm and shoulder and looks as though he is in pain.

5. Now that Tony has given you his name, why is it also important to quickly ask whether he knows where he is and the day of the week?

_____

6. Tony states, "I'm on Main Street, and it's Friday. I was looking forward to the weekend." What would you decide his mental status is?

_____

GZQ **7.** Tony's airway is open, and he is talking but in pain. He has nothing in his mouth, so you ask him to take a deep breath to determine whether his pain is worsened by his breathing. Why do this now?

_____

8. Tony's breathing is a little faster than normal, but he is able to talk in full sentences, and the pain is not from his chest but may be from a fractured clavicle. Next you palpate his radial pulse. It is strong and fast, which you attribute to his heart pumping from fright and pain right now. What else should you check as part of your circulation assessment?

_____

GZQ **9.** You decide that Tony would be a high priority. Why?

_____

©2021 Pearson Education, Inc.
Emergency Care, 14th Ed.

Vital Signs and Monitoring Devices

Core Concepts

- How to obtain vital signs, including pulse, respirations, blood pressure, skin, temperature, and pupils
- How to document vital signs on a prehospital care report
- How to use various monitoring devices

Outcomes

After reading this chapter, you should be able to:

13.1 Explain the contribution of vital signs to the patient assessment process. (pp. 340–359)
- Describe the physiologic processes indicated by each vital sign.
- Explain causes of abnormal vital signs.
- Describe modifications of assessing circulation in children.
- Compare vital signs of infants and children with those in adults.
- Describe the techniques for assessing each of the vital signs.
- Integrate vital signs with other assessment findings to refine the patient's priority.
- Recognize characteristics that can lead to difficulty or false readings when obtaining vital signs.
- Compare auscultation, palpation, and automatic blood pressure monitor approaches to obtaining blood pressure.

13.2 Explain the contribution of information from monitoring devices to patient assessment. (pp. 359–365)
- Identify patients for whom the use of a monitoring device will provide useful information.
- Outline the steps of using various monitoring devices.
- Interpret findings of pulse oximetry.
- Recognize blood glucose level normal ranges.
- Identify situations that can lead to difficulty or false readings when using a monitoring device.

Match Key Terms

Part A

A. The pressure remaining in the arteries when the left ventricle of the heart is relaxed and refilling.

B. A slow pulse; any pulse rate below 60 beats per minute.

C. The force of blood against the walls of the blood vessels.

D. The pulse felt along the large artery on either side of the neck.

E. Assessing the patient through touch or feeling with the hands.

F. The number of pulse beats per minute.

G. The changing size of the pupils when light is shown into them.

H. The rhythmic beats felt as the heart pumps blood through the arteries.

I. The rhythm (regular or irregular) and force (strong or weak) of the pulse.

J. The major artery of the upper arm.

K. The black center of the eye.

L. The act of listening with a stethoscope to auscultate for characteristic sounds.

M. Get larger in diameter.

N. Get smaller in diameter.

O. The pulse felt at the wrist.

_____ 1. Auscultation

_____ 2. Blood pressure

_____ 3. Brachial artery

_____ 4. Bradycardia

_____ 5. Carotid pulse

_____ 6. Constrict

_____ 7. Dilate

_____ 8. Diastolic blood pressure

_____ 9. Palpation

_____ 10. Pulse

_____ 11. Pulse quality

_____ 12. Pulse rate

_____ 13. Pupil

_____ 14. Radial pulse

_____ 15. Reactivity

Part B

A. The number of breaths taken in one minute.

B. The normal or abnormal (shallow, labored, or noisy) character of breathing.

C. A rapid pulse; any pulse rate above 100 beats per minute.

D. The pressure created when the heart contracts and forces blood out into the arteries.

E. The regular or irregular spacing of breaths.

F. The ratio of the amount of oxygen present in the blood to the amount that could be carried, expressed in a percentage.

G. The act of breathing in and breathing out.

H. The cuff and gauge used to measure blood pressure.

I. Outward signs of what is going on inside the body, including respiration; pulse; skin color, temperature, and condition (plus capillary refill in infants and young children); pupils; and blood pressure.

_____ 1. Respiratory quality

_____ 2. Respiratory rate

_____ 3. Respiratory rhythm

_____ 4. Oxygen saturation

_____ 5. Respiration

_____ 6. Sphygmomanometer

_____ 7. Systolic blood pressure

_____ 8. Tachycardia

_____ 9. Blood pressure monitor

_____ 10. Pulse oximeter

_____ 11. Vital signs

_____ 12. Brachial pulse

©2021 Pearson Education, Inc.
Emergency Care, 14th Ed.

J. The pulse felt in the upper arm.

K. An electronic device for determining the amount of oxygen carried in the blood, known as the oxygen saturation or SpO_2.

L. A machine that automatically inflates a blood pressure cuff and measures blood pressure.

Multiple-Choice Review

_____ **1.** You are treating a 35-year-old male who was involved in a fall. The components of the vital signs you will be measuring include all of the following *except*:
- **A.** respiratory rate and quality.
- **B.** skin color and condition.
- **C.** pulse rate and quality.
- **D.** blood sugar level.

_____ **2.** A sign that gives important information about the patient's condition but is *not* considered a vital sign is:
- **A.** blood pressure.
- **B.** mental status.
- **C.** pulse rate.
- **D.** respiratory rhythm.

_____ **3.** Why is it essential that vital signs be recorded as they are obtained?
- **A.** To avoid having to take them more than once
- **B.** To prevent forgetting them and to note trends in the condition.
- **C.** To give the patient a chance to calm down
- **D.** Because they will always change quickly

_____ **4.** You are assessing a 24-year-old female who was involved in a multiple-car crash. You take her pulse, and the rate exceeds 100 beats per minute. This is called:
- **A.** normal.
- **B.** regular.
- **C.** bradycardia.
- **D.** tachycardia.

_____ **5.** On the basis of the pulse alone, a sign that something may be seriously wrong with a patient could be:
- **A.** a sustained rate below 48 beats per minute.
- **B.** a sustained rate above 126 beats per minute.
- **C.** a rate above 150 beats per minute.
- **D.** all of these.

_____ **6.** In addition to the answer to multiple-choice question 5, another serious indicator found in the pulse may be a(n):
- **A.** regular strong rhythm.
- **B.** irregular rhythm.
- **C.** athlete with a pulse of 54.
- **D.** an increase in rate during exercise.

_____ **7.** Assessing the quality of the pulse includes determining the:
- **A.** rhythm and rate.
- **B.** rate and force.
- **C.** rhythm and force.
- **D.** presence and balance.

_____ **8.** A 50-year-old male patient who sustained serious trauma from an ATV crash is described as having a "thready" pulse. This patient most likely has a(n) _____ pulse.
- **A.** strong
- **B.** irregular
- **C.** weak
- **D.** infrequent

_____ **9.** The normal pulse rate for a school-age child (6–10 years) is:
   A. 120 to 160.   **C.** 65 to 120.
   B. 60 to 100.   **D.** 80 to 120.

_____ **10.** When assessing the pulse rate of a typical adult who is not in distress, you would expect to obtain a rate of:
   A. 60 to 100.   **C.** 80 to 120.
   B. 70 to 110.   **D.** 90 to 140.

_____ **11.** The pulse at the thumb side of the wrist is referred to as the _____ pulse.
   A. femoral   **C.** carotid
   B. radial   **D.** brachial

_____ **12.** When assessing the carotid pulse, the EMT should:
   A. palpate the artery as hard as possible.
   B. assess both sides at exactly the same time.
   C. be aware that excessive pressure can slow the heart.
   D. apply pressure until the pulse rate is felt to rise.

_____ **13.** The number of breaths a patient takes in one minute is called the:
   A. minute volume.   **C.** respiratory rate.
   B. minute pressure.   **D.** all of these.

_____ **14.** The respiratory rate is classified as:
   A. normal, slow, or rapid.   **C.** labored, quick, or noisy.
   B. noisy, shallow, or normal.   **D.** weak, thready, or full.

_____ **15.** If the EMT is treating a patient with a sustained respiratory rate above _____ or below _____ breaths per minute, this is serious and high-concentration oxygen should be considered.
   A. 20; 10   **C.** 24; 8
   B. 20; 12   **D.** 24; 10

_____ **16.** Your partner obtains a set of vitals and tells you that the 45-year-old male patient has a normal respiratory rate. The patient's rate at rest should be:
   A. 12 to 24.   **C.** 20 to 30.
   B. 12 to 20.   **D.** 20 to 40.

_____ **17.** The normal respiration rate for a toddler (1–3 years) is:
   A. 12 to 24.   **C.** 20 to 30.
   B. 12 to 20.   **D.** 24 to 40.

_____ **18.** Shallow breathing occurs when:
   A. there is only slight movement of the chest or abdomen.
   B. there is stridor or grunting on expiration.
   C. there is a complete obstruction.
   D. the chest muscles fully expand with each breath.

_____ **19.** Many resting people breathe more with their _____ than with their _____ muscles.
   A. diaphragm; pelvic   **C.** chest; neck
   B. diaphragm; chest   **D.** chest; pelvic

_____ **20.** Signs of labored breathing include all of the following *except*:
   A. an increased respiratory rate.
   B. use of accessory muscles.
   C. retractions above the collarbones.
   D. delayed capillary refill.

_____ **21.** A high-pitched, harsh sound when the patient inhales is called:
   A. nasal flaring.   **C.** crowing.
   B. stridor.   **D.** gurgling.

_____ **22.** When the quality of a patient's respirations is abnormal because something is blocking the flow of air, this is referred to as _____ breathing.
    A. normal   **C.** noisy
    B. shallow   **D.** patent

_____ **23.** You are treating a 28-year-old male patient who was found unconscious in an alley. During your primary assessment, you hear an airway sound that usually indicates the need for suction. This sound is called:
    A. gurgling.   **C.** stridor.
    B. crowing.   **D.** wheezing.

_____ **24.** Two of the best places to assess circulation by skin color in adults are:
    A. under the chin and the nostrils.
    B. the inside of the cheek and the nail beds.
    C. the nail beds and the upper chest.
    D. the toes and the earlobes.

_____ **25.** Your patient sustained a significant blood loss from an injury. This condition may result in skin that is:
    A. flushed.   **C.** pale.
    B. gray.   **D.** jaundiced.

_____ **26.** A patient with a lack of oxygen in the red blood cells resulting from inadequate breathing or inadequate heart function will exhibit a bluish discoloration known as _____ skin.
    A. pink   **C.** flushed
    B. pale   **D.** cyanotic

_____ **27.** On interviewing your 45-year-old male patient, you are told that he has a liver abnormality. This may help explain why his skin appears:
    A. flushed.   **C.** pale.
    B. mottled.   **D.** jaundiced.

_____ **28.** A passerby called the ambulance for the homeless patient you are now assessing. The woman noticed a male in his thirties lying in the parking lot of the supermarket, and she thought he was unconscious. You note that he has cold, dry skin, which is frequently associated with:
    A. high fever and/or heat exposure.
    B. exposure to cold.
    C. shock and anxiety.
    D. a body that is losing heat.

_____ **29.** Hot, dry skin is frequently associated with:
    A. high fever and heat exposure.
    B. exposure to cold.
    C. shock and anxiety.
    D. heat loss.

_____ **30.** You are doing CPR on a patient and see a sudden increase in end-tidal CO_2 on capnography. This is a signal that you should:
    A. switch from nasal cannula to bag-valve-mask.
    B. stop compressions and check for a pulse.
    C. print out the capnograph of the past 30 seconds.
    D. apply a pulse oximeter.

_____ **31.** The reading on the device to test blood sugar level is reported in:
    A. percentage of oxygen in the hemoglobin.
    B. percentage of CO_2 in the exhaled air.
    C. milligrams of glucose per deciliter of blood.
    D. none of these.

_____ **32.** It is a bright, sunny day, and you are treating a 17-year-old woman who fell off her road bike. She is lying supine on the sidewalk. When you assess her pupils, you should:
  A. use a very bright light that is similar to the environmental light.
  B. cover the patient's eyes for a few moments, then uncover one eye at a time.
  C. apply a cold towel to the patient's eyelids for 10 seconds.
  D. move the patient indoors to an area that has dimmer light.

_____ **33.** The pupils may be unequal as a result of any of the following conditions *except*:
  A. stroke.   **C.** eye injury.
  B. head injury.   **D.** shock.

_____ **34.** Fright, blood loss, drugs, and treatment with eye drops may cause the patient's pupils to become:
  A. constricted.   **C.** unequal.
  B. dilated.   **D.** unreactive.

_____ **35.** When the left ventricle of the heart is in the relaxation and refilling phase, the pressure in the arteries is called the _____ pressure.
  A. diastolic   **C.** ventricular
  B. carotid   **D.** systolic

_____ **36.** The pulse oximeter should be used routinely with:
  A. patients who have carbon monoxide poisoning.
  B. patients who complain of respiratory problems.
  C. any patient who is hypothermic.
  D. any patient suffering from severe shock.

_____ **37.** The pulse oximeter is helpful because it:
  A. helps the EMT properly titrate oxygen therapy.
  B. can still read accurately in shock states.
  C. indicates when a patient is about to become hypothermic.
  D. indicates that the patient is a heavy smoker.

_____ **38.** You are treating a firefighter in the rehab sector at a house fire. Your partner reminds you that the pulse oximeter produces falsely high readings in patients with:
  A. hypoxia.
  B. barbiturate poisoning.
  C. carbon monoxide poisoning.
  D. croup.

_____ **39.** Chronic smokers may have a pulse oximeter reading that is:
  A. lower than normal.
  B. higher than the actual oxygen saturation.
  C. 20% to 25% off.
  D. difficult to read.

_____ **40.** In a healthy person, one would expect the oximeter reading to be:
  A. 86% to 90%.   **C.** 96% and above.
  B. 91% to 94%.   **D.** none of these.

_____ **41.** To determine a patient's skin temperature, the EMT often:
  A. holds a thermometer in the patient's axilla for 30 seconds.
  B. has the patient exhale onto a warming device.
  C. feels the patient's skin with the back of the hand.
  D. listens carefully with a stethoscope.

_____ **42.** The normal blood glucose meter reading is usually at least:
  A. 30 to 50 mg/dL.   **C.** 70 to 100 mg/dL.
  B. 50 to 70 mg/dL.   **D.** 100 to 120 mg/dL.

_____ **43.** The systolic blood pressure is:
   A. created when the heart contracts.
   B. listed as the lower number in the BP fraction.
   C. created when the heart relaxes.
   D. seldom used in prehospital care.

_____ **44.** You are treating a patient who was assaulted, and the bar where the fight occurred is still noisy. In a situation like this, it makes sense to take the patient's BP by _____, revealing only the _____ pressure.
   A. auscultation; systolic   **C.** palpation; systolic
   B. auscultation; diastolic   **D.** palpation; diastolic

_____ **45.** Serious hypotension in an adult patient is normally defined as a systolic below _____ mmHg.
   A. 200   **C.** 90
   B. 140   **D.** 60

_____ **46.** In assessing a patient who has an altered mental status, it is not uncommon for the EMT to utilize:
   A. a glucose meter.   **C.** a pulse oximeter.
   B. a BP cuff and stethoscope.   **D.** all of these.

_____ **47.** When a child is under 3 years-old, the blood pressure may be difficult to assess in the field. More useful information about the condition can be obtained by observing for:
   A. respiratory distress.   **C.** unconsciousness.
   B. sick appearance.   **D.** all of the above.

_____ **48.** When assessing the skin of a child under the age of _____ you should also evaluate capillary refill.
   A. 4   **C.** 8
   B. 6   **D.** 10

Complete the Following

1. List the six vital signs assessed by the EMT.

   A. _____

   B. _____

   C. _____

   D. _____

   E. _____

   F. _____

2. List some potential causes of the following:

   A. High blood pressure: _____

   B. Low blood pressure: _____

   C. Cool, clammy skin: _____

   D. Cold, moist skin: _____

E. Cold, dry skin: _____

F. Hot, dry skin: _____

G. Hot, moist skin: _____

H. Dilated pupil: _____

I. Unequal pupils: _____

3. List three different methods used to measure blood pressure.

A. _____

B. _____

C. _____

4. List three methods of measuring temperature.

A. _____

B. _____

C. _____

Label the Diagram

TABLE 13-1   Pulse

Normal Pulse Rates (Beats Per Minute, at Rest)

Adult	60 to 100
Adolescent 11 to 18 years	#1
School age 6 to 10 years	65 to 120 (awake; slightly lower when asleep)
#2	70 to 120 (awake; slightly lower when asleep)
Toddler 1 to 3 years	#3
Infant 0 to 12 months	#4
Newborn	#5
Pulse Quality	**Significance/Possible Causes**
Rapid, regular, and full	Exertion, fright, fever, high blood pressure, first stage of blood loss
Rapid, regular, and thready, irregular	Shock, later stages of blood loss #6
Slow	Head injury, drugs, some poisons, some heart problems, lack of oxygen in children
No pulse	#7

©2021 Pearson Education, Inc.
Emergency Care, 14th Ed.

Fill in the missing information below:

1. _____

2. _____

3. _____

4. _____

5. _____

6. _____

7. _____

Case Study: "Man Down" in the Alley

You are dispatched to a call for a "man down" in the alley behind an auto repair shop in the downtown district. This location has seen considerable trouble before, so the police are dispatched also. As you arrive on the scene, the patrol car pulls up in front of you. A male patient in his thirties is lying by a dumpster, and everyone recognizes him as an alcoholic whom you have transported many times in the past. Although you know his name and a lot of his history, you remember that your EMT instructor said always to begin with the primary assessment and not to cut any corners until you are sure the A-B-Cs are properly assessed and managed.

1. What must be assessed in the primary survey?

_____

2. If you hear gurgling when the patient breathes, what piece of equipment should you have at his side?

_____

As you attempt to place an oral airway, the patient gags and then wakes up. He is a bit drowsy, and you decide to assess his mental status. He seems to know his name, but he has no idea of the day of the week. He does know that he is in the "his" alley behind the auto repair shop, where on occasion he drinks antifreeze often stored in drums for the recycling companies to pick up.

3. What would you say his mental status is?

_____

You decide that the primary assessment does not reveal any life threats, so you move on to obtain some baseline vital signs.

GZQ 4. What would be considered a normal set of vital signs for an adult male patient in his thirties?

_____

5. You recall that this patient has a history of hypertension and diabetes. Given his altered mental status, what additional testing would you consider?

_____

The patient says that he has been eating and actually just had some bread with his "fine" wine. The reading on the glucometer is 60 mg/dL.

6. In your EMS system, you have authorization to administer oral glucose to diabetic patients with low blood sugar as long as the patient has a gag reflex. Would this patient be a candidate for the oral glucose?

_____

7. How often should you reassess the patient's vital signs on the way to the hospital?

_____

©2021 Pearson Education, Inc.
Emergency Care, 14th Ed.

14

Principles of Assessment

Core Concepts

- How examinations are conducted
- History-taking techniques
- Physical examination techniques
- Body system examinations
- Critical thinking concepts for the EMT

Outcomes

After reading this chapter, you should be able to:

14.1 Explain techniques that are useful in obtaining the patient history. (pp. 370–377)
- Distinguish between circumstances when collecting a complete history is better facilitated by open-ended or closed-ended questions.
- Apply the OPQRST mnemonic to gain additional information about a complaint.
- Apply the SAMPLE mnemonic to organize information gathering.

14.2 Describe the general techniques of physical examination. (pp. 377–391)
- Compare the type of information that can be obtained through each general technique of physical examination.
- Provide the information you anticipate getting from different body systems when deciding to use a general technique of physical examination.

14.3 Analyze your approach to decision making in EMS scenarios. (pp. 391–398)
- Compare EMTs' process of diagnosis with that of emergency physicians.
- Explain the impact of experience on diagnostic processes.
- Given a short description of an EMT setting, recognize common cognitive biases.

14.4 Evaluate your approach to decision making in EMS scenarios. (pp. 398–400)
- Compare the features of experienced physicians' thinking with EMTs' thinking.
- Evaluate your approach to thinking like an EMT.

Match Key Terms

A. The grating sound or feeling of broken bones rubbing together.

B. Bulging of the neck veins.

C. A question requiring only a "yes" or "no" answer.

D. A description or label for a patient's condition that assists a clinician in further evaluation and treatment.

E. A memory aid in which the letters stand for elements of the past medical history.

F. A memory aid in which the letters stand for questions asked to get a description of the present illness.

G. The patient's statement that describes the symptom or concern associated with the primary problem the patient is having.

H. A list of potential diagnoses compiled early in the assessment of the patient.

I. Information gathered regarding the patient's health problems in the past.

J. Information gathered regarding the symptoms and nature of the patient's current concern.

K. A question requiring more than just a "yes" or "no" answer.

_____ **1.** Chief complaint

_____ **2.** Crepitation

_____ **3.** Diagnosis

_____ **4.** Past medical history (PMH)

_____ **5.** Closed-ended question

_____ **6.** Differential diagnosis

_____ **7.** SAMPLE

_____ **8.** Jugular vein distention

_____ **9.** Open-ended questions

_____ **10.** History of the present illness (HPI)

_____ **11.** OPQRST

Multiple-Choice Review

_____ **1.** When obtaining a history, it is best to begin with a/an _____ question.
   A. leading.
   B. open-ended.
   C. closed-ended.
   D. summative.

_____ **2.** When taking a history of a patient with multiple problems in the field, your immediate goal is to answer the question:
   A. what is wrong with the patient?
   B. why does this patient skip their medicines?
   C. why does this patient have so many problems?
   D. what does this patient need?

_____ **3.** An example of a closed-ended question would be:
   A. "What are the medications you take?"
   B. "What do you do when you have breathing difficulty?"
   C. "Do you feel like you are going to pass out?"
   D. "Can you describe the pain to me?"

_____ **4.** From a general perspective, _____ can usually be interviewed if you take your time and keep your language simple.
   A. toddlers
   B. preschoolers
   C. school-aged children
   D. adolescents

©2021 Pearson Education, Inc.
Emergency Care, 14th Ed.

_____ **5.** When evaluating a patient during the physical exam, three common techniques the EMT will use are:
  A. auscultate, observe, and visualize.
  C. observe, auscultate, and palpate.
  B. inspect, percuss, and palpate.
  D. visualize, rotate, and percuss.

_____ **6.** When a patient tells you that he called because he cut his wrist with a razor, this is called the:
  A. primary assessment.
  C. SAMPLE history.
  B. chief complaint.
  D. secondary assessment.

_____ **7.** The history of the present illness and PMH includes interviewing bystanders to ask about each of the following _except_:
  A. whether the patient complained of anything before this happened.
  B. how the patient could have prevented the illness from occurring.
  C. whether the patient has any known illnesses or problems.
  D. if the patient is a minor, whether the parent or guardian has been contacted.

_____ **8.** The "M" in the memory aid SAMPLE refers to:
  A. mental status.
  C. mean arterial pressure.
  B. medications.
  D. multiple patients.

_____ **9.** The "P" in the mnemonic OPQRST refers to:
  A. provocation.
  C. priapism.
  B. palpation.
  D. pain.

_____ **10.** All of the following are key questions to answer in taking a patient history, regardless of the type of medical or traumatic complaint, _except:_
  A. Does the patient walk down this street often?
  B. Does the patient take any medications?
  C. When did the patient last eat or take anything by mouth?
  D. Does the patient have any existing medical problems?

_____ **11.** In conducting your body system examination during the secondary assessment of a patient with a respiratory complaint, which of the following questions would the EMT least likley to ask?
  A. Has the patient checked his or her blood glucose recently?
  B. Does the patient have a productive cough?
  C. Does the patient have difficulty breathing when lying down?
  D. Is it increasingly difficult for the patient to catch his or her breath after exertion?

_____ **12.** The mental status assessment is key to the physical examination of patients with:
  A. immune and musculoskeletal system complaints.
  B. genitourinary and reproductive system complaints.
  C. respiratory and neurologic system complaints.
  D. endocrine and gastrointestinal system complaints.

_____ **13.** When a patient with a respiratory complaint states that she has breathing difficulty when lying down, this is called:
  A. paradoxical breathing.
  C. eupnea.
  B. orthopnea.
  D. hypopnea.

_____ **14.** When assessing the abdomen of an adult male critical trauma patient, the EMT should inspect and palpate for _____ in addition to wounds and deformities.
  A. pain
  C. crepitation
  B. colostomy and/or ileostomy
  D. paradoxical motion

_____ **15.** The cardiovascular assessment includes checking for a narrowing pulse pressure. This is defined as the:
  A. difference between the systolic and diastolic pulse pressure.
  B. difference in pulse rate due to normal breathing.
  C. pressure in the arteries when the heart is relaxing.
  D. difference between the fast and slowest pulse the patient has.

_____ **16.** Your patient is an alert 58-year-old male who is complaining of chest pain. The components of the secondary assessment for a medical patient with a cardiovascular system complaint include all of the following *except:*
   A. looking for jugular venous distention.
   B. asking the SAMPLE history questions.
   C. obtaining baseline vital signs.
   D. performing the Cincinnati Prehospital Stroke Scale.

_____ **17.** Many memory aids are used during the secondary assessment. OPQRST is a memory aid to help the EMT remember the:
   A. questions to ask about the past medical history.
   B. questions that expand on the history of the present illness.
   C. status of the patient's condition.
   D. levels of the patient's mental status.

_____ **18.** When you ask a male patient with back pain, "How bad is the pain?" you are questioning him about:
   A. quality.   **C.** time.
   B. severity.   **D.** radiation.

_____ **19.** Why is it important for the EMT to determine the "T" in OPQRST when questioning a 58-year-old male with a chief complaint of chest pain?
   A. The patient's temperature could be a contributing factor.
   B. The patient may have fallen and injured his tibia.
   C. It is helpful to determine the time when the pain began.
   D. The patient may have sustained a tension pneumothorax.

_____ **20.** The 58-year-old male continues to discuss his condition with you. His chief complaint is chest pain. When you ask, "Do you have nausea or have you been vomiting?" you are questioning him about his:
   A. signs and symptoms.   **C.** allergies.
   B. medication history.   **D.** pertinent past history.

_____ **21.** The alert 58-year-old male who is complaining of chest pain goes on to describe other recent hospitalizations and the medical condition for which his doctor is treating him. In the SAMPLE history, this information is considered:
   A. unnecessary information.
   B. pertinent past history.
   C. the provocation, or cause of today's event.
   D. the reason the ambulance was called.

_____ **22.** When you ask an elderly female patient, "How have you been feeling today?" you are asking her about the:
   A. pertinent past history.
   B. signs and symptoms.
   C. events leading to the current illness.
   D. last oral intake.

_____ **23.** When interviewing a patient who has a neurologic system complaint, during your assessment you should examine the patient's mental status and:
   A. auscultate the lungs for breath sounds.
   B. look for a colostomy bag.
   C. assess movement and sensation of the extremities.
   D. observe the neck for JVD.

_____ **24.** In conducting a body system examination of the patient with a GI system complaint, which of the following questions would be most appropriate to ask?
   A. How much soda do you usually drink?
   B. Have you had a bowel movement recently?
   C. Do you carry an epinephrine self-injector?
   D. Are you taking any blood-thinning medications?

©2021 Pearson Education, Inc.
Emergency Care, 14th Ed.

_____ **25.** When assessing a 28-year-old female patient who has a medical complaint involving the endocrine system, be sure to ask whether the patient:
   A. has had a previous TIA.
   B. carries an epinephrine self-injector.
   C. is currently sick.
   D. has taken a medicine for chest pain.

_____ **26.** When conducting a physical exam of an unconscious adult patient with a suspected medical problem, you see a medical bracelet on the patient's wrist. This is important because it may:
   A. reveal the patient's name.
   B. give clues to the patient's home address.
   C. reveal the patient's medical condition.
   D. be the cause of the emergency.

_____ **27.** Your patient is a young child who was injured. During the reassessment, which of the following should you do and why?
   A. Be sure to avoid eye contact at all times because it will scare the child.
   B. Try to stand above the patient so that the patient can look up at you and see you at all times.
   C. Speak in a loud voice so that the patient can hear every one of your instructions.
   D. Use a reassuring voice to help calm the patient.

_____ **28.** When conducting an assessment on a child, the EMT should do each of the following, _except_:
   A. tell the child what will happen next.
   B. take more time and explain if possible.
   C. use the same terms you do for adults.
   D. consider use of toy to distract small children.

_____ **29.** If you must expose the small child in order to conduct a physical exam, remember to:
   A. protect the child from stares of onlookers.
   B. quickly cover the child after the exam.
   C. do not rush the child into accepting all that is happening.
   D. all of the above.

_____ **30.** Which is not considered a part of the body system exam of a patient with a cardiac complaint:
   A. orthostatic blood pressure.   **C.** breath odors.
   B. JVD.   **D.** blood pressure.

_____ **31.** The analytical process that assists the EMT in reaching a field diagnosis is referred to as:
   A. active assessment.   **C.** critical thinking.
   B. passive assessment.   **D.** detailed assessment.

_____ **32.** The basic approach that clinicians use to arrive at a diagnosis includes each of the following _except_:
   A. gathering information.   **C.** considering the possibilities.
   B. administering lab tests.   **D.** reaching a conclusion.

_____ **33.** When a clinician draws up a list of conditions that may be the cause of the patient's condition today, this is referred to as the:
   A. admission diagnosis.   **C.** differential diagnosis.
   B. presenting problem.   **D.** assessment finding.

_____ **34.** A highly experienced physician who reaches an incorrect diagnosis while using heuristics (shortcuts) may have been subject to any of the failings listed here _except_:
   A. search satisfying.   **C.** confirmation bias.
   B. representativeness.   **D.** lack of confidence.

_____ **35.** The traditional approach to diagnosis involves:
   A. narrowing down a long list of possible diagnoses.
   B. jumping to conclusions.
   C. taking lots of shortcuts.
   D. eliminating similar conditions.

_____ **36.** A clinician who is specifically looking for evidence that supports the diagnosis he or she already has in mind is committing a(n) _____ bias.
   A. anchoring
   B. confirmation
   C. satisfying
   D. illusionary

_____ **37.** When a patient does not fit the classic pattern, such as a cardiac patient without crushing chest pain, the EMT has to be careful not to make a(n) _____ error or bias.
   A. confirmation
   B. representativeness
   C. overconfidence
   D. availability

_____ **38.** You recently had a patient with heat stroke. The next time you have a patient in a warm environment, you are more likely to think of a diagnosis of heat stroke instead of more common problems such as dehydration. This bias is referred to as:
   A. overconfidence.
   B. illusory correlation.
   C. confirmation.
   D. availability.

_____ **39.** The EMT should be skeptical about one condition being the actual cause of another condition a patient presents with. Drawing quick conclusions about the cause of a diagnosis can lead to a(n):
   A. anchoring.
   B. illusory correlation.
   C. search satisfying bias.
   D. all of these.

_____ **40.** You are treating a patient who was found on the floor in the nursing home. It seems evident that he has a fractured hip as he lies on the floor in pain. If you stop the search for a diagnosis as soon as you come up with a likely cause of an obvious problem, this can lead to:
   A. missing out on the secondary diagnosis.
   B. overconfidence and misdiagnosis.
   C. confirmation bias.
   D. all of these.

_____ **41.** During your body system exam of a patient, checking the blood glucose is likely associated with a(n) _____ system chief complaint.
   A. respiratory
   B. endocrine
   C. GI/GU
   D. cardiovascular

Complete the Following

1. List questions that are usually asked when using OPQRST to elaborate on the chief complaint.

O. _____

P. _____

Q. _____

R. _____

S. _____

T. _____

2. List questions you might ask when using the SAMPLE history acronym.

S. _____

A. _____

M. _____

P. _____

L. _____

E. _____

3. List six questions you would consider or ask in gathering your history of a patient with a respiratory complaint.

A. _____

B. _____

C. _____

D. _____

E. _____

F. _____

4. List four questions you would consider or ask the patient or bystanders in gathering the history of a patient with a neurologic complaint.

A. _____

B. _____

C. _____

D. _____

5. List four questions you would consider or ask in gathering your history of a patient with a gastrointestinal complaint.

A. _____

B. _____

C. _____

D. _____

6. List eight ways in which an EMT can learn to think like a highly experienced physician.

A. _____

B. _____

C. _____

D. _____

E. _____

F. _____

G. _____

H. _____

Case Study: A Motorcycle Mishap

You are dispatched to a motorcycle collision in an intersection in your community. Apparently, a car made a right turn on red without stopping, and the motorcycle, which had the green light, collided with the left side of the car. On arrival, you conduct a scene size-up. What are four things you should be concerned about in the scene size-up of this collision?

1. _____

2. _____

3. _____

4. _____

You find out from a witness who was standing on the corner at the bus stop that the vehicles were probably traveling 40 mph and the cyclist crashed into the rear left door of the car. He was thrown off the motorcycle onto the roof of the car and then landed on his back in the street. The witness immediately rushed to aid the cyclist and at the same time motioned people in another vehicle to stop traffic and to call 911. The witness stated that the patient was in a lot of pain but never hit his head or lost consciousness. The cyclist was wearing a helmet, which he removed after the collision.

5. How does forming a general impression help you provide emergency care to the patient? On what is the general impression based?

_____

_____

Your general impression reveals a 20-year-old responsive male trauma patient with severe external blood loss. The patient is able to talk with you, although he is experiencing considerable pain in his thighs and lower back. He is able to describe what happened in the collision, knows the day of the week, and is concerned about his new bike. His name is Jesse, and he was on his way to the beach, which explains why he is wearing shorts and a T-shirt.

GZQ **6.** As you question Jesse, what should one of your partners be doing?

_____

_____

©2021 Pearson Education, Inc.
Emergency Care, 14th Ed.

7. What is Jesse's mental status on the AVPU scale?

_____

Jesse keeps crying out, "It's my legs!" They are obviously broken but no longer seriously bleeding. You proceed with the primary assessment, beginning with an assessment of Jesse's airway.

GZQ **8.** Explain why it would be wrong to be distracted by Jesse's pain and immediately begin to treat his broken legs.

_____

9. What should your primary assessment of Jesse consist of?

_____

On the basis of your primary assessment of Jesse, you have determined that he is a high-priority patient, and an ALS unit should be requested if it is not en route already. You found that his airway is open and clear, his breathing is present and adequate, and he is moving air into both sides of his chest equally, but he has a weak, rapid radial pulse, and his skin is pale, cool, and clammy to the touch—possible signs of shock. One of your crew has controlled the bleeding from Jesse's thighs.

10. Why is Jesse a high-priority patient?

_____

11. How long should you wait for an ALS unit to arrive before transporting Jesse?

_____

As one of your crew attends to Jesse's injured legs and then places him onto a long backboard, you continue with the secondary assessment of a patient with musculoskeletal system complaints. Because you have reconsidered the mechanism of injury (MOI), you have decided to provide early transport for Jesse as soon as he is packaged.

12. What would you be looking for as you examine Jesse?

_____

13. In addition to your findings on physical examination, what would be relevant questions to ask Jesse about his musculoskeletal system injuries in your secondary assessment?

_____

14. What vital signs should you assess?

_____

En route to the hospital, you have time to conduct a physical examination. You have provided spinal motion restriction precautions and he is receiving oxygen via nonrebreather mask, the scoop stretcher is in the supine position, and you are keeping the patient warm with a blanket. His vitals are a respiration rate of 20—good quality; a pulse rate of 120—weak and regular; a blood pressure of 110/70 mmHg; SpO_2 90%; and pale, cool, and clammy skin.

15. What would the physical examination include?

_____

15. Secondary Assessment

Core Concepts

- Components of the secondary assessment
- Secondary assessment of the responsive medical patient
- Secondary assessment of the unresponsive medical patient
- Secondary assessment of the trauma patient with minor injury
- Secondary assessment of the trauma patient with serious injury or multisystem trauma
- Detailed physical exam

Outcomes

After reading this chapter, you should be able to:

15.1 Describe the integration of the secondary assessment into the overall patient care process. (pp. 404–407)
- State the purpose of the secondary assessment.
- List the components of secondary assessment.
- Describe modifications to the approach to secondary assessment based on patients' situational factors.

15.2 Describe secondary assessment of medical patients. (pp. 407–419)
- Compare approaches you would take to responsive and unresponsive patients.

15.3 Describe secondary assessment of trauma patient with serious or multisystem injuries. (pp. 420–428)
- Adapt secondary assessment techniques based on the suspected body systems involved.

15.4 Analyze your approach to decision making in EMS scenarios. (pp. 428–450)
- Compare the secondary assessment approaches to trauma patients with minor injuries and those with serious or multisystem injuries.

Match Key Terms

A. A surgical incision into the trachea that is held open by a metal or plastic tube.

B. Movement of part of the chest in the opposite direction to that of the rest of the chest during breathing.

C. Persistent erection of the penis that can result from spinal injury and some medical problems.

D. An assessment of the head, neck, chest, abdomen, pelvis, extremities, and posterior of the body in an injured patient who is unresponsive.

E. Something regarding the patient's condition that the patient tells you.

F. A procedure for detecting changes in a patient's condition after assessment and care has been initiated.

G. A permanent surgical opening in the neck through which the patient breathes.

H. Evidence of the patient's condition that you can see.

I. Information gathered regarding the patient's health problems in the past.

J. Information gathered regarding the symptoms and nature of the patient's current concern.

K. A condition of being stretched, inflated, or larger than normal.

L. An assessment of the head, neck, chest, abdomen, pelvis, extremities, and posterior of the body to detect signs and symptoms of injury.

M. A patient suffering from one or more physical injuries.

N. A patient with one or more medical diseases or conditions.

_____ **1.** Medical patient

_____ **2.** Reassessment

_____ **3.** Past medical history (PMH)

_____ **4.** Detailed physical exam

_____ **5.** Distention

_____ **6.** History of present illness (HPI)

_____ **7.** Symptom

_____ **8.** Sign

_____ **9.** Paradoxical motion

_____ **10.** Priapism

_____ **11.** Rapid trauma assessment

_____ **12.** Stoma

_____ **13.** Tracheostomy

_____ **14.** Trauma patient

Multiple-Choice Review

_____ **1.** Why is the secondary assessment performed after the scene size-up and the primary assessment?
   A. You need to be sure there are no immediate life threats requiring interventions.
   B. You must be sure you are functioning at a safe scene.
   C. You need to have called for all the resources you need.
   D. All of the above.

_____ **2.** A patient suffering from one or more physical injuries is which type of patient?
   A. Medical patient   **C.** Unknown patient
   B. Trauma patient   **D.** none of the above

_____ **3.** When performing a secondary assessment, you will generally complete the:
    A. physical exam.
    B. patient history.
    C. vital signs.
    D. all of the above.

_____ **4.** Which statement is correct about a "sign" and/or a "symptom?"
    A. The patient tells you about a sign.
    B. You can observe a symptom.
    C. You can measure a symptom.
    D. The patient tells you about a symptom.

_____ **5.** When gathering a history from a child the EMT should:
    A. rely only on information obtained from the parents.
    B. kneel or find another way to get on the level of the child.
    C. do not ask about the past medical history.
    D. all of the above.

_____ **6.** A simpler alternative to using the mnemonic DCAP-BTLS suggested by the authors of the textbook would be to remember:
    A. soft tissue, bones, and hollows.
    B. critical, unstable, and stable.
    C. wounds, tenderness, and deformities.
    D. open cuts, contusions, and swelling.

_____ **7.** Which is the correct statement for pediatrics about who should be transported to a hospital that provides trauma care?
    A. Fall > 20 feet (6.1 meters)
    B. Injury to shoulder
    C. Fall > 10 feet (3 meters)
    D. Injury above the knees

_____ **8.** When listening to lung sounds on an infant, use a pediatric stethoscope and:
    A. listen to the back of the chest.
    B. listen in the mid-axillary position.
    C. listen to the front of the chest.
    D. listen at the midclavicular line.

_____ **9.** In the secondary assessment, you will be checking the patient for pain and tenderness. The difference between pain and tenderness is that:
    A. pain occurs only when you squeeze an injury site, whereas tender areas hurt all the time.
    B. pain is considered unbearable, whereas tenderness is usually bearable.
    C. tenderness may not hurt unless the area is palpated, whereas pain is evident without palpation.
    D. pain hurts only for the first 10 minutes, whereas tenderness doesn't go away.

_____ **10.** When assessing the responsive medical patient, the steps include obtaining vital signs and:
    A. gathering the chief complaint and HPI.
    B. gathering a PMH from the patient.
    C. conducting a physical exam.
    D. all of the above.

_____ **11.** You are treating a baseball player who was hit in the face by a pitch. You remember from your EMT training that any blow above the _____ may damage the cervical spine.
    A. clavicles
    B. diaphragm
    C. femur
    D. pelvis

©2021 Pearson Education, Inc.
Emergency Care, 14th Ed.

_____ **12.** If a cervical collar is the wrong size, it may:
  A. cause additional injury to the spine.
  B. obstruct the airway.
  C. prevent the patient from moving his or her neck.
  D. take too much time to adjust and apply correctly.

_____ **13.** What is the correct statement about the typical order of the steps of the secondary assessment of the responsive or the unresponsive medical patient?
  A. the physical exam is done before the history in responsive patients.
  B. the chief complaint and HPI come first in the responsive patient.
  C. the baseline vital signs are done last in the unresponsive patient.
  D. the PMH is obtained before the physical exam in the unresponsive patient.

_____ **14.** What is a sign?
  A. A photograph of the patient's wrecked vehicle
  B. The patient's description of how the injury occurred
  C. An objective finding that you can see, hear, or feel when examining the patient
  D. A subjective finding that the patient tells you about his or her current condition

_____ **15.** When a patient has shortness of breath additional history should include:
  A. fever or chills.   **C.** dyspnea on exertion.
  B. cough.   **D.** all of the above.

_____ **16.** You are treating a patient who was in the front seat of an automobile involved in a collision. You observe a spiderweb crack in the windshield and small facial lacerations on the patient. Most likely the patient:
  A. will have a life-threatening head injury.
  B. did not wear a seat belt or three-point harness.
  C. will also complain of leg injuries.
  D. was involved in a rollover collision.

_____ **17.** When asking about additional history items such as fever, nausea and vomiting, diarrhea, or constipation, you are most likely gathering a history for a medical patient with:
  A. altered mental status.   **C.** abdominal pain.
  B. chest pain.   **D.** shortness of breath.

_____ **18.** When assessing the head of an adult male critical trauma patient, the EMT should inspect and palpate for _____ in addition to wounds, tenderness, and deformities.
  A. hematoma   **C.** crepitation
  B. scalp lacerations   **D.** abrasions

_____ **19.** When assessing the neck of an adult female critical trauma patient, the EMT should inspect and palpate for _____ in addition to wounds and deformities.
  A. jugular vein distention   **C.** lacerations
  B. swelling   **D.** burns

_____ **20.** When assessing the pelvis of an adult male critical trauma patient, the EMT should inspect and palpate for _____ in addition to wounds and tenderness.
  A. paradoxical motion   **C.** distended areas
  B. deformities   **D.** rectal bleeding

_____ **21.** If you are treating a severely injured trauma patient, it may be appropriate to skip the:
  A. secondary assessment.   **C.** baseline vital signs.
  B. detailed physical examination. **D.** primary assessment.

_____ 22. A difference between the detailed physical examination and the rapid trauma assessment is:
   A. skipping the face, ears, eyes, nose, and mouth in the detailed exam.
   B. the detailed examination is usually done en route to the ED.
   C. the lungs are not listened to in a detailed examination.
   D. the extremities and posterior are not assessed in the rapid trauma assessment.

_____ 23. The final step of the detailed physical examination is commonly to:
   A. complete the examination of airway, breathing, and circulation.
   B. make sure that you have notified the ED.
   C. remove the collar and recheck the neck.
   D. roll the patient to examine the posterior of the body.

_____ 24. You are examining a patient who was struck on the head last night. His mental status is altered, and he has a bruise behind one ear. This is referred to as:
   A. raccoon eyes.   C. Battle sign.
   B. orbital hematoma.   D. Cushing reflex.

_____ 25. When performing a rapid assessment of the head in a trauma patient, you note blood in the anterior chamber of the eye. This tells you that the:
   A. patient was wearing contact lenses.
   B. patient has a serious brain injury.
   C. patient's eye is bleeding inside.
   D. all of these.

_____ 26. Clear fluid that is draining from the ears and nose may _____ fluid.
   A. lymphatic   C. chyle
   B. cerebrospinal   D. synovial

_____ 27. In addition to looking for deformities, you should look for all of the following except _____ when examining the mouth.
   A. possible airway obstructions   C. tongue lacerations or swelling
   B. loose or broken teeth   D. crepitation

_____ 28. You will be conducting a rapid physical examination on an unresponsive 54-year-old female medical patient. You should include all of the following steps except:
   A. looking for jugular vein distention.
   B. determining firmness or rigidity of abdomen.
   C. checking for incontinence of urine or feces.
   D. asking the SAMPLE history questions.

_____ 29. Each of the following are high-risk patients (per CDC guidelines) except:
   A. ejection from a vehicle.
   B. death in the same passenger compartment.
   C. a child who fell 2–3 times his/her height.
   D. intrusion > 6 inches into the occupant side of the car.

_____ 30. It is important to realize that people who wear seat belts may sustain injury to:
   A. the neck arteries.   C. abdominal organs.
   B. the bowel.   D. all of the above.

_____ 31. Flat neck veins in a patient who is lying down may be a sign of:
   A. tension pneumothorax.   C. cardiac tamponade.
   B. blood loss.   D. a healthy person.

_____ 32. When conducting the rapid trauma exam of the chest you note the patient has a number of rib fractures broken at both ends. This condition can lead to:
   A. significant blood loss.
   B. paradoxical motion during breathing.
   C. hyperventilating.
   D. cardiac tamponade.

_____ **33.** When examining an infant who sustained trauma you should do each of the following except:
  A. look for blood and clear fluid coming from the nose and ears.
  B. apply pressure to the soft spots on the head to feel for swelling.
  C. check for instability of the pelvis.
  D. check for rigid or tender abdomen.

_____ **34.** The best position to maintain for the injured child's airway would be:
  A. hyperextended.   **C.** neutral position.
  B. hyperflexion.   **D.** all of the above are acceptable.

_____ **35.** The neck veins are usually not visible when the patient is _____:
  A. lying flat.   **C.** supine.
  B. sitting up.   **D.** prone.

Complete the Following

1. List four steps of secondary assessment in their usual order for a responsive medical patient.

  A. _____

  B. _____

  C. _____

  D. _____

2. List four steps of the secondary assessment in their usual order for an unresponsive medical patient.

  A. _____

  B. _____

  C. _____

  D. _____

3. List five significant injuries and signs of significant injuries.

  A. _____

  B. _____

  C. _____

  D. _____

  E. _____

4. When conducting a physical exam/trauma assessment in addition to examining for wounds, tenderness and deformities, what else should be checked for?

  Head - _____

  Neck - _____

Chest - _____

Abdomen - _____

Pelvis - _____

Extremities - _____

5. List four general principles to remember when examining a patient.

A. _____

B. _____

C. _____

D. _____

Case Study: Just a Bit Dizzy

You are dispatched to a shopping mall in your community. The call is for a woman in her forties who was found by mall security sitting in a stairway. You are brought to the patient by another security officer, who states that they are not sure what was wrong with the woman, so they called EMS. You and your partner decide that the scene is safe and notify the dispatcher to keep the medic unit responding to the scene. As you approach the patient, you notice that she is obviously sweating and pale and seems to be shivering. There are no family members or friends with her.

1. After getting a general impression of the patient, what are the components of the primary assessment that you should use to evaluate this patient?

_____

_____

You determine that the patient's name is Linda and she is 44 years old and was busy shopping for her son's sixteenth birthday. She says that her husband and son are out of town at a ball game. You decide that the primary assessment reveals no immediate life threats and that the patient is able to answer all the questions you ask her. She is very pale and clammy and says she that has the chills. You and your partner proceed with the three basic components of the secondary assessment. The dispatcher is advised to keep the medic unit responding but to downgrade the response (no lights and siren).

2. What are the three basic components of the secondary assessment?

_____

_____

_____

From interviewing Linda, you determine she denies any difficulty breathing or pain in her head, chest, or abdomen. She states that when she felt dizzy, she sat down and did not fall or pass out. You also find out that she is a type I diabetic and has an insulin pump. Your partner obtains a full set of vital signs while you ask the appropriate SAMPLE history questions.

3. What does SAMPLE stand for, and what are examples of questions you would ask?

S - _____

A - _____

M- _____

P - _____

L - _____

E - _____

Your partner lets you know that the baseline vital signs are respiration of 20 and regular, pulse of 100 and thready, blood pressure of 108/70 mmHg, and SpO_2 of 98%. Linda told him that her BP is usually low. Because she is an insulin-dependent diabetic, you decide to check her blood sugar, which is 110 mg/dL. She says that she has not had a meal since breakfast (it is about 3:00 p.m. at this point) and that she ate a Snicker's bar about a half hour ago when she first felt dizzy. She did not think to check her own sugar level at that point but thought that it might be a little low.

4. Considering the history you have obtained so far, what body system specific history should you be obtaining in your secondary assessment?

_____

5. What are seven specific questions that would be appropriate to ask Linda on the basis of the body system of her chief complaint at this point?

A. _____

B. _____

C. _____

D. _____

E. _____

F. _____

G. _____

After obtaining a complete secondary assessment and doing the appropriate physical examination, you decide that it would be best to transport Linda to the hospital for an evaluation. The medic unit has arrived, and because her blood sugar has dropped further, they will be starting an IV line and administering glucose en route to the hospital. Mall security lets you know that they were able to contact Linda's neighbor, who will be meeting her at the hospital and contacting Linda's husband.

GZQ **6.** From you best understanding of the information that you obtained from Linda, what may have occurred to her today?

_____

Reassessment

Core Concepts

- Observing trends during reassessment
- Reassessment for stable and for unstable patients

Outcomes

After reading this chapter, you should be able to:

16.1   Analyze the components in your approach to re-evaluating patients in EMS scenarios.
(pp. 454–459)
- Evaluate patient status based on trending assessment findings.
- Compare the approaches to reassessing stable and unstable patients.

Match Key Terms

A. A procedure for detecting changes in a patient's condition. It involves four steps: repeating the primary assessment, repeating and recording vital signs, repeating the physical exam, and checking interventions.

B. Changes in a patient's condition over time, such as slowing respirations or rising pulse rate, that may show improvement.

_____ **1.** Trending

_____ **2.** Reassessment

Multiple-Choice Review

_____ **1.** Which of the following most accurately describes the purpose of performing a reassessment of your patient?
  A. To stabilize the patient's condition or to treat any life threats
  B. To detect and treat life threats and to evaluate the EMS system's effectiveness
  C. To evaluate the EMS system's effectiveness and to detect changes in patient condition
  D. To repeat key elements of assessment procedures already performed to detect changes in patient condition

_____ **2.** Your patient is a young child who was suddenly injured. During the reassessment, which of the following should you do and why?
  A. Be sure to avoid eye contact at all times because it will scare the child.
  B. Try to stand above the patient so that the patient can look up at you and see you at all times.
  C. Speak in a loud voice so that the patient can hear every one of your instructions.
  D. Use a reassuring voice to help calm the patient.

_____ **3.** You are treating a 45-year-old male who sustained multiple injuries in a fall. En route to the hospital, you will be conducting a reassessment, which includes all the following steps *except*:
  A. reassessing vital signs.
  B. repeating the primary assessment for life threats.
  C. repeating the detailed physical exam.
  D. checking interventions.

_____ **4.** En route to the hospital, you will be reassessing your 25-year-old male patient, who sustained a rib fracture. Which of the following is *not* something you should do when performing the reassessment?
  A. Reestablish patient priorities.
  B. Monitor skin color, temperature, and condition.
  C. Maintain an open airway.
  D. Apply a cervical collar.

_____ **5.** During your reassessment of a 22-year-old female who is complaining of abdominal cramps, you note that her pulse is rapid and her skin is cool, pale, and clammy. This may indicate:
  A. deterioration in mental status.
  B. an occluded airway.
  C. heat exhaustion.
  D. the onset of shock.

_____ **6.** You are treating a patient who fell and sustained a laceration to his right arm. The bleeding has been controlled, and there are no other injuries. If the patient has normal vital signs, you would consider his condition to be _____, and the recommended interval for reassessment is every _____ minutes.
  A. stable; 5   **C.** unstable; 10
  B. stable; 15   **D.** unstable; 20

_____ **7.** Examples of subtle changes you should pick up on during reassessment would include:
  A. anxiety.   **C.** sweating.
  B. restlessness.   **D.** all of the above.

_____ **8.** You are transporting an unstable 30-year-old male trauma patient directly to the Regional Trauma Center. How often should you be doing your reassessment?
  A. Every 5 minutes   **C.** Every 15 minutes
  B. Every 10 minutes   **D.** Every 20 minutes

_____ **9.** Your 62-year-old female patient has a fractured ankle. Her only medical history is a past stroke and taking a blood thinner medication. On reassessment her pulse jumped up 20 points. Your next reassessment should be in _____ minutes.

    A. 5   **C.** 15

    B. 10   **D.** 20

Complete the Following

1. List three things you should always evaluate when checking interventions during your patient reassessment.

    A. _____

    B. _____

    C. _____

2. When reassessing your patient, you need to repeat the primary assessment. List the six key steps to recheck:

    A. _____

    B. _____

    C. _____

    D. _____

    E. _____

    F. _____

3. How would the mental status of an unresponsive child or infant be reassessed?

    A. _____

4. List three tips to consider when reassessing a pediatric patient.

    A. _____

    B. _____

    C. _____

Communication and Documentation

Core Concepts

- Radio procedures used at various stages of the EMS call
- Delivery and format of a radio report to the hospital
- Delivery and format of a verbal hand-off report to the hospital
- Communication skills used when interacting with other members of the health care team
- Communication skills used when interacting with the patient
- Components of and procedures for the written prehospital care report
- Legal aspects and benefits of documentation
- Documentation concerns in patient refusal

Outcomes

After reading this chapter, you should be able to:

17.1 Compare public safety radio communications systems to best practices. (pp. 464–469)
- Describe the features of communication system components.
- Describe the impact of each component of a communication system on the delivery of patient care.
- Assess portrayals of radio communication for compliance with basic principles of radio communication.
- Assess portrayals of radio medical reports for the correct use of each of the components of a radio medical report.

17.2 Evaluate the various types of interpersonal communications EMTs have with others. (pp. 469–474)
- Compare the verbal patient report when transferring patient care to hospital personnel to the radio patient report given en route.
- Explain professional ways to overcome a communication problem.
- Describe the importance of communicating with all health care providers involved in patient care at the scene.
- Describe the general guidelines for engaging in therapeutic communication.
- Describe modification of approaches to patients with communication challenges.
- Given a portrayal of an episode of therapeutic communication, identify what went well and what did not go well.

17.3 Generate a written prehospital care report from a portrayal of patient care. (pp. 474–490)
- Describe each of the functions of a prehospital care report.
- Identify the purposes of the National Highway Transportation Safety Administration (NHTSA) data elements.
- Identify the Patient Information and Administrative information elements of the NHTSA minimum data set.
- Identify the minimum NHTSA data required to communicate effectively through the narrative of a prehospital report.
- Explain the importance of each of the required elements of the narrative portion of a written prehospital care report.
- Explain the documentation required when a patient refuses emergency prehospital care and transportation.
- Give examples of how the quality and completeness of your written prehospital care reports can serve you and others, in the near and far future.
- Explain the consequences of falsification of prehospital care report information.
- Describe the proper correction of errors and late entries in prehospital care reports.
- Explain modifications to the EMT's documentation in special situations.

Match Key Terms

A. An abbreviated form of the PCR that an EMS crew can leave at the hospital when there is not enough time to complete the PCR before leaving.

B. A device that picks up signals from lower-power radio units, such as mobile and portable radios, and retransmits them at a higher power.

C. A phone that transmits through the air instead of over wires so that the phone can be transported and used over a wide area.

D. A two-way radio that is used or affixed in a vehicle.

E. A two-way radio at a fixed site such as a hospital or dispatch center.

F. A handheld two-way radio.

G. The process of sending and receiving data wirelessly.

H. The unit of measurement of the output of a radio.

_____ **1.** Base station

_____ **2.** Cell phone

_____ **3.** Mobile radio

_____ **4.** Portable radio

_____ **5.** Repeater

_____ **6.** Watt

_____ **7.** Drop report (or transfer report)

_____ **8.** Telemetry

Multiple-Choice Review

_____ **1.** After arriving in the ED, you should introduce the patient by name, summarize what was in your radio report, and:
  A. provide history that was not given previously.
  B. discuss additional treatment given en route.
  C. update the vital signs taken en route.
  D. all of the above.

_____ **2.** The components of an EMS communications system include:
  A. base stations.   **C.** portable radios.
  B. mobile radios.   **D.** all of these.

_____ **3.** You will need to alert the regional trauma center of the patient's condition directly from the scene. Because your portable radio might not have the power to reach the hospital ED from the scene, you will need to rely on a device that picks up radio signals from lower-powered radios and retransmits them at a higher power. This device is called a:

A. transmitter.   **C.** repeater.
B. cellular.   **D.** portable.

_____ **4.** The U.S. government agency that is responsible for maintaining order on the airwaves is the:

A. FCC.   **C.** FEMA.
B. FAA.   **D.** DOT.

_____ **5.** The reason for always closely following the general principles of radio transmission is to allow everyone to use the frequencies and to:

A. avoid having to repeat orders from medical direction.
B. enable the EMT to talk in code language.
C. prevent delays.
D. do all of these.

_____ **6.** The following is a list of components of a medical radio report: (1) major past illness; (2) chief complaint; (3) unit identification and level of provider; (4) emergency medical care given. In which order they should be stated?

A. 4, 1, 2, 3   **C.** 3, 2, 1, 4
B. 3, 4, 1, 2   **D.** 1, 2, 4, 3

_____ **7.** You arrive at the office of a 52-year-old male. Your unit was alerted because he has had chest pain for the past 45 minutes. The chest pain is referred to as the:

A. major past illness.   **C.** presenting diagnosis.
B. chief complaint.   **D.** call type.

_____ **8.** You are traveling en route to the ED with a 27-year-old female who is in severe pain. During your radio report, you state, "The patient's abdomen feels rigid." You are advising the ED of:

A. the baseline vital signs.
B. the emergency medical care given.
C. the response of the patient to the emergency medical care.
D. pertinent findings of the physical examination.

_____ **9.** During your radio report, you state, "The patient's mental status has not changed during our care." You are attempting to advise the ED of the:

A. baseline vital signs.
B. emergency medical care you have given so far.
C. response of the patient to the emergency medical care you have provided.
D. pertinent findings of the physical examination.

_____ **10.** Your regional or state protocols require a direct medical order to allow you to assist a 22-year-old female with her prescribed bronchodilator device. Whenever you request an order for medical direction over the radio, it is good practice to:

A. repeat the physician's order word for word back to the physician.
B. question all verbal orders that are given.
C. speak quickly because the physician is busy.
D. call the physician back to verify.

_____ **11.** If you receive an order from the on-line physician for ten times the normal dose of a medication (e.g., 1,500 mg of ASA instead of 150 mg), what should you do?

A. Switch to another frequency to find another physician.
B. Question the physician about the order.
C. Follow the physician's order as stated.
D. Ignore the order and do what you believe is correct.

_____ **12.** It is 2:30 a.m., and your partner is interviewing a 25-year-old male who has a minor complaint. You notice that your partner is standing with arms crossed looking down at the patient. What nonverbal message is your partner sending to the patient?

 A. "I am here to help you."
 B. "I am not really interested."
 C. "I can empathize with your problem."
 D. "I am determined to diagnose what's wrong with you."

_____ **13.** You are treating a 35-year-old female who was struck by a car. It is obvious that she has a broken leg because a broken bone end is protruding through the skin. She proceeds to ask you, "Is my leg broken?" What would be the most appropriate response?

 A. "Relax and stay calm. You will be all right."
 B. "I am not qualified to make that determination."
 C. "No, it's a bad cut, and I'll control the bleeding with a bandage."
 D. "Yes, it is, and I will be as gentle as possible in splinting it."

_____ **14.** In treating a 2-year-old who is sitting on the couch crying and complaining of "tummy" pain, the best approach would be to:

 A. kneel down so that you are at the child's level.
 B. speak louder so that the child can hear you above the crying.
 C. stare directly into the child's eyes.
 D. tell the child that you are a friend of his parents.

_____ **15.** The prehospital care report (PCR) has many functions. It serves as a legal document as well as a(n):

 A. press release form for your EMS agency.
 B. receipt for the patient.
 C. aid to research, education, and administrative efforts.
 D. form to report all calls to the local police department.

_____ **16.** Why is it necessary to complete a PCR/drop report if, on each call, you give the ED staff a good oral report?

 A. The QI committee needs something to hold you to.
 B. It provides a means for the ED staff to review the patient's prehospital care.
 C. The ED usually does not listen to oral reports.
 D. Duplication is helpful in emergency call documentation.

_____ **17.** The copy of the prehospital care report (PCR) that is provided to the hospital:

 A. is returned to the state for quality review and follow-up.
 B. is thrown out once it is input into the computer file.
 C. becomes part of the patient's permanent hospital record.
 D. is sent to the regional Emergency Medical Services agency.

_____ **18.** You are called to court to testify about a civil matter involving a patient who is suing the city for an injury that occurred in a public place. Which of the following will best help you recall the events of the call?

 A. The questioning by the defense's attorney
 B. The questioning by the plaintiff's attorney
 C. A complete and accurate prehospital care report (PCR)
 D. Your tape recording of the call dispatch

_____ **19.** The person who completed the prehospital care report (PCR) may be called to a court of law to testify about the:

 A. call in a criminal proceeding.
 B. care provided to the patient.
 C. call in a civil proceeding.
 D. all of these.

_____ **20.** The routine review of prehospital care reports (PCRs) for conformity to current medical and organizational standards is part of a process called:

 A. initial feedback.
 B. quality improvement.
 C. stress debriefing.
 D. system research.

_____ **21.** Each individual box on a prehospital care report (PCR), either paper or electronic, is called a(n):
  A. narrative.   **C.** keypunch.
  B. data element.   **D.** assessment.

_____ **22.** According to the NHTSA, in addition to other data elements, the minimum data set on a prehospital care report (PCR) should include all of the following _except_:
  A. the respiratory rate and effort and skin color and temperature.
  B. the times of incident, dispatch, and arrival at the patient.
  C. the patient's Social Security number.
  D. the capillary refill for patients less than 6 years old.

_____ **23.** The time of incident is an example of _____ data on the PCR.
  A. assessment   **C.** patient
  B. run   **D.** narrative

_____ **24.** The PCR serves a number of purposes for the EMS system and EMTs. An example of patient information on a PCR would be the:
  A. date of birth and age of the patient.
  B. time of arrival at the hospital.
  C. ambulance unit identification number.
  D. ID number of the hospital to which the patient is transported.

_____ **25.** EMTs should consider a good PCR to be one that:
  A. protects them against a QA review.
  B. is vague enough to prevent lawsuits.
  C. paints a picture of the patient.
  D. identifies symptoms overlooked by the patient.

_____ **26.** A statement such as "The patient has a swollen, deformed extremity" on the narrative portion of the PCR is an example of:
  A. subjective information.   **C.** pertinent negative information.
  B. objective information.   **D.** nonstandard abbreviations.

_____ **27.** All the following are examples of information that should be put in quotation marks on the PCR _except_:
  A. bystander statements.   **C.** objective information about the patient.
  B. chief complaint.   **D.** police officer's statements.

_____ **28.** In the narrative section of a PCR, the EMT should:
  A. list his or her conclusions about the situation.
  B. include pertinent negatives.
  C. use the radio codes for each treatment.
  D. list the vital signs and times obtained.

_____ **29.** Medical abbreviations should be used on a PCR:
  A. to save space in the narrative section.
  B. to replace all words you cannot spell.
  C. only if they are standardized.
  D. to ensure correct interpretation by physicians.

_____ **30.** You are treating a 22-year-old male who fell off his motorcycle. He has some road rash and no major injuries and is mostly concerned about his bike. He does not want to go to the hospital and has a friend who can drive him home and take care of him. Before leaving the scene, you should:
  A. document assessment findings and care given.
  B. try again to persuade the patient to go to a hospital.
  C. ensure that the patient is able to make a rational, informed decision.
  D. do all of these.

31. When completing a PCR involving a patient refusal, the EMT should document all of the following *except*:
   A. that the EMT was willing to return if the patient changed his or her mind.
   B. the complete patient assessment.
   C. that alternative methods of care were offered.
   D. the patient's definitive diagnosis.

32. An EMT who forgot to administer a treatment that is required by the state or regional treatment protocols should:
   A. document on the PCR only treatment that was actually given.
   B. be sure to document an excuse for why the treatment was skipped.
   C. record that the patient was given the forgotten treatment.
   D. do none of these things.

33. You are in a rush during a call and did not have time to take a second set of vital signs. Your partner says, "Just write in another set ten minutes after the first one." Falsification of information on a PCR may lead to:
   A. suspension or revocation of your license or certification.
   B. better EMT education.
   C. longer response times.
   D. none of these.

34. To correct an error that is discovered while writing the PCR, you should:
   A. scribble over the error so that it cannot be seen.
   B. draw a line through the error, initial it, and write the correct information.
   C. place your initials over the error.
   D. erase the error completely, and then write the correction.

35. On returning to the station after a call, you have the chance to reread your PCR. If information was omitted by mistake, you should:
   A. prepare another report and substitute that for the earlier one.
   B. notify the service medical director immediately.
   C. add a note with the correct information, date it, and initial it.
   D. do nothing because information should never be added after the call.

36. Occasionally, EMTs have only limited information about the patient to document on the PCR. An example of an instance in which it would *not* be unusual for the EMT to obtain only a limited amount of information is:
   A. during a multiple-casualty incident (MCI).
   B. during an interhospital transfer.
   C. while performing a nonemergency run.
   D. when encountering a child abuse case.

37. You were just on a call about which your service director requires you to complete a special incident report. Special situation (incident) reports:
   A. document events that should be reported to local regulatory authorities.
   B. can be submitted at any time after the call.
   C. need not be accurate or objective.
   D. are required on each call.

38. Ambulance services and EMS personnel are required by _____ to take steps to safeguard patient confidentiality.
   A. OSHA law   C. the NHTSA
   B. HIPAA   D. the U.S. DOT

39. There are laws, both state and federal, that protect patient privacy. An example of a method that an ambulance service would use to safeguard patient confidentiality is:
   A. requiring employees to place completed PCRs in a locked box.
   B. using only patient last names during radio transmissions.
   C. allowing only PCRs with patient names to be distributed during QA meetings.
   D. none of these is an acceptable procedure.

_____ **40.** The policy that an ambulance service develops concerning patient rights and confidentially must take into consideration:

A. state regulations. **C.** HIPAA.

B. local regulations. **D.** all of these.

Complete the Following

1. List six examples of components of a communications system.

A. _____

B. _____

C. _____

D. _____

E. _____

F. _____

2. List six interpersonal communications guidelines to use when dealing with patients, families, friends, and bystanders.

A. _____

B. _____

C. _____

D. _____

E. _____

F. _____

3. List five examples of patient information on a prehospital care report (PCR).

A. _____

B. _____

C. _____

D. _____

E. _____

4. List five examples of situations that may require the use of a special incident report.

A. _____

B. _____

C. _____

D. _____

E. _____

5. List six principles of radio communication.

A. _____

B. _____

C. _____

D. _____

E. _____

F. _____

Case Study: Asleep at the Wheel

You are dispatched to a patient who was involved in a single-vehicle automobile crash. The patient may have fallen asleep at the wheel. There is significant damage to the front end of the vehicle, which struck a tree. On arrival, you conduct a scene size-up. You conclude that the scene is safe, and you have plenty of help. Police officers are on the scene dealing with investigation, making notifications, and controlling traffic.

1. At this point in the call, what two types of radio communication equipment have you most likely already used?

_____

2. You conduct your primary assessment, and there are no immediate life threats present. In the patient's own words, what would be the patient's chief complaint—that is, the reason the ambulance was called to the scene?

_____

3. After determining that there were no life threats, you proceed to interview the patient and conduct the secondary assessment. As a precaution, on the basis of the MOI, what should another EMS provider be doing while you examine the patient?

_____

Aside from a small cut on the head, which has already stopped bleeding, the 28-year-old patient is alert and denies any injuries. He states that he just wants to get home and go to sleep. The police have already done a breathalyzer test, and they tell you that he has not been drinking. You obtain a set of baseline vital signs, and they are all within normal limits. The patient states that he has no medical history, is not under a doctor's care, and takes no medications.

GZQ 4. Should you just let the patient sign off as refusing medical care?

_____

5. Explain why or why not.

_____

6. If the patient simply wants to sign off and go home, what other strategies can you use to attempt to convince him to be seen in the ED?

_____

_____

After a lengthy discussion, you manage to convince the patient it is in his best interest to be seen in the local ED. You and your partner remove the patient from the vehicle while maintaining spinal motion restriction precautions. En route to the hospital, you obtain another set of vital signs and prepare to give a medical radio report.

7. What is an example of the medical radio report that you will be giving to the ED on this patient?

_____

_____

_____

On arrival at the ED, the triage nurse tells you to take the patient to room A-7. Once in the room, you begin to transfer the patient to the hospital stretcher and at the same time give an oral report to the nurse who will be taking over the treatment of the patient.

8. What are some examples of the information that you would pass along in the oral report to the nurse or physician in the ED?

_____

_____

_____

18

General Pharmacology

Core Concepts

- Which medications may be carried by the EMT
- Which medications the EMT may help administer to patients
- What to consider when administering any medication
- The role of medical direction in medication administration
- How the EMT may assist with IV therapy

Outcomes

After reading this chapter, you should be able to:

18.1 Describe medications EMTs may carry on the ambulance and administer. (pp. 496–499)
- Describe the actions of specific medications carried on the ambulance (e.g., aspirin, oral glucose, oxygen, naloxone).
- Identify the reason an EMT would administer a medication carried on the ambulance.
- Identify the routes by which medications carried on the ambulance are administered to the patient by the EMT.
- Identify generic and trade names of all medications carried on the ambulance and those prescribed to patients with which EMTs may assist.

18.2 Describe patients' own prescription medications which EMTs may assist patients in taking. (pp. 499–503)
- Describe the actions of bronchodilators, nitroglycerin, epinephrine auto-injectors, and force protection medication.
- Describe the role of medical direction in assisting with administration of patients' prescribed medications.
- Relate the actions of albuterol and epinephrine to the correction of the pathophysiology of anaphylaxis and asthma.

18.3 Explain general concepts of pharmacology. (pp. 503–510)
- Distinguish between chemical, generic, and trade names of drugs.
- Assess patient and context to determine the indications and contraindications for a medication before you give it.
- Anticipate desired effects, known as side effects, and untoward effects of drugs before you give them.
- Recognize the occurrence of desired effects, untoward effects, and side effects in a patient.

- Describe the importance of clinical judgment in administering medications.
- Compare the two types of medical authorization under which an EMT can administer medications.
- Describe the importance of checking expiration dates and following the Five Rights of medication administration.
- Describe each of the routes of drug administration.
- Describe how pharmacodynamics affect judgments about medication administration.
- Identify the steps of reassessment and documentation required after administering a medication.
- Describe common categories of medications and herbal remedies that you will find used by patients in the field.

18.4 Explain the EMT's role in assisting with intravenous (IV) therapy. (pp. 510–514)
- Identify the parts of the equipment and supplies required for IV therapy.
- Outline the steps of preparing the IV fluid and intravenous tubing.
- Recognize other tasks EMTs can assist with, if asked, when assisting with IV therapy.
- Describe how to troubleshoot an IV that is not running, running too slowly, or running too quickly.

Match Key Terms

A. Specific circumstances under which it is appropriate to administer a drug to a patient.

B. A device with a mouthpiece that contains dry aerosolized form of a medication that a patient can spray into the mouth while they breathe in.

C. The study of drugs, their sources, their characteristics, and their effects.

D. A medication given by mouth to treat an awake patient (who is able to swallow) with an altered mental status and a history of diabetes.

E. A medication used to reduce the clotting ability of blood to prevent and treat clots associated with myocardial infarction.

F. A drug that helps to constrict the blood vessels and relax passages of the airway. It may be used to counter a severe allergic reaction.

G. A gas commonly found in the atmosphere, that is also medication that can be used to treat patients with respiratory distress and hypoxia.

H. A device attached to the end of a syringe that turns liquid medication into fine droplets upon administration.

I. The study of the effects of medications on the body.

J. An unexpected effect of a medication may be potentially harmful to the patient.

K. Any action of a drug other than the desired action.

L. Specific circumstances under which it is not appropriate and may be harmful to administer a drug to a patient.

_____ **1.** Atomizer

_____ **2.** Aspirin

_____ **3.** Contraindication

_____ **4.** Epinephrine

_____ **5.** Indications

_____ **6.** Inhaler

_____ **7.** Nitroglycerin

_____ **8.** Oral glucose

_____ **9.** Oxygen

_____ **10.** Pharmacology

_____ **11.** Pharmacodynamics

_____ **12.** Side effect

_____ **13.** Untoward effect

_____ **14.** Parenteral

_____ **15.** Enteral

_____ **16.** Naloxone

M. A drug that helps to dilate the coronary vessels that supply the heart muscle with blood.

N. An antidote for narcotic overdoses.

O. Referring to a route of medication administration that does not use the gastrointestinal tract, such as an intravenous medication.

P. Referring to a route of medication administration that uses the gastrointestinal tract, such as swallowing a pill.

Multiple-Choice Review

_____ **1.** The study of drugs, their sources, and their effects is referred to as:
   A. anatomy.
   B. physiology.
   C. medicinology.
   D. pharmacology.

_____ **2.** Medications that EMTs can routinely administer or assist with in the field include:
   A. aspirin, oral glucose, and naloxone.
   B. nitroglycerin.
   C. epinephrine and prescribed inhalers.
   D. all of these.

_____ **3.** According to treatment protocols, an EMT in the field would administer aspirin to:
   A. treat headaches.
   B. dilate the coronary arteries.
   C. help prevent clot formation.
   D. eliminate the pain from a serious injury.

_____ **4.** You are considering administering chewable aspirin to your 58-year-old female patient, who is complaining of chest pain. When would aspirin administration be contraindicated?
   A. When no water is available
   B. If the patient has a history of GI bleeding
   C. If the patient may be having a heart attack
   D. All of these

_____ **5.** Your patient is a 13-year-old female with diabetes whose mother states, "She has not accepted her disease and is managing it poorly." Poorly managed diabetes can cause:
   A. hypoxia.
   B. altered mental status.
   C. dilation of the coronary arteries.
   D. absorption of poisons.

_____ **6.** You are treating a 35-year-old diabetic male with an altered mental status. He has a gag reflex, so oral glucose is your treatment, according to your protocols. It is given between the patient's cheek and gum, using a tongue depressor, because:
   A. this method promotes fast absorption into the bloodstream and easy swallowing.
   B. it will not be aspirated if the patient suddenly becomes unconscious.
   C. this area will cause the patient to regurgitate the stomach's contents.
   D. it will assist in dilating the coronary vessels as much as possible.

©2021 Pearson Education, Inc.
Emergency Care, 14th Ed.

_____ **7.** As an important part of your secondary assessment of a 52-year-old male, you must determine whether he is taking any specific medications. Examples of medications he may have in his possession that you may assist him in taking, under the appropriate circumstances, are:

    A. glucose injections and anticonvulsants.

    B. home oxygen, antihypertensives, and anti-inflammatories.

    C. epinephrine auto-injector, a bronchodilator inhaler, and nitroglycerin.

    D. insulin, antihypertensives, and anticonvulsants.

_____ **8.** Your 52-year-old female patient states that she has a long history of asthma and chronic bronchitis. It would be expected that she carry _____ in her purse.

    A. nitroglycerin   **C.** a bronchodilator

    B. an epinephrine auto-injector   **D.** a bronchoconstrictor

_____ **9.** Your 62-year-old male patient has a history of cardiac problems and states that he takes nitroglycerin when he gets chest pain. Nitroglycerin is used to _____ vessels.

    A. dilate the peripheral   **C.** dilate the coronary

    B. constrict the peripheral   **D.** constrict the coronary

_____ **10.** The comprehensive U.S. government publication that lists all drugs is called the:

    A. _Physician's Desk Reference._   **C.** _U.S. Pharmacopoeia (USP)._

    B. _Hazmat Guidebook._   **D.** _National Medicine Guidebook._

_____ **11.** The name that the manufacturer uses in marketing a drug is called the _____ name.

    A. generic   **C.** official

    B. trade   **D.** original

_____ **12.** Your 58-year-old male patient tells you that he is not supposed to take a specific medication when his blood pressure is low or he feels dizzy. A circumstance in which a drug should not be used because it may cause harm to the patient is called a(n):

    A. indication.   **C.** adverse reaction.

    B. side effect.   **D.** contraindication.

_____ **13.** You are administering a medication for a specific purpose according to your treatment protocols. An action of a drug that is other than the desired action is called a(n):

    A. side effect.   **C.** contraindication.

    B. overdose.   **D.** systemic effect.

_____ **14.** Part of your treatment of a seriously ill 45-year-old female will involve administration of a medication. Before administering the medication, you must know all of the following _except_:

    A. the route of administration.

    B. the proper dose to administer.

    C. the actions the medication will take.

    D. both the generic and chemical names.

_____ **15.** You are treating a 29-year-old male who is under a physician's care for chronic low back pain and is taking medication for his condition. Drugs prescribed for pain relief are called:

    A. antidysrhythmics.   **C.** anticonvulsants.

    B. analgesics.   **D.** antihypertensives.

_____ **16.** Your secondary assessment reveals that your 58-year-old male patient takes a medication to control his hypertension. Drugs that are prescribed to reduce high blood pressure are called:
  A. antidysrhythmics.
  B. antiparasympathetics.
  C. anticonvulsants.
  D. antihypertensives.

_____ **17.** Your 55-year-old female patient tells you that she is taking a medication to control her irregular heartbeat. Drugs that are prescribed for heart rhythm disorders are called:
  A. antidiabetics.
  B. bronchodilators.
  C. antidysrhythmics.
  D. anticonvulsants.

_____ **18.** Upon interviewing a 25-year-old female asthmatic, you find that she is taking a drug to treat her disease. Medications that are prescribed to relax the smooth muscles of the bronchial tubes are called:
  A. bronchospasms.
  B. bronchodilators.
  C. anticonvulsants.
  D. bronchoconstrictors.

_____ **19.** Your 28-year-old female patient just had a seizure in her home. On interviewing her after she wakes up, you find that she skipped a couple of doses of her medicine this week. Drugs that are prescribed for prevention and control of seizures are called:
  A. antidiabetics.
  B. antihypertensives.
  C. anticonvulsants.
  D. antidepressants.

_____ **20.** Your 32-year-old male patient is taking a drug that was prescribed to help regulate his emotional activity and keep neurotransmitter levels from dropping too low. This type of drug is called an:
  A. antidepressant.
  B. analgesic.
  C. antidysrhythmic.
  D. anticonvulsant.

_____ **21.** When a patient is administered tiny aerosolized particles of medicine to treat a disease such as asthma, this is considered the _____ route of administration.
  A. intravenous
  B. sublingual
  C. inhaled
  D. oral

_____ **22.** An example of an understanding of the pharmacodynamics of a specific medication is knowing that:
  A. pediatric patients normally require larger doses.
  B. medications may have a longer effect in geriatric patients.
  C. heavier patients require ten times the normal dose.
  D. all of these.

_____ **23.** Your patient may have taken an overdose of an narcotic and is no longer responsive with very slow and shallow breathing. While assisting the ventilations, you should consider administering _____ by the _____ route.
  A. epinephrine: intramuscular
  B. naloxone: intranasal
  C. albuterol: oral
  D. epinephrine: IV

_____ **24.** A powder prepared from charred wood administered by some EMS Systems to the conscious poisoning patient is called:
  A. ipecac.
  B. Zofran.
  C. activated charcoal.
  D. naloxone.

_____ **25.** When assisting an ALS provider in starting an IV on the patient, you notice that the fluid is not flowing thru the drip chamber of the administration set. What could be the problem?
  A. The clamp may be closed on the tubing.
  B. The constricting band was left on the arm.
  C. The tubing may be kinked.
  D. Any of these.

____ **26.** The antidote used in medicine when an overdose of a narcotic has caused a slow respiratory drive is:
   A. albuterol.
   B. oxygen.
   C. naloxone.
   D. activated charcoal.

Pathophysiology: How Medications for Asthma and Anaphylaxis Work

1. When assessing a patient who is having an asthma attack, aside from observing the patient's difficulty in breathing and listening carefully with your stethoscope to the full respiratory cycle, what should you notice?

   _____

2. What is occurring to the airways of the asthmatic patient who is in distress?

   _____

3. What can be trigger an asthma attack?

   _____

4. What medication can be helpful in treating the asthmatic patient and why?

   _____

5. When assessing a patient who is having a severe allergic reaction, such as anaphylaxis, aside from noticing that the patient is experiencing difficulty breathing, what other concerns would you have?

   _____

6. What substance is released from cells of the body during an allergic reaction that can be life-threatening? What is its effect on the body?

   _____

7. What medication do many patients with allergies carry with them that state or regional protocols may allow the EMT to assist the patient in taking?

   _____

8. What is the expected effect of epinephrine on the patient when administered?

   _____

Complete the Following

1. List seven medications that an EMT can administer or assist a patient in taking.

   A. _____

   B. _____

   C. _____

D. _____

E. _____

F. _____

G. _____

2. List the five questions to ask yourself to assure you are addressing the five "rights" when administering a medication.

A. _____

B. _____

C. _____

D. _____

E. _____

3. List eight routes of administration of medications.

A. _____

B. _____

C. _____

D. _____

E. _____

F. _____

G. _____

H. _____

4. List what the following herbal agents are used for.

A. Gingko _____

B. Garlic _____

C. Ginger root _____

D. Evening Primrose oil _____

E. Kava kava _____

Case Study: Altered Mental Status

Your unit is responding to a call for a young male adult who was found in the restroom of the local shopping mall. On your arrival at the closest entrance you are met by the mall security officer who states, "my partner is at the patient's side with the AED and the patient has a pulse." As you arrive at the men's room there are a few people that have gathered but are not in your way. You and your partner decide that the scene is safe and the medic unit should continue to respond at this point. A bystander has already pulled the patient, a 19-year-old male, out of the stall and washed his face off with cold water. It looks like he may have vomited on himself and his shirt.

After taking the appropriate Standard Precautions, you attempt to introduce yourself to the patient and bystanders and find that the patient responds with withdrawal from painful stimuli. Since he is not an obvious cardiac arrest and has no obvious life-threatening bleeding you proceed with the steps of the primary assessment in the "A-B-C" sequence. His airway is open with manual positioning and there is no indication of any trauma to the head or neck so head-tilt, chin-lift works just fine. He is still gurgling a bit so you have your partner quickly suction his mouth. He starts to gag so it is apparent that he will not take an oropharyngeal airway at this point. As you evaluate his breathing you note that first his breathing rate is too slow (approximately 8 times a minute) and his depth or tidal volume is diminished or shallow.

1. When a patient has a slow breathing rate and a shallow rate what is likely to happen if you do not intervene?

2. What would be the most appropriate means of administering oxygen to this patient at this point?

3. Should you continue to have the ALS unit respond to your location?

Suddenly the patient's sister is led into the restroom by a security guard because she has more medical information. His name is Louis and he has struggled with various addictions and depression over the past few years. She says he is on a lot of medications and that he has been taking heroin recently. Your partner checks Louis's pupils and, sure enough, they are pinpoint, so this could account for the respiratory depression. You proceed with the primary assessment. He has a slow pulse, and his skin is pale, clammy, and cool to touch. He has no obvious bleeding that needs to be attended to at this point, although you do note he has many bruises and "track marks" on his arms. You decide he is a high priority, and as your partner continues to assist his ventilations, you both begin to package the patient on the stretcher. The plan has been to alert the medic prior to her arrival on the scene so she is aware the patient may need a dose of naloxone right away.

4. In your secondary assessment of any unresponsive medical patient, what are some of the potential causes of an altered mental state?

5. As it turns out, this patient has a number of medications in a plastic bottle his sister has found in his pocket. What should you do with these medications?

6. His sister also finds a list of the prescribed medications her brother is supposed to be taking for his depression on a piece of paper in his wallet. Aside from writing these meds down on your PCR how might you be able to figure out what these medications are used for?

The patient is loaded into your ambulance and the medic gets a quick history from you and agrees that some naloxone would be appropriate at this point. He proceeds to give 1 mg intramuscular to the patient which is the regional protocol.

7. What effect would you expect to see from administration of this medication?

_____

GZQ 8. Suppose the dose of naloxone did not produce a reaction, given what you have learned and your clinical judgement, what else might be appropriate to try?

_____

After two doses and about ten minutes of assisting the patient's ventilations you start to notice that his mental status is improving and he is fighting the BVM. You decide to switch to a nonrebreather mask and obtain a full set of vital signs. With him breathing on his own and normal vitals you have a moment to check on the other medications he takes using a resource carried on your ambulance. The medic is keeping a close watch on Louis and preparing to call the ED on the radio.

9. What types of medications are the following?

A. Prozac - _____   **B.** Topamax - _____   **C.** OxyContin - _____

©2021 Pearson Education, Inc.
Emergency Care, 14th Ed.

19

Respiratory Emergencies

Core Concepts

- How to identify adequate breathing
- How to identify inadequate breathing
- How to identify and treat a patient with breathing difficulty
- Use of continuous positive airway pressure (CPAP) to relieve difficulty breathing
- Use of a prescribed inhaler and how to assist a patient with one
- Use of a prescribed small-volume nebulizer and how to assist a patient with one

Outcomes

After reading this chapter, you should be able to:

19.1 Explain a patient's breathing status. (pp. 520–522)
- Summarize the coordinated processes required of the cardiopulmonary system to maintain perfusion.
- Outline the assessment procedure for determining the adequacy of respiration.
- Describe the mechanics of inspiration and expiration.

19.2 Distinguish between descriptions of a patient who is breathing adequately and one who is not. (pp. 522–526)
- Discern adequate from inadequate respiratory rate.
- Discern adequate from inadequate respiratory rhythm.
- Discern adequate from inadequate breathing quality.
- Relate the differences in pediatric anatomy and physiology to the differences observed in inadequate breathing in children compared with adults.

19.3 Select the most appropriate intervention sequence for a description of a patient with inadequate breathing. (pp. 526–528)
- Recommend the prioritized treatment for a patient with inadequate breathing.
- Describe the considerations in choosing the means of providing artificial ventilation to a patient.
- Contrast the characteristics of inadequate artificial ventilation with those of adequate artificial ventilation.
- Describe the differences in the respiratory interventions for children versus those for adults.

19.4 Outline the assessment process for a patient complaining of difficulty breathing.
(pp. 528–534)
- Recognize the different ways patients may describe a chief complaint that tells you they are having difficulty breathing.
- Describe immediate observations that give an early means of differentiating between adequate and inadequate breathing in a patient complaining of difficulty breathing.
- Describe the adaptation of the OPQRST mnemonic to a patient with a chief complaint of difficulty breathing.
- Recall symptoms that a patient with shortness of breath may complain of.
- Describe specific observations that EMTs should look for in the assessment of a patient with difficulty breathing.
- Describe the auscultation of the lungs in a patient with difficulty breathing.
- Describe the characteristics of abnormal breath sounds.
- Describe the underlying problem that produces each of the abnormal breath sounds.
- Recognize how vital signs may be altered in a patient with a chief complaint of difficulty breathing.
- Describe how the pulse oximeter should be integrated in assessment of a patient complaining of difficulty breathing.

19.5 Propose a treatment plan for a representation of a patient with breathing difficulty. Describe the components of the general approach to caring for a patient with difficulty breathing.
(pp. 534–538)
- Select the best oxygen administration modality for a patient complaining of difficulty breathing.
- Describe how continuous positive airway pressure (CPAP) works.
- List the indications for treating a patient with CPAP.
- List the contraindications for treating a patient with CPAP.
- Describe the procedure for treating a patient with CPAP.
- Describe how different complications of CPAP can be recognized.

19.6 Recommend a diagnosis-based treatment plan for a patient with difficulty breathing.
(pp. 538–546)
- Describe the features of chronic obstructive pulmonary disease (COPD).
- Describe the features of asthma.
- Describe the features of pulmonary edema.
- Describe the features of pneumonia.
- Describe the features of spontaneous pneumothorax.
- Describe the features of pulmonary embolism.
- Describe the features of epiglottitis.
- Describe the features of croup.
- Describe the features of bronchiolitis.
- Describe the features of cystic fibrosis.
- Describe the features of viral respiratory infections.

19.7 Identify common medications used for patients with difficulty breathing. (pp. 546–551)
- Differentiate between the types of inhaled medications EMTs may give to a patient with difficulty breathing and those they may not give.
- List the indications for assisting a patient with a metered-dose inhaler.
- List the contraindications of treating a patient with a metered-dose inhaler.
- Provide the instructions a patient needs to use the inhaler.
- Recall the rights of medication administration.
- List the side effects of the inhaled medications EMTs assist with.
- Describe the steps in assisting a patient with using prescribed inhaler.
- Compare the use of a small-volume nebulizer with that of a metered-dose.

Match Key Terms

A. An active process in which the intercostal (rib) muscles and the diaphragm contract, expanding the size of the chest cavity and causing air to flow into the lungs.

B. Another term for inspiration.

C. Abnormal narrowing of the smaller airways of the lungs from conditions such as allergies or pulmonary conditions.

D. Another term for expiration.

E. A form of noninvasive positive pressure ventilation (NPPV) consisting of a mask and a means of blowing oxygen or air into the mask to prevent airway collapse or to help alleviate difficulty breathing.

F. A passive process in which the intercostal (rib) muscles and the diaphragm relax, causing the chest cavity to decrease in size and force air from the lungs.

_____ 1. Bronchoconstriction

_____ 2. Exhalation

_____ 3. Expiration

_____ 4. Inhalation

_____ 5. Inspiration

_____ 6. Continuous positive airway pressure (CPAP)

Multiple-Choice Review

_____ 1. You are assessing a 45-year-old male who has pain in his upper abdomen and his lower chest. The thin, umbrella-shaped muscle that divides the chest cavity from the abdominal cavity is called the _____ muscle.
A. intercostal
B. sternocleidomastoid
C. diaphragm
D. inguinal

_____ 2. In the mechanical process of breathing, expiration is a(n) _____ process that involves the _____.
A. active; relaxation of the intercostal muscles and the diaphragm
B. passive; relaxation of the intercostal muscles and the diaphragm
C. active; contraction of the intercostal muscles and the diaphragm
D. passive; contraction of the intercostal muscles and the diaphragm

_____ 3. You are assessing a 36-year-old female who has asthma. Her chief complaint is breathing difficulty. Which of the following assessment parameters would be least helpful in determining if she is breathing adequately?
A. presence of breath sounds.
B. chest expansion.
C. depth of respirations.
D. breathing rhythm.

_____ 4. You are assessing an unresponsive 58-year-old male who has only a few shallow gasps per minute. Aside from quickly checking his pulse, your treatment of this patient should involve:
A. oxygen given via nasal cannula.
B. immediate transport to a medical facility.
C. immediate ventilation with supplemental oxygen.
D. oxygen given via nonrebreather mask.

_____ 5. Your patient is a 60-year-old male who is having difficulty breathing, and he appears to be working very hard to breathe. He is using the muscles in his neck and abdomen to assist his breathing. These muscles are referred to as the _____ muscles of breathing.
A. extra
B. accessory
C. subdiaphragmatic
D. smooth

_____ 6. Oxygenation of the body's tissue is reduced in a patient with inadequate breathing, so the skin may be _____ in color and feel _____.
   A. pale; dry and cool   C. yellow; dry and warm
   B. red; clammy and hot   D. blue; clammy and cool

_____ 7. You are treating an unresponsive 38-year-old female. If she is making _____ sounds, she may have a serious airway problem requiring your immediate intervention.
   A. snoring or gurgling   C. sniffling
   B. slight wheezing   D. whistling or grunting

_____ 8. Of the following causes of death, statistically, the leading killer of infants and children is:
   A. motor vehicle collisions.   C. respiratory conditions.
   B. heart attacks.   D. infection.

_____ 9. Your patient is a 4-year-old child who is having difficulty breathing. You need to recall that the structure of an infant's or child's airway is different from an adult's in each of the following ways *except*:
   A. all airway structures are smaller and more easily obstructed.
   B. their tongues are proportionately larger than an adult's.
   C. the trachea is softer and more flexible.
   D. the cricoid cartilage is more rigid.

_____ 10. Because the chest wall is softer in infants and children, they:
   A. must inhale twice the amount of air to breathe.
   B. depend more heavily on the diaphragm for breathing.
   C. grunt and gurgle whenever they breathe.
   D. expend less energy than adults do when breathing.

_____ 11. In infants and children, signs of inadequate breathing include all of the following *except*:
   A. nasal flaring.   C. seesaw breathing.
   B. grunting.   D. lip quivering.

_____ 12. To move air, the respiratory system changes pressure within the chest cavity. _____ is used to move air in and _____ is used to move air out.
   A. Excessive pressure: relaxation
   B. Negative pressure: positive pressure
   C. Positive pressure: negative pressure
   D. Low pressure: high pressure

_____ 13. The appropriate rate of artificial ventilations for a nonbreathing adult who still has a pulse is _____ breaths per minute.
   A. 8 to 10   C. 12 to 16
   B. 10 to 12   D. 16 to 20

_____ 14. The appropriate rate of artificial ventilations for a nonbreathing infant or child who still has a palpable pulse is _____ breaths per minute.
   A. 8 to 10   C. 12 to 20
   B. 10 to 12   D. 20 to 26

_____ 15. If an infant or a child has _____ in the setting of a respiratory emergency, this usually indicates trouble.
   A. a fever   C. a slow pulse
   B. cold skin   D. a rapid pulse

_____ **16.** A respiratory rate of _____ would be considered adequate for a child.
   A. 12 to 20   **C.** 30 to 60
   B. 18 to 30   **D.** all of the above.

_____ **17.** In observing the breathing of a 45-year-old female, all of the following are important observations for you to make *except*:
   A. the patient's positioning.
   B. the lung sounds.
   C. unusual anatomy such as a barrel chest.
   D. pale, cyanotic, clammy skin.

_____ **18.** In neonates and infants, the rib cage flares outward at the bottom as compared to an adult's rib cage which flares inward. What is the problem posed by this difference in anatomy?
   A. A thicker diaphragm provides too much positive pressure in children.
   B. A flatter diaphragm makes it more difficult for infant to generate negative pressure.
   C. The infant needs to rely more on strong chest muscles to breathe.
   D. The adult rarely uses the diaphragm to aid in breathing.

_____ **19.** You are talking to a 62-year-old female who is speaking in short, choppy sentences. This could be an indication that she:
   A. has a language problem.
   B. is unable to hear you clearly.
   C. is experiencing breathing difficulty.
   D. is afraid of you.

_____ **20.** One of your first observations on arrival at the scene is the patient's position. You note that she is seated in the tripod position. This means that she is:
   A. holding herself up by two legs and one arm.
   B. leaning forward with hands resting on knees.
   C. in the recovery position.
   D. supine with knees flexed against the chest.

_____ **21.** Which pair of signs/symptoms is *not* commonly associated with breathing difficulty?
   A. Crowing/restlessness   **C.** Increased pulse/tightness in chest
   B. Retractions/shortness of breath   **D.** Vomiting/headache

_____ **22.** You are treating a 45-year-old male who has a chief complaint of breathing difficulty and nausea. During your assessment, you decide that he is breathing adequately. If oxygen is administered, it should be given via:
   A. CPAP.
   B. nonrebreather mask.
   C. pocket face mask.
   D. bag mask device with supplemental oxygen.

_____ **23.** If a 62-year-old male is experiencing breathing difficulty and is breathing adequately, it is usually best to place him in the _____ position.
   A. tripod   **C.** sitting-up
   B. supine   **D.** none of these

_____ **24.** Infants and children are subject to respiratory infections that may cause swelling of airway passages. The care of these patients includes all of the following *except*:
   A. administer oxygen.
   B. check the airway with a tongue depressor.
   C. provide ventilations as needed.
   D. transport to most appropriate facility.

_____ 25. Your patient is a 37-year-old male with a history of breathing distress. He has his prescribed inhaler with him. Once you receive permission from medical direction to assist a patient with an inhaler, make sure that you have all of the following *except*:
A. the right dose.
B. an inhaler that has not expired.
C. a large enough syringe.
D. a patient who is alert enough to cooperate.

_____ 26. Before coaching the patient from question 25 in the use of his inhaler, you should:
A. shake the inhaler vigorously.
B. test the unit by spraying into the air.
C. ensure that the patient is no longer alert.
D. call the patient's personal physician.

_____ 27. To ensure that the most medication is absorbed when using an inhaler, encourage the patient to:
A. take short, shallow breaths.
B. hold the breath as long as possible.
C. inhale slowly.
D. hyperventilate.

_____ 28. Using CPAP on a patient with respiratory distress is a means of:
A. preventing the alveoli from collapsing at the end of inhalation.
B. pushing fluid out of the alveoli and back into the capillaries.
C. providing artificial ventilation to the apneic patient.
D. all of these.

_____ 29. A physician realizes that the patient may become anxious and use the inhaler improperly. To help improve the volume of the medication that the patient is able to self-administer when in distress, the physician may prescribe a:
A. tranquilizer.   C. spacer device.
B. decongestant.   D. heat treatment.

_____ 30. Of the prescribed inhalers listed below, which is *not* considered a medication that would be used in an emergency to reverse airway constriction because its use is intended to prevent attacks by reducing inflammation?
A. Ventolin   C. Proventil
B. Advair   D. Albuterol

_____ 31. When assessing the lungs of a 55-year-old male complaining of respiratory distress, you hear a fine bubbling sound on inspiration. This sound, caused by fluid in the alveoli, is called:
A. wheezes.   C. rhonchi.
B. stridor.   D. crackles.

_____ 32. Although CPAP is frequently effective in relieving a patient's difficulty with breathing, it can have a side effect of:
A. producing hypotension.   C. gastric distention.
B. pneumothorax.   D. any of these.

_____ 33. If a patient who has been treated with CPAP for the past 10 minutes starts to experience a decrease in mental status, the EMT should:
A. turn up the pressure.
B. remove CPAP and ventilate with a BVM.
C. lower the level of pressure in the CPAP device.
D. administer a bronchodilator treatment per medical control.

_____ **34.** Your 58-year-old female patient has a chronic respiratory disease that has episodic exacerbations or flares. She is most likely suffering from:

A. pulmonary edema.

B. asthma.

C. pneumonia.

D. emphysema.

_____ **35.** You are standing by at the finish line of a 5-kilometer road race when a runner crosses the line and suddenly appears in distress. He is 30 years old, is very thin and tall, and complains of a sudden sharp unilateral chest pain with each breath. What is his most likely respiratory condition?

A. Spontaneous pneumothorax

B. Pulmonary embolism

C. Cystic fibrosis

D. A viral respiratory infection

_____ **36.** The use of CPAP may be indicated if the patient who you suspect has _____ also has stable vital signs.

A. a viral respiratory infection

B. epiglottitis

C. acute pulmonary edema

D. spontaneous pneumothorax

_____ **37.** You are treating a 52-year-old female who just came off an airplane from Australia. A respiratory condition that may be caused by a deep vein thrombosis (DVT) after sitting for a very long flight is called:

A. epiglottitis.

B. asthma.

C. acute pulmonary edema.

D. pulmonary embolism.

_____ **38.** A respiratory condition that used to be prominent with children but has been virtually eliminated by vaccination of infants is:

A. epiglottitis.

B. croup.

C. asthma.

D. emphysema.

_____ **39.** For a child with a suspected respiratory infection you should transport quickly if they have:

A. wheezing, stridor, or grunting.

B. flared nostrils or retracted muscles of breathing.

C. pale or cyanotic lips or mouth.

D. any of the above.

_____ **40.** By inhaling and exhaling against the flow of air created by CPAP, patients increase their:

A. ventilation volume.

B. dead space.

C. PEEP.

D. NPPV.

_____ **41.** Of the following signs of respiratory distress in a child, which is not an early sign?

A. Nasal flaring

B. Decreased heart rate

C. Retraction of the muscles above, below and between the sternum and ribs

D. Stridor (high-pitched, harsh sound)

_____ **42.** Your patient has a respiratory disease in which the walls of the alveoli break down, reducing surface area for respiratory exchange. What condition is most likely?

A. Pneumonia

B. Emphysema

C. Chronic bronchitis

D. Cystic fibrosis

_____ **43.** A condition common in children where small airways become inflamed because of viral infections is most likely:

A. cystic fibrosis.

B. walking pneumonia.

C. bronchiolitis.

D. croup.

Complete the Following

1. List eight observations during your primary and secondary assessment of the patient with breathing difficulty and inadequate breathing.

   A. _____

   B. _____

   C. _____

   D. _____

   E. _____

   F. _____

   G. _____

   H. _____

2. List three of the prehospital indications for CPAP.

   A. _____

   B. _____

   C. _____

3. List and describe four of the common abnormal lung sounds.

   A. _____

   B. _____

   C. _____

   D. _____

4. Oxygen should be administered to all patients with severe respiratory distress, regardless of their oxygen saturation readings. The oximeter reading in a normal, healthy person is typically (A) _____. An oximeter reading below (B) _____ indicates hypoxia.

   A. _____

   B. _____

5. List the indications and contraindications and side effects of albuterol.

   A. Indications - _____

   B. Contraindications - _____

   C. Side effects - _____

Label the Diagrams

Fill in each phase of respiration on the line provided.

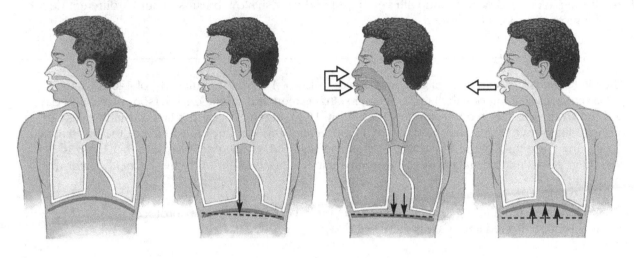

1. _____ 2. _____ 3. _____ 4. _____

Case Study: The Three A.M. Call: "Mom Simply Cannot Breathe"

Your unit and the police are dispatched to a private residence in a suburban neighborhood. It is 3 a.m., and you find the house easily because it is the only one with a front porch light on and a police car out front. You are met at the front door by the patient's daughter, who nervously states, "Mom simply cannot breathe well." She leads you to a bedroom, which is upstairs in the rear of the home.

1. As you approach the patient, what Standard Precautions should you take?

_____

2. When would you consider using an N-95 mask?

_____

3. If the patient with a chief complaint of breathing difficulty is awake and alert, in what position would it be best for her to be treated and transported?

_____

You begin your assessment by introducing yourself, and you find out that the patient's name is Linda. She states that she is 72 years old, and she tells you that she cannot catch her breath. You notice that she is talking in short, choppy sentences. Your partner starts oxygen administration, and you ask a few more interview questions and obtain a set of baseline vital signs.

4. What is the significance of speaking in short, choppy sentences?

_____

5. What appliance is most appropriate for the initial oxygen administration to this patient?

_____

GZQ **6.** If the patient had been found with very rapid and very shallow breaths, would a different device be more appropriate to use?

_____

The vital signs are respirations of 24 and labored, pulse of 110 and irregular, BP of 140/82, and a pulse oximeter reading of 94%. Linda's mental status is alert and oriented to person, place, and day, and the oxygen has started to calm her down a bit. Her daughter states that Linda usually uses her bronchodilator twice a day but has recently been feeling run down from "a touch of the flu." Linda denies any chest pain but is a little weak when she sits up. Her daughter also says that Linda is allergic to penicillin and sulfa drugs. Apparently, she has not thought to try her bronchodilator this morning.

   7. If Linda has albuterol prescribed to her and you have a standing order protocol to assist her, how is this administered and what is the usual dose?

_____

GZQ **8.** If Linda's medication was not immediately available but her daughter's medication was available because the daughter is asthmatic, could you just administer her medication to Linda?

_____

You are preparing to assist Linda in taking her medication by following your protocol. When you reassess her after a few minutes, she seems to be breathing better, she is talking in full sentences, and she is apologizing profusely for waking you and your partner up so early in the morning. You still insist that she take the ride to the hospital for follow-up care and possibly some additional tests. She is happy to go along with your plan.

   9. If Linda's daughter handed you a spacer device, what would you be able to say about why and how it is used?

_____

   10. What side effects should you expect to see when you administer albuterol?

_____

Cardiac Emergencies

Core Concepts

- Aspects of acute coronary syndrome (ACS)
- Conditions that may lead to a cardiac emergency

Outcomes

After reading this chapter, you should be able to:

20.1 Explain the anatomy and physiology of the cardiovascular system. (pp. 557–558)
- Describe the flow of blood through the heart's chambers.
- Describe the flow of blood from the heart, to the body, and back to the heart.

20.2 Explain the concept of acute coronary syndrome (ACS). (pp. 558–559)
- Recognize the signs and symptoms of acute coronary syndrome.
- Describe the concept of cardiac compromise.

20.3 Outline management when presented with a portrayal of a patient presenting with signs and symptoms of acute coronary syndrome. (pp. 559–569)
- Evaluate the patient's signs any symptoms against those for ACS.
- Describe the role of positioning for a patient with ACS.
- Describe the practice for administering oxygen to a patient with suspected ACS.
- Describe the pharmacology of medications that EMTs can administer to patients with suspected ACS.
- Describe the EMT's responsibilities with respect to administering aspirin to a patient with suspected ACS.
- Describe the EMT's responsibilities with respect to administering nitroglycerin to a patient with suspected ACS.
- Identify criteria for immediate transport of a patient with ACS signs and symptoms.
- Explain the teamwork required to carry out interventions while transporting an ACS patient to the hospital.
- Explain the advantage of prehospital 12-lead electrocardiograms (ECGs).

20.4 Illustrate how the underlying pathophysiology of the various causes of cardiac conditions poses threats to the patient. (pp. 570–577)
- Describe the relationship between coronary artery disease, angina pectoris, and acute myocardial infarction (AMI).
- Describe the concept of a dysrhythmia.
- Relate the pathophysiology of heart failure to its presenting signs and symptoms.
- Describe the concept of an aneurysm.
- Identify conditions that interfere with the mechanical work of the heart.

Match Key Terms

Part A

A. Another term for acute coronary syndrome.

B. Shortness of breath; labored breathing or difficult breathing.

C. Diseases that affect the blood vessels of the heart.

D. A blanket term used to represent any symptoms related to lack of oxygen (ischemia) in the heart muscle.

E. The dilation, or ballooning, of a weakened section of the wall of an artery.

F. Pain in the chest occurring when blood supply to the heart is reduced and a portion of the heart muscle is not receiving enough oxygen.

G. The condition in which a portion of the heart muscle dies as a result of occlusion; often called a heart attack by laypersons.

H. When the heart rate is slow, usually below 60 beats per minute.

I. The heart and the blood vessels.

J. A disturbance in the heart rate and/or rhythm.

_____ **1.** Acute coronary syndrome (ACS)

_____ **2.** Acute myocardial infarction (AMI)

_____ **3.** Angina pectoris

_____ **4.** Aneurysm

_____ **5.** Bradycardia

_____ **6.** Cardiovascular system

_____ **7.** Cardiac compromise

_____ **8.** Coronary artery disease (CAD)

_____ **9.** Dyspnea

_____ **10.** Dysrhythmia

Part B

A. The failure of the heart to pump efficiently.

B. Accumulation of fluid in the lungs.

C. A medication that dilates the blood vessels.

D. Accumulation of fluid in the feet or ankles.

E. A clot formed of blood and plaque attached to the inner wall of an artery or vein.

F. A heart rate of more than 100 beats per minute.

G. Blockage, as of an artery by fatty deposits.

H. Blockage of a vessel by a clot or foreign material brought to the site by the blood current.

_____ **1.** Embolism

_____ **2.** Nitroglycerin

_____ **3.** Occlusion

_____ **4.** Pedal edema

_____ **5.** Pulmonary edema

_____ **6.** Heart failure (HF)

_____ **7.** Tachycardia

_____ **8.** Thrombus

Multiple-Choice Review

_____ **1.** Your 58-year-old male patient is going to be admitted to the hospital for ACS. ACS (acute coronary syndrome) is a blanket term that refers to:
   A. a mild heart attack.
   B. sudden death of the cells in the heart muscle.
   C. any time the heart may not be getting enough oxygen.
   D. a period of time when the heart stops beating.

_____ **2.** Chest discomfort from the heart is typically described by the patient as a "squeezing sensation." It is also often described as any of the following _except_:
   A. pressure.   **C.** tearing.
   B. aching.   **D.** radiating to jaw/neck.

_____ **3.** Your 55-year-old male patient states that his pain seems to radiate from the chest. When it is due to a heart problem, pain commonly radiates to the:
   A. arms and jaw.   **C.** stomach and lower abdomen.
   B. feet and head.   **D.** right arm and lower abdomen.

_____ **4.** In addition to chest pain or discomfort, the patient with ACS may also complain of:
   A. diarrhea.   **C.** dyspnea.
   B. shivering.   **D.** headache.

_____ **5.** Patients with heart problems may complain of any of the following _except_:
   A. pain in the center of the chest.
   B. mild chest discomfort.
   C. sudden onset of sharp abdominal pain.
   D. difficulty breathing.

_____ **6.** Early in your assessment of a 56-year-old male who presents with chest pain, you take his pulse. This is a very important vital sign because if the heart is beating too fast or too slow, the patient with ACS may also:
   A. have stomach pain.   **C.** have a seizure or convulsion.
   B. lose consciousness.   **D.** have right-side weakness.

_____ **7.** You are evaluating a 59-year-old female patient who you suspect may be exhibiting the signs and symptoms of acute coronary syndrome. Her signs and symptoms may include any of the following _except_:
   A. difficulty breathing and abnormal pulse rate.
   B. sudden onset of sweating with nausea or vomiting.
   C. sharp lower abdominal pain and a fever.
   D. pain in the chest or upper abdomen.

_____ **8.** You are treating a 62-year-old male patient who is complaining of crushing substernal chest pain and shortness of breath. His pulse is fast, his BP is high, and his pulse oximetry is in the low 90s. The EMT management of the patient with a suspected acute coronary syndrome should include all of the following _except_:
   A. administering chewable aspirin per your protocols.
   B. administering oxygen by nonrebreather mask or nasal cannula.
   C. administering CPAP.
   D. assisting the patient with nitroglycerin administration if medical direction authorizes it.

_____ **9.** An interruption to the heart's supply of oxygenated blood can result in significant problems. This is because:
   A. the heart is the last organ to receive oxygenated blood.
   B. having no reserve of oxygen, heart muscle needs a constant supply of oxygenated blood.
   C. the heart can rely on anaerobic metabolism for lengthy times.
   D. all of the above.

_____ 10. You should consider using nitroglycerin when a 65-year-old female patient:
  A. is hypertensive and has a headache.
  B. has her own nitroglycerin and has crushing chest pain.
  C. loses consciousness after feeling dizzy.
  D. has chest pain for over 5 minutes and is hypotensive.

_____ 11. Which of the following is the best description of the role of medical direction in the treatment of a 55-year-old male who you suspect has acute coronary syndrome?
  A. Authorizing the EMT to administer oxygen via nonrebreather mask
  B. Prescribing nitroglycerin that the EMT can then assist the patient in taking
  C. Authorizing the EMT to assist the patient in taking his prescribed nitroglycerin
  D. Contacting the patient's physician to ensure that the patient's nitroglycerin prescription is not out of date

_____ 12. A patient is complaining of chest pain. For the EMT to administer nitroglycerin, all the following conditions must be met _except_ that:
  A. medical direction authorizes its administration.
  B. the patient's physician has prescribed the medication.
  C. the patient's blood pressure is at least 80 mmHg systolic.
  D. the patient has a history of cardiac problems.

_____ 13. The maximum number of doses of nitroglycerin routinely given by the EMT with medical direction permission or taken by the patient at the advice of his or her physician is:
  A. one.   C. three.
  B. two.   D. four.

_____ 14. Nitroglycerin is contraindicated for a patient who has:
  A. an obvious head injury and altered mental state.
  B. a systolic blood pressure of 110.
  C. not yet taken the maximum dose.
  D. been complaining of pain for at least 20 minutes.

_____ 15. You are treating a 62-year-old male patient who has a chief complaint of chest pain. You are considering administering aspirin to the patient. Of the following considerations, which would _not_ be pertinent to administering this medication?
  A. The patient has had recent surgery.
  B. The patient has a history of emphysema.
  C. The patient has taken Viagra.
  D. The patient has a stomach ulcer.

_____ 16. You have administered aspirin to the patient with chest pain per your protocols. The patient has her own prescribed nitroglycerin and a stable BP, so you decide to assist her in administering one of her prescribed pills. After administering the nitroglycerin, it is important for you to:
  A. immediately administer the next dose.
  B. discontinue the oxygen therapy.
  C. reassess the blood pressure.
  D. lay the patient down.

_____ 17. When conducting a physical exam of a suspected ACS patient, you should look for findings such as:
  A. Levine's sign.   C. pale or gray skin.
  B. sweating.   D. any of the above.

_____ 18. When managing a pediatric patient who appears to be suffering from an unknown or unclear cardiac condition you should:
  A. transport to a facility capable of managing the patient's condition.
  B. ask caregivers how this condition differs from normal (baseline) for the child.
  C. manage primary assessment issues in the same way you would for other children.
  D. all of the above.

©2021 Pearson Education, Inc.
Emergency Care, 14th Ed.

_____ **19.** A condition that is often the result of the buildup of fatty deposits on the inner walls of the arteries is called:

A. pulmonary embolism.

C. obesity.

B. coronary artery disease.

D. congestive heart failure.

_____ **20.** Factor(s) that put a person at risk for developing coronary artery disease (CAD) include:

A. age.

C. obesity.

B. cigarette smoking.

D. all of these.

_____ **21.** Which of the following risk factors can be modified to reduce the risk of coronary artery disease?

A. Age

C. Hypertension

B. Heredity

D. None of these

_____ **22.** Most cardiac-related medical emergencies result from:

A. changes of the inner walls of arteries.

B. cardiac arrest.

C. loss of consciousness.

D. breathing difficulty.

_____ **23.** Angina pectoris means, literally:

A. a small heart attack.

C. paralyzed chest muscles.

B. a pain in the chest.

D. breathing difficulty.

_____ **24.** Why is nitroglycerin administered to the patient with chest pain?

A. It increases blood flow to the brain.

B. It dilates the blood vessels and decreases the work of the heart.

C. It constricts the blood vessels and raises the blood pressure.

D. It is easy to administer to unconscious patients.

_____ **25.** A condition in which a portion of the myocardium dies as a result of oxygen starvation is known as:

A. coronary occlusion.

C. myocardial starvation.

B. acute myocardial infarction.

D. acute angina attack.

_____ **26.** A cardiac arrest that occurs within 2 hours of the onset of cardiac symptoms is referred to as:

A. prehospital death.

C. sudden death.

B. prehospital arrest.

D. ventricular tachycardia.

_____ **27.** Your 70-year-old female patient has a cardiovascular disorder that stems from weakened sections in the arterial walls. These weak spots begin to dilate to form a condition that is known as a(n):

A. thrombosis.

C. inflammation.

B. aneurysm.

D. infarction.

_____ **28.** You are treating a 55-year-old male patient who has a history of three past myocardial infarctions (MIs) and angina. Because of his difficulty breathing and normally sedentary lifestyle, you suspect that he may be experiencing heart failure (HF). HF is:

A. clotting of the coronary artery.

B. failure of the heart to pump blood with normal efficiency.

C. an infection in the heart that makes it difficult to oxygenate the blood.

D. a chronic lung condition that requires a low concentration of oxygen administration.

_____ **29.** Damage to the left ventricle causes blood to back up into the lungs. Fluid shifting into the lungs is referred to as:

A. pedal edema.

C. fibrinolytics.

B. pulmonary edema.

D. diaphoresis.

_____ **30.** If your patient has HF and presents with acute pulmonary edema the prehospital management should include:
- **A.** contacting ALS immediately.
- **B.** CPAP if the patient is alert.
- **C.** nitroglycerin if your protocols allow.
- **D.** all of the above.

_____ **31.** You are treating a 59-year-old male patient whose wife called EMS because he had difficulty breathing and was acting anxious and confused. He is diaphoretic and cyanotic, and his vitals are rapid respirations, tachycardia, and hypertension. He has swollen ankles and is coughing up pink sputum. What do you suspect is wrong with this patient?
- **A.** He is having an asthma attack.
- **B.** He is having angina pectoris.
- **C.** He has HF affecting both the right and left heart.
- **D.** He is in the end stage of emphysema.

_____ **32.** A patient with pulmonary edema is likely to have each of the following in the field *except*:
- **A.** crackles in the lungs.
- **B.** dyspnea.
- **C.** flat neck veins.
- **D.** pedal edema.

_____ **33.** If a young child has a cardiac history it is likely to be:
- **A.** due to an overdose or poisoning.
- **B.** congenital, due to a birth defect.
- **C.** caused by multiple heart attacks.
- **D.** passed on from generation to generation.

Complete the Following

1. List the nine signs and symptoms that are often associated with ACS:

A. _____

B. _____

C. _____

D. _____

E. _____

F. _____

G. _____

H. _____

I. _____

2. List the four steps recommended for 12-lead ECG placement:

A. _____

B. _____

C. _____

D. _____

©2021 Pearson Education, Inc.
Emergency Care, 14th Ed.

Case Study: The Patient Was "Just Stacking Wood."

Your unit and the police are dispatched to a private camp in a rural community on the outskirts of your small village. It is 6 p.m., and you find the house down a long winding dirt road. The police arrive moments after you, and you both pull into the parking area. You are met at the front door by the patient's wife, who nervously states, "Bill has been stacking wood all afternoon." She says she just got home and her husband is having chest pain. She leads you to a back porch area where you see piles of firewood and a middle-aged man sitting on a bench. He is holding his closed fist to his chest, sweating profusely, and seeming to have some difficulty breathing.

1. As you approach the patient, what are your immediate concerns?

_____

2. When would you consider administering oxygen to the patient?

_____

3. If the patient with a chief complaint of chest pain is awake and alert, in what position would it be best for him to assess and manage him?

_____

You begin your assessment by introducing yourself, and you find out that the patient's name is Bill. He states that he is 56 years old, and he tells you that he has been working all afternoon on this once-a-year project. The pain in his chest began about 30 minutes ago. When his wife came home she decided to call 911. You notice that he is talking in short, choppy sentences. His airway is open and clear, and a quick listen to his lungs reveals he is moving air in both lungs. You tell Bill that your partner is going to give him some oxygen and get his vital signs as you proceed to ask him a few questions about his pain. You also note that the ALS unit is en route to your location.

4. What line of questioning would help to elaborate on the chief complaint?

_____

5. What oxygen device is most appropriate for the initial oxygen administration to this patient?

_____

GZQ 6. If the patient is believed to have cardiac "ischemic" chest pain, which equipment should be available at your side?

_____

The vital signs are respirations of 22 and labored, pulse of 100 and irregular, BP of 150/82, and a pulse oximeter reading of 95% on oxygen via cannula. Bill's mental status is alert and oriented to person, place, and day, and the oxygen has started to calm him down a bit. His wife states that Bill usually takes an aspirin each morning, Lisinopril 10 mg for hypertension and has nitroglycerin from the last time he had chest pain a few months ago. Bill denies any dizziness and is a little nauseous. His wife also says that Bill is allergic to Novocain. Apparently, he has not thought to take a nitro as yet.

7. If Bill has his own nitroglycerin prescribed to him and you have a standing order protocol to assist him, how is this administered and what is the usual dose?

_____

GZQ **8.** Your protocol is to acquire a quick 12-lead ECG to assist in the transport/hospital destination decision. Why is this an important procedure that should be done quickly?

_____

You are assisting Bill in taking his nitroglycerin following your protocol. When you reassess him after a few minutes, his pain went from a 7/10 to 5/10 and he seems to be breathing better. You have moved him to your unit as the medic arrives on the scene. The medic jumps in with some additional equipment and in moments you are all headed to the hospital. The wife plans to follow along in her personal vehicle.

9. If Bill's vitals are still similar to the initial set, will the medic consider another nitroglycerin?

_____

10. The medic reviews the ECG and states the patient is having a ST-elevation myocardial infarction (STEMI). How does this affect the hospital destination?

_____

172   **Section 4 | Medical Emergencies**

©2021 Pearson Education, Inc.
Emergency Care, 14th Ed.

Resuscitation

Core Concepts

- Cardiac arrest and the chain of survival
- Management of a cardiac arrest patient
- Use of an automated external defibrillator (AED)
- Special considerations in AED use
- Use of mechanical cardiopulmonary resuscitation (CPR) devices

Outcomes

After reading this chapter, you should be able to:

21.1 Explain the pathophysiology of cardiac arrest. (pp. 583–589)
- Describe conditions that may trigger cardiac arrest.
- Identify key signs of cardiac arrest.

21.2 Summarize the importance of EMS systems' use of the chain of survival as a means of improving outcomes from cardiac arrest. (pp. 589–612)
- Explain the features of each component of the chain of survival.
- Explain how each component of the chain of survival is intended to improve cardiac arrest outcomes.
- Describe the treatment sequence by which EMTs manage a patient in cardiac arrest.
- Identify circumstances when a mechanical CPR device is advantageous.
- Compare the two types of mechanical CPR devices an EMT may use.
- Describe types and operation of automated external defibrillators (AEDs).
- Explain the integration of CPR and AED use in a patient in cardiac arrest.
- Explain how roles change during the transition of patient care.
- Describe the EMT's approach to different patient responses to treatment, including regaining a pulse and going back into cardiac arrest.
- Describe modifications to cardiac arrest management for pediatric patients.

21.3 Summarize the EMT's obligations with respect to terminating resuscitative efforts before arriving at the hospital. (p. 612)
- Identify the circumstances of the cardiac arrest that must be present prior to an individual EMT's stopping resuscitative efforts.
- Identify the criteria that must be reported to medical direction when requesting an order to cease resuscitative efforts.

21.4 Identify special circumstances in resuscitation that the EMT may encounter. (pp. 612–616)
- Explain the teamwork required to carry out interventions in coordination with others or where transporting a patient with ACS to the hospital.
- Describe the significance to cardiac arrest management of cardiac implants and surgeries.

Match Key Terms

A. The amount of time chest compressions are being performed compared with the total time of patient contact.

B. A cardiac arrest dysrhythmia cause by acute blunt force trauma to the chest.

C. A condition in which the heart's electrical rhythm remains relatively normal, yet the mechanical pumping activity of the heart fails, causing cardiac arrest.

D. A cardiac dysrhythmia originating in the larger chambers of the heart, that if rapid enough, will not allow for sufficient pumping of blood to meet the body's needs.

E. Irregular, gasping breaths that precede apnea or death.

F. A condition in which the heart's electrical impulses are disorganized, preventing the heart muscle from contracting normally.

G. No breathing.

H. A cardiac arrest occurring due to the abrupt onset of a dysrhythmia.

I. A cardiac arrest caused by systemic hypoxia, typically due to a respiratory disorder, airway occlusion, or significant impedance of the bellows action of the chest.

J. The heart beating again after successful resuscitation.

K. A condition in which the heart has ceased generating electrical impulses. Commonly called flatline.

L. An electrical disturbance in heart rate and/or rhythm.

M. A state in which the heart is no longer pumping blood.

N. Delivery of an electrical shock to stop the fibrillation of heart muscles and restore a normal heart rhythm.

O. Actions taken to revive a person by keeping the person's heart and lungs working artificially.

P. A metaphor that describes the key elements of cardiac arrest management. A representation of different but interconnected interventions that optimize care for cardiac arrest patients.

_____ **1.** Agonal breathing

_____ **2.** Apnea

_____ **3.** Asphyxial cardiac arrest

_____ **4.** Asystole

_____ **5.** Cardiac arrest

_____ **6.** Cardiopulmonary resuscitation (CPR)

_____ **7.** Chain of survival

_____ **8.** Commotio cordis

_____ **9.** Compression fraction

_____ **10.** Defibrillation

_____ **11.** Dysrhythmia

_____ **12.** Pulseless electrical activity (PEA)

_____ **13.** Return of spontaneous circulation (ROSC)

_____ **14.** Sudden cardiac arrest

_____ **15.** Ventricular fibrillation (VF)

_____ **16.** Ventricular tachycardia (VT)

Multiple-Choice Review

_____ 1. The most common mechanical reason the heart ceases to function correctly is:
   A. blunt trauma.
   B. loss of normal heart muscle structure.
   C. loss of blood volume.
   D. a penetrating injury.

_____ 2. When a patient is in cardiac arrest and the monitor shows an organized ECG rhythm, this is referred to as:
   A. asystole.
   B. pulseless electrical activity (PEA).
   C. ventricular fibrillation.
   D. electromechanical non-association.

_____ 3. If the heart's electrical system fails completely and no electricity is created, this would show as _____ on a cardiac monitor.
   A. PEA   C. asystole
   B. ventricular fibrillation   D. ventricular tachycardia

_____ 4. The five elements of the chain of survival include early activation and all of the following links _except_:
   A. immediate high-quality CPR.
   B. rapid defibrillation.
   C. basic and advanced emergency medical care.
   D. hyperthermia therapy.

_____ 5. Poor blood supply to a portion of the heart muscle can lead to irritability causing a _____ which in turn can lead to life-threatening ECG rhythms including:
   A. dysrhythmia, commotio cordis.
   B. seizures, bradycardia.
   C. dysrhythmia, ventricular fibrillation (VF).
   D. cardiac arrest, PEA.

_____ 6. Which of the following steps is _not_ necessary to ensure that CPR can be delivered earlier to cardiac arrest victims?
   A. Send CPR-trained professionals to patients faster.
   B. Ensure that heart specialists are involved in CPR training.
   C. Train the public in CPR.
   D. Have EMDs instruct rescuers in how to perform hands-only CPR.

_____ 7. You just treated a 17-year-old male who was struck in the chest with a baseball and went into sudden cardiac arrest. What was this condition likely caused by?
   A. Commotio cordis   C. Asphyxial cardiac arrest
   B. Exhaustion or dehydration   D. A metabolic condition

_____ 8. When the heart stops pumping due to issues related to systemic hypoxia this is referred to as a/an:
   A. sudden cardiac arrest.   C. flatline.
   B. heart attack.   D. asphyxial cardiac arrest.

_____ 9. When the heart stops the brain may still send messages to the muscles of breathing as a primal reflex to the cardiac arrest. This reflex is not always present but called _____ and should be treated with:
   A. sudden arrest, ventilations.
   B. asphyxia, defibrillation.
   C. agonal breathing, CPR.
   D. agonal gasps, applying oxygen.

_____ **10.** When providing a notification to the family that your resuscitation efforts have been terminated, per medical direction, you should:

A. use straightforward language and no vague terms.

B. allow the family some time with the deceased.

C. do not suggest you know how they feel.

D. all of the above are appropriate.

_____ **11.** The key elements of quality CPR in an adult patient include:

A. hand placement on lower third of the sternum.

B. compression depth of 2 inches (5 cm), allowing full chest recoil.

C. compression rate of 100–120 per minute.

D. all of the above.

_____ **12.** When doing compressions on an infant there are two acceptable methods: the _____ and the _____ techniques.

A. two-finger, two-thumb encircling hands

B. heel-of-hand, two-finger

C. two-thumb encircling hands, three-finger

D. Lucus-2®, heel of hand

_____ **13.** The shockable rhythms include all of the following *except*:

A. PEA.

B. ventricular fibrillation.

C. pulseless ventricular tachycardia.

D. ventricular tachycardia.

_____ **14.** A nonshockable but electrically organized rhythm that can be the result of a heart with mechanical problems or severe blood loss is called:

A. pulseless electrical activity.

B. ventricular tachycardia.

C. asystole.

D. ventricular fibrillation.

_____ **15.** A nonshockable rhythm that is commonly called flatline is named:

A. pulseless electrical activity.

B. ventricular tachycardia.

C. asystole.

D. ventricular fibrillation.

_____ **16.** When the AED is analyzing the patient's heart rhythm, the EMT must:

A. continue the CPR compressions.

B. avoid touching the patient.

C. hyperventilate the patient.

D. reassess for a carotid pulse.

_____ **17.** High-quality CPR includes a minimum of pauses in compressions. All efforts should be made to provide a compression fraction of _____ percent during a resuscitation.

A. 50

B. 70

C. 90

D. 100

_____ **18.** After the first shock, the patient seems to move, and you assess a strong carotid pulse. The patient is also breathing adequately. You should then _____ and transport.

A. give high-concentration oxygen via bag-valve mask

B. provide artificial ventilations with high-concentration oxygen

C. use pulse oximeter to titrate oxygen to at least 95% saturation.

D. administer two more shocks

_____ **19.** When a cardiac arrest patient has ROSC, you should prepare to transport to:

A. the nearest ED.

B. the closest immediate care facility.

C. the most appropriate receiving hospital.

D. the local trauma center.

_____ **20.** Which of the following is *not* a general principle of AED use?
  A. Hook up oxygen before beginning defibrillation.
  B. Avoid contact with the patient during rhythm analysis.
  C. Be sure everyone is "clear" before delivering each shock.
  D. Avoid defibrillation in a moving ambulance.

_____ **21.** Of the cardiac arrest patients listed below, assuming they are in ventricular fibrillation, which one should be defibrillated immediately?
  A. A soaking-wet patient lying in the rain.
  B. A trauma patient with severe hypothermia.
  C. A patient on a metal deck being cradled by another person.
  D. A patient with an implanted defibrillator.

_____ **22.** If a patient is wearing a nitroglycerin or other medication patch, you should carefully remove it before defibrillating because:
  A. the patch's adhesive can burn and may impede defibrillation.
  B. defibrillation can force adhesive from the patch into the pores of the skin and poison the patient.
  C. the patch can melt and run down the chest, redirecting the defibrillation current.
  D. it is hard to make a defibrillation pad stick on top of a plastic patch.

_____ **23.** If a 55-year-old patient with an implanted cardiac pacemaker needs to be defibrillated, the EMT should:
  A. perform the procedure as he or she would for other cardiac patients.
  B. remove the pacemaker before defibrillation.
  C. position the pad several inches away from the pacemaker battery.
  D. double the power setting on the AED.

_____ **24.** You are assessing a 59-year-old male patient who has a serious cardiac condition, and you notice that he has no palpable pulses or blood pressure despite being conscious and alert. What device does he likely have?
  A. An automatic implantable cardiac defibrillator
  B. A demand pacemaker installed in his chest
  C. A left ventricular assist device (LVAD)
  D. An atrial pacemaker designed for electrical capture

_____ **25.** When assessing the pulse of an infant, use the _____ pulse.
  A. radial   **C.** carotid
  B. brachial   **D.** apical

_____ **26.** The causes of a sudden unexplained infant death syndrome (SUIDS) may include any of the following *except*:
  A. sudden infant death syndrome.
  B. unknown causes.
  C. accidental suffocation and strangulation in bed.
  D. trauma to the head.

_____ **27.** If you suspect a SUIDS, you should attempt a resuscitation unless there is:
  A. a long transport time.   **C.** rigor mortis or lividity.
  B. no ALS backup.   **D.** no pediatric AED available.

_____ **28.** Often the public is trained in hands-only CPR. Once EMS arrives, ventilations should play a role in the resuscitation especially in:
  A. suspected asphyxia arrest.   **C.** suspected opiate arrest.
  B. pediatric patients.   **D.** all of the above.

_____ **29.** When using an AED on a pediatric patient under 8 years old, you can:
  A. place pads in anterior-posterior configuration.
  B. use pediatric pads.
  C. use adult pads if they are only ones available.
  D. all of the above.

_____ **30.** Resuscitation is a team effort and the likelihood of success is increased when:
   A. high-quality CPR is performed.
   B. rescuers are rotated to minimize fatigue.
   C. the team is well practiced.
   D. all of the above.

_____ **31.** You are assessing a 2-year-old female child who was found in her bedroom unconscious by a parent. Her heart rate is 56, and she is hypotensive. What are your priorities?
   A. Begin assisting ventilations with oxygen.
   B. Start CPR compressions if pulse does not increase.
   C. Alert ALS and prepare for transport.
   D. All of the above.

_____ **32.** If you are responding alone on a rapid response unit and arrive at a home where there is a 7 year-old boy who was found unresponsive and pulseless. What should you do next?
   A. Load and go to the ED.
   B. Immediately begin chest compressions and ventilations.
   C. Immediately apply the AED to the patient.
   D. Apply the Lucas-2® or Thumper® to the patient.

Complete the Following

1. Once you have started resuscitation, you must continue to provide resuscitation (CPR, defibrillation) until:

   A. _____

   B. _____

   C. _____

   D. _____

   E. _____

2. List the five links in the adult chain of survival:

   A. _____

   B. _____

   C. _____

   D. _____

   E. _____

3. List five suggestions to consider when making a death notification to family members after an unsuccessful resuscitation.

A. _____

B. _____

C. _____

D. _____

E. _____

Diabetic Emergencies and Altered Mental Status

Core Concepts

- General approaches to assessing the patient with an altered mental status
- Understanding the causes, assessment, and care of diabetes and various diabetic emergencies
- Understanding the causes, assessment, and care of seizure disorders
- Understanding the causes, assessment, and care of stroke
- Understanding the causes, assessment, and care of dizziness and syncope

Outcomes

After reading this chapter, you should be able to:

22.1 Explain the concepts of altered mental status (AMS). (pp. 622–624)
- Recall the role of the reticular activating system in level of responsiveness.
- List factors that can interfere with the function of the reticular activating system.
- Identify the range of changes that are considered alterations in mental status.
- Recognize the reason why a patient presenting with altered mental status is considered an emergency.
- Describe the emphasis on using the AVPU mnemonic in patients with AMS.
- Describe how the determination to use blood glucose monitoring is made in the assessment of a patient with AMS.
- Compare the assessment of the level of responsiveness in pediatric patients with limited verbal skills with that of adults.
- State the importance of interpreting trends in repeated assessments of the level of responsiveness.

22.2 Summarize the application of concepts of diabetes to patient care. (pp. 624–634)
- Describe the physiology of normal glucose breakdown and use by the body.
- Compare the pathophysiology of type 1 and type 2 diabetes.
- Describe causes of diabetic emergencies.
- Compare the effects of hypoglycemia on the body with those of hyperglycemia.
- Describe the pathophysiology of diabetic ketoacidosis.
- Differentiate through assessment findings between hypoglycemia and hyperglycemia.
- Describe the determination of blood glucose levels by glucometer.
- Interpret glucometer readings.
- Identify the indications and contraindications for administering oral glucose.

- Describe how to prioritize the administration of oral glucose with other interventions for a diabetic patient with AMS.
- Recall the key pharmacology of oral glucose.
- Describe the decision-making process in giving oral glucose to a diabetic patient in whom the EMT cannot distinguish between hypoglycemia and hyperglycemia.

22.3 Summarize the application of concepts of seizures to patient care. (pp. 634–638)
- Differentiate between partial and generalized seizures.
- Describe the phases of tonic-clonic generalized seizures.
- Identify common causes of seizures.
- Apply knowledge of causes of seizures to assessment findings to identify correctible causes of seizures.
- Explain why status epilepticus requires priority transport.
- Formulate questions to ask of witnesses about a patient who has had a seizure.
- Use the information attained in the clinical reasoning process to establish the patient's priority for transportation.
- Identify situations in which requesting advanced life support providers should be considered in the management of a patient having a seizure.
- Justify a treatment plan based on assessment findings.
- Compare the nature of pediatric seizures with that of seizures in adults.

22.4 Summarize the application of the concepts of stroke to patient care. (pp. 639–643)
- Compare the mechanisms of stroke caused by blood vessel obstruction and by hemorrhagic stroke.
- Describe how a stroke scale, such as the Cincinnati Prehospital Stroke Scale, is used to identify patients whose signs and symptoms may be caused by a stroke.
- Use clinical reasoning to determine whether your patient is likely to be having a stroke.
- Describe considerations in transporting a patient to a stroke center.

22.5 Summarize the application of concepts of dizziness and syncope to patient care. (pp. 643–647)
- Give examples of questions to ask a patient to clarify whether what was experienced was dizziness or syncope.
- Recognize potentially life-threatening causes of dizziness and syncope.
- Outline specific steps in the care of a patient with dizziness or syncope.

Match Key Terms

A. A form of sugar, the body's basic source of energy.

B. The medical condition brought about by decreased insulin production or the inability of the body cells to use insulin properly.

C. A hormone produced by the pancreas that facilitates the transport of the glucose into the body's cells.

D. Fainting.

E. A prolonged seizure or the situation in which a person suffers two or more convulsive seizures without regaining full consciousness.

F. Low blood sugar.

G. A medical condition that causes seizures.

H. High blood sugar.

_____ **1.** Diabetes mellitus

_____ **2.** Epilepsy

_____ **3.** Glucose

_____ **4.** Hyperglycemia

_____ **5.** Hypoglycemia

_____ **6.** Insulin

_____ **7.** Seizure

_____ **8.** Status epilepticus

_____ **9.** Stroke

_____ **10.** Syncope

I. A sudden change in sensation, behavior, or movement. Capable of producing violent muscle contractions called convulsions.

J. A condition of altered function caused when an artery in the brain is blocked or ruptured, disrupting the supply of oxygenated blood or causing bleeding into the brain.

K. A sensation experienced by a seizure patient right before the seizure that might be a smell, sound, or general feeling.

L. A condition that occurs as the result of high blood sugar (hyperglycemia), characterized by dehydration, altered mental status, and shock.

M. A seizure that affects both sides of the brain.

N. A seizure that affects only one part or one side of the brain.

O. The period of time immediately following a tonic-clonic seizure in which the patient goes from full loss of consciousness back to a normal mental status.

P. A series of neurologic circuits in the brain that control the functions of staying awake, paying attention, and sleeping.

Q. A generalized seizure in which the patient loses consciousness and has jerking movements of paired muscle groups.

_____ **11.** Aura

_____ **12.** Diabetic ketoacidosis (DKA)

_____ **13.** Generalized seizure

_____ **14.** Partial seizure

_____ **15.** Postictal phase

_____ **16.** Reticular activating system

_____ **17.** Tonic-clonic seizure

Multiple-Choice Review

_____ **1.** The relationship between glucose and insulin is often described as:
   A. oppositional.
   B. adversarial.
   C. a lock-and-key mechanism.
   D. antagonistic.

_____ **2.** You are treating a 27-year-old female whose signs and symptoms result from a condition described as a "decrease in insulin production." This condition is known as:
   A. diabetes mellitus.
   B. hypotension.
   C. hypoglycemia.
   D. stroke.

_____ **3.** Your 38-year-old male patient has a history of diabetes. You were called to his home because his family feels that his mental status is altered "again." The most common medical emergency related to diabetes is:
   A. diabetes mellitus.
   B. hypotension.
   C. hypoglycemia.
   D. stroke.

_____ **4.** You are treating a 24-year-old female triathlete who seems to have overdone her exercise routine today. She has a medical alert bracelet that reads "Type 1 Diabetes." She is a little confused about where she is and the day of the week. She has most likely developed:
   A. hypoglycemia.
   B. hyperglycemia.
   C. diabetes mellitus.
   D. a hemorrhagic stroke.

_____ **5.** The hypoglycemia that EMTs see in the field has many causes. Which of the following is *not* a cause of hypoglycemia?
   A. The patient may have taken too much insulin by mistake.
   B. The patient ate a box of candy too fast.
   C. The patient has been vomiting.
   D. The patient has been fasting.

6. If sugar is not replenished quickly for the patient described in question 4, she:
  A. may sustain permanent brain damage.
  B. may go into pulmonary edema.
  C. will have chest pain.
  D. suffer a stroke resulting in an altered mental status.

7. You are treating a 45-year-old male who was found unconscious for an unknown reason. The clues that he may be a diabetic may include all of the following *except*:
  A. a medical alert bracelet that specifies diabetes.
  B. the presence of insulin in the refrigerator.
  C. nonlactose ice cream in the freezer.
  D. information provided by family members.

8. In the patient found with an altered mental status, you should always consider _____ before proceeding with assessment and transport.
  A. hypothermia
  B. an airway or breathing problem
  C. that the patient may have had a seizure
  D. scene safety

9. When suffering a diabetic emergency, the diabetic can present with all of the following signs and symptoms *except*:
  A. cold, clammy skin.   **C.** anxiety.
  B. decreased heart rate.   **D.** combativeness.

10. Typical prehospital protocols state that for an EMT to administer oral glucose, the patient must have an altered mental status and have a:
  A. history of diabetes and be awake enough to swallow.
  B. prescribed medication and have an absent gag reflex.
  C. history of seizures and be awake.
  D. medical alert tag that says "diabetes".

11. You are treating a diabetic patient who has low blood sugar as documented on your glucometer. When reassessing the patient after you administered oral glucose, you notice that the patient's condition has not improved. What action should you take next?
  A. Call the patient's personal physician.
  B. Give glucose in orange juice.
  C. Consult medical direction about whether to administer more glucose.
  D. Administer oxygen by nasal cannula.

12. Which statement about children with the disease diabetes is *most* accurate?
  A. Children are more likely than adults to eat correctly.
  B. Children are less likely than adults to exhaust blood sugar levels.
  C. Children are more at risk than adults for developing hypoglycemia.
  D. Children have a lower risk for medical emergencies than do adults.

13. Which of the following would *most* likely indicate an alteration in the patient's blood sugar level?
  A. Right lower abdominal pain
  B. Nausea and vomiting
  C. Change in mental status
  D. Rigid abdomen on palpation

14. Your 42-year-old female patient is going to need oral glucose. Before and after administering the medication, you should make sure to:
  A. check for distal pulses in both arms.
  B. document the patient's mental status.
  C. increase the oxygen flow rate by 5 liters per minute.
  D. have the patient drink a glass of water.

_____ **15.** A trade name for the medication oral glucose is:
  A. D₅W.
  B. lactose.
  C. insulin.
  D. Insta-glucose.

_____ **16.** Your 22-year-old male patient is very confused and disoriented. Before deciding that he has a behavioral problem, you should consider all of the following *except*:
  A. a potential head injury.
  B. a brain tumor.
  C. hypoxia.
  D. glucose allergy.

_____ **17.** People with diabetes routinely test the level of sugar in their blood using a(n):
  A. capnograph.
  B. glucose meter.
  C. urinal.
  D. oximeter.

_____ **18.** Complications of diabetes can include:
  A. kidney failure.
  B. heart disease.
  C. blindness.
  D. any of these.

_____ **19.** The reading on a glucometer is reported in:
  A. grams of sugar per liter of blood.
  B. centimeters of blood per decimeter of sugar.
  C. milligrams of glucose per deciliter of blood.
  D. none of these.

_____ **20.** A diabetic who is symptomatic and has a sugar level below _____ is considered hypoglycemic.
  A. 90 mg/dL
  B. 80 mg/dL
  C. 70 mg/dL
  D. 60 mg/dL

_____ **21.** A diabetic who is symptomatic and has a sugar level above _____ is considered hyperglycemic.
  A. 140 mg/dL
  B. 120 mg/dL
  C. 100 mg/dL
  D. 80 mg/dL

_____ **22.** You are assessing a 22-year-old male who just had a seizure. The *most* common cause of seizures in adults is:
  A. taking a double dose of antiseizure medication.
  B. taking a small dose of antiseizure medication.
  C. not taking prescribed antiseizure medication.
  D. use of illicit street drugs.

_____ **23.** Seizures are commonly caused by all of the following *except*:
  A. exposure to cold.
  B. a high fever.
  C. a brain tumor.
  D. an infection.

_____ **24.** Your patient has been diagnosed with idiopathic seizures. Which of the following is *not* a characteristic of idiopathic seizures?
  A. They last longer than 10 minutes.
  B. They occur spontaneously.
  C. The cause is unknown.
  D. They often start in childhood.

_____ **25.** You are responding to a call for a 37-year-old male patient who has had a seizure. Convulsive seizures may be seen with:
  A. epilepsy or hypoglycemia.
  B. hyperventilation or AMI.
  C. anaphylaxis or pulmonary embolism.
  D. hyperglycemia or asthma.

_____ **26.** You are interviewing a family member of a 35-year-old female patient who just had a seizure. The most common condition that results in seizures is:
  A. a stroke.
  B. epilepsy.
  C. measles.
  D. eclampsia.

_____ **27.** The _____ is a part of the brain responsible for staying awake, paying attention, and sleeping.
A. cerebrum
B. hypothalamus
C. reticular activating system
D. pineal gland

_____ **28.** In obtaining the medical history from a seizure patient, also interview the bystanders to find out each of the following *except*:
A. how long did the seizure last?
B. what the patient did after the seizure?
C. what the patient was doing before the seizure started?
D. what the family's reaction was to the seizure?

_____ **29.** You are treating a 28-year-old male who is actively seizing. His skin color is turning cyanotic. As the convulsions end, what action should you take?
A. Wait for the patient's color to return to normal.
B. Place a nonrebreather mask with oxygen on the patient.
C. Provide artificial ventilations with supplemental oxygen.
D. Monitor the pulse closely for 2 minutes.

_____ **30.** The most common cause of seizures in infants and toddlers is:
A. traumatic brain injury.
B. a high fever.
C. toxins.
D. stroke.

_____ **31.** A seizure will normally last no more than _____ minutes.
A. 2 to 3
B. 4 to 6
C. 7 to 10
D. 30

_____ **32.** You are treating a 68-year-old female who has just had two back-to-back seizures without regaining consciousness. This is a serious condition called _____, and the treatment will include _____.
A. repeating seizure; ventilation
B. status epilepticus; possible ALS intercept
C. status asthmaticus; the recovery position
D. convulsions; oxygen administration

_____ **33.** If you suspect that a conscious 49-year-old female has had a stroke, you should transport her in the _____ position and pay close attention to her _____.
A. recovery; heart rate
B. supine; breathing rate
C. prone; skin color
D. semi-sitting airway

_____ **34.** When assessing your 53-year-old male patient, you determine that he is having difficulty saying what he is thinking, even though he clearly understands you. This condition found in stroke patients is called:
A. receptive aphasia.
B. expressive aphasia.
C. miscommunication.
D. confusion.

_____ **35.** When assessing your 42-year-old female patient, you determine that she can speak clearly but cannot understand what you are saying. This is called:
A. expressive aphasia.
B. hyperactivity.
C. receptive aphasia.
D. petit mal seizure.

_____ **36.** You are assessing a 58-year-old female who you suspect may have had a stroke. If this was a hemorrhagic stroke, a symptom that you would expect her to exhibit is:
A. tingling in both legs.
B. diminished urine flow.
C. low blood pressure.
D. headache.

_____ **37.** You are treating a 58-year-old male patient who you suspect may be having a stroke. The signs and symptoms might include:
A. vomiting.
B. seizures.
C. loss of bladder control.
D. all of these.

_____ **38.** The 62-year-old male patient who presented with a number of the signs and symptoms of a stroke was taken to the ED yesterday. When talking with your Medical Director about the call, he tells you that the signs and symptoms were completely resolved within 24 hours. This patient was most likely suffering a(n):
  A. altered mental status (AMS).
  B. transient ischemic attack (TIA).
  C. acute myocardial infarction (AMI).
  D. hypoglycemic incident.

_____ **39.** You are treating a patient who passed out while waiting in a long line to get into a concert. When a patient faints, the medical term to describe this is usually a(n) _____, and the treatment would involve:
  A. hypoglycemic incident; oxygen administration.
  B. stroke; Fowler position.
  C. syncopal episode; oxygen administration.
  D. hyperglycemic incident; supine position.

_____ **40.** When you are assessing your 85-year-old female patient, she says that she feels lightheaded. Lightheadedness or dizziness is a symptom that is often due to:
  A. too much blood being circulated to the brain.
  B. poor perfusion to the brain.
  C. too much fluid intake in too short a period of time.
  D. standing erect for too long a period of time.

_____ **41.** If a patient demonstrates one of the three findings of the Cincinnati Prehospital Stroke Scale, they have a _____ percent chance of having an acute stroke.
  A. 25   **C.** 70
  B. 45   **D.** 90

_____ **42.** If you can determine the exact time your suspected stroke patient was normal, you may have up to _____ for them to be administered thrombolytic drugs if they are a candidate.
  A. 1 hour   **C.** 3 hours
  B. 2 hours   **D.** 5 hours

Pathophysiology: Hypoglycemia

1. When the sympathetic division of the autonomic nervous system engages, what occurs?

_____

2. What are some signs and symptoms of the hypoglycemic patient?

_____

Pathophysiology: Hyperglycemia

1. As the blood sugar level creeps up, what volume changes occur in the patient's body?

_____

2. What is the cause of the acetone or fruity smell on the diabetic's breath?

_____

©2021 Pearson Education, Inc.
Emergency Care, 14th Ed.

Pathophysiology: Tonic-Clonic Seizure

1. What happens in the tonic phase of a seizure?

_____

2. What happens in the clonic phase?

_____

3. What is the postictal phase?

_____

Complete the Following

1. List nine signs and symptoms associated with a diabetic emergency.

A. _____

B. _____

C. _____

D. _____

E. _____

F. _____

G. _____

H. _____

I. _____

2. Give four reasons why a diabetic may develop hyperglycemia.

A. _____

B. _____

C. _____

D. _____

3. List ten causes of seizures.

A. _____

B. _____

C. _____

D. _____

E. _____

F. _____

G. _____

H. _____

I. _____

J. _____

4. List the four categories of causes of dizziness and syncope.

A. _____

B. _____

C. _____

D. _____

5. List ten signs or symptoms of a stroke.

A. _____

B. _____

C. _____

D. _____

E. _____

F. _____

G. _____

H. _____

I. _____

J. _____

Case Study: Call for a "Man Down"

You respond to an alleyway in an area of town where there are a number of factories. It is early evening, and this area is usually not heavily traveled on the weekends. The police are on the scene of an approximately 35-year-old male who was found unconscious by some children who were riding by on their bikes. The scene is safe, and you begin your primary assessment.

1. You do not see any apparent trauma. How would you open the patient's airway?

_____

2. If the patient is breathing, but very shallowly and very slowly, what should you do?

_____

In a couple of moments, the patient wakes up and is a bit nasty and combative. One of the police officers says that he remembers this guy. He has some medical problems and never takes his medicine.

3. You notice that the patient has urinated on himself. What may have caused this?

_____

4. With the assistance of the police, you carefully go through the patient's pockets, and you come across an empty medicine bottle of dilantin. How does this contribute to the history?

_____

5. Is it safe to decide that this patient had a seizure and simply transport him?

_____

You decide to get a full set of baseline vital signs, administer some oxygen, and check the patient's blood sugar with the glucometer. Your partner goes back to the ambulance to get the stretcher.

GZQ 6. Why would you be doing all this when it may just be a seizure?

_____

GZQ 7. The glucometer reads 60. What could this mean? Will this patient need immediate treatment?

_____

At this point, the medics arrive, and you share all the information you have with them. Because the patient is still "altered" and all of you are not confident in his gag reflex, the decision is made to start an IV and administer dextrose by an IV infusion. Very soon thereafter, the patient becomes alert and tells you that he has developed type 2 diabetes in the last few years because of his poor eating habits and other factors.

8. What is type 2 diabetes? Do patients with this type of diabetes always have to take insulin?

_____

23

Allergic Reaction

Core Concepts

- How to identify a patient experiencing an allergic reaction
- Differences between a mild allergic reaction and anaphylaxis
- How to treat a patient experiencing an allergic reaction
- Who should be assisted with an epinephrine auto-injector

Outcomes

After reading this chapter, you should be able to:

23.1 Summarize the concepts of the spectrum of mild allergic reactions to anaphylactic shock. (pp. 651–656)
- Describe how the interaction of the immune system with a substance leads to allergic reactions.
- List substances commonly implicated in allergic reactions.
- Describe the special considerations involved with latex allergies.
- Relate the signs and symptoms of allergic reactions to their underlying pathophysiologic processes.

23.2 Summarize the application of prehospital management for patients with allergic reactions. (pp. 656–666)
- Recognize assessment findings that point toward an allergic reaction.
- Distinguish the severity of patient allergic reactions.
- Explain the importance of communicating with medical direction based on the patient's history and current presentation.
- Describe decision making for assisting a patient with a prescribed epinephrine auto-injector.
- Describe decision making for administering epinephrine carried by the EMT.
- Outline the pharmacology of epinephrine.
- Compare the features of different kinds of epinephrine auto-injectors patients may have.
- List the priority of the administration of epinephrine with other patient interventions.
- Determine whether calling for paramedic assistance will benefit a patient.

Match Key Terms

A. Red, itchy, raised blotches on the skin that often result from an allergic reaction.

B. A severe or life-threatening allergic reaction in which the blood vessels dilate, causing a drop in blood pressure, and the tissues lining the respiratory system swell, interfering with the airway.

C. Something that causes an allergic reaction.

D. A hormone produced by the body. As a medication, it constricts blood vessels and dilates respiratory passages, and is used to relieve severe allergic reactions.

E. A syringe preloaded with medication that has a spring-loaded device and pushes the needle through the skin to deploy the medication when the tip of the device is pressed firmly against the body.

F. An exaggerated immune response.

_____ **1.** Allergen

_____ **2.** Allergic reaction

_____ **3.** Anaphylaxis

_____ **4.** Auto-injector

_____ **5.** Epinephrine

_____ **6.** Hives

Multiple-Choice Review

_____ **1.** A 27-year-old male's exaggerated response of his body's immune system to any substance is called a(n) _____ reaction.
  A. vasoconstricting
  B. immune
  C. allergic
  D. syncopal

_____ **2.** You are treating a 22-year-old female who you suspect is having an anaphylactic reaction. Why would a person with an anaphylactic reaction be treated as a high-priority patient?
  A. The patient can vomit.
  B. The patient can become covered with hives.
  C. An anaphylactic reaction can speed up the heart rate.
  D. An anaphylactic reaction can cause airway obstruction.

_____ **3.** The first time a person is exposed to an allergen, the person's immune system:
  A. reacts violently.
  B. shuts down.
  C. forms antibodies.
  D. ignores the allergen.

_____ **4.** The second time a person is exposed to the same allergen, the body reactions may include all of the following *except*:
  A. destruction of antibodies.
  B. difficulty breathing.
  C. massive swelling.
  D. dilation of the blood vessels.

_____ **5.** When interviewing a 23-year-old male, you should consider the common causes of allergic reactions, which include all of the following *except*:
  A. hornet stings.
  B. eggs and milk.
  C. poison ivy and penicillin.
  D. red fruits and vegetables.

_____ **6.** It is possible for a patient to be allergic to peanuts and not to walnuts or almonds because:
  A. walnuts have a protective quality to them.
  B. almonds cause vasoconstriction of the arteries.
  C. peanuts are legumes and not nuts.
  D. all of these.

_____ 7. You are treating a 35-year-old male patient who you suspect is having a life-threatening anaphylactic reaction. He was stung by a few bees when mowing the lawn. Respiratory signs and symptoms of anaphylactic shock include all of the following *except*:

A. rapid breathing.
B. hives.
C. cough.
D. stridor.

_____ 8. The effects on the cardiac system of an allergic reaction for a 35-year-old male could include _____ heart rate and _____ blood pressure.

A. decreased; decreased
B. increased; increased
C. decreased; increased
D. increased; decreased

_____ 9. For an immune response to be considered a severe allergic reaction, the patient must have signs and symptoms of shock or:

A. a history of allergies.
B. massive swelling.
C. respiratory distress.
D. increased blood pressure.

_____ 10. You are assessing a 43-year-old male who is experiencing a severe allergic reaction. He believes that he meets the protocol criteria and has his own auto-injector. After you administer epinephrine by auto-injector, you should:

A. prepare to administer another dose if condition worsens.
B. reassess the patient after 2 minutes.
C. decrease the oxygen being administered.
D. allow the patient to remain at home.

_____ 11. When capillaries become leaky, fluid moves into the tissue and appears as swelling, called _____, especially around the site of an injection (or sting) and to the face—including eyes, lips, ears, and tongue—and the airway.

A. hives
B. angioedema
C. pruritis
D. urticaria

_____ 12. Your 22-year-old male patient has an epinephrine auto-injector in his backpack. Besides helping him take his medication, you should:

A. ask the patient whether he has any spare auto-injectors for the trip to the hospital.
B. call the patient's physician and request another dosage of the medication.
C. determine whether other family members have a history of allergic reactions.
D. take the insect or substance that caused the reaction to the hospital.

_____ 13. You are treating a 40-year-old male who you suspect is having a severe allergic reaction. He has an EpiPen® on him for situations like this. The recommended location for injection with an epinephrine auto-injector is the:

A. center of the back.
B. lateral mid-thigh.
C. buttocks.
D. biceps.

_____ 14. Your patient is a 5-year-old preschooler who has a history of peanut allergies. He has an epinephrine auto-injector that is held by the school nurse. What is the epinephrine dose contained in the child sized auto-injector?

A. 0.05 mg.
B. 0.15 mg.
C. 0.5 mg.
D. 1.0 mg.

_____ 15. Which statement is *true* regarding allergies and anaphylactic reactions in infants and children?

A. Infants frequently experience anaphylactic reactions.
B. Many children outgrow allergies as they mature.
C. Anaphylactic reactions are common in younger children.
D. Parents seldom can provide useful information about the child's medical history.

_____ **16.** Which of the following is a sign of a patient experiencing a minor allergic reaction?
   A. The patient has generalized hives.
   B. The patient has local swelling.
   C. The patient has tachycardia and hypotension.
   D. The patient is wheezing.

Pathophysiology: Allergic or Anaphylactic Reaction?

1. List the signs and symptoms of a minor allergic reaction in each category below:

   A. Respiratory complaints - _____

   B. Respiratory sounds - _____

   C. Skin findings - _____

   D. Swelling - _____

   E. Vital signs - _____

   F. Mental status - _____

2. List the signs and symptoms of an anaphylactic reaction in each category below:

   A. Respiratory complaints - _____

   B. Respiratory sounds - _____

   C. Skin findings - _____

   D. Swelling - _____

   E. Vital signs - _____

   F. Mental status - _____

Complete the Following

1. List fourteen signs and symptoms of allergic reaction or anaphylactic shock.

   A. _____

   B. _____

   C. _____

   D. _____

   E. _____

F. _____

G. _____

H. _____

I. _____

J. _____

K. _____

L. _____

M. _____

N. _____

2. List eight side effects of epinephrine auto-injector.

A. _____

B. _____

C. _____

D. _____

E. _____

F. _____

G. _____

H. _____

3. During your secondary assessment of a patient with a chief complaint of allergic reaction. What six questions should you ask?

A. _____

B. _____

C. _____

D. _____

E. _____

F. _____

Label the Diagrams

Fill in the name of each substance type that may cause an allergic reaction on the line provided.

1. _____

2. _____

3. _____

4. _____

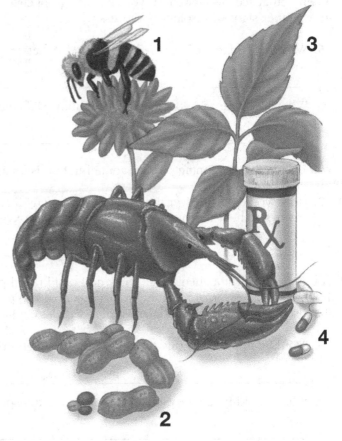

Case Study: The Lakefront Emergency

You respond to a call from a woman having difficulty breathing while at a camp on a lake. On your arrival, you ensure that the scene is safe, and you find a woman in her forties who is clutching her chest and is having obvious breathing difficulty.

1. Is there a need for another ambulance?

_____

2. Should you call for an ALS unit to respond?

_____

After taking Standard Precautions, you begin your primary assessment. There is no reason to suspect trauma, and the patient has an open airway. She is responsive, although she talks in short, choppy sentences. She knows her name, where she is, and the day of the week.

3. Why is she talking in short, choppy sentences?

_____

4. What would be your assessment of her level of responsiveness (mental status)?

_____

When you auscultate her chest, you hear a high-pitched musical tone as the patient breathes. She shows other signs of respiratory distress.

5. What is the name of her breathing sound? What are some of the potential causes of this sound?

_____

6. What are some additional signs of breathing difficulty that you may observe in this patient?

_____

You decide that beginning oxygen administration is an appropriate thing to do at this time.

GZQ **7.** How would you deliver the oxygen? How many liters per minute would you administer? Is there any assessment parameters that can guide your oxygen administration?

_____

You notice that the patient has a weak and rapid radial pulse. There is no reason to suspect any life-threatening external bleeding in this instance. The patient is very pale and is sweating profusely. She also complains of chest tightness and dizziness, which she denies that she has ever had before.

8. Would you prioritize this patient as a low or high priority? Why?

_____

9. What would be the best position in which to transport the patient? Why?

_____

As you begin to prepare the patient for transport, you start to obtain a secondary assessment, history, and physical examination. The patient has chest tightness and breathing difficulty, which she states "came on suddenly." The pain is across the upper chest, doesn't radiate, and is constant. Nothing the patient does makes the pain go away. She states that it is a 7 on a scale of 1 to 10, where 10 is the worst pain she ever had. The pain has been present for approximately 15 to 20 minutes. You assign a crew member to obtain a complete set of baseline vital signs. She has a weak and rapid pulse at 110, respirations are labored at 26 per minute, and her blood pressure is 88/50 mmHg.

10. As you load the patient into the ambulance, what additional history should you obtain?

_____

Your patient states that she was cleaning out the gutter and may have been stung by a bee. She previously reacted severely to a bee sting and carries a bee-sting kit.

GZQ **11.** What medicine is usually in these kits? Should you help her take the medicine?

_____

12. Is it necessary to call medical director? What must be checked before administering the medicine?

_____

As you leave the scene, the driver arranges for an ALS intercept on the way to the hospital. Other than reassessing the patient after administering the medication, you continue to monitor her. About 5 minutes en route, your driver pulls the ambulance to the side of the road momentarily to let the ALS paramedic jump in with his equipment. Then you proceed to the hospital.

13. What would be your quick report to the paramedic on the patient's chief complaint, your assessment of the situation, and the treatment you have given?

_____

14. What care would you expect to see the paramedic provide en route to the hospital?

_____

24

Infectious Diseases and Sepsis

Core Concepts

- Pathophysiology of infectious diseases and sepsis
- How infectious diseases spread
- recognition and management of patients with infectious diseases
- Recognition and management of the possibly septic patient

Outcomes

After reading this chapter, you should be able to:

24.1 Identify key factors involved in transmission of infectious diseases. (pp. 671–674)
- Describe the factors that determine whether exposure to a communicable disease results in infection.
- Define the terms incubation period, bacteria, viruses, sepsis, and septic shock.
- List the two most effective methods of preventing the spread of disease.

24.2 Explain the pathophysiology and progression of sepsis. (pp. 674–677)
- Describe how exposure to a disease can progress to septic shock.
- Identify common causes of sepsis.
- List criteria for recognizing sepsis using the systemic inflammatory response syndrome criteria.
- Given a patient description, determine whether you should notify the emergency department of a sepsis alert.

24.3 List the common patient presentation, treatment, standard precautions and postexposure actions for each of the following diseases: (pp. 677–691)
- Chickenpox
- Measles
- Mumps
- Hepatitis
- HIV/AIDS
- Influenza
- Croup
- Pertussis
- Pneumonia

©2021 Pearson Education, Inc.
Emergency Care, 14th Ed.

- Tuberculosis
- Meningitis
- Sexually transmitted infections (STIs)
- Diseases carried by ticks

24.4 Discuss reactions among the public and health care providers when a potentially deadly infectious disease is discovered or rediscovered. (pp. 691–692)

Match Key Terms

A. Diseases that can be passed from one individual to another, through either direct contact or contact with secretions from an infected person.

B. A life-threatening condition resulting from an abnormal and counterproductive response by the body that causes damage to tissues and organs after the body is invaded by a pathogen.

C. Diseases that can be spread by bacteria, viruses, and other microbes.

_____ **1.** Infectious diseases

_____ **2.** Communicable diseases

_____ **3.** Sepsis

Multiple-Choice Review

_____ **1.** Of the many types of microbes that can transmit diseases, only _____ are not cells and need to be in a host cell to reproduce.
   A. bacteria   **C.** fungi
   B. viruses   **D.** protozoa

_____ **2.** When an EMT is exposed to a sick patient and contracts an infectious microbe, the EMT:
   A. may or may not become sick.
   B. will eventually become sick.
   C. will require antibiotic therapy for two weeks.
   D. must go through diagnostic testing.

_____ **3.** When a minor infection worsens and spreads to the bloodstream it can cause:
   A. food poisoning.   **C.** a painful rash on the chest.
   B. hypertension.   **D.** life-threatening conditions.

_____ **4.** _____ is an infection in the lungs that may lead to sepsis.
   A. Croup   **C.** Mumps
   B. Hepatitis A   **D.** Pneumonia

_____ **5.** _____ is an infection that causes inflammation of the tissues surrounding the brain and spinal cord.
   A. Varicella   **C.** Meningitis
   B. Measles   **D.** Pertussis

_____ **6.** To prevent the spread of very contagious chickenpox, the patient should be isolated until:
   A. all lesions are dried and crusted.
   B. all the rashes have disappeared.
   C. three days after a post-exposure vaccination.
   D. a mask is worn by the patient.

_____ 7. Which of the following infectious diseases is often considered a childhood disease, but can return in adults in a different form?
   A. Varicella
   B. Measles
   C. Influenza
   D. Croup

_____ 8. A young adult patient is complaining of headache, muscle aches, loss of appetite, and painful swelling of the cheeks. What precautions should the EMT take?
   A. Isolate the patient.
   B. Wear a N-95 mask.
   C. Wear gloves, eye protection, and gown.
   D. Avoid contact with the patient's saliva.

_____ 9. The EMT is transporting a patient from a nursing facility whose urinary catheter has come out. The patient has a fever and new onset of altered mental status. The EMT should notify the hospital:
   A. of a stroke alert.
   B. that the patient may be septic.
   C. that the patient will need a new catheter.
   D. that the patient may have low blood sugar.

_____ 10. When entering the home of a sick patient, which of the following should alert the EMT to a potential infectious or communicable risk?
   A. Coughing and sneezing.
   B. The smell of vomitus.
   C. The smell of urine.
   D. An older adult patient with altered mental status.

_____ 11. In addition to getting recommended vaccinations, the best way to prevent the spread of disease while on the job is to:
   A. reduce the risk of exposure.
   B. get plenty of sleep.
   C. lose weight and avoid fast foods.
   D. avoid being in close contact with sick patients.

_____ 12. Lyme disease typically presents with:
   A. a bull's-eye rash and itching two weeks after a tick bite.
   B. no symptoms initially, but a bull's-eye rash months to years after a tick bite.
   C. bull's-eye rash within a week and possible neurologic complications months to years later.
   D. fever, bull's-eye rash, nausea and vomiting within 24 hours after a tick bite.

_____ 13. _____ is a bacterial illness that can infect the lungs, as well as other organs and tissues.
   A. Hepatitis
   B. Pertussis
   C. Tuberculosis
   D. Lyme disease

_____ 14. Which types of hepatitis are spread by the fecal-oral route?
   A. A and E
   B. B and C
   C. A and D
   D. E and B

_____ 15. A six-year-old child has rubeola and was never vaccinated for the disease. The symptoms of rubeola begin with:
   A. rash on the torso.
   B. stiffness in the neck.
   C. muscle aches.
   D. fever and coughing.

_____ 16. Which type(s) of hepatitis has(have) an effective and specific treatment but no vaccination?
   A. A
   B. B
   C. C
   D. D, E

17. The treatment for a person who has HIV/AIDS is:
   A. antibiotic medications.
   B. antiviral medications.
   C. supportive care for symptoms.
   D. only available in the United States.

18. The risk for the EMT of sustaining a significant exposure to HIV/AIDS on the job is primarily associated with exposure to:
   A. urine.
   B. airborne droplets.
   C. fecal matter.
   D. blood.

19. Influenza can be caused by:
   A. less than one dozen bacteria.
   B. more than two dozen viruses.
   C. both viruses and bacteria.
   D. flu vaccinations.

20. Pertussis is a respiratory infection that begins with cold symptoms, worsens to coughing fits, then:
   A. resolves without medication.
   B. persists for 1 to 2 months.
   C. is no longer communicable.
   D. resolves but lingers in the body, reactivating later.

Complete the Following

1. List ten communicable diseases discussed in the text and their mode of transmission.

   A. _____

   B. _____

   C. _____

   D. _____

   E. _____

   F. _____

   G. _____

   H. _____

   I. _____

   J. _____

2. In an adult with suspected infection, what are the assessment criteria used to determine if the patient may also have sepsis?

   A. _____

   B. _____

   C. _____

   D. _____

   E. _____

   F. _____

3. List eight examples of emerging new infectious diseases:

A. _____

B. _____

C. _____

D. _____

E. _____

F. _____

G. _____

H. _____

Case Study: "Just Another Rash"

Your unit was dispatched to a private residence for a call involving a 7-year-old boy who woke up with "just a rash." The mother is home and states that she kept him home from school today and yesterday because he was not feeling well. Today he seems to be covered with a red blotchy rash that started on the face and now has spread to the chest. She tells you that she has no transportation to the local emergency department and wanted him checked out. She leads you to a den, where the child is on the couch watching the television.

1. As you approach the patient, what Standard Precautions should you take?

_____

2. With this rash expanding over time from the face to the chest, could this be serious?

_____

3. Why would it make sense to inquire who else lives in the home?

_____

You begin your assessment by introducing yourself, and you find out that the patient's name is Tommy. He is oriented to person, place, and day so you decide he is alert. He states that he is 7 years old and seems to be enjoying the vacation from school. He does complain that the rash or pimples are very itchy. His mother says that he had a low-grade fever the other day and has been coughing and complaining of irritated eyes. She kept him home from school because she thought he had "pink eye." Mom says she did not want the school to send him home because she has been arguing with the school nurse for the past few weeks.

You determine the primary assessment reveals no problems and proceed to get a set of vital signs.

4. Should you inquire what the school nurse's concerns have been about Tommy?

_____

5. The mother tells you that her husband has very strong opinions about not having vaccinations for their children. Could this information be relevant to the secondary assessment?

_____

©2021 Pearson Education, Inc.
Emergency Care, 14th Ed.

The vital signs are respirations of 20 and regular, pulse of 90 and regular, BP of 110/72, and a pulse oximeter reading of 97%. Tommy is warm to touch but denies the chills. He does have a nonproductive cough and his eyes are no longer itchy but the rash certainly is. You are careful not to touch the rash and instruct him to put on a tee shirt over it for now. His mom tells you Tommy takes no meds, has no medical history aside from a broken ankle two years ago, and has no allergies. You complete the rest of your OPQRST and SAMPLE and decide it is time for a quiet ride to the hospital. Tommy is cooperative although he would rather just watch the end of his TV show.

6. What disease do you suspect Tommy might have?

_____

7. Who might be at high-risk of contracting this disease?

_____

8. Is any special notification needed before arriving at the ED?

_____

25

Poisoning and
Overdose Emergencies

Core Concepts

- How to know if a patient has been poisoned
- Assessment and care for ingested poisons
- Assessment and care for inhaled poisons
- Assessment and care for absorbed poisons
- Types of injected poisons
- Assessment and care for alcohol abuse
- Assessment and care for substance abuse

Outcomes

After reading this chapter, you should be able to:

25.1 Summarize concepts of poisoning. (pp. 697–699)
- Describe ways that poisons can damage the body.
- Describe the routes of exposure to poison.
- Explain the effects of commonly ingested poisons.
- Determine when a poisonous substance should be transported with the patient.
- Prioritize the specific steps in the care of patients with poisoning with other needed interventions.

25.2 Explain how to incorporate management relevant to ingested poisoning into the patient care process. (pp. 700–707)
- State the rationale for the specific questions that EMTs should ask of each type of poisoned patient.
- Identify the EMT's key decision points in the care of poisoned patients.
- Describe the steps that can minimize exposure to food poisoning.
- Outline the pharmacology of activated charcoal.
- Explain why syrup of ipecac is rarely used for ingested-poisoning emergencies.
- Explain the reason why many state legislatures have amended laws to allow laypeople to administer naloxone.
- Outline the process of using dilution as a treatment for ingested poisoning.
- Explain the extra consideration for avoiding direct mouth-to-mouth contact with a patient who has ingested poison and who requires positive pressure ventilation.

- State the reasons that the pediatric population is especially prone to ingested poisoning.
- Outline the pharmacology of naloxone.
- Paraphrase the concerns with acetaminophen overdose.

25.3 Explain how to incorporate management of inhaled poison into the patient care process. (pp. 708–712)
- Describe the observations that should make an EMT suspect carbon monoxide inhalation.
- Describe the special concerns associated with smoke inhalation.
- Recognize indications of hydrogen sulfide gas exposure.

25.4 Explain how to incorporate management of absorbed poison into the patient care process. (pp. 712–714)
- Describe the potential risks to EMTs of entering a scene involving absorbed poisons.
- Identify the additional resources that may be required at the scene before an EMT can provide treatment for a patient with absorbed poison.
- Describe the proper way of decontaminating patients of exposures to absorbed poisons.
- Describe special considerations in the scene size-up for poisoned patients.
- Recall sources of information about specific kinds of poisons.
- Identify situations in which additional resources are required for poisoning situations.

25.5 Summarize concepts of alcohol and substance abuse. (pp. 715–716)
- Describe the role of professionalism in increasing the substance abuse patient's cooperation with your interactions.
- Compare the acute and chronic effects of common substances of abuse.
- Explain the need for careful assessment of patients who are acutely intoxicated.
- Anticipate the potential for violence toward EMTs when caring for patients who have a substance abuse issue.
- Explain the considerations for restraining a substance abuse patient.

25.6 Apply knowledge of the effects of alcohol to the patient care process. (pp. 716–717)
- Explain clinical reasoning to identify problems that may be incorrectly attributed to alcohol intoxication.
- Recognize signs of alcohol intoxication.
- Recognize signs and symptoms of the spectrum of withdrawal from alcohol.
- Explain the reason why reassessment is especially important in the care of a patient with acute alcohol intoxication.
- Describe the risks of turning over an intoxicated patient without apparent injury or illness to law enforcement.
- Apply medical-legal and ethical principles to decision making regarding a patient's ability to consent under the influence of a substance.

25.7 Apply knowledge of the effects of a variety of substances of abuse to the patient care process. (pp. 717–722)
- Identify substance abuse as an illness.
- Outline the characteristics of the different categories of commonly abused substances.
- Relate a patient's presentation to the category of substance most likely to cause observed signs and symptoms.
- Recognize indications of substance withdrawal.
- Describe priorities in the care of patients with substance abuse.

Match Key Terms

A. Any substance that can harm the body by altering cell structure or functions.	_____ **1.** Absorbed poisons
	_____ **2.** Activated charcoal
B. Stimulants, such as cocaine and methamphetamine that affect the central nervous system to excite the user.	_____ **3.** Antidote
C. Referring to alcohol or drug withdrawal in which the patient's body reacts severely when deprived of an abused substance.	_____ **4.** Delirium tremens (DTs)

D. Poisons that are taken into the body through unbroken skin

E. Depressants, such as benzodiazepines, that depress the central nervous system, and which are often used to bring on a more relaxed state of mind.

F. Poisons that are swallowed.

G. A class of drugs that affect the nervous system and change many normal body activities. Their legal use is for relief of pain; illicit use is to produce an intense state of relaxation.

H. A substance that adsorbs many poisons and prevents them from being absorbed by the body.

I. Thinning down or weakening a poison by mixing with something else.

J. Poisons that are inserted through the skin, for example, by needle, snake fangs, or insect stinger.

K. A severe reaction that can be part of alcohol withdrawal, characterized by sweating, trembling, anxiety, and hallucinations.

L. Poisons that are breathed in.

M. Mind-affecting or mind-altering drugs that act on the central nervous system to produce excitement and distortion of perceptions.

N. A poisonous substance secreted by bacteria, plants, or animals.

O. Vaporized compounds, such as cleaning fluid, that are breathed in by an abuser to produce a "high."

P. A substance that will neutralize the poison or its effects.

_____ **5.** Dilution

_____ **6.** Downers

_____ **7.** Hallucinogens

_____ **8.** Ingested poisons

_____ **9.** Inhaled poisons

_____ **10.** Injected poisons

_____ **11.** Narcotics

_____ **12.** Poison

_____ **13.** Toxin

_____ **14.** Uppers

_____ **15.** Volatile chemicals

_____ **16.** Withdrawal

Multiple-Choice Review

_____ **1.** You are on the scene of a 28-year-old female who you suspect may have been poisoned. Which of the following is an environmental clue at the scene that can be used to help you determine whether she has been poisoned?
   A. She appears to have been vomiting.
   B. There is an empty pill bottle on her night table.
   C. The patient has an altered mental status.
   D. The patient states that she has a headache.

_____ **2.** The most accurate definition of a poison would be that it is any:
   A. substance that can potentially harm the body.
   B. foreign substance swallowed by the patient.
   C. substance that could kill the patient if it is injected into the body.
   D. substance labeled with a hazardous material placard or label.

_____ **3.** Most of the more than two million poisonings in the United States each year are due to:
   A. suicide attempts by adults.
   B. attempts to murder someone.
   C. accidents involving young children.
   D. teenagers using illicit drugs.

_____ **4.** Any substance secreted by plants, animals, or bacteria that is poisonous to humans is called a:
   A. chemical.
   B. toxin.
   C. narcotic.
   D. pathogen.

_____ **5.** Because of the poisons they produce, _____ can be dangerous to humans.
   A. mistletoe
   B. mushrooms
   C. rubber plants
   D. all of these

_____ **6.** Bacteria may produce toxins that cause deadly diseases such as:
   A. HIV.
   B. botulism.
   C. tuberculosis.
   D. covid-19.

_____ **7.** The body's reaction to poisonous substances is often most severe in:
   A. the evening hours.
   B. the elderly and the ill.
   C. smaller concentrations.
   D. the summer.

_____ **8.** Poisons may enter the body through any of the following routes _except_:
   A. inhalation.
   B. ingestion.
   C. injection.
   D. excretion.

_____ **9.** Carbon monoxide, chlorine, and sulfur are examples of _____ poisons.
   A. ingested
   B. injected
   C. inhaled
   D. swallowed

_____ **10.** You suspect that your 28-year-old male patient was exposed to a poison that was absorbed. Examples of absorbed poisons include:
   A. insecticides and agricultural chemicals.
   B. carbon monoxide and chlorine.
   C. insect stings and snake bites.
   D. aspirin and LSD.

_____ **11.** The venom of a bite from a rattlesnake is an example of an _____ poison.
   A. ingested
   B. injected
   C. inhaled
   D. absorbed

_____ **12.** You are treating a 32-year-old female who was found unconscious by her roommate when the roommate got home late at night. If it is being assumed that she was poisoned, why is it important to determine when the ingestion of a poison occurred?
   A. Different poisons act on the body at different rates.
   B. Poison ingested in the evening is more likely to cause vomiting.
   C. Dilution of the poison is not effective after ten minutes.
   D. The antidote works more effectively once the poison is in the intestines.

_____ **13.** The most common findings of ingesting a poison are:
   A. altered mental status and diarrhea.
   B. nausea and vomiting.
   C. abdominal pain and diarrhea.
   D. chemical burns around the mouth and stomach pain.

_____ 14. You are having a discussion with medical direction about an order to use activated charcoal for a conscious patient who ingested a poison. Activated charcoal is used to:
A. act as an antidote.
B. dilute the poisonous substance.
C. reduce the amount of poison absorbed by the body.
D. speed up the digestion of most chemicals in the body.

_____ 15. The decision on when to use activated charcoal is best made:
A. en route to the hospital.
B. on arrival at the emergency department (ED).
C. with medical direction or consultation with the poison control center.
D. in consultation with the patient's family physician.

_____ 16. You are treating a 28-year-old male who accidentally ingested a poison. Activated charcoal is _not_ routinely used with ingestion of:
A. caustic substances.   C. strong alkalis.
B. strong acids.   D. any of these.

_____ 17. Your 8-year-old male patient has ingested a caustic substance that he should not have been able to access. Examples of caustic substances include all of the following _except_:
A. lye.   C. toilet bowl cleaner.
B. venom.   D. oven cleaner.

_____ 18. Your patient is a 22-year-old male who has been stealing fuel from his neighbors' cars at night. Tonight he may have sucked in and inhaled too much gasoline vapor, and his friend called 911 because the patient continued to cough violently after the ingestion. The appropriate treatment for this patient should:
A. not include activated charcoal.
B. not include oxygen administration.
C. include immediate transportation.
D. be to treat him like a patient with an airway obstruction.

_____ 19. When a physician orders dilution of an ingested substance, in most cases you can use either water or:
A. a cola drink.   C. milk.
B. coffee.   D. apple juice.

_____ 20. Your patient is a 32-year-old female who is having signs and symptoms of poison inhalation. The most commonly inhaled substance at poisonous levels is:
A. carbon dioxide.   C. carbon monoxide.
B. nitrogen.   D. phosgene.

_____ 21. As you approach a 35-year-old male patient who has passed out while cleaning a large industrial tank, you smell an unusual odor. What should you do?
A. Stand back and attempt to learn more about the chemical involved.
B. Rapidly remove the patient from the area, using a drag maneuver.
C. Ignore the smell, which is probably a normal odor around industrial sites.
D. Ask the patient's coworkers to bring him to your ambulance.

_____ 22. The principal prehospital treatment of a 40-year-old female patient who has inhaled poison is:
A. administering activated charcoal to the patient.
B. administering high-concentration oxygen.
C. providing spine motion restriction precautions.
D. administering an antidote.

_____ **23.** Besides motor vehicle exhaust, where else might you find carbon monoxide?
  A. In the patient compartment of your ambulance
  B. Wherever you can smell its odor
  C. Around an improperly vented wood-burning stove
  D. Around the foundation of a house

_____ **24.** Your patient is one of the five members of a family who may have been exposed to a faulty heating system leaking carbon monoxide into the home. How does carbon monoxide affect the body?
  A. It causes severe respiratory burns.
  B. It impairs the normal carrying of oxygen by the red blood cells.
  C. It causes the tissues in the airway to swell, making breathing difficult.
  D. It stimulates the central nervous system to decrease breathing.

_____ **25.** You are treating a family whose fireplace may not have been properly vented to the outside of their home. Given this scenario, which of the findings would least likely be present in those affected?
  A. cyanosis.   C. dizziness.
  B. nausea.   D. cherry-red lips.

_____ **26.** You are treating a 22-year-old male who has powdered fertilizer all over his arms and legs. After ensuring your own safety with PPE, you should:
  A. brush off as much of the powder as possible, then irrigate.
  B. immediately start irrigation with very cold water.
  C. leave the powder in place and transport immediately.
  D. irrigate with water for 20 minutes.

_____ **27.** You have responded to a call where a 32-year-old female seems to have mixed a couple of cleaning agents and is now unconscious. There is a strong smell of rotten eggs in the air. What would you suspect?
  A. The mixture produced large quantities of chlorine.
  B. The mixture may have produced hydrogen sulfide, which can be deadly.
  C. The mixture contains cyanide because that chemical causes unconsciousness.
  D. One of the chemicals was dish soap, which is often deadly when mixed with salts.

_____ **28.** Which of the following signs and symptoms is _not_ seen with alcohol abuse but _is_ seen in a diabetic emergency?
  A. Acetone breath
  B. Hallucinations
  C. Slurred speech
  D. Swaying and unsteadiness of movement

_____ **29.** The sweating, trembling, anxiety, and hallucinations that are found in the patient experiencing alcohol withdrawal are called:
  A. intoxication signs.   C. delirium tremens.
  B. seizures.   D. Parkinsonian tremors.

_____ **30.** It is important to determine an infant or child's _____ and estimated amount of substance in cases of pediatric poisonings.
  A. height: ingested.   C. height: injected.
  B. weight: ingested.   D. weight: inhaled.

_____ **31.** Your patient is a 35-year-old female who is very anxious and jittery. She has taken an overdose of a drug that stimulates the nervous system, causing extreme excitement. These drugs are called:
  A. uppers.   C. narcotics.
  B. downers.   D. antihypertensives.

_____ 32. The 48-year-old female you are treating states that she has difficulty sleeping, so she takes tranquilizers. These pills are examples of:
A. uppers.
B. downers.
C. narcotics.
D. hallucinogens.

_____ 33. You are treating a 29-year-old male who has taken an overdose of a drug called GHB. These types of drugs are called:
A. uppers.
B. downers.
C. narcotics.
D. hallucinogens.

_____ 34. You are evaluating a 40-year-old male who has taken an overdose of a drug that is capable of producing stupor or sleep. The drug is also normally used to relieve pain. These types of medications are called:
A. uppers.
B. downers.
C. narcotics.
D. hallucinogens.

_____ 35. Your 25-year-old male patient has taken a mind-altering drug designed to act on the nervous system and produce intense excitement or distortion of the patient's perceptions. This drug was most likely a(n):
A. upper.
B. downer.
C. narcotic.
D. hallucinogen.

_____ 36. Your patient is a 16-year-old female who was found sniffing (huffing) a rag drenched in chemicals. Cleaning fluid, glue, and model cement are examples of:
A. hallucinogens.
B. volatile chemicals.
C. controlled substances.
D. narcotics.

_____ 37. A 21-year-old female who has overdosed on an upper may have signs and symptoms such as:
A. excitement, increased pulse and breathing rates, dilated pupils, and rapid speech.
B. sluggishness, sleepiness, and lack of coordination of body and speech.
C. fast pulse rate, dilated pupils, flushed face, and seeing or hearing things.
D. reduced pulse rate and rate and depth of breathing, constricted pupils, and sweating.

_____ 38. Your 22-year-old male patient has overdosed on phenobarbital, according to his significant other. You can expect to observe signs and symptoms such as:
A. excitement, increased pulse and breathing rates, dilated pupils, and rapid speech.
B. sluggishness, sleepiness, and lack of coordination of body and speech.
C. fast pulse rate, dilated pupils, flushed face, and seeing or hearing things.
D. increased pulse rate and slowing respirations, constricted pupils, and sweating.

_____ 39. A 32-year-old female patient who has overdosed on psilocybin (magic mushrooms) may have signs and symptoms such as:
A. excitement, increased pulse and breathing rates, dilated pupils, and rapid speech.
B. sluggishness, sleepiness, and lack of coordination of body and speech.
C. fast pulse rate, dilated pupils, flushed face, and seeing or hearing things.
D. reduced pulse rate and rate and depth of breathing, constricted pupils, and sweating.

_____ 40. Your 52-year-old male patient has been taking double to triple doses of his pain relief medication, but that is not even touching the pain for him. If he has overdosed on the narcotic he takes, he might have signs and symptoms such as:
A. excitement, increased pulse and breathing rates, dilated pupils, and rapid speech.
B. seizures, sleepiness, and exaggerated reflexes of the body.
C. fast pulse rate, dilated pupils, flushed face, and "seeing" or "hearing" things.
D. reduced pulse rate and rate and depth of breathing, pinpoint pupils, and sweating.

_____ 41. If a patient who took a "handful" of pills told you he had second thoughts and then took ipecac, you should be careful to plan for:
A. vomiting.
B. a potential for aspiration.
C. a potential for airway obstruction.
D. all of the above.

_____42. Which of the following would not indicate an airway that was injured by smoke inhalation?
   A. Coughing.
   B. Black residue in the sputum.
   C. Singed nose hairs.
   D. Pinpoint pupils.

Pathophysiology: Acetaminophen Overdose

1. The patient who overdoses on acetaminophen is likely to have what type of internal organ damage?

_____

2. What are some common signs and symptoms of an acetaminophen overdose?

_____

Complete the Following

1. What are the steps in the care of the patient who has ingested a poison?

   A. _____

   B. _____

   C. _____

   D. _____

   E. _____

   F. _____

2. List at least eight signs and symptoms of alcohol abuse.

   A. _____

   B. _____

   C. _____

   D. _____

   E. _____

   F. _____

   G. _____

   H. _____

3. What is the phone number for the poison control center?

_____

Label the Diagrams

Fill in the way in which each type of poison enters the body

1. _____

2. _____

3. _____

4. _____

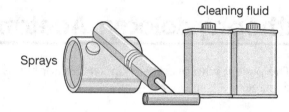

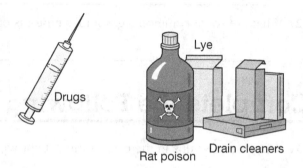

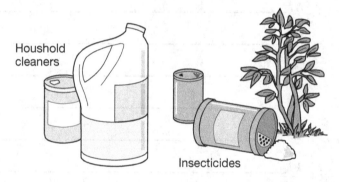

Complete the Chart

On the lines provided, write whether each of these commonly abused drugs is classified as an upper, downer, narcotic, mind-altering drug, or volatile chemical.

Amphetamine   1. _____

Codeine   2. _____

DMT LSD   3. _____

Psilocybin   4. _____

Gasoline   5. _____

Secobarbital   6. _____

Methaqualone   7. _____

Cocaine   8. _____

Dextroamphetamine   9. _____

Chloral Hydrate	10. _____
Mescaline	11. _____
Morning Glory Seeds	12. _____
STP	13. _____
Heroin	14. _____
Butyl Nitrate	15. _____
PCP	16. _____
Fentanyl	17. _____
Methadone	18. _____
Barbiturates	19. _____
Demerol	20. _____
Phenobarbital	21. _____
Marijuana	22. _____
Opium	23. _____
Amyl Nitrate	24. _____

Case Study: Not a Fun Party for Everyone

Your ambulance responds to a private home in a suburban neighborhood. The police are on the scene, trying to sort out the details of a party that seems to have been thrown by a teenager whose parents are away on a cruise. On your arrival, it is clear that the scene is safe, although quite a few detectives are attempting to question the ten teenagers who are still at the house. There are literally piles of beer cans all over the place, and the house is obviously a mess. Apparently, the police were called because a fight broke out.

1. Your patient is a 16-year-old female who is unconscious and appears to have vomited all over herself. What is your first assessment and treatment priority?

   _____

GZQ 2. Her friend states that the patient drank about a six-pack of beer and smoked some pot. That was the last the friend saw the patient until the police arrived a few hours later. The patient's name is Sofia, and she does not respond to her name or to painful stimuli. You notice that she has a raspy cough, and there is still some gurgling when she breathes. What should you do?

   _____

3. Would an ALS unit be helpful for this patient?

   _____

Your partner obtains a fast and faint radial pulse and very shallow respirations at about 8 to 10 per minute. You decide to begin ventilations with a BVM attached to high-concentration oxygen. You also decide to get the patient packaged and head for the hospital. You will be trying to meet with the ALS unit on the way to the ED.

4. What is this patient's priority status?

_____

5. What is the likely prehospital diagnoses for this patient?

_____

About 5 minutes after you leave the residence, your partner pulls into a gas station where the medic unit is waiting. The medic climbs into your unit along with some of her portable equipment, and off you go to the ED.

GZQ **6.** Why is it important not to delay this patient's arrival at the ED?

_____

7. Is this a patient for whom activated charcoal would be indicated? Why or why not?

_____

Abdominal Emergencies

Core Concepts

- Understanding the nature of abdominal pain or discomfort
- Becoming familiar with abdominal conditions that may cause pain or discomfort
- How to assess and care for patients with abdominal pain or discomfort

Outcomes

After reading this chapter, you should be able to:

26.1 Summarize the anatomy and physiology of abdominal organs. (pp. 727–729)
- Describe the mechanism for visualizing abdominal quadrants.
- Describe the structure of the peritoneum.
- Match abdominal organs with their descriptions.
- Given a visual image, identify the abdominal organs.
- Differentiate between abdominal and retroperitoneal organs.
- List the internal female reproductive organs found in the pelvis.

26.2 Outline the pathophysiology of abdominal emergencies. (pp. 730–734)
- Compare the characteristics of different patterns of abdominal pain.
- Give examples of problems associated with describing abdominal pain.
- Describe characteristics of common causes of abdominal conditions.
- Identify nonabdominal causes of abdominal pain.

26.3 Explain how to prioritize specific steps of managing patients with abdominal pain.
(pp. 734–742)
- Recognize elements of the scene size-up that can be clues to abdominal emergencies.
- Identify the significance of a patient's position in suspecting abdominal pain.
- Describe the reason why a thorough history and exam of the patient with abdominal pain are critical, despite limitations in identifying the exact problem.
- Anticipate complications of abdominal conditions that may change the sequence of an EMT's planned approach to care.
- Adapt the approach to history taking to account for a complaint of abdominal pain.

- Adapt the approach to history taking for abdominal complaints to a female patient.
- Recognize complicating factors when assessing geriatric patients with abdominal complaints.
- Outline the approach to physical examination of the abdomen.
- Describe the limitations of palpating for pulsating abdominal masses.
- Describe the approach to reassessment of the patient with abdominal complaints.
- Describe how to make a patient with abdominal pain as comfortable as possible.

Match Key Terms

A. Pain that is felt in a location other than where the pain originates.

B. Sharp pain that feels as if body tissues are being ripped apart.

C. A poorly localized, dull, or diffuse pain that arises from the abdominal organs, or viscera.

D. A localized, intense pain that arises from the outer layer of the lining of the abdominal cavity.

E. The two thin membranes that line the abdominal cavity and covers the organs within it.

F. The area between the peritoneum and the back.

_____ **1.** Parietal pain

_____ **2.** Peritoneum

_____ **3.** Referred pain

_____ **4.** Tearing pain

_____ **5.** Visceral pain

_____ **6.** Retroperitoneal space

Multiple-Choice Review

_____ **1.** The membrane that covers the abdominal organs is called the _____ peritoneum.
　　A. pleural　　　　　　　**C.** parietal
　　B. visceral　　　　　　 **D.** serous

_____ **2.** The organs outside the peritoneum that are found between the abdomen and the back are in the _____ space.
　　A. posterior pelvic　　　**C.** retroperitoneal
　　B. subxiphoid　　　　　**D.** dorsal back

_____ **3.** Your 22-year-old male patient has pain in the lower right quadrant. Pain felt in a location other than where it originated is called:
　　A. somatic.　　　　　　**C.** referred.
　　B. parietal.　　　　　　 **D.** visceral.

_____ **4.** You are assessing a 35-year-old female who has abdominal pain that is coming from an organ. This pain is often described as intermittent and:
　　A. dull.　　　　　　　　**C.** diffuse.
　　B. achy.　　　　　　　　**D.** any of these.

_____ **5.** You are assessing a 23-year-old female who has colicky pain. This pain is often _____ pain from a _____ organ in the abdomen.
　　A. tearing; hollow　　　 **C.** visceral; hollow
　　B. referred; solid　　　　**D.** parietal; solid

©2021 Pearson Education, Inc.
Emergency Care, 14th Ed.

_____ 6. You are treating a 40-year-old male patient who states that he is having another gallbladder attack. He says that he has pain in his right shoulder blade. Why might the pain in right shoulder blade be a symptom of gallbladder problems?
   A. The gallbladder is located under the right shoulder blade in most adult patients.
   B. Nerve pathways from the gallbladder return to the spinal cord by way of shared pathways with the shoulder.
   C. The muscle that holds the gallbladder in position is attached to the right scapula.
   D. The pain travel up the phrenic nerve, which is also the nerve that scapular pain travels up.

_____ 7. Your 16-year-old male patient is complaining of abdominal discomfort. Why is his last oral intake an important part of your SAMPLE history for this patient?
   A. The food may have been spoiled or related to current complaint.
   B. Food can lead to altered mental state in many instances.
   C. Visceral pain is more severe on an empty stomach.
   D. Referred pain is more severe on a full stomach.

_____ 8. You are treating a 22-year-old female with a chief complaint of lower abdominal discomfort. It would be appropriate to ask her where she is in her menstrual cycle to:
   A. file a complete PCR.
   B. begin to focus on the possibility of an ectopic pregnancy.
   C. definitively rule out an ectopic pregnancy.
   D. rule out the possibility that the patient could be pregnant.

_____ 9. You are assessing a 25-year-old male who states that he has abdominal pain in his upper right quadrant. When you palpate his abdomen, be sure to palpate the area with the pain:
   A. last.   C. second.
   B. first.   D. third.

_____ 10. You are treating a 45-year-old male patient who has a chief complaint of abdominal discomfort. He denies any difficulty breathing yet has a pulse of 110 regular, a BP of 98/68 mmHg, and an SpO$_2$ of 91%. You should:
   A. transport him in a semi-Fowler position.
   B. administer 10–15 lpm oxygen by nonrebreather mask.
   C. contact medical direction for permission to administer activated charcoal.
   D. contact medical direction for permission to assist the patient with a nitroglycerin dose.

_____ 11. When a 61-year-old male patient tells you that he has a tearing sensation in his lower back and denies any recent injury, you should suspect:
   A. acute appendicitis.
   B. urinary tract infection.
   C. an abdominal aortic aneurysm.
   D. a flare-up of pancreatitis.

_____ 12. Your 35-year-old female patient is experiencing a severe and sudden epigastric pain that seems to radiate to her right shoulder. She says that it gets worse when she eats. Of the following choices, which is the most likely cause?
   A. Ectopic pregnancy   C. A hernia
   B. Cholecystitis   D. Renal colic

_____ 13. You are assessing a 25-year-old male who has no primary assessment issues but is writhing in pain. He cannot seem to find a comfortable position because of pain in the lower back and flank. What would you suspect is the most likely problem?
   A. Peritonitis   C. An abdominal aortic aneurysm
   B. A hernia   D. Renal colic

_____ 14. You have responded to the local high school physical education center, where a 17-year-old male is complaining of lower abdominal pain. On palpation, you discover a lump that he is concerned about. Because this came on suddenly during exercising, you suspect that it could be:
  A. a tension pneumothorax.
  B. a hernia.
  C. a spontaneous embolism.
  D. an abdominal aortic aneurysm.

_____ 15. Your 55-year-old male patient called the ambulance because he has been feeling weak and dizzy most of the day. He states that he has no chest pain or difficulty breathing, but he is nauseated and has had very dark-colored diarrhea all day. What do you suspect is his most likely problem?
  A. An acute myocardial infarction
  B. An abdominal aneurism
  C. A bleeding ulcer
  D. Food poisoning

_____ 16. When assessing a geriatric patient, you may find difficulty obtaining a history of pain from the abdomen due to:
  A. an existing heart problem.
  B. decreased ability to perceive pain.
  C. a history of tachycardia.
  D. all of the above.

_____ 17. When a patient has a hole in the muscle layers of the abdominal wall that allows intestine to protrude this is called (a):
  A. esophageal varices.
  B. hernia.
  C. appendicitis.
  D. AAA.

_____ 18. Common abdominal conditions in the pediatric patient include:
  A. gastroenteritis.
  B. appendicitis.
  C. constipation.
  D. all of the above.

_____ 19. A serious condition that can involve pain in the epigastric area radiating to the back and made worse by chronic alcohol use is:
  A. renal colic.
  B. stomach ulcer.
  C. pancreatitis.
  D. inguinal hernia.

_____ 20. When a patient with abdominal pain is found with the knees drawn up and arms across the abdomen this is called the _____ position.
  A. tripod
  B. guarding
  C. semi-Fowler
  D. referred

Complete the Following

1. List four solid structures (organs) found in the abdomen.

  A. _____

  B. _____

  C. _____

  D. _____

2. List six hollow structures (organs) found in the abdomen.

  A. _____

  B. _____

  C. _____

©2021 Pearson Education, Inc.
Emergency Care, 14th Ed.

D. _____

E. _____

F. _____

3. When doing an assessment on a female patient with a chief complaint of abdominal pain, what are six important questions to ask?

A. _____

B. _____

C. _____

D. _____

E. _____

F. _____

Label the Diagrams

Fill in the name of each structure on the line provided.

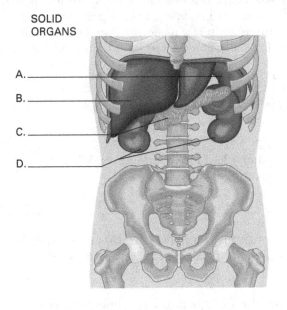

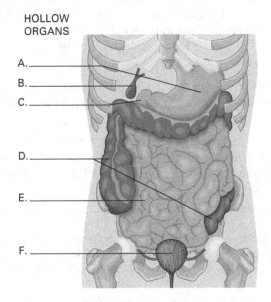

Solid Organs

A. _____

B. _____

C. _____

D. _____

Hollow Organs

A. _____

B. _____

C. _____

D. _____

E. _____

F. _____

Case Study: Just a Belly Ache

Your unit is responding to a call in a suburban community for a middle-aged male patient with abdominal pain. It is about midnight on a weeknight, and the houses on the street are dark, with the exception of the patient's home. As you pull up, his wife is opening the garage door to let you in. The scene seems safe at this point, so you introduce yourselves and proceed into the house. The woman states that her name is Angela and her husband Calvin could not get to sleep because of pain in his belly. She leads you to the family room in the back of the first floor, where the patient is lying on the couch in fetal position. There is a bucket nearby, and it is apparent that he has been vomiting. He sits up and seems embarrassed that his wife "bothered the EMS guys," but he is willing to answer your questions. You quickly determine that his mental status is alert, his airway is open and clear, and his breathing rate and depth are within normal range. His skin is pale, warm, and clammy, and he has no obvious external bleeding. It is obvious that he is having a lot of pain in his abdomen, as he is holding the area with his forearm. He also states that he has vomited a few times in the last few hours. When asked about the vomit, he said that it looked like it was just his dinner from 7 p.m. and then bile. There was no obvious blood that he could see. Because Calvin is a responsive medical patient, you decide to ask a few more questions to elaborate on his chief complaint as your partner obtains a set of baseline vital signs.

1. From your observations of the patient, even if he did not come right out and say that his abdomen hurts, what are indications of a potential abdominal problem?

   _____

2. Why would it be appropriate to inquire whether the patient had looked at the vomit before dumping the bucket into the toilet, had he done so before EMS arrived?

   _____

Your partner reports that the patient's pulse is 100 and regular, his respirations are 20 and normal, his blood pressure is 110/70 mmHg and his SpO_2 is 97%. You begin to ask specific questions about the chief complaint (OPQRST) and obtain a SAMPLE history.

3. The patient describes his pain as having started around his belly button a few hours earlier but states that now it is mostly in his right lower abdominal area. What would you suspect on the basis of this description?

   _____

4. The patient states that he is having chills and requests another blanket as you carefully move him onto your stretcher. What could be the cause of the chills?

   _____

©2021 Pearson Education, Inc.
Emergency Care, 14th Ed.

During your history, you find out that the patient has no history of problems with stomach ulcers or his gallbladder, and he denies any chest pain or cardiac history. He is allergic to sulfa drugs, and he takes medicine to control his cholesterol and an antihypertensive medication. He states that he is still nauseated but probably has nothing left in him to vomit. You still keep an emesis basin handy, as you have learned that lesson the hard way.

GZQ **5.** Using your clinical judgment, the information you have obtained from the patient so far, and a physical examination revealing intense pain in the lower right quadrant, do you think a medic unit should be called?

_____

6. The patient states that he is "very thirsty." Would it be appropriate to give him a glass of water?

_____

27

Behavioral and Psychiatric Emergencies and Suicide

Core Concepts

- The nature and causes of behavioral and psychiatric emergencies
- Emergency care for behavioral and psychiatric emergencies
- Emergency care for potential or attempted suicide
- Emergency care for aggressive or hostile patients
- When and how to restrain a patient safely and effectively
- Medical/legal considerations in behavioral and psychiatric emergencies

Outcomes

After reading this chapter, you should be able to:

27.1 Summarize the concepts of behavioral emergencies. (pp. 747–751)
- Describe the factors that interact to determine if a patient's behavior constitutes an emergency.
- Identify the contribution of psychiatric conditions to the incidence of behavioral emergencies.
- Identify the rationale for prescribing drugs that affect neurotransmitters.
- Describe the pathophysiology by which physical conditions can result in altered behavior.
- Recognize signs of hostility and potential for violence against the patient's self or others.
- Describe approaches to preventing patients who are hostile or violent from harming themselves or others.
- Recognize common presentations that indicate psychiatric emergencies.

27.2 Integrate knowledge of behavioral emergencies into the overall care of specific patients. (pp. 751–755)
- Explain how to safely and compassionately treat a patient with behavioral emergencies.
- Give examples of how a thorough history can contribute to determining the underlying cause of a behavioral emergency.
- Recognize risk factors for suicide.
- Describe the priorities of care for patients who have attempted suicide.
- Explain the decision making related to care of a patient with a behavioral emergency.

©2021 Pearson Education, Inc.
Emergency Care, 14th Ed.

27.3 Explain the decision-making process in the use of patient restraints. (pp. 755–760)
- Identify public safety personnel who may be required to assist with restraint procedures.
- Describe the concept of using reasonable force in restraint.
- Distinguish between safe and unsafe restraint procedures.
- Describe how restraint can lead to positional asphyxia.
- Describe the actions to be taken after a patient is restrained.
- Identify reasons the EMT should avoid being alone with patients with behavioral and psychiatric emergencies.

Match Key Terms

A. Bizarre and/or aggressive behavior, shouting, paranoia, panic, violence toward others, insensitivity to pain, unexpected physical strength, and hyperthermia.

B. The manner in which a person acts.

C. Inadequate breathing or respiratory arrest caused by a body position that restricts breathing.

D. When a patient's actions are not typical for the situation; is unacceptable or intolerable to the patient, the patient's family, or the community; or when the patient may harm self or others.

E. A mental disorder that affects how a person thinks, feels, and behaves. People may seem like they have lost touch with reality.

F. Chemicals within the body that transmit a message in the brain from the distal end of one neuron to the proximal end of the next neuron.

_____ **1.** Behavior

_____ **2.** Behavioral emergency

_____ **3.** Excited delirium

_____ **4.** Schizophrenia

_____ **5.** Neurotransmitters

_____ **6.** Positional asphyxia

Multiple-Choice Review

_____ **1.** You are doing an assessment on a 46-year-old male whom you suspect is exhibiting altered behavior as observed by his neighbors. The physical causes of altered behavior include all of the following *except*:
   A. inadequate blood flow to the brain.
   B. mind-altering substances.
   C. excessive heat or cold.
   D. differing lifestyles.

_____ **2.** Your 56-year-old male patient is exhibiting altered behavior ranging from irritability to altered mental status. This behavior can be due to any of the following *except*:
   A. lack of oxygen.   **C.** hypoactivity.
   B. head trauma.   **D.** hypoglycemia.

_____ **3.** You are assessing a 34-year-old male who you suspect is experiencing a stress reaction. To calm this patient, you should consider:
   A. completing your assessment as quickly as possible.
   B. allowing the patient to control the situation.
   C. explaining things to the patient honestly in a calm tone.
   D. restraining the patient quickly.

_____ 4. You are assessing a 25-year-old female whose family members called the ambulance because they felt that she was having an acute psychosis episode. Which one of the following is *not* usually a common presentation for such a patient?
   A. Paranoia
   B. A calm and neat appearance
   C. Severely erratic behavior.
   D. Hallucinations of visions or voices.

_____ 5. You are responding to a call involving a 22-year-old male who has attempted suicide previously. Today, he has a handgun and is threatening to kill himself. Your first concern should be:
   A. how you will restrain the patient.
   B. your personal safety.
   C. determining the patient's method for suicide.
   D. the patient's and family's safety.

_____ 6. The highest suicide rates occur in the _____ age group.
   A. 15- to 25-year-old
   B. 25- to 30-year-old
   C. 30- to 35-year-old
   D. 35- to 40-year-old

_____ 7. As you arrive on the scene. the police officer tells you that the 32-year-old female patient has been exhibiting self-destructive activity and making suicidal threats. Which one of the following is *not* an example of a risk factor for suicide?
   A. Verbalizing a defined lethal plan of action
   B. Giving away many personal possessions
   C. Denial of suicidal thoughts when you ask
   D. Previous suicide threats

_____ 8. You are assessing a 36-year-old female who has a long history of depression and suicidal gestures and attempts. The family member who called 911 states that the patient has actually been exhibiting a sudden improvement from depression over the past few days. In this case, you should consider that the patient is:
   A. no longer suicidal.
   B. now ready to accept care.
   C. still at risk for suicide.
   D. none of these.

_____ 9. When assessing an aggressive patient for a possible threat to you or your crew, take all of the following actions *except*:
   A. trying to determine the patient's history of aggressive behavior.
   B. paying attention to the patient's speech and movement.
   C. noting the patient's posturing.
   D. assessing the patient in the kitchen.

_____ 10. If your 35-year-old male patient stands in a corner of the room with his fists clenched, screaming obscenities, you should:
   A. request police backup and keep the doorway in sight.
   B. raise your voice to a higher level than the patient's.
   C. challenge the patient in an attempt to calm him.
   D. explain that you would respond in the same way.

_____ 11. Use of reasonable force to restrain a patient should involve an evaluation of all of the following *except* the:
   A. patient's size and strength.
   B. family's ability to pay for your services.
   C. patient's mental status.
   D. available methods of restraint.

_____ 12. In some instances, the EMT may have to utilize force. The use of force by an EMT is generally allowed:
   A. to defend against an attack by an emotionally disturbed patient.
   B. only when the police are present.
   C. whenever a patient refuses any of your treatments.
   D. whenever you suspect the patient has been drinking.

_____ 13. Once the decision has been made to restrain your 22-year-old male patient, which one of the following steps should be avoided?
   A. Use multiple straps to restrain the patient.
   B. Reassure the patient throughout the procedure.
   C. Reassess the patient's distal circulation frequently.
   D. Use two rescuers to secure the patient.

_____ 14. You have physically restrained a patient who is combative to you and your crew. After he is safely secured, he begins to spit at you and your partner. This behavior can be managed best by:
   A. placing the patient in a prone position on the stretcher.
   B. wrapping the patient's mouth with roller gauze.
   C. placing 3-inch tape across the patient's mouth.
   D. placing a surgical mask on the patient's face.

_____ 15. You are treating a 28-year-old male patient who you feel is becoming a danger to himself or the people around him and will need to be transported against his will. You should:
   A. restrain the patient immediately.
   B. transport the patient with the family's assistance.
   C. contact the police for assistance.
   D. contact the patient's physician.

_____ 16. You are treating a 48-year-old male patient who you feel is exhibiting inappropriate behavior and has an altered mental status. Which of the following is not considered a cause of altered mental status?
   A. Low blood sugar
   B. Nervousness when speaking to a large group
   C. A lack of oxygen as in a stroke
   D. Blunt trauma to the head

_____ 17. The patient who has excited delirium is likely to have unexpected physical strength and:
   A. hypotension.   C. a narcotic overdose.
   B. hyperthermia.   D. bradycardia.

_____ 18. The care of the patient with a behavioral or psychiatric emergency should include each of the following, except:
   A. using good eye contact.
   B. encouraging patients to discuss what's troubling them.
   C. talking in a calm, reassuring voice.
   D. going along with their hallucinations.

_____ 19. Substance abuse, such as cocaine or amphetamines, can be associated with bizarre and/or aggressive behavior referred to as:
   A. positional asphyxia.   C. excited delirium.
   B. depression.   D. anxiety disorder.

_____ 20. Your patient is exhibiting an almost complete noninteraction with the environment and you have no reason to believe there is a medical cause for this behavior. What is this called?
   A. A delusion   C. A thought disorder
   B. Catatonia   D. Anxiety burnout

Pathophysiology: Neurotransmitters

1. What is the purpose of a neurotransmitter?

_____

2. Medications such as Prozac®, Paxil®, Zoloft®, and Celexa® are in a class of medications called selective serotonin reuptake inhibitors. What are these medications used for and why?

_____

Complete the Following

1. List nine factors that are associated with a risk for suicide.

A. _____

B. _____

C. _____

D. _____

E. _____

F. _____

G. _____

H. _____

I. _____

2. When a patient acts as if he or she may hurt himself or herself or others, your first concern must be your own safety. List three precautions you should take.

A. _____

B. _____

C. _____

3. List behaviors that you may expect to see in an aggressive or hostile patient.

A. _____

B. _____

C. _____

D. _____

E. _____

4. List seven common presentations, or signs and symptoms, of patients experiencing a psychiatric emergency.

A. _____

B. _____

C. _____

D. _____

E. _____

F. _____

G. _____

Case Study: Today Is Not the Day to Die

You respond to a call for a 36-year-old male who is bleeding severely. It is late at night, the call is to a private residence, and the police are also responding. On your arrival, a police officer meets your crew at the door and tells you that the patient had a razor and has slashed both of his wrists numerous times. They talked him into dropping the razor, but he is going to require medical care. As you approach the patient, you introduce yourself and see that there is a blood trail all over the floor.

1. Since you can talk with the patient, what are the next steps of the primary assessment?

_____

_____

GZQ **2.** The patient still has a considerable amount of bleeding from the right wrist. What should you do?

_____

_____

3. Blood is oozing from some wounds and flowing from others. What types of vessels did the patient likely cut?

_____

_____

After beginning to control the bleeding wounds, you are able to engage the patient to say what happened. It seems that he is very upset because his wife left him after months of his being unemployed. He also has no money and way too many bills, so their family needs to file bankruptcy.

4. Would it be appropriate to ask the patient whether he was trying to take his own life?

_____

_____

5. The patient says that he does not want to go to the hospital because he does not want his wife to find out what happened here tonight. What should you do?

_____

_____

After further questioning, the patient starts to get very agitated and insists that he will not go to the hospital. You feel strongly that he needs to go for wound care, stitches, a tetanus shot, and a mental health assessment. The police officer calls you aside and states that he and his fellow officers will help you restrain the patient if you feel that he needs to go.

GZQ **6.** If you need to restrain the patient, how should restraint be done?

_____

_____

Hematologic and Renal Emergencies

Core Concepts

- Disorders of the hematologic system.
- Disorders of the renal system.

Outcomes

After reading this chapter, you should be able to:

28.1 Explain the anatomy and physiology of the blood as an organ. (pp. 765–766)
- Describe the overall functions of the blood.
- Identify the elements required for normal blood clotting.

28.2 Summarize the characteristics of disorders of the blood. (pp. 766–767)
- Describe the spectrum of coagulopathies.
- Recognize causes of coagulopathies.

28.3 Describe the EMT care approach to patients with coagulopathies. (pp. 767–770)
- Identify patients in whom coagulopathies may be a factor in their stability.
- Describe EMT decision making that provides coagulopathy patients with the best potential outcomes.
- Compare the characteristics of different types of anemia.
- Relate the pathophysiology of sickle cell anemia to presentations of the disease.

28.4 Describe the EMT care approach to patients with sickle cell anemia. (p. 770)
- State the importance of clarifying whether a patient has sickle cell anemia or sickle cell trait.
- Identify the signs and symptoms of sickle cell anemia emergencies.
- Identify the role of oxygen in treating sickle cell emergencies.
- Recognize factors that influence an EMT's decision to request ALS when caring for a patient with sickle cell anemia.

28.5 Summarize the anatomy and physiology of the kidneys. (pp. 771–772)
- Describe the function of each structure of the renal system.
- Describe the role of the kidneys in maintaining the proper balance of substances in the blood.
- Explain the kidneys' reactions to differences in hydration.

28.6 Summarize features of diseases of the renal system. (pp. 771–776)
- Identify the risk associated with inadequately treated urinary tract infections.
- Identify the circumstances when kidney stones become painful.
- Recognize reasons why patients may use urinary catheters.

- Describe the pathophysiology of renal failure.
- Recognize causes of acute renal failure.
- State causes of chronic renal failure.
- Compare the processes of hemodialysis and peritoneal dialysis in patients with renal failure.

28.7 Summarize the EMT care approach to patients with medical emergencies related to end-stage renal disease. (pp. 776–779)
- List complications of end-stage renal disease.
- Explain the consequences of missing dialysis appointments.
- Recognize complications of dialysis.
- Propose care plans for a variety of portrayals of dialysis complications.
- Describe the considerations in caring for a kidney transplant patient.

Match Key Terms

A. Irreversible renal failure to the extent to which the kidneys can no longer provide adequate filtration and fluid balance to sustain life.

B. A mechanical process for dialysis in which a machine fills and empties the abdominal cavity of dialysis solution.

C. A gravity exchange process for dialysis in which a bag of dialysis fluid is raised above the level of an abdominal catheter to fill the abdominal cavity and then is lowered below the level of the abdominal catheter to drain the fluid out.

D. Deficiency in the number of red blood cells in the circulation.

E. The process by which toxins and excess fluid are removed from the body by a medical system independent of the kidneys.

F. An abnormally low number of RBCs in the circulation due to sickle cell disease.

G. Loss of the kidneys' ability to filter the blood and remove toxins and excess fluid from the body, the condition may be reversible depending on cause.

H. A vibration felt on gentle palpation, such as that which typically occurs within an arterial-venous fistula.

I. Infection within the peritoneal cavity.

J. One cycle of filling and draining the peritoneal cavity in peritoneal dialysis.

K. Loss of the normal ability to form a blood clot with internal or external bleeding.

L. An inherited disease in which patients have a genetic defect in their hemoglobin that results in an abnormal structure of the red blood cell.

M. An infection that begins in the urinary tract and ascends up the ureter into the kidney.

N. A drainage tube placed into the urinary system to allow the flow of urine out of the body.

_____ **1.** Anemia

_____ **2.** Continuous ambulatory peritoneal dialysis (CAPD)

_____ **3.** Continuous cycle assisted peritoneal dialysis (CCPD)

_____ **4.** Dialysis

_____ **5.** End-stage renal disease (ESRD)

_____ **6.** Exchange

_____ **7.** Peritonitis

_____ **8.** Renal failure

_____ **9.** Sickle cell anemia (SCA)

_____ **10.** Thrill

_____ **11.** Coagulopathy

_____ **12.** Urinary catheter

_____ **13.** Pyelonephritis

_____ **14.** Sickle cell disease (SCD)

Multiple-Choice Review

_____ **1.** The medical specialty concerned with diseases that affect the kidneys is:
A. neurology.
B. nephrology.
C. histology.
D. hematology.

_____ **2.** The purpose of blood is to do each of the following, _except_:
A. remove oxygen from the cells.
B. control bleeding by clotting.
C. deliver waste products to the kidneys and the liver.
D. remove carbon dioxide from the cells.

_____ **3.** You are obtaining a history from a 48-year-old male who tells you that he has a blood disorder. The medical specialty concerned with the blood disorders is:
A. nephrology.
B. neurology.
C. hematology.
D. histology.

_____ **4.** A component of the blood that is critical to the body's response to infection is:
A. red blood cells.
B. platelets.
C. white blood cells.
D. hemoglobin.

_____ **5.** A component of the blood that is designed to aggregate as a response to a bleeding injury is:
A. red blood cells.
B. platelets.
C. white blood cells.
D. hemoglobin.

_____ **6.** The liquid in which the blood cells and platelets are suspended is called:
A. interstitial fluid.
B. plasma.
C. lymph (fibrinolytic).
D. coumadin.

_____ **7.** You are assessing a 45-year-old male who tells you that he has chronic anemia. He is pale and complains of fatigue. This condition could be due to:
A. and increase in blood iron and hemoglobin levels.
B. a slow GI bleed.
C. a disease that affects the white blood cells.
D. all of these.

_____ **8.** Your 32-year-old female patient tells you that she has a genetic disease, but she does not specify what it is. She goes on to say that she had to have her spleen removed a few years ago. She called the ambulance today because she has severe pain in her arms, legs, and abdomen. What condition is likely given this information?
A. A stroke
B. A pulmonary embolism
C. A sickle cell crisis
D. A blood clot in the aorta

_____ **9.** A complication that may be found in a 35-year-old male, in respiratory distress, who has sickle cell anemia is:
A. destruction of the spleen.
B. acute chest syndrome.
C. priapism.
D. all of these.

_____ **10.** During the general management of a patient with sickle cell disease, you should be prepared to provide:
A. high-flow supplemental oxygen.
B. monitoring for a high fever.
C. treatment for shock.
D. all of these.

_____ **11.** Your 58-year-old female patient has a long history of ineffectively controlled diabetes and hypertension. What life-ending disease is highly likely to occur in this patient?
A. GI bleeding
B. Renal failure
C. Brain hemorrhage
D. COPD

_____ 12. Patients who are taking medications such as: Coumadin®, Pradaxa®, Xarelto®, and Eliquis® often have a medical history of:
- **A.** atrial fibrillation.
- **B.** stroke.
- **C.** heart attack.
- **D.** any of the above.

_____ 13. The process by which an external medical system independent of the kidneys is used to remove toxins and excess fluid from the body is called:
- **A.** excretion.
- **B.** dehydration.
- **C.** dialysis.
- **D.** resuscitator.

_____ 14. Your 56-year-old male patient tells you that he has kidney problems and must go to the clinic three times a week. The reason he goes there is probably to:
- **A.** do blood tests.
- **B.** take blood transfusions.
- **C.** receive hemodialysis.
- **D.** undergo peritoneal dialysis.

_____ 15. A vibration that can be palpated at the fistula in the arm of the dialysis patient is called a(n):
- **A.** thrill.
- **B.** aneurism.
- **C.** hematoma.
- **D.** embolism.

_____ 16. A winter storm over the last few days has closed the schools and affected road travel. You are called to the home of a 62-year-old female patient who states that she missed dialysis twice this week because of the storm. What are the symptoms that she may exhibit?
- **A.** Shortness of breath
- **B.** Fluid in the lungs
- **C.** Swollen ankles, hands, and face
- **D.** All of these

_____ 17. The most commonly transplanted organ(s) is (are) the:
- **A.** kidneys.
- **B.** liver.
- **C.** lungs.
- **D.** spleen.

_____ 18. You are treating a 58-year-old female who states that she is not feeling well after returning home from her dialysis treatment. All of the following are complications of dialysis *except*:
- **A.** development of an aortic aneurism.
- **B.** bleeding from the site of the A-V fistula.
- **C.** clotting and loss of function of the A-V fistula.
- **D.** a bacterial infection of the blood.

_____ 19. The most common serious complication of ESRD patients on peritoneal dialysis is:
- **A.** pulmonary edema.
- **B.** peritonitis.
- **C.** kidney rejection.
- **D.** stroke.

_____ 20. When encountering an ESRD patient who missed dialysis and is experiencing problems, the EMT should do each of the following *except*:
- **A.** consider CPAP in severe respiratory distress.
- **B.** be prepared for a cardiac arrest.
- **C.** check the BP on the arm with the fistula.
- **D.** administer high-flow oxygen if in respiratory distress.

Complete the Following

1. List the two types of peritoneal dialysis.

   A. _____

   B. _____

2. What is the difference between the two types of peritoneal dialysis?

A. _____

B. _____

3. List seven steps in the assessment and care of ESRD patient who has missed dialysis.

A. _____

B. _____

C. _____

D. _____

E. _____

F. _____

G. _____

Case Study: Simply No Comfortable Position

Your unit is responding to a call from a freeway rest stop for an unknown situation in the men's restroom. When you and your partner arrive at the rest stop, there is already a state trooper on the scene who says that there is a 25-year-old male in severe pain in one of the stalls. The scene is safe, so you all proceed into the restroom and introduce yourself to a young adult, who identifies himself as Darryl.

The patient has been trying to urinate unsuccessfully. He appears very uncomfortable, as if he cannot find a position to sit still for even a moment. The trooper pulls your partner aside and asks, "Is this guy on drugs?" Your partner says, "Not sure. Let's evaluate him and see what's up."

Darryl's mental status is alert and very anxious. His airway is open and clear, and his breathing is normal. He is a bit pale, cool, and clammy, and there is no external bleeding. You decide, because of the severe pain, that he is a high priority, and you continue with the secondary assessment of a responsive medical patient. Aside from being nauseated and having vomited once, Darryl's chief complaint is pain described as a 10 on a scale of 1 to 10. Your partner states that the medic unit should be on the scene in about five minutes. You decide to get a quick set of baseline vital signs and try to find a comfortable position for the patient on your stretcher. Then you can meet the medic outside in the ambulance to save some time.

Darryl's pain is unilateral flank pain on the right side. He denies any other painful areas in his head, chest, or abdomen. He also says that he felt a little dizzy when he was trying to urinate but did not actually pass out. You manage to get him onto the stretcher, and your partner reports that his vital signs are pulse 100 and regular, respirations 20 and normal, a blood pressure of 118/72 mmHg, and SpO_2 of 98%.

1. From the history you have obtained so far, what do you suspect is the patient's problem?

_____

2. Darryl does mention that he always carries a water bottle but forgot to get one at the last gas station, which was a few hours ago. How might this be relevant?

_____

You begin to ask specific questions about the chief complaint (OPQRST) and obtain a SAMPLE history. It seems that the patient is not on any specific medication but has been told by his doctor to stay away from foods that are high in calcium. He says that he had a kidney stone about five years ago and this pain is very similar.

3. If Darryl tells you that he had a kidney stone before and this pain is similar, does that end your assessment?

_____

4. Do you think it is necessary to put Darryl on high-concentration oxygen at this point?

_____

GZQ 5. Using your clinical judgment and the information you have obtained from the patient so far, should you cancel the medic unit and take a slow ride to the emergency department, since his baseline vital signs are all within normal range?

_____

Interim Exam 2

Use the answer sheet provided to complete this exam. It is perforated, so it can be removed easily from this workbook.

1. The scene size-up begins as you approach the location of the EMS call and:
   A. continues throughout the entire call.
   B. ends when you arrive at the patient.
   C. includes assessing airway, breathing, and circulation.
   D. helps you discover all possible dangers at the scene.

2. At the scene of a motor vehicle collision the EMT identifies multiple patients. The next action the EMT takes is to:
   A. triage all the patients.
   B. begin treatment on the most critical patient.
   C. separate the patients by severity of injury.
   D. contact dispatch for additional ambulances.

3. After forming a general impression, the next part of the primary assessment is:
   A. assessing breathing.
   B. assessing mental status.
   C. determining the priority of the patient.
   D. assessing the airway.

4. The "V" in AVPU stands for:
   A. virtual.   C. verbal.
   B. visible.   D. vertex.

5. The "P" in AVPU stands for:
   A. pulse.   C. prior.
   B. painful.   D. past history.

6. If a patient's level of responsiveness is lower than "Alert," and breathing is inadequate, you should:
   A. apply a cervical collar.
   B. administer high-concentration oxygen.
   C. place the patient in a recovery position.
   D. assist ventilations.

7. If a patient is talking or crying, assume that the patient:
   A. is in little pain.
   B. has no life-threatening bleeding.
   C. has an open airway.
   D. has an "A" mental status.

8. Pale clammy skin often indicates:
   A. nervous system damage.
   B. shock.
   C. an extremely high temperature.
   D. an airway problem.

9. When opening the airway of an unresponsive infant, the EMT should:
   A. tilt the head and lift the chin.
   B. place the head in a neutral position.
   C. perform a jaw thrust maneuver.
   D. have suction ready.

10. Tuberculosis is a respiratory infection that includes a cough, fever, night sweats, and weight loss. Special considerations with this disease should include:
    A. chronic untreated infection can lead to cirrhosis.
    B. EMTs should wear N-95 respirators when treating this patient.
    C. adult males can develop inflammation of the testicles.
    D. can be fatal to infants so vaccination of adults is very important.

11. When evaluating the circulation in an infant, the EMT should use the:
    A. femoral pulse.
    B. distal pulse check.
    C. capillary refill test.
    D. radial pulse.

12. When assessing the pupils, the EMT may shine a light into the eyes looking for:
    A. size and color.
    B. size, equality, and reactivity.
    C. foreign objects.
    D. ocular pressure.

13. The EMT documents that the patient with chest pain denies shortness of breath. This is most appropriately termed:
    A. an informative objective.
    B. advisory information.
    C. a pertinent negative.
    D. run data information.

14. The device that measures the proportion of oxygen in the blood is a:
    A. $EtCO_2$ wave form monitor.
    B. CO-oximeter.
    C. pulse oximeter.
    D. end-tidal CO detector.

15. Which statement best describes an important concept of documentation?
    A. Always fill out a continuation sheet.
    B. If it is not written down, you did not do it.
    C. It should include plenty of medical terms.
    D. Document everything you see.

©2021 Pearson Education, Inc.
Emergency Care, 14th Ed.

16. If the patient does not want to go to the hospital, the EMT should:
    A. document with a refusal-of-care form.
    B. take the patient to the hospital anyway.
    C. end the assessment immediately.
    D. call for another crew to subdue the patient.

17. An important part of the assessment or care was not performed. This is called an error of:
    A. submission.   C. inhibition.
    B. omission.   D. commission.

18. If an EMT makes up a set of vitals for inclusion on the prehospital care report (PCR), this is called:
    A. assault.   C. falsification.
    B. libel.   D. battery.

19. The EMT writes, "The patient is alert and oriented" on the prehospital care report (PCR) This is an example of:
    A. objective information.
    B. interpreted information.
    C. subjective information.
    D. nonfactual information.

20. When you are documenting exactly what a patient told you on the prehospital care report (PCR), you should:
    A. paraphrase for brevity.
    B. summarize the key points.
    C. use medical terminology.
    D. use quotes around the statement.

21. After establishing the patient's mental status, the next part of the primary assessment is to:
    A. ensure an open airway.
    B. check for adequate breathing.
    C. check for circulation.
    D. look for profuse bleeding.

22. Which of the following is a true vital sign?
    A. Nausea
    B. Skin temperature
    C. Level of responsiveness
    D. Age

23. The normal pulse rate for an adult at rest is between _____ beats per minute.
    A. 50 and 70   C. 65 and 95
    B. 60 and 100   D. 80 and 100

24. During the determination of vital signs, the initial pulse rate for patients 1 year of age and older is normally taken at the _____ pulse.
    A. carotid   C. pedal
    B. femoral   D. radial

25. When the force of the pulse is weak and thin, it is described as:
    A. shallow.   C. partial.
    B. full.   D. thready.

26. Normal at-rest respiration rates for adults vary from _____ breaths per minute.
    A. 5 to 10   C. 15 to 30
    B. 12 to 20   D. 20 to 32

27. A noisy, harsh sound heard during inhalation that indicates a partial airway obstruction is:
    A. gurgling.
    B. snorting.
    C. stertorous respirations.
    D. crowing.

28. The systolic blood pressure indicates the arterial pressure that is created when the:
    A. artery contracts.   C. heart contracts.
    B. artery relaxes.   D. heart relaxes.

29. Diastolic blood pressure indicates the arterial pressure that is created as the:
    A. heart contracts.
    B. heart refills.
    C. artery contracts.
    D. artery relaxes.

30. Determining the blood pressure by palpation is:
    A. not as accurate as by the auscultation method.
    B. used when there is no noise around a patient.
    C. documented as the "palp/diastolic."
    D. used whenever the patient is hypertensive.

31. Information that you can see, hear, feel, or smell is called a(n):
    A. sign.   C. symptom.
    B. sensation.   D. assessment.

32. When you ask your patient, "Have you recently had any surgery or injuries?" you are inquiring about the:
    A. patient's medications.
    B. patient's pertinent past history.
    C. events leading up to the illness.
    D. allergies that the patient may have.

33. A young child has croup, which is an upper respiratory infection including dyspnea and:
    A. rash on the torso.
    B. stiffness in the neck.
    C. a bark-like cough.
    D. ringing in the ears.

34. An acronym that is used to remember what questions to ask about the patient's present problem and past history is:
A. AVPU. C. SAMPLE.
B. DCAP-BTLS. D. PEARL.

35. In the prehospital setting using a blood glucose meter, a normal blood glucose level is usually:
A. less than 100 mg/dL.
B. more than 100 mg/dL.
C. 70-100 mg/dL.
D. 120-140 mg/dL.

36. Capnography is often used when EMS is performing CPR because it:
A. helps to identify a return of pulse.
B. measures the amount of oxygen in the blood.
C. measures the amount of carbon dioxide in capillary blood.
D. helps to determine when to start CPR.

37. When assessing an alert pediatric patient, the EMT may have to modify the physical exam by:
A. singing to the child.
B. assessing extremities first.
C. letting the parent do the exam with your instruction.
D. observing only, not touching.

38. The term for having difficulty breathing when lying down is:
A. hypoxia. C. tachypnea.
B. dyspnea. D. orthopnea.

39. In taking a patient's blood pressure, the stethoscope is placed over the _____ artery.
A. carotid C. brachial
B. radial D. femoral

40. A 32-year-old male adult patient is complaining of nausea, loss of appetite, malaise, abdominal pain, and jaundice. What precautions should the EMT take?.
A. Isolate the patient.
B. Wear an N-95 mask.
C. Wear a gown if you will do direct lifting.
D. Avoid contact with the patient's blood.

41. When there are no apparent hazards at the scene of a collision, the danger zone should extend _____ feet in all directions from the wreckage.
A. 25 C. 75
B. 50 D. 100

42. An elderly woman fell and as a result has some minor bruising to her head, and she has a headache. She has a history of an irregular heartbeat for which she takes medication. Which medication makes you think that this patient should be transported to the hospital right away?
A. antihypertensive C. blood thinner
B. beta blocker D. insulin

43. The purpose of the primary assessment is to:
A. take the patient's vital signs.
B. gather information about the collision.
C. discover and treat life-threatening conditions.
D. obtain the patient's history.

44. Anemia is a blood disorder in which the number of _____ is deficient.
A. white blood cells
B. red blood cells
C. platelets
D. clotting factors

45. The "S" in OPQRST stands for:
A. SAMPLE. C. severity.
B. situation. D. scene.

46. A 42-year-old male with a complaint of severe abdominal pain has baseline vital signs that are respiratory rate of 20 nonlabored, pulse of 100 and regular, blood pressure 88/60. When should his vital signs be assessed next?
A. After oxygen is administered.
B. When the patient is in the ambulance.
C. About every 15 minutes.
D. About every 5 minutes.

47. Which of the following is *true* of the rapid trauma assessment?
A. It begins with examination of the posterior body and ends with examination of the head.
B. It evaluates areas of the body where the greatest threats to the patient are likely to be.
C. It is performed on a trauma patient who has no significant mechanism of injury.
D. It includes careful examination of the face, eyes, ears, nose, and mouth.

48. On which type of patient is the detailed secondary assessment most often performed?
A. A trauma patient with a significant mechanism of injury
B. A trauma patient with no significant mechanism of injury
C. A responsive medical patient
D. An unresponsive medical patient

©2021 Pearson Education, Inc.
Emergency Care, 14th Ed.

49. To obtain a history of a patient's present illness:
   A. ask the OPQRST questions.
   B. conduct the subjective interview.
   C. ask the SAMPLE questions.
   D. use the look, listen, feel, and smell method.

50. The "P" in OPQRST stands for:
   A. punctures.   C. provocation.
   B. penetrations.   D. pulses.

51. For a stable patient, you should perform the reassessment every _____ minutes.
   A. 5   C. 15
   B. 10   D. 20

52. During your reassessment, whenever you believe there may have been a change in the patient's condition, you should:
   A. repeat the primary assessment.
   B. transport the patient immediately.
   C. document trends in vital signs.
   D. repeat the rapid trauma assessment.

53. Pale, clammy skin in a middle-aged male most likely indicates:
   A. high fever.
   B. exposure to cold.
   C. mild fever.
   D. shock.

54. The overriding concern of the EMT at all times is:
   A. the patient's safety.
   B. the safety of patients and bystanders.
   C. the patient's life.
   D. personal safety.

55. The chief complaint of your patient is:
   A. what you find in the primary assessment.
   B. what you find in the secondary assessment.
   C. what the patient tells you is the matter.
   D. obtained when getting a patient history.

56. Infants and young children under the age of _____ years are primarily abdominal breathers.
   A. 2   C. 8
   B. 4   D. 12

57. At the scene of a motor vehicle collision, you are assessing a patient who is sitting up behind the steering wheel in her vehicle. You see that she has jugular vein distention (JVD) which could be an indication that:
   A. her heart is not pumping effectively.
   B. she has a head injury.
   C. she is about to go into cardiac arrest.
   D. there is no problem this is a normal finding.

58. Which of the following is an appropriate interpersonal communication technique?
   A. Standing above a patient
   B. Avoiding eye contact
   C. Directly facing a patient
   D. Standing with arms crossed

59. What is the *first* item given to the hospital in your medical radio report to the receiving facility?
   A. The patient's age and sex
   B. Unit identification and level of provider
   C. Estimated time of arrival
   D. Emergency medical care given

60. Pediatric patients with a traumatic injury are susceptible to spinal cord injury because:
   A. their bones fracture easily.
   B. neck muscles are underdeveloped.
   C. the spinal cord is proportionately larger than adults.
   D. they have soft spots in the skull.

61. Which of the following is *true* of the medical radio report?
   A. The EMT uses codes to communicate patient information.
   B. The EMT makes sure to give his or her patient diagnosis.
   C. The EMT paints a picture of the patient's problem in words.
   D. The EMT speaks rapidly to limit transmission time.

62. When listening to lung sounds in the infant, the EMT should place a stethoscope:
   A. on the sides of the chest.
   B. on the back.
   C. over the middle of the neck.
   D. over the top of the lungs.

63. Any action of a drug other than the desired action is called a(n):
   A. contraindication.
   B. indication.
   C. reflex.
   D. side effect.

64. When a drug is administered subcutaneously, it is:
   A. dissolved under the tongue.
   B. injected into a vein.
   C. rubbed into a muscle.
   D. injected under the skin.

65. In the prehospital setting the EMT may give aspirin to a patient with suspected cardiac chest pain because it:
   A. can reduce pain.
   B. it is easy to administer.
   C. no one is allergic to aspirin.
   D. can reduce blood clotting.

66. The adequate rate of artificial ventilations for a nonbreathing adult with a pulse patient is _____ breaths per minute.
- **A.** 6–8
- **B.** 10–12
- **C.** 14–16
- **D.** 18–20

67. The adequate rate of artificial ventilations for a nonbreathing infant or child patient with a pulse is _____ breaths per minute.
- **A.** 8–16
- **B.** 10–18
- **C.** 12–20
- **D.** 16–24

68. Which of the following respiratory sounds made by an unresponsive adult most likely indicates a serious airway problem that requires immediate intervention?
- **A.** Snoring or gurgling
- **B.** Slight wheezing
- **C.** Sniffling
- **D.** Whistling or grunting

69. The skin of a patient with inadequate breathing will most likely be:
- **A.** pale, cool, and dry.
- **B.** red, hot, and clammy.
- **C.** yellow, warm, and dry.
- **D.** blue, cool, and clammy.

70. If a patient is experiencing breathing difficulty but is breathing adequately, it is usually best to place the patient in the _____ position.
- **A.** bipod
- **B.** supine
- **C.** sitting-up
- **D.** recovery

71. Which of the following is a name for adult chest pain due to a decreased blood supply to the heart muscle?
- **A.** Stroke
- **B.** Dysrhythmia
- **C.** Congestive heart failure
- **D.** Angina pectoris

72. Most heart attacks are caused by the narrowing or occlusion of a _____ artery.
- **A.** cephalic
- **B.** brachial
- **C.** coronary
- **D.** carotid

73. Which of the following is the condition in which a portion of the myocardium dies because of oxygen starvation?
- **A.** Angina pectoris
- **B.** Mechanical pump failure
- **C.** Cardiogenic shock
- **D.** Acute myocardial infarction

74. An irregular heart rhythm is called:
- **A.** bradyrhythmia.
- **B.** dysrhythmia.
- **C.** hyperrhythmia.
- **D.** eurhythmia.

75. Which of the following terms applies to an adult pulse rate that is slower than 60 beats per minute?
- **A.** Bradycardia
- **B.** Ventricular fibrillation
- **C.** Tachycardia
- **D.** Atrial fibrillation

76. An adult at-rest heartbeat that is faster than 100 beats per minute is referred to as:
- **A.** bradycardia.
- **B.** ventricular fibrillation.
- **C.** tachycardia.
- **D.** atrial fibrillation.

77. Which of the following is the name for a condition caused by excessive fluid buildup in the lungs because of the inadequate pumping of the heart?
- **A.** Heart failure
- **B.** Acute lung failure
- **C.** Acute myocardial infarction
- **D.** Chronic angina pectoris

78. A diabetic with a weak, rapid pulse and cold, clammy skin who complains of hunger is suffering from:
- **A.** hypoglycemia.
- **B.** cardiogenic shock.
- **C.** hyperglycemia.
- **D.** ulcers.

79. Which of the following conditions frequently results in an acetone smell on the patient's breath?
- **A.** Stroke
- **B.** Hyperglycemia
- **C.** Ulcers
- **D.** Hypoglycemia

80. A conscious hypoglycemic patient who is able to swallow is frequently administered:
- **A.** oral glucose.
- **B.** insulin.
- **C.** nitroglycerin.
- **D.** epinephrine.

81. You are treating a 25-year-old female diabetic patient. If you cannot administer glucose gel because she is not alert enough to swallow, you should:
- **A.** wait until her mental status improves.
- **B.** contact medical direction immediately.
- **C.** treat her like any other patient with altered mental status.
- **D.** place her in a position of comfort.

82. The first time a person is exposed to an allergen, the immune system:
- **A.** reacts violently.
- **B.** shuts down.
- **C.** forms antibodies.
- **D.** ignores the allergen.

©2021 Pearson Education, Inc.
Emergency Care, 14th Ed.

83. To be considered a severe allergic reaction, a patient must have signs and symptoms of shock and/or:
    A. a history of allergies.
    B. massive swelling.
    C. respiratory distress.
    D. increased blood pressure.

84. A 21-year-old male patient who has no history of allergies is having his first allergic reaction. What action should you take?
    A. Consult with medical direction.
    B. Treat for shock and transport immediately.
    C. Administer epinephrine via auto-injector.
    D. Attempt to determine the cause.

85. Carbon monoxide, chlorine, and ammonia are examples of _____ poisons.
    A. ingested
    C. inhaled
    B. injected
    D. absorbed

86. It is important for the EMT to determine when the ingestion of a poison occurred because:
    A. different poisons act on the body at different rates.
    B. people who ingest poison in the evening tend to vomit frequently.
    C. dilution of the poison is ineffective after ten minutes.
    D. the antidote is more effective once the poison reaches the stomach.

87. The principal prehospital treatment of a patient who has inhaled poisonous gas is:
    A. administering activated charcoal.
    B. administering high-concentration oxygen.
    C. rapidly administering an antidote.
    D. irrigating the respiratory tract with water.

88. Drinking alcohol along with taking beta blockers can result in:
    A. uncontrolled shivering.
    B. depressed vital signs.
    C. extreme agitation.
    D. all of these.

89. Most cases of poisoning:
    A. are intentional.
    B. involve elderly patients.
    C. involve young children.
    D. lead to disability or death.

90. Poisons that are swallowed are _____ poisons.
    A. absorbed
    C. ingested
    B. inhaled
    D. injected

91. When assessing a small child who is having difficulty breathing, which of the following is a late sign of respiratory distress?
    A. Nasal flaring
    B. Tachycardia
    C. Bradycardia
    D. Stridor

92. The physical exam of an older adult woman reveals swelling in both feet, ankles and lower legs. This finding is associated with a/an:
    A. allergic reaction.
    B. cardiac history.
    C. endocrine disorder.
    D. pancreatitis.

93. The administration of nitroglycerin to a patient with suspected cardiac chest pain will:
    A. increase the workload of the heart.
    B. decrease the workload of the heart.
    C. cause nausea and vomiting.
    D. increase the blood pressure.

94. In which of the following patients should the EMT begin chest compressions?
    A. Unresponsive infant with a heart rate of 50.
    B. Unresponsive adult with a heart rate of 40.
    C. An adult who is not breathing but has a pulse.
    D. An unconscious elderly patient who has an implanted defibrillator that is discharging.

95. The most serious condition of the kidneys is:
    A. pyelonephritis.
    B. urinary tract infection.
    C. kidney stones.
    D. renal failure.

96. The organs that are found outside the peritoneum and between the abdomen and the back are in the:
    A. posterior pelvic compartment.
    B. retroperitoneal space.
    C. periumbilical region.
    D. posterior buttocks.

97. The spleen is located in the _____ quadrant.
    A. upper right
    B. lower right
    C. upper left
    D. lower left

98. Your 60-year-old male patient tells you that he has a tearing sensation going into the middle of his back. He states that he has no back problems and has a history of hypertension. What is possibly wrong with him?
A. A kidney stone
B. Acute pulmonary edema
C. Acute appendicitis
D. An aortic aneurysm

99. Your 32-year-old male patient has a history of alcoholism and is complaining of stomach pains and feeling weak and dizzy. He states that he vomited a coffee ground emesis twice and has had very dark, foul-smelling diarrhea all day. What is the likely cause of today's problem?
A. He also has diabetes and needs insulin.
B. He has a bleeding ulcer.
C. He is having a stroke.
D. His spleen is malfunctioning.

100. Your first step when called to care for any attempted suicide victim is to:
A. gain access to the patient.
B. wait for police assistance.
C. survey the patient for behavioral changes.
D. ensure your own safety.

101. You are on the scene of a patient with whom the police have been talking for quite some time. They were originally called to the patient's home because a neighbor thought she had heard shots fired. No one was injured, but there are weapons in the home. You are unable to perform normal assessment and care procedures because the patient is aggressive and hostile. What action should you take?
A. Restrain the patient immediately.
B. Ask a family member to assist you.
C. Seek advice from medical direction.
D. Call the patient's physician.

102. A disease that interferes with the body's ability to transport glucose into cells is:
A. sickle cell anemia.
B. diabetes.
C. hepatitis A.
D. meningitis.

103. When a patient presents with more than one condition or with a familiar condition but under unusual circumstances, the EMT should:
A. call medical direction right away.
B. call for an ALS unit right away.
C. assess the patient as usual and then seek guidance.
D. assign a higher priority to the patient.

104. A patient with acute abdominal pain and a history of alcoholism also has referred pain to the back and shoulders. What condition do you suspect?
A. Pancreatitis
B. Abdominal aortic aneurysm
C. Appendicitis
D. Kidney stones

105. During the physical exam of the patient with abdominal pain it is recommended that the EMT:
A. rapidly transport to the trauma center.
B. do not touch a guarded abdomen.
C. palpate the area with pain first.
D. palpate the area with pain last.

106. Your 59-year-old female patient has slurred speech. She may have had:
A. a stroke.
B. an overdose.
C. a seizure.
D. any of these.

107. The function of the kidneys is to:
A. produce clotting factors.
B. filter blood and remove wastes.
C. maintain normal levels of hemoglobin.
D. prevent anemia.

108. When assessing a dialysis patient with a surgically created fistula in their arm, the EMT should:
A. obtain a blood pressure below the fistula.
B. obtain a blood pressure above the fistula.
C. avoid taking a blood pressure in the same arm.
D. palpate the fistula for a thrill.

109. You are dispatched to a call for a possible stroke. When you arrive on scene you find a patient who has no distress. Her daughter called 9-1-1 because mother was unable to speak or move for 10 minutes, but now is feeling better. What do you suspect is happening?
A. The patient is having a psychiatric problem.
B. The patient had a stroke.
C. The patient may be having a mini-stroke or TIA.
D. The patient may be a diabetic.

110. The conclusion that you make about a patient's condition after assessing that patient is called your:
A. field diagnosis.
B. EMT diagnosis.
C. EMS diagnosis.
D. all of these are correct.

111. The analytical process that assists you in reaching a field diagnosis is referred to as:
    A. active assessment.
    B. passive assessment.
    C. critical thinking.
    D. detailed assessment.

112. Epinephrine is the drug of choice for severe allergic reaction because it:
    A. is a naturally occurring hormone.
    B. constricts airway passages.
    C. constricts blood vessels.
    D. dilates blood vessels.

113. You are on the scene of a 60-year-old female patient who is complaining of difficulty breathing and a fever. The list of conditions that may be the cause of her problems is referred to as the:
    A. admission diagnosis.
    B. presenting problem.
    C. differential diagnosis.
    D. assessment finding.

114. Which of the following is most accurate about anaphylaxis and the pediatric patient?
    A. Infants do not experience hypotension as adults do.
    B. The dose of epinephrine is less than an adult dose.
    C. The dose of epinephrine is 0.3 mg.
    D. Severe allergic reactions are common in older children.

115. A slow pulse, excessive salivation, nausea, vomiting and diarrhea are signs and symptoms associated with poisoning from:
    A. aspirin.
    B. antihistamines.
    C. petroleum products.
    D. insecticides.

116. The traditional approach to clinical diagnosis involves:
    A. narrowing down a long list.
    B. jumping to conclusions.
    C. taking lots of shortcuts.
    D. eliminating similar conditions.

117. When an EMT is specifically looking for evidence that supports the diagnosis he or she already has in mind, the EMT is committing a(n) _____ bias.
    A. anchoring
    B. confirmation
    C. satisfying
    D. illusionary

118. You once treated a 50-year-old female with heat stroke. The next time you have a female patient and you are in a warm environment you may be more likely to think of heat stroke as the diagnosis than more common problems such as dehydration. This bias is referred to as:
    A. overconfidence.
    B. illusory correlation.
    C. confirmation.
    D. availability.

119. The primary concern for the EMT treating a patient who has absorbed a poison through the skin is:
    A. maintaining the patient's airway.
    B. preventing exposure to the substance.
    C. to determine how much substance is on the patient.
    D. preventing shock.

120. You are treating a patient who was found lying on the floor in the basement of his son's house. He is in a lot of pain, and it seems evident that he has a fractured hip. If you stop the search for a diagnosis as soon as you note the fractured hip, this can lead to:
    A. missing out on the secondary diagnosis.
    B. overconfidence and misdiagnosis.
    C. overestimating the frequency of the problem.
    D. all of these.

121. You are treating a respiratory patient who is conscious, alert, and in severe distress. He took an albuterol treatment before your arrival on the scene. At this point, you have been administering CPAP for about 10 minutes. You notice that his mental status is rapidly diminishing. What should you do next?
    A. Administer another bronchodilator treatment per medical control.
    B. Remove the CPAP and ventilate the patient with a BVM device.
    C. Lower the level of pressure in the CPAP device considerably.
    D. Turn up the pressure of the oxygen going into the CPAP device.

122. You receive a high-priority call to meet an incoming airplane on the tarmac at the regional airport. A 60-year-old female patient with a history of deep vein thrombosis and 35 years of smoking a pack a day of cigarettes is acutely short

of breath. This shortness of breath began about 20 minutes ago. The duration of the flight was approximately 6 hours. What do you suspect is the patient's prehospital diagnosis?

A. An acute exacerbation of her COPD
B. The development of epiglottitis
C. A pulmonary embolism
D. Acute pulmonary edema

123. You arrive on the scene of a family who is very anxious because the 45-year-old father and his 17-year-old daughter were taking wood from the woodpile when they disturbed a beehive. They both have numerous stings. The daughter is experiencing signs of an anaphylactic reaction, while the father is experiencing a simple allergic reaction. You will most likely find that:

A. the daughter has hypotension.
B. the father has hypertension.
C. the daughter has hives.
D. the father has swelling of the airway structures.

124. You respond to a call for a woman who was described as sleeping in her car. The police have arrived and have broken a car window to gain access to the 35-year-old female because the doors were locked, and she is unconscious. As you enter the vehicle, there is a strong smell of rotten eggs. What should you suspect happened?

A. The exhaust fumes were not well vented on the vehicle, causing a CO_2 leak.
B. She may have attempted suicide by mixing chemicals to produce hydrogen sulfide.
C. There was a cyanide leak into the vehicle.
D. She may have taken an overdose of a strong sleeping pill.

125. The complications of sickle cell disease can include all of the following *except*:

A. destruction of the pancreas.
B. acute chest syndrome.
C. priapism.
D. stroke.

©2021 Pearson Education, Inc.
Emergency Care, 14th Ed.

Interim Exam 2 Answer Sheet

Fill in the correct answer for each item. When scoring, note that there are 125 questions valued at 0.8 point each.

1. [ ] A	[ ] B	[ ] C	[ ] D	**36.** [ ] A	[ ] B	[ ] C	[ ] D
2. [ ] A	[ ] B	[ ] C	[ ] D	**37.** [ ] A	[ ] B	[ ] C	[ ] D
3. [ ] A	[ ] B	[ ] C	[ ] D	**38.** [ ] A	[ ] B	[ ] C	[ ] D
4. [ ] A	[ ] B	[ ] C	[ ] D	**39.** [ ] A	[ ] B	[ ] C	[ ] D
5. [ ] A	[ ] B	[ ] C	[ ] D	**40.** [ ] A	[ ] B	[ ] C	[ ] D
6. [ ] A	[ ] B	[ ] C	[ ] D	**41.** [ ] A	[ ] B	[ ] C	[ ] D
7. [ ] A	[ ] B	[ ] C	[ ] D	**42.** [ ] A	[ ] B	[ ] C	[ ] D
8. [ ] A	[ ] B	[ ] C	[ ] D	**43.** [ ] A	[ ] B	[ ] C	[ ] D
9. [ ] A	[ ] B	[ ] C	[ ] D	**44.** [ ] A	[ ] B	[ ] C	[ ] D
10. [ ] A	[ ] B	[ ] C	[ ] D	**45.** [ ] A	[ ] B	[ ] C	[ ] D
11. [ ] A	[ ] B	[ ] C	[ ] D	**46.** [ ] A	[ ] B	[ ] C	[ ] D
12. [ ] A	[ ] B	[ ] C	[ ] D	**47.** [ ] A	[ ] B	[ ] C	[ ] D
13. [ ] A	[ ] B	[ ] C	[ ] D	**48.** [ ] A	[ ] B	[ ] C	[ ] D
14. [ ] A	[ ] B	[ ] C	[ ] D	**49.** [ ] A	[ ] B	[ ] C	[ ] D
15. [ ] A	[ ] B	[ ] C	[ ] D	**50.** [ ] A	[ ] B	[ ] C	[ ] D
16. [ ] A	[ ] B	[ ] C	[ ] D	**51.** [ ] A	[ ] B	[ ] C	[ ] D
17. [ ] A	[ ] B	[ ] C	[ ] D	**52.** [ ] A	[ ] B	[ ] C	[ ] D
18. [ ] A	[ ] B	[ ] C	[ ] D	**53.** [ ] A	[ ] B	[ ] C	[ ] D
19. [ ] A	[ ] B	[ ] C	[ ] D	**54.** [ ] A	[ ] B	[ ] C	[ ] D
20. [ ] A	[ ] B	[ ] C	[ ] D	**55.** [ ] A	[ ] B	[ ] C	[ ] D
21. [ ] A	[ ] B	[ ] C	[ ] D	**56.** [ ] A	[ ] B	[ ] C	[ ] D
22. [ ] A	[ ] B	[ ] C	[ ] D	**57.** [ ] A	[ ] B	[ ] C	[ ] D
23. [ ] A	[ ] B	[ ] C	[ ] D	**58.** [ ] A	[ ] B	[ ] C	[ ] D
24. [ ] A	[ ] B	[ ] C	[ ] D	**59.** [ ] A	[ ] B	[ ] C	[ ] D
25. [ ] A	[ ] B	[ ] C	[ ] D	**60.** [ ] A	[ ] B	[ ] C	[ ] D
26. [ ] A	[ ] B	[ ] C	[ ] D	**61.** [ ] A	[ ] B	[ ] C	[ ] D
27. [ ] A	[ ] B	[ ] C	[ ] D	**62.** [ ] A	[ ] B	[ ] C	[ ] D
28. [ ] A	[ ] B	[ ] C	[ ] D	**63.** [ ] A	[ ] B	[ ] C	[ ] D
29. [ ] A	[ ] B	[ ] C	[ ] D	**64.** [ ] A	[ ] B	[ ] C	[ ] D
30. [ ] A	[ ] B	[ ] C	[ ] D	**65.** [ ] A	[ ] B	[ ] C	[ ] D
31. [ ] A	[ ] B	[ ] C	[ ] D	**66.** [ ] A	[ ] B	[ ] C	[ ] D
32. [ ] A	[ ] B	[ ] C	[ ] D	**67.** [ ] A	[ ] B	[ ] C	[ ] D
33. [ ] A	[ ] B	[ ] C	[ ] D	**68.** [ ] A	[ ] B	[ ] C	[ ] D
34. [ ] A	[ ] B	[ ] C	[ ] D	**69.** [ ] A	[ ] B	[ ] C	[ ] D
35. [ ] A	[ ] B	[ ] C	[ ] D	**70.** [ ] A	[ ] B	[ ] C	[ ] D

71. [ ] A   [ ] B   [ ] C   [ ] D   99. [ ] A   [ ] B   [ ] C   [ ] D

72. [ ] A   [ ] B   [ ] C   [ ] D   100. [ ] A   [ ] B   [ ] C   [ ] D

73. [ ] A   [ ] B   [ ] C   [ ] D   101. [ ] A   [ ] B   [ ] C   [ ] D

74. [ ] A   [ ] B   [ ] C   [ ] D   102. [ ] A   [ ] B   [ ] C   [ ] D

75. [ ] A   [ ] B   [ ] C   [ ] D   103. [ ] A   [ ] B   [ ] C   [ ] D

76. [ ] A   [ ] B   [ ] C   [ ] D   104. [ ] A   [ ] B   [ ] C   [ ] D

77. [ ] A   [ ] B   [ ] C   [ ] D   105. [ ] A   [ ] B   [ ] C   [ ] D

78. [ ] A   [ ] B   [ ] C   [ ] D   106. [ ] A   [ ] B   [ ] C   [ ] D

79. [ ] A   [ ] B   [ ] C   [ ] D   107. [ ] A   [ ] B   [ ] C   [ ] D

80. [ ] A   [ ] B   [ ] C   [ ] D   108. [ ] A   [ ] B   [ ] C   [ ] D

81. [ ] A   [ ] B   [ ] C   [ ] D   109. [ ] A   [ ] B   [ ] C   [ ] D

82. [ ] A   [ ] B   [ ] C   [ ] D   110. [ ] A   [ ] B   [ ] C   [ ] D

83. [ ] A   [ ] B   [ ] C   [ ] D   111. [ ] A   [ ] B   [ ] C   [ ] D

84. [ ] A   [ ] B   [ ] C   [ ] D   112. [ ] A   [ ] B   [ ] C   [ ] D

85. [ ] A   [ ] B   [ ] C   [ ] D   113. [ ] A   [ ] B   [ ] C   [ ] D

86. [ ] A   [ ] B   [ ] C   [ ] D   114. [ ] A   [ ] B   [ ] C   [ ] D

87. [ ] A   [ ] B   [ ] C   [ ] D   115. [ ] A   [ ] B   [ ] C   [ ] D

88. [ ] A   [ ] B   [ ] C   [ ] D   116. [ ] A   [ ] B   [ ] C   [ ] D

89. [ ] A   [ ] B   [ ] C   [ ] D   117. [ ] A   [ ] B   [ ] C   [ ] D

90. [ ] A   [ ] B   [ ] C   [ ] D   118. [ ] A   [ ] B   [ ] C   [ ] D

91. [ ] A   [ ] B   [ ] C   [ ] D   119. [ ] A   [ ] B   [ ] C   [ ] D

92. [ ] A   [ ] B   [ ] C   [ ] D   120. [ ] A   [ ] B   [ ] C   [ ] D

93. [ ] A   [ ] B   [ ] C   [ ] D   121. [ ] A   [ ] B   [ ] C   [ ] D

94. [ ] A   [ ] B   [ ] C   [ ] D   122. [ ] A   [ ] B   [ ] C   [ ] D

95. [ ] A   [ ] B   [ ] C   [ ] D   123. [ ] A   [ ] B   [ ] C   [ ] D

96. [ ] A   [ ] B   [ ] C   [ ] D   124. [ ] A   [ ] B   [ ] C   [ ] D

97. [ ] A   [ ] B   [ ] C   [ ] D   125. [ ] A   [ ] B   [ ] C   [ ] D

98. [ ] A   [ ] B   [ ] C   [ ] D

Bleeding and Shock

Core Concepts

- Signs, symptoms, and care of a patient in shock
- Recognizing hemorrhage
- How to evaluate the severity of external bleeding
- How to control external bleeding
- Signs, symptoms, and care of a patient with internal bleeding

Outcomes

After reading this chapter, you should be able to:

29.1 Summarize the significance of bleeding in trauma. (pp. 786–788)
- Explain the impact on the body when a significant amount of blood escapes the vascular system due to injury.
- Explain the impact of modern battlefield injuries on the importance of immediate hemorrhage control in saving lives.
- Describe the interaction of the components of the circulatory system to maintain perfusion.

29.2 Summarize concepts of shock. (pp. 788–797)
- Describe how failure of any of the components of the cardiovascular system can lead to hypoperfusion.
- Describe the characteristics of the major classifications of shock.
- Compare compensated and decompensated shock.
- Compare the pediatric patient's presentation in shock with that of adults.
- Explain the role of time to definitive care in survival from hemorrhagic shock.
- Relate signs and symptoms of shock to the body's attempts to compensate for the amount of blood lost.

29.3 Summarize the EMT care approach to the patient in shock. (pp. 798–799)
- Prioritize the interventions for specific portrayals of patients in shock.
- Describe the decision-making process for transporting a patient in shock.

29.4 Summarize the EMT care approach to the patient with external bleeding. (pp. 799–818)
- Distinguish the characteristics of venous, arterial, and capillary bleeding.
- Identify assessment procedures required to ensure all external bleeding is found.
- Describe the team approach to caring for a patient with massive external bleeding.
- Explain the prioritization of external bleeding control in the overall context of the patient's presentation.

- Identify the rationale for selecting methods of controlling external hemorrhage.
- Outline the steps of the various approaches to external bleeding control.
- Describe the modified approaches to managing bleeding from head injuries and nose bleeds.

29.5 Summarize the EMT care approach to the patient with internal bleeding. (pp. 818–820)
- Recognize indications of internal bleeding.
- Outline the priorities of care for a patient with internal bleeding.

Match Key Terms

A. Hypoperfusion caused by a spinal cord injury that results in systemic vasodilatation.

B. When the patient is developing shock, but the body is still able to maintain perfusion.

C. Bleeding which is characterized by a slow, oozing flow of blood.

D. Shock resulting from blood or fluid loss.

E. When the body can no longer compensate for a shock state which results in hypotension and death. Late signs such as decreasing blood pressure become evident.

F. The medical term for body's inability to adequately circulate blood to the body's cells to supply them with oxygen and nutrients.

G. Bleeding which is characterized by bright red blood and is rapid, profuse, and difficult to control.

H. Shock or lack of perfusion brought on not by blood loss but by the heart's inadequate pumping action.

I. Substances applied as powders, dressings, gauze, or bandages to open wounds to stop bleeding.

J. Bleeding, especially severe bleeding.

K. Shock resulting from blood loss.

L. Bleeding which is characterized by dark red or maroon blood and a steady, easy-to-control flow.

M. A device used for bleeding control that constricts all blood flow to and from an extremity.

N. The supply of oxygen to, and removal of wastes from, the cells and tissues of the body as a result of blood flow through the capillaries.

O. A bulky dressing held in position with a tightly wrapped bandage, which applies pressure to help control bleeding.

P. A general or lay term used to describe the inability to adequately circulate blood to the body's cells in order to supply them with oxygen and nutrients.

Q. A type of shock in which the heart cannot pump blood due to a blockage of blood flow into or out of the heart.

R. Hypoperfusion due to a lack of blood vessel tone.

_____ **1.** Arterial bleeding

_____ **2.** Capillary bleeding

_____ **3.** Cardiogenic shock

_____ **4.** Compensated shock

_____ **5.** Decompensated shock

_____ **6.** Hemorrhage

_____ **7.** Hemorrhagic shock

_____ **8.** Hemostatic agents

_____ **9.** Hypoperfusion

_____ **10.** Hypovolemic shock

_____ **11.** Neurogenic shock

_____ **12.** Perfusion

_____ **13.** Pressure dressing

_____ **14.** Shock

_____ **15.** Tourniquet

_____ **16.** Venous bleeding

_____ **17.** Distributive shock

_____ **18.** Obstructive shock

Multiple-Choice Review

_____ **1.** Blood that has been depleted of oxygen and loaded with carbon dioxide and other wastes empties into the _____, which carry it back to the heart.
    A. arteries   **C.** capillaries
    B. veins   **D.** tissues

_____ **2.** Cells and tissues of the brain, spinal cord, and _____ are the _most_ sensitive to inadequate perfusion.
    A. spleen   **C.** liver
    B. lungs   **D.** heart

_____ **3.** Your 26-year-old male patient was stabbed multiple times in a bar fight. Police are on the scene, and it is now safe for you to begin your assessment and treatment. The use of _____ is essential whenever bleeding is discovered or simply anticipated.
    A. full protective gear   **C.** universal isolation precautions
    B. Standard Precautions   **D.** Tyvek overalls

_____ **4.** The process of substances such as hormones, water, and enzymes that are transported by the blood and control the body's functions is referred to as:
    A. transportation.   **C.** regulation.
    B. nutrition.   **D.** excretion.

_____ **5.** Which statement about arterial bleeding is correct?
    A. Clot formation takes place rapidly.
    B. Arterial bleeding is often rapid and profuse.
    C. Arterial bleeding is the least difficult type of bleeding to control.
    D. Arterial bleeding causes the blood pressure to rise.

_____ **6.** Your 38-year-old female patient has sustained an injury to her right lower leg. There is a steady flow of dark red blood, which is most likely a result of _____ bleeding.
    A. arterial   **C.** capillary
    B. venous   **D.** femoral

_____ **7.** Your 22-year-old male patient has a large area of road rash from sliding along the highway when he crashed his motorcycle. Bleeding described as oozing is usually a result of _____ bleeding.
    A. arterial   **C.** capillary
    B. venous   **D.** bronchiole

_____ **8.** When a patient is losing blood, _____ shock begins to occur. When blood is lost so are the _____ which affect the patient's ability to clot, and _____ which affects the blood's oxygen carrying ability.
    A. obstructive; RBCs; toxins
    B. hemorrhagic; platelets; hemoglobin
    C. septic; platelets; fight infection
    D. hemorrhagic; WBCs; transport

_____ **9.** Pediatric patients are excellent compensators when confronted with blood loss from trauma. All of the following are reasons why children are so successful in compensating, _except_:
    A. They are very effective at shunting blood to the core.
    B. They rely on their heart rate when compensating.
    C. They can produce very forceful heart contractions.
    D. They are able to maintain their BP even with up to 40% blood loss.

_____ **10.** Each of the following is an example of distributive shock, except:
   A. anaphylactic shock.
   B. obstructive shock.
   C. neurogenic shock.
   D. septic shock.

_____ **11.** Of the following, which is *not* a cause of an obstructive type of shock?
   A. brain hemorrhage
   B. tension pneumothorax
   C. cardiac tamponade
   D. pulmonary embolism

_____ **12.** When a patient cuts a blood vessel, the body attempts to protect the patient even before a bandage is applied. The body's natural responses to bleeding are constriction of the injured blood vessel and:
   A. cobbling.
   B. slowing of the heart rate.
   C. compensation.
   D. clotting.

_____ **13.** You are treating a 19-year-old female who experienced a series of lacerations. Your assessment of external bleeding includes all of the following *except*:
   A. estimating the amount of blood lost to predict potential shock.
   B. waiting for signs and symptoms of shock to appear before beginning treatment.
   C. prioritizing which bleeding location should be treated first.
   D. identifying during the primary assessment any bleeding that must be treated.

_____ **14.** The major methods that are used to control massive external extremity bleeding include all of the following *except*:
   A. direct pressure.
   B. hemolytic dressing.
   C. tourniquet on extremities.
   D. wound packing.

_____ **15.** Why is administration of supplemental oxygen an important treatment for the trauma patient?
   A. It enhances blood clotting.
   B. It improves oxygenation of the tissues.
   C. It constricts the blood vessels.
   D. It is important for all of these reasons.

_____ **16.** You are treating a 28-year-old female who sustained several deep lacerations when she fell off her scooter and was thrown into a guardrail. The most common and effective way to control massive external extremity bleeding is by:
   A. cold application.
   B. elevation.
   C. tourniquet.
   D. direct pressure.

_____ **17.** The patient has already bled through a small pile of gauze pads. You will be applying some additional sterile pads to the injury. The initial layer of dressing should not be removed from a bleeding wound because it:
   A. can become a biohazard.
   B. takes too long to remove.
   C. is a necessary part of clot formation.
   D. may increase the chance of infection.

_____ **18.** Wound packing can be effective, especially when hemostatic gauze is used, for the following areas:
   A. extremities and junctional areas.
   B. chest penetrating injuries.
   C. abdominal eviscerations.
   D. open chest injury.

_____ **19.** When you suspect that a patient is in a late stage of shock, an additional sign of late shock may be:
   A. a rise in blood pressure.
   B. constricted pupils.
   C. cyanosis around the lips and nail beds.
   D. widening of pulse pressure.

_____ **20.** Your patient is a 9-year-old male who fell off his skateboard and has numerous injuries to both of his legs. You should be especially careful when evaluating pediatric patients for shock because children:
   A. cannot be administered oxygen at low flow rates.
   B. may display few signs until a large percentage of blood volume is lost.
   C. can decompensate for blood loss very quickly.
   D. may exhibit erratic capillary refill times.

_____ **21.** A 39-year-old female, who was dressing the mannequins in a clothing store display, fell through the store window and has sustained a large cut. Blood is flowing from her forehead. What method of bleeding control should you use?
   A. A tourniquet will need to be applied to control the bleeding.
   B. Direct pressure with a dressing and bandage should be applied.
   C. Apply cold directly to the wound right away.
   D. Lower the patient's head below her heart, and the bleeding will stop.

_____ **22.** You are treating a 22-year-old male who has a deep laceration that is continuing to bleed. Use of direct pressure may _not_ be effective if the wound:
   A. was caused by an impaled object.
   B. was accompanied by spinal injury.
   C. is at the distal end of a limb.
   D. involves a profusely bleeding artery.

_____ **23.** You are going to use an air splint to manage the bleeding on the lower leg of a 22-year-old male patient. Which of the following is _true_ about the use of an air splint?
   A. It is effective for controlling venous and capillary bleeding.
   B. It should be used only if there is suspected bone injury.
   C. It is most effective for controlling arterial bleeding.
   D. It should be used before other manual methods of bleeding control.

_____ **24.** Which of the following is _not_ a guideline for supplementing bleeding control with cold application?
   A. Wrap the ice pack in a cloth or towel.
   B. Pour ice chips directly into the open skin.
   C. Do not leave the cold pack in place for more than 20 minutes.
   D. Cold application should be accompanied by other manual techniques.

_____ **25.** When attempting to control a deep laceration across the entire right buttock of a 22-year-old ski racer, you note that the cut goes down to the bone and will not stop bleeding. The best treatment would be to utilize _____ while beginning to transport the patient by Medevac to the regional trauma center.
   A. elevation of the wound
   B. hemostatic gauze into the wound
   C. ice packs into the wound
   D. a commercial tourniquet

_____ **26.** You are treating a 29-year-old female factory worker who was involved in an accident in which a machine has amputated her right forearm. Bleeding from a clean-edged amputation is usually cared for initially with:
   A. a pressure dressing.   **C.** a tourniquet.
   B. cold application.   **D.** an air splint.

_____ **27.** When the body has lost the battle to maintain perfusion to the organ systems and the systolic BP begins to drop, the patient is experiencing _____ shock.
   A. delayed   **C.** decompensated
   B. compensated   **D.** reversible

_____ **28.** You have decided that the most appropriate method of bleeding control for your patient is to apply a tourniquet. Once a tourniquet is in place, it must:
   A. not be removed or loosened unless ordered by medical direction.
   B. be covered immediately to keep the wound warm.
   C. be loosened every 15 minutes to dislodge clots.
   D. be packed in ice and a pressure dressing.

_____ **29.** Early signs of shock that are actually the body's compensating mechanisms include all of the following *except*:
   A. increased heart rate.
   B. increased respirations.
   C. pale, cool skin.
   D. shorter capillary refill time in children.

_____ **30.** Your 20-year-old female patient fell off her mountain bike and has a head injury. If you note bleeding or leakage of cerebrospinal fluid (CSF) from the patient's ears or nose, you should:
   A. apply direct pressure to the skull.
   B. apply direct pressure to the ears and nose.
   C. apply cold packs to the ears and nose.
   D. allow the drainage to flow freely.

_____ **31.** You are treating a 58-year-old male who has had a nosebleed for the last hour. The medical term for a nosebleed is:
   A. hemorrhage.
   B. epistaxis.
   C. epihemorrhage.
   D. nostrium.

_____ **32.** You are treating a 59-year-old female patient who called the ambulance because her nose has been bleeding for quite a while. To stop or control a nosebleed, try each of the following *except*:
   A. having the patient sit down and lean forward.
   B. applying direct pressure to the fleshy skin around the nostrils.
   C. keeping the patient calm and quiet.
   D. applying cold packs to the bridge of the nose and face.

_____ **33.** The leading cause of internal injuries and bleeding is:
   A. blunt trauma.
   B. penetrating trauma.
   C. auto collisions.
   D. large lacerations.

_____ **34.** Which of the following is not *typically* considered a cause of a penetrating trauma?
   A. A blast injury
   B. A gunshot wound
   C. A knife wound
   D. An ice pick wound

_____ **35.** After interviewing a 52-year-old male patient, you suspect that he may have internal bleeding. Signs of internal bleeding include all of the following *except*:
   A. vomiting a coffee-ground-like substance.
   B. bradycardia and a flushed face.
   C. dark, tarry stools.
   D. a tender, rigid, or distended abdomen.

_____ **36.** A 28-year-old male patient fell off the roof of a two story house and landed on a pile of firewood. You suspect that he has sustained an injury that is causing internal bleeding. Internal bleeding may be signaled by all of the following *except*:
   A. painful, swollen, or deformed extremities.
   B. signs and symptoms of shock.
   C. bright red blood from the rectum.
   D. bleeding from a laceration to the forearm.

_____ 37. Because of internal bleeding, the patient is developing inadequate tissue perfusion. This condition is referred to as:
A. hyperperfusion.
B. hypoxia.
C. hypoperfusion.
D. hypotension.

_____ 38. Which cause is least likely to result in a state of shock or hypoperfusion?
A. pump failure.
B. lost blood volume.
C. dilated blood vessels.
D. a closed injury to the head.

_____ 39. The most common mechanism of shock for a heart attack patient is:
A. vasoconstriction.
B. fluid loss.
C. pump failure.
D. vasodilation.

_____ 40. Your patient was involved in an automobile crash. She is unable to move her lower extremities, and you suspect that she is in shock. Shock caused by the failure of the nervous system to control the diameter of blood vessels is called _____ shock.
A. hypovolemic
B. cardiogenic
C. neurogenic
D. reversible

_____ 41. Your 46-year-old male patient is in shock, yet his body is still able to maintain perfusion to his vital organs, and his systolic BP is still 120 mmHg. This is often referred to as _____ shock.
A. compensated
B. decompensated
C. delayed
D. constricted

_____ 42. You are treating a 45-year-old female patient who has sustained considerable blood loss after slicing her hand while preparing food. She states that she feels nauseated. What is causing this symptom of feeling nauseated?
A. Blood is diverted from the digestive system.
B. Blood rushes rapidly to the digestive system.
C. Shock increases the production of digestive juices.
D. The patient has swallowed a large amount of blood.

_____ 43. The pulse rate in a female who has cut herself and is in an early stage of shock will be?
A. decreased.
B. absent.
C. increased.
D. irregular.

_____ 44. The patient in question 42 has a drop in her systolic blood pressure. This is:
A. an early sign of shock.
B. an early sign of shock in a child.
C. always present in shock.
D. a late sign of shock.

Pathophysiology: Fight-or-Flight

1. What happens to a patient when the blood vessels constrict?

_____

2. What happens to a patient when the blood vessels in the kidneys constrict?

_____

3. What happens to a patient when the blood vessels in the GI tract constrict?

_____

Complete the Following

1. List four categories of shock and their key interventions.

   A. _____

   B. _____

   C. _____

   D. _____

2. List five signs of shock.

   A. _____

   B. _____

   C. _____

   D. _____

   E. _____

3. List seven principles of care for the patient with external hemorrhage.

   A. _____

   B. _____

   C. _____

   D. _____

   E. _____

   F. _____

   G. _____

Label the Diagram

Fill in the name of the appropriate term on the line provided.

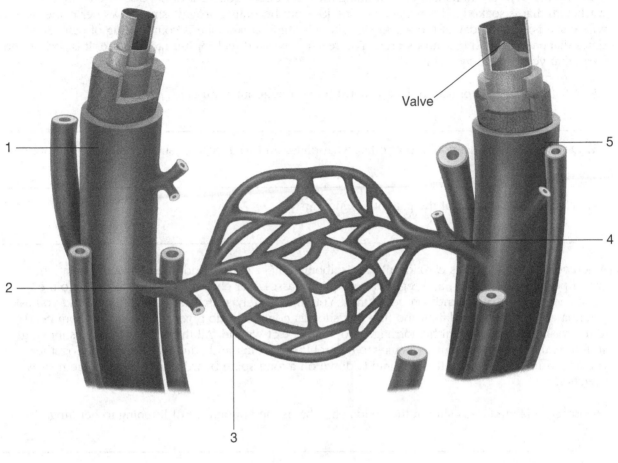

Valve

1.

2.

3.

4.

5.

1. _____

2. _____

3. _____

4. _____

5. _____

Case Study: Convenience Store Shooting

You respond to a local convenience store where there has been an armed robbery. The call was dispatched as a shooting. The police are reporting that the scene is secure and asking for a rush on the ambulance. A bystander who pulled up to the store just as the shooter was running out the front door and down the street told the police that he found the injured clerk sitting on the floor behind the counter, clutching her stomach.

1. What is the importance of a witness stating that the shooter ran away?

_____

2. As you enter the store, what scene size-up procedures are important?

_____

You find the 21-year-old female clerk holding the right upper quadrant of her abdomen with a washcloth that is soaked in blood. She is conscious but becoming groggy, she knows her name, where she is, and the day of the week. Her name is Miranda, and she is complaining of pain. She states that she is very thirsty and scared. You reach down and feel for her radial pulse. It is so fast and weak that you can barely feel it.

3. What important information have you just found out about Miranda?

_____

4. On the basis of what you know so far, what phase and what type of shock is your patient in?

_____

5. What is the relevance of the patient's being thirsty?

_____

When you check Miranda's carotid pulse, it is about 120 per minute and thready. Her respirations are 24 per minute, shallow, and regular. You quickly assess her chest. You find no entry into the chest and equal breath sounds on both lungs. You immediately search for other injuries, and you ask Miranda about other complaints and find that she has none. You do a very quick search from head to toe for additional external hemorrhage and a bullet exit wound. All the while, Miranda is moving all four extremities. Your partner begins to control the bleeding and administers oxygen. Together, you and your partner carefully lay Miranda down on a long spine board to move her to the nearby stretcher.

6. Because Miranda was shot in the abdomen, what is the importance of listening to her lungs?

_____

7. What device should first be used to administer oxygen to Miranda? If her ventilations become inadequate, what oxygen-delivery device would you switch to?

_____

GZQ **8.** Should an ALS unit be requested if one was not dispatched with you? If so, should you wait on the scene for ALS or arrange an intercept?

_____

The patient is very pale and sweating profusely. She is beginning to get anxious about dying. You and your partner rapidly move her to the ambulance.

9. On a call like this, what is the maximum time you should spend on the scene?

_____

10. To give the surgeons a good chance to save Miranda's life, what is the maximum time you should spend in assessment and transportation of the patient to the trauma center? How can you be sure that they will be ready for your arrival?

_____

©2021 Pearson Education, Inc.
Emergency Care, 14th Ed.

After you load the patient in the ambulance, you reassess her level of responsiveness. She is responding only to painful stimuli. ALS will intercept you en route.

11. Aside from reassessing the vitals, what airway care should be considered at this time?

_____

GZQ **12.** Would spinal immobilization be indicated for this patient?

_____

13. Is this patient critical?

_____

You meet the ALS unit. The paramedics board your ambulance with their portable equipment. The driver quickly continues to the hospital.

GZQ **14.** What procedures would an ALS unit be likely to do en route to the hospital?

_____

15. The patient initially told you that she has no allergies, takes no medications, and has been healthy. Her last meal was lunch a few hours ago. The paramedics establish two large-bore IVs and prepare to intubate the patient endotracheally. Her pulse oximeter reading is 85%, and her ECG is sinus tachycardia at a rate of 136 with no ectopy (irregular beats). Briefly write down the radio report that you would give to the hospital en route.

_____

_____

_____

_____

30 Soft-Tissue Trauma

Core Concepts

- Understanding closed wounds and emergency care for closed wounds
- Understanding open wounds and emergency care for open wounds
- Understanding burns and emergency care for burns
- Understanding electrical injuries and emergency care for electrical injuries
- How to dress and bandage wounds

Outcomes

After reading this chapter, you should be able to:

30.1 Summarize concepts of soft-tissue injuries. (pp. 825–835)
- List the soft tissues in the body.
- Describe the anatomy and physiology of the skin.
- Relate the potential for complications to the mechanisms that cause soft-tissue injuries.
- Distinguish between closed and open soft-tissue wounds.
- Recognize the characteristics of specific types of soft-tissue wounds.
- Relate soft-tissue injuries to the potential for trauma to underlying structures.

30.2 Integrate the steps of caring for soft-tissue injuries into the overall care of specific patients. (pp. 835–845)
- Relate the mechanism of injury to steps in caring for the patient.
- Compare the general approach to closed soft-tissue wounds with the approach to open soft-tissue wounds.
- Outline the specific considerations in managing a patient with penetrating trauma.
- Outline the specific considerations for treating an injury with an impaled object.
- Compare the approaches to managing partial and complete avulsions.
- Describe the care of amputations.
- Describe the approach to managing a patient with injuries to the genitalia.

30.3 Summarize the concepts of burn injuries. (pp. 845–863)
- Outline the prioritization for care for a variety of portrayals of burn patients.
- Identify the agents of burns.
- Identify the sources of burns.
- Classify portrayals of burn injuries by depth.
- Classify the severity of a variety of portrayals of burn injuries.

- Explain the classification of burn severity for patients of different age groups.
- Differentiate the steps in the approaches to treating specific types of burns.
- Explain complications commonly sustained with different types of burns.
- Match specific injury characteristics to the most appropriate dressing and bandaging techniques.

Match Key Terms

Part A

A. A swelling caused by the collection of blood under the skin or in damaged tissues as a result of an injured or broken blood vessel.

B. The outer layer of the skin.

C. Any material used to hold a dressing in place.

D. A cut.

E. An injury in which the skin is interrupted, exposing the tissue beneath.

F. An internal injury with no open pathway from the outside.

G. A burn in which all the layers of the skin are damaged. There are usually areas that are charred black or areas that are dry and white.

H. The tearing away of a piece or flap or other soft tissue. This term also may be used for an eye pulled from its socket or a tooth dislodged from its socket.

I. Any material (preferable sterile) used to cover a wound that will help control bleeding and prevent additional contamination.

J. An injury caused when force is transmitted from the body's exterior to its internal structures, often causing massive internal injuries and bone fractures.

K. Any dressing that forms an airtight seal.

L. The inner (second) layer of the skin found beneath the epidermis. It is rich in blood vessels and nerves.

M. A bruise.

N. A scratch or scrape to the skin.

O. The surgical removal or traumatic severing of a body part, usually an extremity.

_____ **1.** Abrasion

_____ **2.** Amputation

_____ **3.** Avulsion

_____ **4.** Bandage

_____ **5.** Closed wound

_____ **6.** Contusion

_____ **7.** Crush injury

_____ **8.** Dermis

_____ **9.** Dressing

_____ **10.** Epidermis

_____ **11.** Full-thickness burn

_____ **12.** Hematoma

_____ **13.** Laceration

_____ **14.** Occlusive dressing

_____ **15.** Open wound

Part B

A. A bulky dressing.

B. A method for estimating the extent of larger burns.

C. A method for estimating the extent of smaller burns.

D. A burn that involves only the epidermis, the outer layer of the skin. It is characterized by reddening of the skin and perhaps some swelling.

E. A burn in which the epidermis (first layer of skin) is burned through and the dermis (second layer) is damaged. Burns of this type cause reddening, blistering, and a mottled appearance.

F. An open wound that tears through the skin and destroys underlying tissues. This type of wound can be shallow or deep.

G. The layers of fat and soft tissues found below the dermis

H. A dressing applied tightly to control bleeding.

_____ **1.** Partial-thickness burn

_____ **2.** Pressure dressing

_____ **3.** Puncture wound

_____ **4.** Rule of nines

_____ **5.** Rule of palm

_____ **6.** Subcutaneous layers

_____ **7.** Superficial burn

_____ **8.** Universal dressing

Multiple-Choice Review

_____ **1.** The soft tissues of the body include all of the following *except*:
- **A.** skin, fatty tissue, and muscles.
- **B.** blood vessels and bones.
- **C.** teeth and cartilage.
- **D.** nerves, membranes, and glands.

_____ **2.** Which of the following is *not* a function of the skin?
- **A.** Protection
- **B.** Shock absorption
- **C.** Temperature regulation
- **D.** White blood cell production

_____ **3.** The layers of the skin include all of the following *except*:
- **A.** epidermis.
- **B.** dermis.
- **C.** subcutaneous.
- **D.** epithelial.

_____ **4.** The outermost _____ is the layer of the skin that is composed of dead cells, which are rubbed or sloughed off and are replaced continuously.
- **A.** epidermis
- **B.** dermis
- **C.** subcutaneous
- **D.** epithelial

_____ **5.** Specialized nerve endings in the _____ are involved in the senses of touch, cold, heat, and pain.
- **A.** epidermis
- **B.** dermis
- **C.** subcutaneous layers
- **D.** epithelial cells

_____ **6.** Shock absorption and insulation are major functions of the _____ layer of the skin.
- **A.** epidermis
- **B.** dermis
- **C.** subcutaneous
- **D.** epithelial

_____ **7.** You are treating a 35-year-old male who sustained an injury from an impact with a blunt object. There is no external bleeding. This wound is called a _____ injury.
- **A.** stabbing
- **B.** laceration
- **C.** closed
- **D.** perforation

_____ **8.** A patient has experienced a closed wound involving tissue damage and a collection of blood at the injury site. This is called a:

A. crush injury.
B. hematoma.
C. contusion.
D. penetration.

_____ **9.** A patient has experienced a soft-tissue injury from a force that caused a rupture or bleeding of internal organs. This injury is called a closed _____ injury.

A. contusion
B. hematoma
C. crush
D. high-force

_____ **10.** An 8-year-old female patient crashed her bike and slid along the road on the rainy pavement. The oozing of blood from her capillary beds is from an injury called a(n):

A. amputation.
B. abrasion.
C. laceration.
D. puncture.

_____ **11.** A 28-year-old male sustained a cut on his hand while slicing carrots for a stew. The wound that he sustained is called a(n):

A. abrasion.
B. puncture.
C. laceration.
D. avulsion.

_____ **12.** When a sharp or pointed object, such as an ice pick or a bullet, passes through the skin or other tissue, a(n) _____ wound has occurred.

A. abrasion
B. puncture
C. amputation
D. crush injury

_____ **13.** You are treating a 30-year-old male patient who was involved in a knife fight. The tip of his nose was almost completely cut off by the knife. This is a(n) _____ injury.

A. avulsion
B. penetration
C. crush
D. amputation

_____ **14.** You are on the scene of a local bar where there was just a shooting. The police are there, and the scene is considered "safe at this point." Various types of guns, when fired at close range, can cause all of the following _except_:

A. burns around the entry wound.
B. injection of air into the tissues.
C. large contusion to the tissue.
D. significant cold injuries.

_____ **15.** You are treating a 38-year-old female who has a large shard of glass impaled in her right leg. Emergency care in the field for this patient includes:

A. stabilizing the object in place.
B. using direct pressure on the site.
C. leaving the object alone and transporting rapidly.
D. carefully removing the object.

_____ **16.** Which of the following is _not_ correct about an injury caused by an impaled object?

A. The object may plug bleeding from a major artery.
B. Removal of the object may cause further injury to the nerves, muscles, and soft tissue.
C. Pressure should be applied to the object to stabilize it.
D. All of these are incorrect.

_____ **17.** You are assessing an 18-year-old male who was running with a sharp tool and tripped, impaling the tool in his right cheek. Which of the following is _false_ about this impaled object?

A. It should never be removed.
B. It can create an airway obstruction.
C. It can cause nausea and vomiting.
D. It is pulled out in the direction it entered.

_____ **18.** If a 22-year-old female patient has an impaled object in her right eye, the care that you provide should include use of a:
   A. pressure bandage placed over the eye.
   B. loose bandage placed over the eye.
   C. combination of 4 × 4s and a paper cup.
   D. combination of 3-inch gauze and a Styrofoam cup.

_____ **19.** Your 33-year-old male patient fell off a fence and sustained an injury that tore open his left leg. There is no break in the bone, but a large avulsed flap of tissue has been torn loose. You should do all of the following *except*:
   A. fold the skin back to its normal position.
   B. control bleeding and dress the wound.
   C. clean the wound surface.
   D. tear off the remainder of the flap and cool it during transport.

_____ **20.** You are treating a 37-year-old female patient who stuck her hand in the chute of an operating snow blower. She was severely injured, and all of her fingers are severed. The amputated parts torn from her body should be wrapped and placed in a:
   A. cup of dry ice placed in an airtight container.
   B. plastic bag filled with ice.
   C. plastic bag on top of a sealed bag of ice.
   D. saline and ice solution.

_____ **21.** You are treating a 35-year-old male whose lower leg has been amputated by a train. The most effective treatment for an amputation is to:
   A. apply a tourniquet and cool the lower leg.
   B. place the amputated part in ice.
   C. place a snug pressure dressing over the stump.
   D. apply ice over the stump.

_____ **22.** Your 19-year-old male patient has sustained a very serious injury, and it will be necessary to apply an occlusive dressing to the wound. An occlusive dressing is used to:
   A. form an airtight seal.   **C.** control severe bleeding.
   B. stabilize an impaled object.   **D.** secure sprain injuries.

_____ **23.** The primary injuries that occur from a blast are caused by:
   A. superheated gases.   **C.** patient displacement.
   B. a pressure wave.   **D.** exposure to hazardous materials.

_____ **24.** You are treating a male patient who sustained blunt trauma to the genitals. Your treatment should include each of the following, except:
   A. consider that the injury suggests a more serious internal injury.
   B. control bleeding as you would for other soft tissue injuries.
   C. pack his genitals on ice as soon as possible.
   D. display a calm professional manner to maintain the patient's dignity.

_____ **25.** The victim of an electrical accident may have the following signs and symptoms:
   A. elevated BP or low BP with shock signs and symptoms.
   B. seizures.
   C. muscle tenderness or twitching.
   D. any of the above.

_____ **26.** You are dispatched to the scene of an explosion. On arrival, you find a 35-year-old female who bystanders say was in an area of the explosion. In terms of injuries, you expect to find a(n):
   A. mixture of open and closed injuries.
   B. series of penetrating objects.
   C. impaled object.
   D. amputation.

_____ **27.** You are evaluating a 52-year-old male patient who was the driver of a vehicle that was involved in a head-on collision. He was not wearing his seat belt. When he pitched forward, he smashed his chest into the steering column, causing internal tissue damage and bleeding. This type of injury is called:
A. torn lung injury.　　　　　　　　**C.** crush injury.
B. penetrating trauma.　　　　　　　**D.** puncture trauma.

_____ **28.** Blast injuries often include all of the following *except*:
A. potentially infectious disease.
B. tertiary injuries such as avulsions.
C. primary lacerations and abrasions.
D. secondary projectile injuries.

_____ **29.** Your patient has serious thermal burns to her face and forearm. In addition to the physical damage caused by burns, patients often suffer:
A. heart attacks.
B. emotional and psychological problems.
C. diabetic emergencies.
D. delayed reactions such as developing skin cancer.

_____ **30.** When caring for a 22-year-old male who was burned:
A. do not neglect assessment in order to begin burn care.
B. transport immediately.
C. take the patient to the closest hospital.
D. run cold water on the patient for at least 20 minutes.

_____ **31.** Examples of agents that can cause burns include all of the following *except*:
A. AC current.　　　　　　　　　　**C.** dry lime.
B. hydrochloric acid.　　　　　　　**D.** distilled water.

_____ **32.** A burn that involves only the epidermis is called a(n) _____ burn.
A. superficial　　　　　　　　　　**C.** full thickness
B. partial-thickness　　　　　　　**D.** epi-thickness

_____ **33.** Which of the following types of burns will result in deep, intense pain; blisters; and mottled skin?
A. Superficial　　　　　　　　　　**C.** Full thickness
B. Partial thickness　　　　　　　**D.** Medium layer

_____ **34.** To distinguish between a partial-thickness burn and a full-thickness burn, look for _____, which indicate(s) a full-thickness burn.
A. blisters　　　　　　　　　　　　**C.** charred or dry and white areas
B. mottled skin　　　　　　　　　　**D.** swelling

_____ **35.** Your patient is a 22-year-old male who sustained an electrical burn when improperly installing an outlet. Electrical burns are of special concern because they:
A. cause respiratory burns if superheated gas is inhaled.
B. pose a great risk of severe internal injuries.
C. may remain on the skin and continue to burn for hours.
D. cause the patient to lose hair over time.

_____ **36.** A patient who was working in a chemistry lab sustained a burn when a beaker of a strong acid spilled all over her. Chemical burns are of special concern because the chemicals:
A. cause respiratory burns if superheated gas is inhaled.
B. pose a great risk of internal injury.
C. may remain on the skin and continue to burn for hours.
D. jump from one extremity to another.

_____ **37.** Burns to the face are of special concern because they:
  A. tend to cause extensive muscle damage.
  B. can cause heart irregularities.
  C. increase the potential for shock.
  D. may involve airway injury.

_____ **38.** You are treating a 35-year-old male patient who has partial-thickness burns to his entire left arm, chest, face, and neck. Using the rule of nines, approximate the size of the burn area.
  A. 18%   **C.** 27%
  B. 22%   **D.** 32%

_____ **39.** You are treating a 45-year-old female patient who has partial-thickness burns totally covering her legs, and the anterior surface of her chest and abdomen. Using the rule of nines, approximate the size of the burn area.
  A. 18%   **C.** 45%
  B. 36%   **D.** 54%

_____ **40.** Your patient has sustained a burn injury that is about the size of five of his palms. This burn would cover approximately _____ of the patient's total body surface area.
  A. 5%   **C.** 15%
  B. 10%   **D.** 20%

_____ **41.** The age of the patient is an important factor in burns. Patients under _____ and over _____ years of age have the most severe body responses to burns.
  A. 3; 50   **C.** 10; 65
  B. 5; 55   **D.** 15; 70

_____ **42.** Burn center criteria includes all of the following _except_:
  A. partial thickness greater than 10% BSA.
  B. inhalation burns.
  C. burns complicated by musculoskeletal injuries.
  D. partial thickness burns on the wrist.

_____ **43.** A 22-year-old male patient who has a partial-thickness burn to the entire back should be:
  A. wrapped in a dry, sterile burn sheet.
  B. cooled down with ice for 15 minutes.
  C. wrapped in moist sterile dressings.
  D. dried and wrapped in an airtight dressing.

_____ **44.** The primary care for a patient with a chemical burn to the eyes is to:
  A. wrap the patient in a dry, sterile burn sheet.
  B. wash away the chemical with flowing water.
  C. dry the patient and wrap him or her in an airtight dressing.
  D. wrap the patient with moist sterile dressings.

_____ **45.** You are treating a 22-year-old female patient who was burned. She is having visual difficulties, is restless and irritable, and has an irregular pulse rate and muscle tenderness. This patient probably suffered a(n) _____ burn.
  A. chemical   **C.** electrical
  B. thermal   **D.** radiation

_____ **46.** If _____ is the burn agent, brush it from the patient's skin and then flush the patient's skin with water.
  A. dry lime   **C.** road tar
  B. radiation   **D.** acid

Pathophysiology: Acids and Alkalis

1. Why should an alkali burn be irrigated for a longer time than an acid burn?

_____

2. Which acid is the exception to the rule addressed in question 1? Why?

_____

Complete the Following

1. List three ways that burns can be classified.

A. _____

B. _____

C. _____

2. List the eleven parts of the adult body that account for 9% each, using the rule of nines.

A. _____

B. _____

C. _____

D. _____

E. _____

F. _____

G. _____

H. _____

I. _____

J. _____

K. _____

3. List seven criteria for patients who should be treated at a burn center.

A. _____

B. _____

C. _____

D. _____

E. _____

F. _____

G. _____

Label the Diagram

Fill in the name of each type of burn on lines 1, 2, and 3. Fill in how the skin is damaged on lines 4, 5, and 6.

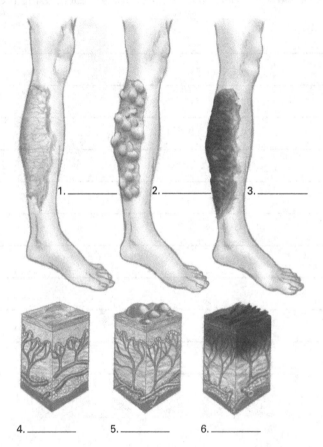

1. _____ 2. _____ 3. _____

4. _____ 5. _____ 6. _____

Case Study: No Patience for Lighter Fluid

Your unit and the police are dispatched to the scene of an adult male burned in the backyard of a private suburban residence. It is around 5:00 p.m. on a warm summer day. On arrival, the scene is safe, and a family member leads you, your crew, and a police officer to the rear of the home. It is obvious the family and a few friends have been celebrating an event most of the day. You see a 25-year-old male standing in a T-shirt and shorts. He appears to be in a lot of pain. According to a family member, the patient's name is Emilio and he was planning to cook some hot dogs and hamburgers on the grill. Evidently, the charcoal did not start fast enough for him, although there may have been some slowly burning coals. Emilio decided to switch to a different accelerant. He filled a paper cup with some gasoline, and as he moved close enough to pour it on the charcoals, the fumes exploded. On closer observation, you find that Emilio has blistered skin on his right and left palms, the anterior and posterior surfaces of his right and left arms, and his entire chest. Fortunately, he instinctively raised his hands to shield his face—a movement that caused burns on both the fronts and backs of his forearms. Although this protective movement prevented burns to the skin of his face, his eyebrows and moustache are singed a bit.

1. On the basis of information you have so far, approximately what percentage of the patient's total body surface area is burned?

   _____

2. What is the significance of the singed facial hair?

   _____

3. From a commonsense point of view, why was there an explosion in this case?

   _____

You immediately assess the patient's mental status and find that he is alert and oriented and can follow instructions. You instruct him to remove the remains of the clothing he is wearing, and your partner goes to get the stretcher and burn sheets. Emilio's radial pulse rate is 100 and strong at this point. Because his upper arms are not burned, you proceed to determine his blood pressure is 110/70 mmHg and his SpO_2 is 97%. You assist him in removing his watch and rings as your partner arrives with the stretcher for the patient to sit on the sterile burn sheet.

4. Because most of the burned area is already blistered, what type of burn is this?

   _____

GZQ 5. Fortunately, Emilio protected his face and airway, and the slight singing of eyebrows and mustache are not severe. Is there any other reason for you to consider transport to the regional burn center?

   _____

6. How should you manage Emilio's injuries?

   _____

7. Why was it so important to take the time to remove Emilio's watch and rings?

   _____

After placing the patient in the supine position on the burn sheet and obtaining a full set of baseline vital signs, you determine that the most appropriate action will be to transport him to the local high school football field, where the fire department is already setting up a landing zone for the helicopter that will be taking the patient to the regional burn center. You explain this to the patient, obtain a SAMPLE, and complete your physical examination. The patient states that he takes no medications but is allergic to sulfa drugs and did have a "couple of beers this afternoon." A paramedic, who will be going along with you to meet the flight crew, sets up to start a large bore IV on the patient. The paramedic asks you to start some oxygen with a nasal cannula and to hook up the electrodes for the ECG monitor.

8. This patient has a straightforward SAMPLE history. What would be a serious concern that you might identify in this patient that could change the course of his management?

_____

9. Why would it be smart to listen to this patient's lung sounds?

_____

GZQ **10.** With the patient's chest entirely burned, where do you put the electrodes?

_____

©2021 Pearson Education, Inc.
Emergency Care, 14th Ed.

Chest and Abdominal Trauma

Core Concepts

- Understanding chest injuries and emergency care for chest injuries
- Understanding abdominal injuries and emergency care for abdominal injuries

Outcomes

After reading this chapter, you should be able to:

31.1 Summarize the concepts of chest injuries. (pp. 869–875)
- Review the anatomy and physiology of the chest.
- Review the anatomy and physiology of the abdomen.
- Relate mechanisms of injury to the potential for specific chest injuries.
- Compare the characteristics of closed (blunt) and open (penetrating) chest wounds.
- Relate the pathophysiology of specific types of chest injuries to patient assessment findings.

31.2 Summarize the management decisions required in the case of patients with chest injuries. (pp. 875–885)
- Select the approach to addressing gas exchange based on the adequacy of the patient's respiration.
- Describe how the treatment indicated for specific injuries helps mitigate the underlying problem.
- Outline the steps in designing the interventions for specific chest injuries.
- Explain how to prioritize management decisions for portrayals of a variety of patients with chest trauma.
- Compare the characteristics of pneumothorax, tension pneumothorax, hemothorax, and hemopneumothorax.
- Describe the processes by which specific types of chest injuries interfere with cardiopulmonary system function.

31.3 Summarize the concepts of abdominal injuries. (pp. 885–887)
- Relate mechanism of injury to the potential for closed or open abdominal injuries.
- Relate mechanism of injury to the potential for specific organ injury.
- Compare the characteristics of injury to solid abdominal organs with those of injury to hollow abdominal organs.

31.4 Summarize the management decisions required in the care of patients with abdominal injuries. (pp. 887–889)
  - Prioritize the care of specific abdominal injuries among the other interventions for trauma patients.
  - Use assessment findings to inform measures to minimize the pain of abdominal injury.
  - Describe how to address the concerns for vomiting by the patient with an abdominal injury.
  - Describe the special bandaging techniques for specific open abdominal wounds.
  - Apply assessment and EMS system characteristics to make decisions about patient transportation.

Match Key Terms

A. Movement of ribs in a flail segment that is opposite to the direction of movement of the rest of the chest cavity.

B. Air in the chest cavity.

C. A type of chest injury in which air that enters the chest cavity is prevented from escaping causing the lung to collapse and the heart to shift.

D. An intestine or other internal organ protruding through a wound in the abdomen.

E. An open chest wound in which air is "pulled" into the chest cavity during inhalation.

F. Fracture of two or more adjacent ribs in two or more places that allows for free movement of the fractured segment.

_____ **1.** Tension pneumothorax

_____ **2.** Sucking chest wound

_____ **3.** Evisceration

_____ **4.** Flail chest

_____ **5.** Pneumothorax

_____ **6.** Paradoxical motion

Multiple-Choice Review

_____ **1.** Of the over 150,000 traumatic injury deaths in 2018, over 75% were associated with:
  A. chest trauma.
  B. penetrating trauma.
  C. blunt trauma.
  D. chest and abdominal trauma.

_____ **2.** A 25-year-old male patient was in a fight in which he was kicked numerous times when he was down on the ground. Three consecutive ribs were fractured in at least two places each. This patient has a(n):
  A. sternal contusion.
  B. tension pneumothorax.
  C. flail chest.
  D. anterior wall injury.

_____ **3.** When the patient with the large flail segment takes a breath, the EMT may notice that he is exhibiting:
  A. hyperventilation.
  B. paradoxical motion.
  C. periods of apnea.
  D. an injury to his kidneys.

_____ **4.** When a penetrating injury to the heart causes blood to flow into the pericardial sac and to compress the heart, this injury is called:
  A. traumatic asphyxia.
  B. cardiac tamponade.
  C. commotio cordis.
  D. aortic dissection.

_____ **5.** Your patient, who is a 22-year-old female, has sustained an open chest wound. A chest cavity that is open to the atmosphere is referred to as a(n):
  A. flail chest.
  B. hemothorax.
  C. sucking chest wound.
  D. rib fracture.

©2021 Pearson Education, Inc.
Emergency Care, 14th Ed.

_____ **6.** The treatment for a patient with an open chest wound includes all of the following *except*:

    A. maintaining an open airway.
    B. binding the chest tightly.
    C. administering high-concentration oxygen.
    D. sealing the open wound.

_____ **7.** When air becomes trapped in the chest cavity, it can affect the body in all of the following ways *except* by

    A. putting pressure on the unaffected lung and heart.
    B. reducing cardiac output.
    C. affecting oxygenation of the blood.
    D. increasing the ventilatory volume of the chest.

_____ **8.** The signs of pneumothorax or tension pneumothorax include all of the following *except*:

    A. tracheal deviation to the uninjured side.
    B. distended neck veins.
    C. uneven chest wall movement.
    D. increased depth of respiration.

_____ **9.** Which of the following is *not* a sign of traumatic asphyxia?

    A. Distended neck veins
    B. Wide pulse pressure
    C. Head, neck, and shoulders that appear dark blue
    D. Bloodshot and bulging eyes

_____ **10.** When you are taping an occlusive dressing in place for a patient with penetrating chest trauma:

    A. have the patient inhale as you tape.
    B. have the patient exhale as you tape.
    C. tape the dressing in place quickly because this is a life-threatening situation.
    D. have the patient hold his or her breath while taping.

_____ **11.** An open wound to the abdomen that is so large and deep that organs protrude through the opening is called a(n):

    A. impaled object.
    B. evisceration.
    C. avulsion.
    D. amputated intestine.

_____ **12.** Potential signs of an abdominal injury include all of the following *except*:

    A. lacerations and puncture wounds to the lower back.
    B. large bruises on the abdomen.
    C. indications of developing shock.
    D. contusions over the upper ribs.

_____ **13.** Your patient was skiing in a closed zone of the mountain. Suddenly, there was a snow avalanche, and he was covered by about three feet of snow. Fortunately, another skier quickly called for help and located your patient. Of the following injuries, which is most likely the reason why his upper body is blue and he is in cardiac arrest?

    A. Tension pneumothorax
    B. Hemothorax
    C. Traumatic asphyxia
    D. Cardiac tamponade

_____ **14.** How would you consider positioning a patient who has an abdominal injury?

    A. Prone, with arms outstretched
    B. Supine, with legs flexed at the knees
    C. In the left lateral recumbent position
    D. Supine, with legs straight

_____ **15.** When covering an exposed abdominal organ, the EMT should apply a(n) _____ directly over the wound site.

    A. sheet of plastic wrap from a sterile roll of Saran wrap
    B. occlusive dressing that is warm and dry
    C. sterile saline-moistened dressing and then an occlusive dressing
    D. aluminum foil wrapping over sterile saline

_____ **16.** Your patient is a healthy 17-year-old female lacrosse player with no past medical history who suddenly collapsed after being hit in the chest with the lacrosse ball. What is her likely condition?
   A. Pneumothorax
   B. Tension pneumothorax
   C. Traumatic asphyxia
   D. *Commotio cordis*

_____ **17.** You are evaluating a 25-year-old male patient whose abdomen was slashed open. The treatment of an evisceration should *never* include:
   A. using an occlusive dressing.
   B. cutting away the clothing.
   C. replacing or touching the exposed organ.
   D. applying a sterile, saline-soaked dressing.

_____ **18.** Common signs of abdominal injury include each of the following, except:
   A. cramps and distended abdomen.
   B. nausea and vomiting blood.
   C. headache and photophobia.
   D. thirst and weakness.

_____ **19.** When a small child (typically younger than 8 years old) is compared to an adult, the child would have:
   A. abdominal organs that are more exposed to injury.
   B. a more pliable chest.
   C. less calcified bones.
   D. all of the above.

_____ **20.** When would it be appropriate to consider using a flutter valve dressing?
   A. When the patient has a closed chest injury
   B. When the patient has a large exit wound in the chest wall
   C. When you suspect a buildup of pressure from a punctured lung
   D. When the patient has sustained a flail chest

Pathophysiology: The Path of the Bullet

1. A patient has a gunshot wound in the lower rib with an exit at the same level in the back. Is it possible for this to be both a chest injury and an abdominal injury? If so, how?

_____

2. Refer to the patient in question 1. Is there a way in which the spleen or liver, which are abdominal organs, may have been injured?

_____

Complete the Following

1. Explain what the following injuries are.

   A. *Commotio cordis:* _____

   B. Cardiac tamponade: _____

   C. Traumatic asphyxia: _____

   D. Hemothorax: _____

E. Pneumothorax: _____

F. Aortic injury: _____

2. List seven signs of a tension pneumothorax.

  A. _____

  B. _____

  C. _____

  D. _____

  E. _____

  F. _____

  G. _____

3. For each organ below, list the location, type and primary function.

  A. Gallbladder:_____

  B. Intestine (large and small):_____

  C. Kidneys:_____

  D. Liver:_____

  E. Pancreas:_____

  F. Spleen:_____

  G. Stomach:_____

  H. Urinary bladder:_____

  I. Uterus and ovaries:_____

Case Study: Assault with an Ice Pick

Your unit is sitting in front of a local coffee shop, where you are on break between calls. You are having a nice conversation with neighborhood residents when suddenly a teenager runs into the coffee shop yelling, "Where are the EMT's?" As you move out to the street, you note that the traffic is starting to back up, and you figure there must have been a car crash. You question the boy and learn that he witnessed a man being robbed and stabbed in the chest just a block up the street. He said that he had often seen the ambulance sitting at the coffee shop, so he ran here to get help. You jump into the ambulance and notify dispatch of the reported incident as well as the need for police backup. Once your lights go on, the traffic starts to make a path for you, and it is not far to the location, where a couple of bystanders are hovering over a 45-year-old well-dressed male who is lying unconscious on the ground. They tell you that he is a local merchant who was on his way to drop the day's deposits at the bank. One bystander said that he witnessed a struggle and that Nick, the patient, was stabbed in the left side of the chest with an ice pick. Then the assailant ran off with a packet that the bystander said was probably full of money.

1. On the basis of the information you have so far, is the scene safe?

_____

2. If the police have not arrived yet, should you leave the scene?

_____

3. On finding an unconscious patient, what is your first priority in patient care after scene safety?

_____

The police have arrived, and you pass along what you know while doing your primary assessment and preparing to move the patient into your ambulance. The police are helpful in dealing with the small crowd of people who are now watching your every move. You find that the patient has an open airway, is breathing shallowly about 24 times a minute, and has a very weak and rapid radial pulse. He has lung sounds on the right, but they are difficult to hear on the left. Your partner is getting the stretcher while you look more closely at the location of the wounds. There is a small amount of bleeding, but it is under control. You ask one of the witnesses whether the patient fell to the ground and struck his head. The witness states that he collapsed to his knees after he was stabbed at least twice in the chest. You quickly do a check for any head or neck trauma. Your partner returns, and you tell her that you find no injuries to the head, neck, or back of the chest but two to the front, which you sealed with occlusive dressings. You suggest that you need to get going right away.

GZQ **4.** On the basis of the information you have so far, is it appropriate not to provide full spine motion restriction precautions?

_____

5. From the information you have so far, what types of injuries do you suspect that this patient has sustained (i.e., what is your differential field diagnosis)?

_____

6. What is the significance of the very weak radial pulse?

_____

After placing the patient in the supine position on the stretcher and into the back of the ambulance, which was about thirty steps away, you apply a nonrebreather mask and reassess the vital signs. The BP is 90/70 mm Hg, and the pulse is about 120, weak and thready, with shallow respirations of 28. The medic unit is arriving, and after you give a quick report, the medic decides to ride along. You switch to a BVM ventilation assist, and she hooks up the monitor and reassesses the lung sounds. Fortunately, the hospital is only about ten minutes away.

7. Why was it a good decision to switch from the nonrebreather mask to the BVM assist?

_____

8. This patient is critical at this point and getting worse. The wounds have been sealed, but the medic suspects that the stab wound may have nicked his heart. What would be the essential information to tell the emergency department to give them early warning of your arrival?

_____

_____

_____

_____

32

Musculoskeletal Trauma

Core Concepts

- Knowledge of bones, muscles, and other elements of the musculoskeletal system
- Knowledge of general guidelines for emergency care of musculoskeletal injuries
- Purposes and general procedures for splinting
- Assessment and care of specific injuries to the upper and lower extremities

Outcomes

After reading this chapter, you should be able to:

32.1 Summarize concepts of the musculoskeletal system. (pp. 894–904)
- Describe the functions of the musculoskeletal system.
- Identify the anatomy of bone.
- Relate the nature of bones as living tissue to the implications of skeletal injury.
- Describe the function of joints.
- Identify each of the bones of the skeletal system.
- Apply knowledge of the forces that produce musculoskeletal injuries to the anticipation of specific patterns of injury.
- Identify fractures with high potential for emergency complications.
- Distinguish the anatomy and physiology of muscles, cartilages, ligaments, and tendons.
- Relate the anatomy of musculoskeletal injuries to the potential for underlying organ injury.
- Match different types of musculoskeletal injuries to their descriptions.
- Relate the anatomy and physiology of structures adjacent to bone to complications of musculoskeletal injury.

32.2 Summarize the management decisions required in the care of patients with musculoskeletal injuries. (pp. 904–943)
- Outline the general assessment findings associated with musculoskeletal injuries.
- Relate specific findings to the potential for specific types of musculoskeletal injuries.
- Explain the importance of serial checks of the distal circulation, sensation, and motor function (CSM) in the care of extremity injuries.
- Explain how to prioritize steps in caring for patients with musculoskeletal injuries.
- Explain how and when traction may be used in caring for patients with musculoskeletal injuries.
- Recognize the signs of compartment syndrome.
- Describe the role of splinting in managing musculoskeletal injuries.

- Identify the principles of splinting musculoskeletal injuries.
- Associate musculoskeletal injuries with the most appropriate type of splint.
- Explain how to make transport decisions by placing musculoskeletal injuries in the overall context of the patient's condition.

Match Key Terms

A. Tissues or fibers that cause movement of body parts and organs.

B. The disruption or "coming apart" of a joint.

C. An injury in which the skin has been broken or torn through from the inside or from the outside.

D. A splint that applies constant pull along the length of the lower extremity to help stabilize the fractured bone and to reduce muscle spasms in the limb; used primarily on femoral shaft fractures.

E. A grating sensation or sound that is made when fractured bone ends rub together.

F. Tissues that bind muscles to bones.

G. Any break in a bone.

H. The portions of the skeleton that include the clavicles, scapulae, arms, wrists, and hands and the pelvis, thighs, legs, ankles, and feet.

I. Tough tissue that covers the joint ends and bones and helps to form certain body parts, such as the outer ear.

J. Muscle injury caused by overstretching or overexertion of the muscle.

K. The process of applying tension to straighten and realign a fractured limb before splinting.

L. Places where bones articulate, or meet.

M. The stretching and tearing of ligaments.

N. Connective tissues that connect bone to bone.

O. An incomplete fracture from excessive bending force.

P. A fracture in which the broken bone segments are at an angle to each other.

Q. An injury to an extremity with no associated opening in the skin.

R. Hard but flexible living structures that provide support for the body and protection to vital organs.

S. A fracture in which the bone is broken in several places.

T. Injury caused when tissues such as blood vessels and nerves are compressed from swelling or because of a tight dressing or cast.

_____ **1.** Angulated fracture

_____ **2.** Bones

_____ **3.** Cartilage

_____ **4.** Closed extremity injury

_____ **5.** Comminuted fracture

_____ **6.** Compartment syndrome

_____ **7.** Crepitus

_____ **8.** Dislocation

_____ **9.** Extremities

_____ **10.** Fracture

_____ **11.** Greenstick fracture

_____ **12.** Joints

_____ **13.** Ligaments

_____ **14.** Manual traction

_____ **15.** Muscles

_____ **16.** Open extremity injury

_____ **17.** Sprain

_____ **18.** Strain

_____ **19.** Tendons

_____ **20.** Traction splint

Multiple-Choice Review

_____ **1.** As we age, our bones become _____, resulting in bones that are more brittle and easier to break.
   A. deficient in magnesium   **C.** high in iron
   B. deficient in calcium   **D.** high in potassium

_____ **2.** The strong white fibrous material that covers the bones is called the:
   A. perineum.   **C.** periosteum.
   B. marrow.   **D.** fascia.

_____ **3.** In children, the majority of long bone growth occurs in the:
   A. bone marrow.   **C.** periosteum.
   B. growth plate.   **D.** growth shaft.

_____ **4.** Musculoskeletal injuries are caused by direct, indirect, and _____ force.
   A. positive   **C.** negative
   B. sliding   **D.** twisting

_____ **5.** Fractures of the pelvis typically cause a _____-pint blood loss over the first 2 hours.
   A. 1/2   **C.** 2
   B. 1   **D.** 3

_____ **6.** The death rate from closed fracture of the femur dropped from 80% to under 20% in the post–World War I period as a result of the invention of the:
   A. air splint.   **C.** traction splint.
   B. IV bag.   **D.** tourniquet.

_____ **7.** The objective of realignment of a deformed extremity is to:
   A. prevent future infection.
   B. assist in restoring effective circulation.
   C. eliminate the pain of the injury.
   D. improve movement of the joint.

_____ **8.** You are managing a 32-year-old male patient who is suffering from a stretching or tearing of a ligament. This injury is called a:
   A. dislocation.   **C.** sprain.
   B. fracture.   **D.** strain.

_____ **9.** A break in the continuity of the skin of a fractured extremity is considered a(n) _____ bone or joint injury.
   A. simple   **C.** closed
   B. open   **D.** grating

_____ **10.** Your 29-year-old female patient fell while skiing. You suspect that she broke her right tibia with a comminuted fracture. Proper splinting of this closed fracture is:
   A. done with an air splint and gentle traction.
   B. not possible because of the boot.
   C. designed to prevent closed injuries from becoming open ones.
   D. completed in the hospital by a surgeon.

_____ **11.** The signs and symptoms of a bone or joint injury include all of the following _except_:
   A. grating.   **C.** vomiting.
   B. swelling.   **D.** bruising.

_____ **12.** Your 19-year-old female patient was snowboarding when she injured her right shoulder. The head of the humerus appears to move in front of the shoulder. This is a sign of a possible:

A. anterior dislocation.

B. posterior dislocation.

C. fractured clavicle.

D. sprained humerus.

_____ **13.** Which procedure is done at least twice whenever a splint is applied?

A. Elevation of the injured extremity

B. Manual stabilization of the injured extremity

C. Assessment for circulation, sensation, and motor function (CSM) distal to the injury

D. Application of gentle manual traction

_____ **14.** You are treating an 18-year-old male who you suspect has sustained a fracture to his right elbow. In what order will you take the following steps?

1. Assess CSM.

2. Secure the splint.

3. Reassess CSM.

4. Manually stabilize the extremity.

A. 2, 3, 4, 1

B. 4, 1, 2, 3

C. 3, 2, 4, 1

D. 1, 4, 2, 3

_____ **15.** Your 50-year-old female patient had just stepped off a curb into the street when a large truck cut the corner too closely and ran her over. She has numerous fractures and is in a great deal of pain. Multiple fractures, especially of the _____, can cause life-threatening external and internal bleeding.

A. radius

B. ulna

C. femur

D. tibia

_____ **16.** After splinting and treating the patient with multiple lower extremity fractures, you decide en route to the emergency department to apply cold too. Applying cold packs to fractures:

A. helps to reduce the swelling.

B. stops bleeding from the bone.

C. eliminates the need for a pressure bandage.

D. stops all the pain and discomfort.

_____ **17.** You are treating a 26-year-old male who fell off the roof of his house. Your primary assessment of this patient with multiple musculoskeletal injuries reveals that he is unstable. Care should include all of the following *except*:

A. managing the A-B-Cs.

B. moving the patient on a long board.

C. transporting the patient immediately.

D. splinting each injury individually.

_____ **18.** You are treating a 28-year-old female who fell on an outstretched arm. A splint properly applied to a closed bone injury should help prevent all of the following *except*:

A. damage to muscles, nerves, or blood vessels.

B. an open bone injury.

C. motion of bone fragments.

D. prevent circulation to the extremity.

_____ **19.** Fracture management is not generally the highest priority compared to other problems that are identified during the primary survey of the patient. However, fractures can introduce complications, which may include all of the following *except*:

A. excessive bleeding.

B. increased pain from movement.

C. paralysis of the extremity.

D. increased distal sensation.

_____ 20. You are treating a 45-year-old male patient who has a grossly deformed ulnar and radius fracture that will need to be properly splinted. A properly applied splint should do each of the following, *except*:
A. minimize blood loss.
B. decrease the patient's pain.
C. restrict movement of adjacent joints.
D. prevent the need for surgery.

_____ 21. You are treating a 65-year-old female patient who fell down the basement stairs. She did not strike her head, but she is in a lot of pain from lower-extremity fractures. There is a severe deformity of the right extremity about midway between the knee and the ankle, and the extremity distal to this injury lacks sensation. You should:
A. align with manual traction before splinting.
B. apply a pillow splint to the extremity.
C. delay splinting until you are en route to the hospital.
D. contact medical direction immediately.

_____ 22. What are the three basic types of splints?
A. Rigid, formable, and traction
B. Pillow, board, and ladder
C. Padded, soft, and anatomical
D. Air, cardboard, and vacuum

_____ 23. Which of the following is *not* true about rigid splints?
A. They require that the limb be moved into anatomic position.
B. They tend to provide the greatest support.
C. They are ideally used to splint long bones.
D. They are preferred for immobilizing joint injuries in the position found.

_____ 24. Your patient has a serious fracture to which you will be applying a traction splint. Which bone is most likely fractured?
A. Pelvis
B. Humerus
C. Femur
D. Clavicle

_____ 25. When applying a traction splint, the EMT should:
A. first move the patient to a stretcher.
B. leave any open leg wounds exposed so that bleeding can be monitored.
C. replace protruding bones as soon as priorities are arranged.
D. first manually stabilize the leg and then apply manual traction distally.

_____ 26. Your 55-year-old male patient has sustained a fracture to his right tibia. To ensure proper stabilization and increase comfort when applying a rigid splint, you should:
A. place him on a stretcher before splinting.
B. place him on a long spine board before splinting.
C. pad the spaces between the body part and the splint.
D. ensure that the splint conforms to his body curves.

_____ 27. The method of splinting should be dictated by the:
A. time when the injury occurred.
B. severity of the patient's condition and the priority decision.
C. distance to the destination hospital.
D. presence or absence of pain.

_____ 28. The 39-year-old female patient you are treating for lower extremity musculoskeletal injuries is unstable. You should do all of the following *except*:
A. care for life-threatening problems first.
B. align the injuries in an anatomical position.
C. provide spine motion restriction precautions with a long spine board or scoop stretcher.
D. apply two traction splints before securing the patient on a long spine board.

_____ 29. Hazards of improper splinting may include:
   A. aggravation of a bone or joint injury.
   B. reduced distal circulation.
   C. delay in transport of the patient with a life-threatening injury.
   D. all of these.

_____ 30. You are treating a 35-year-old male who was the front-seat, unrestrained passenger in a rear-end collision. His right tibia struck the lower dashboard of the car. If his lower leg is cyanotic or lacks a pulse when a knee joint injury is assessed, you should:
   A. splint the knee joint in the position in which it was found.
   B. transport the patient to the hospital immediately.
   C. realign the knee joint with gentle traction if no resistance is met.
   D. call for assistance from a paramedic unit.

_____ 31. Examples of bipolar traction splints include all of the following _except_:
   A. Hare.   C. Fernotrac.
   B. Sager.   D. half-ring.

_____ 32. The amount of traction that the EMT should pull when applying a Sager traction splint is:
   A. to the point at which the patient verbalizes relief.
   B. about 10% of the patient's body weight up to 15 pounds (6.8 kg).
   C. minimal because it doesn't require traction.
   D. about 15% of the patient's body weight up to 30 pounds.

_____ 33. The indications for a traction splint are a possible midshaft femur fracture with:
   A. either knee or ankle involvement.
   B. no joint or lower leg injury.
   C. extensive blood loss.
   D. an open fracture.

_____ 34. You are treating a 19-year-old female who twisted her left knee playing racquet ball. The signs and symptoms of a knee injury may include any of the following _except_:
   A. pain and tenderness.   C. deformity.
   B. swelling.   D. discoloration to the thigh.

_____ 35. Elderly patients are more susceptible to _____ fractures from falls because of brittle bones or bones weakened by disease.
   A. hip   C. heel
   B. tibia   D. clavicle

_____ 36. You are treating a 62-year-old male who was found on the floor in the hallway at the county extended care facility. You suspect that he had a syncopal episode and sustained a fractured hip. Your suspicion of a fractured hip is based on the injured limb appearing:
   A. slightly warm.
   B. shorter than the other extremity.
   C. longer than the other extremity.
   D. mottled and cold.

_____ 37. Your 36-year-old female patient had a serious fall. She is complaining of an unexplained sensation of having to empty her bladder. She may have experienced a _____ fracture.
   A. femur   C. pelvic
   B. hip   D. rib

_____ 38. Your 59-year-old male patient was crushed by a vehicle. You suspect that he has a pelvic injury. When stabilizing him, you should do all of the following _except_:
   A. assume that there is a spinal injury.
   B. determine distal function.
   C. closely monitor the vitals for shock.
   D. raise the lower legs.

Complete the Following

1. List eight signs and symptoms of musculoskeletal injury.

   A. _____

   B. _____

   C. _____

   D. _____

   E. _____

   F. _____

   G. _____

   H. _____

2. List eight signs and symptoms of a hip fracture.

   A. _____

   B. _____

   C. _____

   D. _____

   E. _____

   F. _____

   G. _____

   H. _____

3. List the "six Ps" in assessing compromise to an extremity:

   A. _____

   B. _____

   C. _____

   D. _____

   E. _____

   F. _____

Label the Diagram

Fill in the name of each bone on the line provided.

Skeletal System

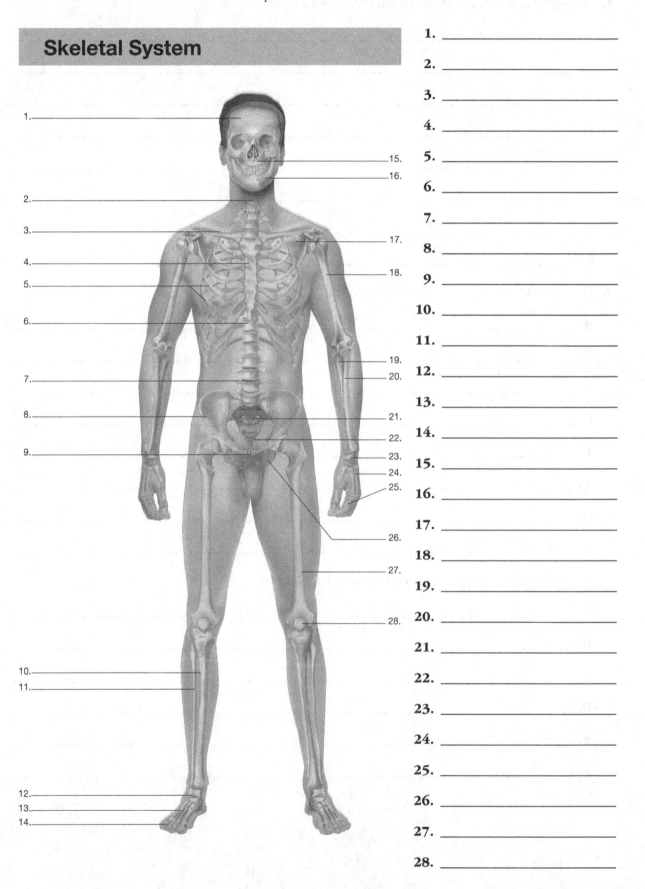

1. _____
2. _____
3. _____
4. _____
5. _____
6. _____
7. _____
8. _____
9. _____
10. _____
11. _____
12. _____
13. _____
14. _____
15. _____
16. _____
17. _____
18. _____
19. _____
20. _____
21. _____
22. _____
23. _____
24. _____
25. _____
26. _____
27. _____
28. _____

©2021 Pearson Education, Inc.
Emergency Care, 14th Ed.

Pathophysiology: Fracture or No Fracture?

1. Why do patients who experience a long bone fracture often experience shock?

_____

2. Why should the EMT splint on suspicion of a fracture rather than confirming the presence of a fracture?

_____

3. What is the significance of the swelling when a patient has a suspected fracture?

_____

Case Study: Just a Slip on Ice

Your unit is responding to a call for an older adult patient who slipped on the ice in her driveway on a winter morning. Upon your arrival, you find a neighbor comforting the patient, who is lying covered with a blanket in the middle of the driveway. The neighbor says that she was in her kitchen looking out the window and happened to notice Mrs. Smith walking out to check her mail. The neighbor says that she saw Mrs. Smith slip and fall, so she grabbed a blanket and cell phone and rushed right out to help her. You introduce yourself to the patient and find that she has pain in both of her wrists and forearms. Apparently, when she started to slip, she fell on her outstretched arms. Your partner quickly gets the stretcher as you assess Mrs. Smith's mental status and the rest of the primary assessment. She is confused about the day of the week, is shivering, and is very cold already.

1. In addition to her mental status, what else should be checked as a part of your primary assessment of Mrs. Smith?

_____

GZQ **2.** Would it be appropriate to quickly move the patient into your ambulance?

_____

3. Once you determine that the patient has an open airway, breathing, and a pulse, what examination should you be conducting on her?

_____

The patient has no complaints of back pain or neck pain and did not strike her head. You carefully move her to the stretcher, being alert to the injuries in both arms. Once she is in the ambulance, you turn on the heat and obtain a complete set of baseline vital signs. The rapid trauma examination revealed scrapes to both elbows, a bloody nose, and two closed wrist fractures. You begin applying splints to the injured arms. The vitals are pulse 70 and regular, respirations 20 and regular, BP 110/70 mmHg, and SpO_2 97%.

4. Before and after splinting the patient's arms, what additional assessment should be done and documented?

_____

5. On the basis of your assessment and vital signs obtained so far, do you believe that the patient is in shock from the injuries?

_____

6. What information should you ask in reference to the patient's medical history that may be relevant to this case?

_____

The dispatcher notifies you that a medic unit might not be available for another 15 minutes because of heavy call volume due to the weather. You then plan to transport and confirm that you will not be waiting on the scene for the medic unit. The nearest hospital that can handle orthopedic injuries is only 10 minutes away. As she warms up, the patient stops shivering and is able to explain her entire medical history to you. She had a stroke two years ago and did not sustain any long-term deficits. She is occasionally a little unstable on her feet, and the icy driveway caused her to fall. She can recall the entire incident and is very thankful that her neighbor came right out to her aid. You have a nice conversation on the way to the hospital, although you know Mrs. Smith's arms must be hurting her a lot.

7. What is the relevance of a previous stroke in this case?

_____

GZQ **8.** What can you do to help to minimize the patient's pain, in the absence of an ALS unit to administer medication?

_____

33

Trauma to the Head, Neck, and Spine

Core Concepts

- Understanding the anatomy of the nervous system, head, and spine
- Understanding skull and brain injuries and emergency care for skull and brain injuries
- Understanding wounds to the neck and emergency care for neck wounds
- Understanding spine injuries and assessment and emergency care for spine injuries
- Understanding spinal motion restriction issues and how to immobilize various types of patients with potential spine injury

Outcomes

After reading this chapter you should be able to:

33.1 Summarize concepts of injuries to the head and spine. (pp. 950–958)
- State the consequences to society of brain and spine injuries.
- Explain the overall purposes served by the nervous system.
- Describe how the structures and functions of the central and peripheral divisions of the nervous system work together.
- Identify the anatomy of the skull.
- Explain the relationship between the components of the central nervous system and the structures that protect them.
- Describe the pathophysiologic consequences of injuries to the brain and spinal cord.
- Explain how the presence of injuries of the soft tissues, skull, and spinal column relates to injuries to the central nervous system.
- Relate mechanisms of injury to the potential for injuries to the head and spine.
- Categorize the features of different types of traumatic brain injuries.
- Describe the pathophysiology that increases intracranial pressure.

33.2 Summarize management considerations in the care of a patient with an injury to the head and spine. (pp. 958–963)
- Explain the attention required for the assessment of an intervention with a patient's airway and breathing.
- Relate abnormal assessment findings to the potential for central nervous system injury.
- Apply the Glasgow Coma Scale to the assessment of level of responsiveness.

- Explain how to prioritize the steps of management for patients who have sustained injuries to the head or spine.
- Justify transportation decision making with interpretation of the patient condition in the context of the EMS system.

33.3 Summarize concepts of injuries to the face, jaw, and soft tissues of the neck. (pp. 963–966)
- Recognize how injuries of facial and soft tissues of the neck are associated with potential brain and spinal cord injuries.
- Explain the relationship between injuries to the face, jaw, and soft tissues of the neck and life-threatening injuries of associated structures.
- Recommend a prioritized plan of treatment for patients with injuries to the face, jaw, and soft tissues of the neck.

33.4 Summarize concepts of spinal injuries. (pp. 966–993)
- Distinguish between spinal injury and spinal cord injury.
- Identify mechanisms of injury with potential for injury to the spine and spinal cord.
- Outline the steps for assessing for a suspected injury of the spine and spinal cord.
- Identify signs and symptoms of spine and spinal cord injuries.
- Describe the application of the NEXUS algorithm in assessing for spinal cord injury.
- Identify patients who are candidates for spinal motion restriction procedures.
- Prioritize spinal motion restriction among the patient's needs.
- Match various portrayals of patients with the devices most suited to achieve spinal motion restriction.
- Outline the steps of applying each type of spinal motion restriction device to a patient.
- Explain how to adapt steps of spinal motion restriction to special circumstances.

Match Key Terms

Part A

A. All of the body's nerves with the exception of the brain and spinal cord.

B. Mild closed head injury without detectable damage to the brain. Complete recovery usually expected but effects may linger for weeks, months, even years.

C. Provides overall control of thought, sensation, and the voluntary and involuntary motor functions of the body. The components of this system are the brain and spinal cord as well as the nerves that enter and exit the brain and spinal cord and extend to various parts of the body.

D. The cheek bone. Also called the zygomatic bone.

E. The bony bump on a vertebra.

F. The bones of the spinal column (singular vertebra).

G. The movable joint formed between the mandible and the temporal bones.

H. The bony structure making up the forehead, top, back, and sides of the skull.

I. The fluid that surrounds the brain and spinal cord.

J. A bruised brain caused when the force of a blow to the head is great enough to rupture blood vessels.

K. The brain and spinal cord.

_____ 1. Autonomic nervous system

_____ 2. Central nervous system

_____ 3. Cerebrospinal fluid (CSF)

_____ 4. Concussion

_____ 5. Contusion

_____ 6. Cranium

_____ 7. Orbits

_____ 8. Peripheral nervous system

_____ 9. Spinous process

_____ 10. Temporal bones

_____ 11. Temporomandibular joint (TMJ)

_____ 12. Laceration

L. The bones that forms part of the sides of the skull.

M. The bones that form the upper third, or bridge, of the nose.

N. The bony structures around the eye sockets.

O. A state of shock (hypoperfusion) caused by nerve paralysis that sometimes develops from spinal injuries.

P. Controls involuntary functions.

Q. The lower jaw bone.

R. In brain injuries, a cut to the brain.

_____ **13.** Malar

_____ **14.** Mandible

_____ **15.** Vertebrae

_____ **16.** Nasal bones

_____ **17.** Nervous system

_____ **18.** Neurogenic shock

Part B

A. The opening at the base of the skull through which the spinal cord passes from the brain.

B. Pressure inside the skull.

C. The two fused bones forming the upper jaw.

D. Pushing of a portion of the brain down towards the foramen magnum as a result of increased intracranial pressure.

E. In a head injury, a collection of blood within the skull or brain.

F. An area of the skin that is innervated by a single spinal nerve.

G. A blockage in the blood circulation of the lung caused by a air bubble.

H. A bubble of air in the bloodstream.

I. Limiting the movement of the spine to prevent additional injury.

J. A pattern of irregular and unpredictable breathing commonly caused by brain injury.

K. A distinct pattern of breathing characterized by quickening and deepening respirations followed by a period of apnea.

L. A pattern of rapid and deep breathing caused by injury to the brain.

_____ **1.** Dermatome

_____ **2.** Foramen magnum

_____ **3.** Hematoma

_____ **4.** Herniation

_____ **5.** Intracranial pressure (ICP)

_____ **6.** Maxillae

_____ **7.** Spinal motion restriction

_____ **8.** Cheyne-Stokes breathing

_____ **9.** Pulmonary air embolism

_____ **10.** Air embolism

_____ **11.** Ataxic respirations

_____ **12.** Central neurogenic hyperventilation

Multiple-Choice Review

_____ **1.** The function of the spinal column is to:
   A. produce cerebrospinal fluid.
   B. protect the spinal cord.
   C. allow for back movement in all directions.
   D. manufacture platelets.

2. The spine is made up of _____ vertebrae.
   A. 35   C. 33
   B. 23   D. 38

3. You are assessing a 38-year-old male who was struck on the head with a beer bottle in a bar fight. When a patient has a scalp injury, the EMT should:
   A. expect minimal bleeding.   C. expect profuse bleeding.
   B. determine the wound depth.   D. palpate the site with the fingertips.

4. You are assessing a who was involved in a bar fight earlier this evening. It is now 4 a.m., and the family called the ambulance because he has been vomiting. You notice that he has a bruise behind the ear. This is called:
   A. Cushing syndrome.   C. Battle sign.
   B. raccoon eyes.   D. posturing syndrome.

5. While assessing a patient with blunt trauma to the head, your assessment reveals that he also has discoloration of the soft tissues under both eyes. This finding is called:
   A. Cushing syndrome.   C. Battle sign.
   B. raccoon eyes.   D. LaFort fracture.

6. You suspect that your 41-year-old female patient may have a traumatic brain injury after a significant blow to the head. Her signs and symptoms may include:
   A. blood or fluid flowing from the ears and/or nose.
   B. yellow discoloration in the eyes.
   C. bruising around the base of the nose.
   D. pain at the base of the neck.

7. Traumatic brain injury may result in:
   A. airway swelling and dizziness.
   B. altered mental status and unequal pupils.
   C. difficulty moving below the waist.
   D. headache and hypoperfusion.

8. Which of the following is a late sign of traumatic brain injury?
   A. A temperature increase (fever)   C. Slow breathing
   B. Bleeding from the nose   D. Constricted pupils

9. Which of the following is generally *not* a sign of traumatic brain injury, except in infants?
   A. Bleeding from the nose and ears   C. Hypoperfusion
   B. Unequal pupils   D. Seizures

10. Based on the NEXUS study, the current spinal assessment used in the field should incorporate:
   A. determining if the patient is reliable.
   B. determining if there are distracting injuries.
   C. close attention to the MOI in younger children.
   D. all of the above.

11. You are treating a 32-year-old female who was not wearing a helmet and struck her head when she fell off her bike. In some EMS systems, she would be taken to a trauma center if her Glasgow Coma Scale (GCS) score was less than:
   A. 8.   C. 12.
   B. 10.   D. 14.

12. You are treating a 45-year-old male construction worker who has a four-foot steel rod penetrating his skull. You should:
   A. shorten lengthy objects, using any appropriate tools to minimize vibration.
   B. elevate the patient's legs immediately.
   C. remove the object and quickly control the bleeding.
   D. stabilize the object with bulky dressings and transport immediately.

©2021 Pearson Education, Inc.
Emergency Care, 14th Ed.

_____ **13.** You are treating a 19-year-old female who was found at the bottom of a stairway in a pool of blood. Her face has multiple fractures, her nose is broken, and her jaw may be fractured. The primary concern for emergency care of a facial fracture or jaw injury is the:

  A. external bleeding.   **C.** loss of teeth.
  B. patient's airway.   **D.** basilar skull fracture.

_____ **14.** You are treating a 35-year-old male who has an injury to one of his spinal vertebrae. The _____ vertebrae are the vertebrae most susceptible to injury because they are not supported by other bony structures.

  A. lumbar and sacral   **C.** coccygeal and thoracic
  B. thoracic and cervical   **D.** cervical and lumbar

_____ **15.** When the spine is excessively pulled, which commonly occurs during a hanging, this is called a(n) _____ injury.

  A. excessive rotation   **C.** distraction
  B. lateral bending   **D.** compression

_____ **16.** On your size-up of an automobile collision, you notice that both sides of the windshield have a spiderweb crack. In calling for a backup ambulance you should report that both the driver and passenger:

  A. have probably sustained abdominal injuries.
  B. are in critical condition.
  C. may require spinal motion restriction.
  D. will require multiple EMS personnel to properly extract them from the vehicle.

_____ **17.** Which of the following would be least likely to cause a spine injury?

  A. A motorized recreational vehicle crash.
  B. A fall from a roof that causes open fractures to the ankles.
  C. A trauma patient who was shot in the abdomen.
  D. A diving injury into the shallow end of the pool.

_____ **18.** All of the following are examples of cervical-spine injuries that can result from a diving accident *except*:

  A. excessive extension.   **C.** excessive flexion.
  B. compression.   **D.** lateral bending.

_____ **19.** The patient does not complain of any spinal pain. It is important to remember that a lack of spinal pain does not rule out the possibility of spinal-cord injury because:

  A. spinal injuries seldom cause pain.
  B. other distracting painful injuries may mask it.
  C. spinal injuries are not painful until shock sets in.
  D. a patient may feel the pain but not be able to verbalize it.

_____ **20.** When assessing a suspected spine-injured patient, you note excessive abdominal motion with each breath but no chest wall motion. This is likely a result of damage to the nerves that control the:

  A. intercostal muscles.   **C.** abdomen.
  B. diaphragm.   **D.** lungs.

_____ **21.** When a child who was in a car seat needs to be taken to the hospital after a high-speed motor vehicle collision, the best procedure is to:

  A. keep the child in the car seat.
  B. use the rapid extrication from car seat procedure.
  C. lay down the car seat on your stretcher.
  D. lift the child out of the seat and place on your stretcher.

_____ **22.** You are treating a 52-year-old male who was involved in a serious high-speed collision. If the patient is up and walking around at the scene, you should:
  A. assess for a potential spinal injury.
  B. check with medical direction for orders.
  C. check with bystanders about the patient's mental status.
  D. assume that the patient is uninjured.

_____ **23.** If a responsive patient has the mechanism of injury for a spinal injury, the EMT should do all of the following *except*:
  A. assess for spinal pain by asking the patient to move.
  B. keep the patient still while asking him or her questions.
  C. assess for sensation in the extremities.
  D. assess for tingling in the extremities.

_____ **24.** After performing the primary assessment on a patient found in the supine position that you suspect has a spinal cord injury, your next step is to:
  A. apply an appropriately sized rigid cervical collar.
  B. administer high-concentration oxygen.
  C. secure the patient's head.
  D. reassess the patient's distal CSM.

_____ **25.** You are assessing a 27-year-old male who you suspect has a spine injury. If he complains of pain when you attempt to place his head in a neutral inline position, you should:
  A. pad the neck before immobilizing.
  B. steady the head in the position found.
  C. continue with the stabilization procedure.
  D. contact medical direction immediately.

_____ **26.** When treating a patient, who you suspect has a spine injury, one EMT on your crew should:
  A. strap the patient's head, then the torso, to the long spine board.
  B. maintain manual inline spine motion restriction until the patient is secured.
  C. assess for range of cervical spine motion.
  D. pad the neck before stabilizing.

_____ **27.** Which of the following statements about the rigid cervical collar is *false*?
  A. A collar of an incorrect size can hyperextend the neck.
  B. Maintain manual spine motion restriction when applying a rigid cervical collar.
  C. The collar completely eliminates neck movement.
  D. The collar should never obstruct the airway.

_____ **28.** If a stable 22-year-old male patient is found in a sitting position in a car and is complaining about severe back pain, the EMT should:
  A. apply a cervical collar and rapidly transport the patient.
  B. guide and lower the patient to a long spine board.
  C. use a "big splint" due to multiple injuries.
  D. perform a rapid take-down procedure with a long spine board.

_____ **29.** You are treating a 45-year-old female who was involved in a high-speed car crash and has multiple fractures. You have decided to use the long spine board, which is typically used in all of the following situations *except* when:
  A. moving a patient rapidly from an unsafe scene.
  B. a stable, low-priority patient must be immobilized.
  C. a more seriously injured patients must be accessed.
  D. moving a high-priority patient to the stretcher.

_____ **30.** When immobilizing a 6-year-old or younger child on a long backboard:
  A. provide padding beneath the shoulder blades.
  B. it is unnecessary to apply a cervical collar.
  C. place a chin cup or chin strap on the patient.
  D. secure the head first and then secure the torso.

_____ **31.** Your patient is a 19-year-old male who was involved in a motorcycle crash. You should consider keeping the helmet on the patient:
  A. if it interferes with breathing management.
  B. if it has a snug fit that allows no head movement.
  C. by using a two-rescuer procedure.
  D. if it hinders immobilization.

_____ **32.** Which is the correct order of steps for applying a vest-type extrication device?
  1. Secure the device to the patient's torso.
  2. Secure the patient's head to the device.
  3. Position the device behind the patient.
  4. Reassess distal CSM.

  A. 3, 2, 1, 4   **C.** 4, 3, 1, 2
  B. 3, 1, 2, 4   **D.** 3, 4, 1, 2

_____ **33.** Before and after immobilization, the EMT should assess:
  A. pulses in all extremities.
  B. motor function in all extremities.
  C. sensation in all extremities.
  D. all of these.

_____ **34.** You are treating a patient who fell backward and struck his head after being shot. You suspect that he is developing increased ICP. The time it takes to develop the symptoms from an increased ICP depends on the location of the bleed and:
  A. the rate of bleeding into the head.
  B. the type of weapon used.
  C. the age of the patient
  D. all of these.

_____ **35.** You are treating a 22-year-old female who was assaulted with a knife. The attacker slashed the patient's throat. Initially, there was considerable blood, but you were able to control it and bandage the wound. The patient went into sudden cardiac arrest. What is the most likely cause?
  A. A stroke   **C.** An air embolism
  B. A heart attack   **D.** Infection from the wound

Pathophysiology: Dysfunction from Spine Injury

1. Your 35-year-old male patient was involved in a car crash and sustained an injury to the third, fourth, or fifth cervical vertebrae. He may have an injury to which nerve? What would be the expected effect on the patient?

_____

2. At a point in the development of this patient's injury, as described in question 1, the patient begins to exhibit hypotension. Why does this develop?

_____

3. Why doesn't this patient's pulse increase like that of most other patients who are in shock?

_____

Complete the Following

1. List fifteen signs of a skull fracture or brain injury.

   A. _____

   B. _____

   C. _____

   D. _____

   E. _____

   F. _____

   G. _____

   H. _____

   I. _____

   J. _____

   K. _____

   L. _____

   M. _____

   N. _____

   O. _____

2. List five high-risk mechanisms for spinal injury.

   A. _____

   B. _____

   C. _____

   D. _____

   E. _____

3. List the missing descriptions for the number value in the Glasgow Coma
   Scale below:

   A. Eye Opening: 4 _____

   B. Eye Opening: 3 _____

C. Eye Opening: 2 _____

D. Eye Opening: 1 _____

E. Verbal Response: 5 _____

F. Verbal Response: 4 _____

G. Verbal Response: 3 _____

H. Verbal Response: 2 _____

I. Verbal Response: 2 _____

J. Verbal Response: 1 _____

K. Motor Response: 6 _____

L. Motor Response: 5 _____

M. Motor Response: 4 _____

N. Motor Response: 3 _____

O. Motor Response: 2 _____

P. Motor Response: 1 _____

4. A patient has a significant epidural hematoma after being struck on the side of the head with a baseball. List seven stages in the progression of this patient.

A. _____

B. _____

C. _____

D. _____

E. _____

F. _____

G. _____

Label the Diagram

Fill in the name of each division of the spine on the line provided.

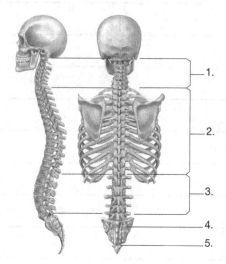

1.
2.
3.
4.
5.

1. _____

2. _____

3. _____

4. _____

5. _____

Case Study: Deep Dive in a Shallow Pool

You respond to a call for an injury in a pool at a private residence. The EMS dispatcher tells you that they have received numerous 911 calls about this incident and are trying to calm someone down to obtain better information. Fortunately, your EMS station is only about a mile from the location. As you pull up in front, you see lots of cars parked outside. A bystander runs up to the ambulance and says, "Please come quickly. He is still in the swimming pool. Can I help you carry anything?" Hearing this, you notify the dispatcher to continue the ALS unit and have the police respond also.

You and your partner are experienced swimmers. As you enter the backyard with your equipment, you ask your partner quickly, "Wet or dry?" She says, "Go. I'll take care of coordinating the poolside activities."

When you first see the patient, he is face up and is being assisted in floating on his back by another person in the pool, who states that his name is Max. He says that he was a lifeguard 15 years ago. The patient, an adult male about 40 years old, is in about 5 feet of water.

You quickly empty your pockets, remove your shoes, and hand the radio to your partner. Then you carefully enter the shallow end of the pool without making any waves.

1. What would you want to know about the patient from Max right away?

_____

2. How would you move the patient from the deep water to the shallow end of the pool?

_____

Seeing that most of the adults are a bit intoxicated and most of the children at poolside are a bit small, you ask your partner to get an ETA on the backup unit. Just then, the members of the backup unit come into the backyard. There are two paramedics and an EMT who is a student in the paramedic course. You ask them to assist with the patient removal if they are good swimmers.

3. What equipment will be needed?

_____

In talking with Max, you learn that the party is a celebration for the children's having won a soccer tournament. The patient, whose name is Tom, is the coach and apparently is not usually a drinker, so after he had two beers he did something he normally would never have done. Apparently, several people were horsing around near the edge of the pool, and Tom flipped head-first into the shallow end. Max reports that the patient was initially unconscious. Max entered the pool and carefully turned him over, as he was trained years ago to do, and Tom regained consciousness after a moment or two. Max said that he did not believe Tom swallowed any water.

4. What other information should you obtain?

_____

As one of the medics and the student enter the water with a long backboard and a rigid collar, you instruct Max to continue to stabilize the patient's head and neck in a neutral position. You assist the patient in floating. The patient is very scared because he is unable to feel his arms or legs.

GZQ **5.** When the patient asks you what are you going to do, what should you tell him?

_____

You carefully float the patient to the shallow end of the pool and do the immobilization there. The voids are padded, and the patient is strapped to the board. By this time, the police have arrived and have asked the soccer team members and their parents to move to the deck area and watch from there. Your partner has found two more helpers who are not intoxicated to assist in the lifting at poolside. Your in-water team lifts the immobilized patient onto the edge of the pool, and the out-of-water team carefully lifts the patient and backboard onto a stretcher.

6. What are some of the initial management steps that your partner should take while you get out of the pool?

_____

Once it is clear that your patient has no movement in his arms and legs, your partner and the paramedic call for a helicopter and ask the police to set up a landing zone. Fortunately, there is an elementary school with a large field about a half-mile away. The patient will be going directly to the regional trauma center, and a paramedic will be going along.

When the patient is loaded into your ambulance, the paramedic inserts an IV, the patient's clothing is cut off, he is covered with a blanket, the pulse oximeter is attached, and ECG electrodes are placed on him. His vital signs are still within normal range at this time (pulse of 62 and regular, respirations of 24, BP of 130/80 mmHg, and SpO_2 of 98%).

You take the patient and the paramedic to the elementary school, where the patient is transferred to the helicopter, and it takes off. The report that is relayed back to you from the helicopter team says that the patient sustained a fracture at C-6 that severed his spinal cord.

7. Before handing in your PCR, is there anything that you should make sure is clearly documented? If so, what?

_____

_____

_____

_____

Multisystem Trauma

Core Concepts

- How to balance the critical trauma patient's need for prompt transport against the time needed to treat all of the patient's injuries at the scene
- How to determine the severity of the trauma patient's condition, priority for transport, and appropriate transport destination
- How to select the critical interventions to implement at the scene for a multiple-trauma patient
- How to calculate a trauma score

Outcomes

After reading this chapter, you should be able to:

35.1 Summarize the approach to patients with multisystem trauma. (pp. 998–1009)
  - Outline the key decisions that must be made with regard to treatment and transport priorities of patients with multisystem trauma.
  - Analyze the combination of physiologic, anatomic, mechanism-of-injury, patient, and situational factors to estimate the patient's severity of injury.
  - Relate specific assessment findings to a potential for critical internal injuries.
  - Describe the emphasis on teamwork required for successful management of multisystem trauma situations.
  - Apply the principles of managing multisystem trauma to descriptions of multisystem trauma situations.
  - Explain the utility of trauma scoring tools in assessing trauma patients.

Match Key Terms

A. One or more injuries that affect more than one body system.

B. A numerical rating system for trauma patients to determine severity.

C. More than one serious injury.

_____ 1. Multiple trauma

_____ 2. Multisystem trauma

_____ 3. Trauma score

Multiple-Choice Review

_____ **1.** You were called to the scene of a motor vehicle collision where two cars collided in an intersection. One of the vehicles pinned a 26-year-old female pedestrian against a tree. She has sustained a fractured right femur and crushed pelvis. She would be considered a _____ patient.
   A. lower-extremity
   B. multiple-trauma
   C. shock
   D. stable

_____ **2.** The driver of one of the vehicles involved in a multi-car MVC is a 52-year-old male who has an obvious angulated forearm. You find him lying unresponsive across the front seat of his vehicle. What is the highest priority for this multiple-trauma patient?
   A. Splinting his arm
   B. Immobilizing his neck
   C. Managing his airway
   D. Assessing his distal pulses

_____ **3.** At what point will an unresponsive 52-year-old male involved in an MVC most likely be considered stabilized?
   A. At the emergency department
   B. Once en route to the trauma center
   C. Once his injured arm is splinted
   D. Once the ALS has been called.

_____ **4.** To save the life of a critical patient, it will be important for the EMT to remember the three "Ts" in the management of a multiple-trauma patient. The three "Ts" are timing, transport, and:
   A. teamwork.
   B. trauma.
   C. treatment.
   D. thorax.

_____ **5.** The guidelines for trauma triage and transport released by the Centers for Disease Control and Prevention take into consideration all of the following factors _except_:
   A. physiologic determinants.
   B. the patient's sex.
   C. MOI.
   D. anatomic criteria.

_____ **6.** A 29-year-old female trauma patient begins to make gurgling sounds as she breathes. What should you do next?
   A. Ventilate her.
   B. Suction the airway.
   C. Hyperextend the neck.
   D. Apply oxygen with a nonrebreather mask.

_____ **7.** Your 31-year-old male patient has numerous fractures in his legs from being run over by a pickup truck. Sometimes a _____ can act as a universal splint when the critical patient must be immobilized quickly.
   A. wheeled stretcher
   B. short Kendrick extrication device
   C. warm blanket
   D. long backboard

_____ **8.** Your 39-year-old male patient was changing his tire on a major highway ramp when another vehicle ran into him and his vehicle. He has two open fractured femurs, a crushed pelvis, and a possible abdominal injury. You should:
   A. not take the time to apply two traction splints.
   B. apply tourniquets to both legs if there is severe bleeding.
   C. set up an ALS intercept en route to the hospital.
   D. do all of these.

_____ **9.** You are treating an unstable multi-system trauma patient and have decided that it is appropriate to minimize your scene care in accordance with your established multisystem trauma protocols. You will most likely perform any or all of the following at the scene _except_:
   A. suctioning the airway.
   B. ventilating with a BVM.
   C. bandaging all of the lacerations.
   D. provide spinal motion restriction.

_____ **10.** Even when you are trying to limit on-scene time for a multiple-trauma patient, the one thing that you do *not* leave out is:
  A. applying traction splints if needed.
  B. the secondary assessment.
  C. ensuring scene safety.
  D. immobilization to a long backboard.

_____ **11.** An example of a patient who requires triage to a higher level of trauma care would be the:
  A. child who has a headache after being struck by a golf ball.
  B. geriatric patient who fell and is on anticoagulant medications.
  C. adolescent with a femur fracture from playing basketball.
  D. middle-aged man who may have fractured his forearm.

_____ **12.** In some EMS systems, the EMTs are asked to assign a number to the severity of the trauma patient, using the trauma score. This will help in determining where the patient should be transported. The scoring system for trauma patients also helps to:
  A. allow the trauma centers to evaluate themselves in comparing trauma patient outcomes.
  B. determine which steps in the primary survey come first.
  C. determine if the patient should only be transported by helicopter EMS from the scene.
  D. all of these.

_____ **13.** All of the following are considered physiologic criteria according to the CDC Trauma Triage Guidelines *except*:
  A. systolic blood pressure <90 mmHg.
  B. Glasgow Coma Scale <14.
  C. two or more proximal long-bone fractures.
  D. adult respiratory rate <10 or >29.

_____ **14.** According to the CDC Trauma Triage Guidelines, all of the following are considered mechanism of injury criteria *except*:
  A. intrusion (including roof) >12 inch (30 cm) occupant site.
  B. crushed, degloved, mangled, or pulseless extremity.
  C. falls (in an adult) >20 feet (6 meters).
  D. ejection (partial or complete) from automobile.

_____ **15.** In the context of multiple trauma, when assessing pediatric patients you will need to consider:
  A. MOI considerations for spinal motion restriction.
  B. additional emotional support.
  C. the need to transport family members together if possible.
  D. all of the above.

_____ **16.** Pediatric trauma patients may compensate for blood loss more effectively than adults. In this situation there may be:
  A. no need for fluid resuscitation.
  B. much faster clotting.
  C. a sudden appearance of decompensation.
  D. all of the above.

Pathophysiology: Internal Injuries

1. A patient is exhibiting an elevated pulse, respiratory distress, and absent lung sounds on the left side of his chest after having been stabbed with an ice pick. With these signs and symptoms you should suspect that he has what type of internal injury?

2. A patient has audible lung sounds on both sides of the chest but has distended neck veins, a narrowing pulse pressure, and increased pulse and respirations after being stabbed with an ice pick. You should suspect that he has what type of internal injury?

_____

Complete the Following

1. List eight examples of treatments that would be appropriate on the scene of a critical trauma patient.

A. _____

B. _____

C. _____

D. _____

E. _____

F. _____

G. _____

H. _____

2. The four principles of multisystem trauma management are the following:

A. _____

B. _____

C. _____

D. _____

3. Fill in the missing information in the Revised Trauma Score chart below:

Characteristic	Criterion	RTS Points
Glasgow Coma Scale	13–15	4
	(A)	3
	6–8	2
	4–5	**(D)**
	3	0
Systolic BP	> 89 mmHg	4
	(B)	3
	50–75 mmHg	2
	1–49 mmHg	1
	0	0

©2021 Pearson Education, Inc.
Emergency Care, 14th Ed.

Characteristic	Criterion	RTS Points
Respiratory Rate	10–29 / min	**(E)**
	(C)	3
	6–9 /min	2
	1–5 /min	1
	0	0
Revised Trauma Score	TOTAL	

A. _____

B. _____

C. _____

D. _____

E. _____

4. Using the Revised Trauma Score, chart and compile the appropriate score for each of the following patients and decide (Yes or No) if each should be transported to the trauma center:

A. An adult male who was involved in an ATV crash who struck his head. He has a GCS of 10 and vitals include a BP of 110/60 and respiratory rate of 30.

B. A child who fell down stairs and has multiple leg fractures and a GCS of 12 with a BP of 70/50 and respiratory rate of 28.

C. An adult who was involved in a motor vehicle crash. You suspect there may have been drug intoxication involved. She was initially unconscious from striking her head and chest. Her GCS is 9 and BP is 88/60 with a respiratory rate of 8 on her own although you are assisting with BVM.

Case Study: A Fastball to the Head

Your ambulance is dispatched to the town park for an unconscious 12-year-old male. The medic unit is also responding from the other side of town. While you are en route to the call, the dispatcher calls you back stating that the "police on the scene are requesting your ETA." As you respond, "we are a minute from the park entrance," you can already see the police car and a crowd surrounding home plate on field number two. A bystander motions you to come quickly, so you park the ambulance and grab your primary bag.

As you and your partner get closer to the field, you can see that about five children and three adults, including the police officer, are trying to attend to the child, who has an obvious injury to the right side of his head and eye. He is bleeding, so you take Standard Precautions. Your partner kneels at the child's head, manually stabilizes the head and neck, and opens the airway using a jaw thrust maneuver.

One of the children steps forward and says, "This is Ali, and we were just playing baseball. Ali was trying to hit my fastball, and he got hit on the side of the head. We called for help right away when we saw his head bleeding and his eye socket got all swollen like that. At first he was talking to us, but he said it hurt a lot. After a couple of minutes, he passed out."

1. Because the scene is safe and ALS is en route, what will be your next steps in the assessment of this injured child?

_____

2. Your partner is able to confirm from a police officer that Ali was conscious but became unconscious just as your unit was pulling into the parking lot. How should you determine Ali's mental status?

_____

GZQ **3.** The bleeding has slowed and does not seem to be a life threat, although the patient's right eye is so swollen that it can no longer be opened. Will it be necessary to use a collar and a long backboard with this patient?

_____

You complete the primary assessment and determine that your major concern at this point is a closed head injury that is causing the patient to be responsive only to painful stimuli. When you squeeze his muscle on top of his shoulder, his legs extend and his arms flex. You remember from your EMT course that this is called "decorticate posturing" and is not a good sign. You and your partner decide that Ali is a high priority, and the plan is to get a set of baseline vitals, do a quick rapid trauma examination while immobilizing him, and head for the ambulance. If the medic unit does not arrive, you will try to arrange a meeting spot on the way to the trauma center. The baseline vitals are respirations 26, shallow and irregular, pulse of 52 and strong, blood pressure of 132/78 mmHg and SpO_2 of 92%.

4. Just as you are packaging Ali onto the long backboard, he begins to vomit. How should you deal with this complication?

_____

GZQ **5.** Apparently, the large blood clot that had formed in Ali's right sinus area has opened up, and he is now bleeding into his airway. Does this change his priority?

_____

After clearing the patient's airway, you decide to assist his ventilations with the BVM and oxygen. This will tie up both you and your partner, but as you move the stretcher into the ambulance, the medic unit pulls up. After a brief update on the patient's condition, the medic begins to assist in airway management and asks your partner to start driving to the trauma center. The medic notes that the area that was struck is the temporal area of the skull. While securing the airway, the medic asks you to call ahead to the trauma center to give them early notice that Ali may have an epidural hematoma and that the patient's parent is being taken directly to the hospital by the police.

6. With a patient who is this critical, when would be the appropriate time for you to calculate the trauma score?

_____

_____

©2021 Pearson Education, Inc.
Emergency Care, 14th Ed.

35

Environmental Emergencies

Core Concepts

- Effects on the body of generalized hypothermia; assessment and care for hypothermia
- Effects on the body of local cold injuries; assessment and care for local cold injuries
- Effects on the body of exposure to heat; assessment and care for patients suffering from heat exposure
- Signs, symptoms, and treatment for drowning and other water-related injuries
- Signs, symptoms, and treatment for bites and stings
- Signs, symptoms, and treatment for high-altitude illness

Outcomes

After reading this chapter, you should be able to:

35.1 Summarize the scope of environmental emergencies. (p. 1015)
- Identify situations in which environmental emergencies may occur.
- List the general types of environmental emergencies.

35.2 Summarize the physiology and limitations of body temperature regulation. (pp. 1015–1016)
- Describe the mechanisms by which the body produces and conserves heat.
- Describe the mechanisms by which the body loses heat.
- Compare the mechanism of local cold injuries with that of generalized hypothermia.
- Describe the mechanisms underlying heat emergencies.

35.3 Recognize the presence of cold-related environmental emergencies. (pp. 1016–1018)
- Analyze environment, patient predisposing factors, and signs and symptoms to establish a suspicion for cold-related emergencies.
- Explain how age influences the suspicion for hypothermia.
- Recognize the potential for patients' becoming hypothermic as a result of another emergency circumstance.
- Differentiate the characteristics of early and late localized cold injuries.

35.4 Summarize the approach to managing patients with cold emergencies. (pp. 1019–1025)
- Explain the significance in decision making of the finding of altered mental status in a patient with hypothermia.
- Explain how to prioritize rewarming procedures with other priorities for treatment as they are impacted by the presence of hypothermia.

- Compare the characteristics of active and passive rewarming techniques.
- Explain precautions in managing a hypothermic patient in proposed treatment plans.
- Explain the adaptation of resuscitative techniques to the severely hypothermic patient.
- Outline the management of localized cold injuries.

35.5 Recognize the presence of heat-related environmental emergencies. (pp. 1025–1026)
- Analyze environment, patient predisposing factors, and signs and symptoms to establish a suspicion for heat-related emergencies.
- Compare the heat-related emergencies most likely in patients who have moist, pale, and normal or cool skin; and those in patients who have hot, either dry or moist skin.

35.6 Summarize the approach to managing patients with heat-related environmental emergencies. (pp. 1027–1029)
- Recognize the importance of skin color and condition in the decision-making process for treating patients with suspected heat-related environmental emergencies.
- Compare the cooling techniques used for patients with cool, pale, moist, or normal skin with those used for patients with hot skin, whether dry or moist.

35.7 Explain the role of EMTs in the rescue of patients in water accidents. (pp. 1029–1031)
- List the conditions under which an EMT might reasonably consider making a water rescue.
- Describe the sequence of rescue attempts for reaching a patient in the water.
- Describe how EMTs may safely reach a patient requiring ice rescue.
- Describe considerations for starting rescue breathing with the patient still in the water.
- Describe the approach for caring for possible spinal injuries in the water.
- Anticipate injuries related to open-water diving emergencies.

35.8 Summarize the pathophysiology of a patient in a water accident. (pp. 1031–1039)
- Anticipate the types of problems that can accompany water-related accidents.
- Explain the mechanism by which drowning occurs.
- Compare the pathophysiology of air embolism and decompression sickness in scuba diving accidents.
- Compare the signs and symptoms of air embolism and decompression sickness in scuba diving accidents.

35.9 Summarize the pathophysiology of altitude illness. (pp. 1039–1041)
- Explain physiologic adaptations to high altitude.
- Describe the signs and symptoms of high-altitude illness.
- Discuss procedures to care for patients with high-altitude illness.

35.10 Differentiate the concepts of bites leading to anaphylaxis and those leading to venomous injection with localized or systemic reactions. (pp. 1041–1047)
- List information that should be gathered at the scene to determine the source of a bite.
- Recognize the assessment findings associated with dry and envenomated bites.
- Describe specific steps that are taken to manage the absorption of venom into the tissues and circulation.

Match Key Terms

Part A

A. The change of a substance from liquid to gas.

B. An increase in the body temperature above normal, which is a life-threatening condition in its extreme.

C. Application of an external heat source to rewarm the body of a hypothermic patient.

D. Carrying away of heat by currents of air, water, or other gases or liquids.

_____ **1.** Active rewarming

_____ **2.** Central rewarming

_____ **3.** Conduction

_____ **4.** Convection

_____ **5.** Decompression sickness

E. Generalized cooling that reduces body temperature below normal, which is a life-threatening condition in its extreme.

F. Gas bubble in the bloodstream.

G. A condition resulting from nitrogen trapped in the body's tissues, caused by coming up too quickly from a deep, prolonged dive.

H. Application of heat specifically to the lateral chest, neck, armpits, and groin of a hypothermic patient.

I. The process of experiencing respiratory impairment from submersion or immersion in liquid, which may result in death.

J. The transfer of heat from one material to another through direct contact.

_____ **6.** Drowning

_____ **7.** Evaporation

_____ **8.** Hyperthermia

_____ **9.** Hypothermia

_____ **10.** Air embolism

Part B

A. Chilling caused by convection of heat from the body in the presence of air currents.

B. Covering a hypothermic patient and taking other steps to prevent further heat loss and help the body rewarm itself.

C. Sending out energy, such as heat, in waves.

D. Refers to the loss of body heat through breathing.

E. Cooling or freezing of particular part of the body.

F. A toxin (poison) produced by certain animals such as snakes, spiders, and some marine life forms.

G. Substances produced by animals or plants that are poisonous to humans.

H. Chilling caused by conduction of heat from the body when the body or clothing is wet.

_____ **1.** Local cooling

_____ **2.** Passive rewarming

_____ **3.** Radiation

_____ **4.** Respiration

_____ **5.** Toxins

_____ **6.** Venom

_____ **7.** Water chill

_____ **8.** Wind chill

Multiple-Choice Review

_____ **1.** Heat will flow from a warmer material to a cooler one. Water conducts heat away from the body _____ than still air.
  A. 25 times faster
  B. 25 times slower
  C. 50 times faster
  D. 50 times slower

_____ **2.** When there is _____ wind, there is _____ heat loss.
  A. more; less
  B. less; greater
  C. more; greater
  D. no; maximum

_____ **3.** Most radiant heat loss occurs from a person's:
  A. arms and legs.
  B. chest and back.
  C. head and neck.
  D. feet and hands.

_____ 4. You are treating a 40-year-old male who you suspect may have been predisposed to hypothermia. The factors that could predispose him include all of the following *except*:
A. burns.
B. diabetes.
C. spinal-cord injuries; spinal trauma.
D. headache.

_____ 5. Which of the following is *not* a reason that infants and children are more prone to hypothermia?
A. They have small muscle mass.
B. They have large skin surface in relation to their total body mass.
C. They are unable to shiver effectively.
D. They have more body fat than adults do.

_____ 6. You are treating a 58-year-old male patient with an open right tibia fracture. He was found lying on his cold garage floor by his son, who states, "He must have been lying there all night." Besides the fracture, you should consider:
A. stroke.
B. hypothermia.
C. pulmonary edema.
D. hyperperfusion.

_____ 7. You are treating a 68-year-old female who was found wandering around intoxicated on a cold evening. She was not wearing a coat, and you determine that her body temperature is below 90°F. With a core body temperature in this range, she:
A. may be shivering uncontrollably.
B. may no longer be shivering.
C. will be pulseless.
D. will suddenly become alert.

_____ 8. All of the following are signs and symptoms of hypothermia *except*:
A. high blood pressure and low pulse.
B. stiff or rigid posture.
C. cool abdominal skin temperature.
D. loss of motor coordination.

_____ 9. You are treating a 68-year-old male who stepped out of his house in his pajamas on a winter morning to grab the newspaper and accidentally locked himself out of the house. He wandered around the neighborhood for 20 minutes until he found a neighbor who would let him in and call 911 for help. Your protocol calls for passive rewarming of this patient. This procedure involves:
A. applying heat packs to the patient.
B. removing wet clothing and covering the patient.
C. administering heated oxygen to the patient.
D. massaging the patient's limbs.

_____ 10. You are assessing a 28-year-old female patient who got caught outdoors in a cold rain for three hours. She is alert and responding, but she is very cold, and you suspect that she is hypothermic. Her treatment may include all of the following *except*:
A. removal of all the patient's wet clothing.
B. actively rewarming the patient during transport.
C. rapidly giving the patient plenty of hot liquids.
D. providing care for shock and providing oxygen as appropriate.

_____ 11. You are actively rewarming a patient. If your medical director has authorized this treatment, you should:
A. apply heat to the chest, neck, armpits, and groin.
B. quickly rewarm the patient.
C. give the patient stimulants to drink.
D. immerse the patient's arms and feet in hot water.

_____ 12. Once the decision has been made to rewarm a hypothermic patient, central rewarming should be used. The reason why you should rewarm the body's core first is to:

    A. prevent blood from collecting in the extremities due to vasodilation.

    B. quickly circulate cold blood throughout the body.

    C. speed up the blood flow to the extremities.

    D. increase blood flow to the brain to prevent unconsciousness.

_____ 13. In a heat emergency, EMT care of a patient with moist, pale, and normal or cool skin includes all of the following _except_:

    A. placing the patient in an air-conditioned ambulance.

    B. fanning the patient so that he or she begins to shiver.

    C. placing patient in supine position.

    D. apply moist towels over cramped muscles.

_____ 14. In a heat emergency, if a patient with moist, pale, and normal or cool skin is responsive but not yet nauseated, you should:

    A. skip the oxygen.

    B. place cold packs in the patient's armpits.

    C. have the patient drink small sips of water.

    D. do all of these.

_____ 15. You are treating an unresponsive 33-year-old female hypothermia patient who is not responding appropriately. You should:

    A. keep her head raised above her feet for transport to the hospital.

    B. place her in a bath of warm for at least 20 minutes.

    C. provide high-concentration oxygen passed through a warm humidifier.

    D. massage her extremities for 35 to 45 seconds.

_____ 16. You are treating a 65-year-old male who was found by his mailbox in the snow. He is unconscious and very cold to your touch. You suspect that he slipped, fell on the ice, and struck his head. Once in the ambulance, you check his core body temperature and find that it is below 80°F. Because patients with extreme hypothermia might not reach biological death for over 30 minutes, the medical philosophy is:

    A. If there is a pulse, start CPR.

    B. They are not dead until they are warm and dead.

    C. Resuscitate for no longer than 30 minutes.

    D. Always resuscitate very aggressively.

_____ 17. A cold injury usually occurring to exposed areas of the body that is brought about by direct contact with a cold object or exposure to cold air is called:

    A. an early or superficial local cold injury.

    B. frostbite.

    C. a superficial late cold injury.

    D. a deep local cold injury.

_____ 18. The skin color of a patient with light skin who has a superficial local cold injury will change from _____ to _____.

    A. red; white   **C.** red; blue

    B. white; red   **D.** white; blue

_____ 19. Your 50-year-old male patient fell on an outstretched arm and sustained a fractured right radius and ulna. While he waited for help to arrive, the arm was exposed, and you suspect that there is a local superficial cold injury. You should:

    A. splint the arm and leave it uncovered.

    B. rub the arm briskly.

    C. not re-expose the injury to cold.

    D. immerse the arm in hot water.

_____ **20.** If the muscles, bones, deep blood vessels, and organ membranes became frozen in the patient exposed to the outside cold elements for a long period of time, this type of injury is referred to as:
  A. a superficial local cold injury.   **C.** a deep local cold injury.
  B. frostnip.   **D.** local cooling.

_____ **21.** In frostbite, the affected area first appears:
  A. black and stiff.   **C.** red and blotchy.
  B. white and waxy.   **D.** blue and abraded.

_____ **22.** Do not allow a frostbite patient to smoke or drink alcohol because:
  A. the patient may suffer altered mental status or fall asleep.
  B. these substances stimulate the patient to move, which could cause further injury.
  C. constriction of blood vessels and decreased circulation to the injured tissues may result.
  D. either could contaminate the frostbitten area.

_____ **23.** You are treating a 22-year-old female who has local deep frostbite injuries to her fingers. You have contacted medical direction and received permission to provide active rewarming of the frozen parts. This procedure:
  A. is seldom recommended in the field.
  B. includes using very hot water.
  C. is performed without removing the patient's clothing.
  D. includes covering the patient's face.

_____ **24.** When assessing an unconscious adult patient who you suspect is in extreme hypothermia, check the carotid pulse for at least _____ seconds.
  A. 10   **C.** 45
  B. 25   **D.** 60

_____ **25.** The environmental condition(s) associated with hyperthermia include heat and:
  A. high winds.   **C.** high humidity.
  B. light rain.   **D.** low humidity.

_____ **26.** You hear on the news that today will be both very hot and very humid. The higher the humidity, the:
  A. less you perspire.
  B. less your perspiration evaporates.
  C. less you radiate heat.
  D. more heat you lose from your body.

_____ **27.** When the body loses salts through sweating, the patient may have all of the following *except*:
  A. muscle cramps.   **C.** dizziness or periods of faintness.
  B. weakness or exhaustion.   **D.** fluid buildup in the lungs.

_____ **28.** You are treating a 45-year-old male who was installing a new roof on a very hot day. You suspect that he may have heat exhaustion, which means that he is likely to have:
  A. dry, hot skin.
  B. moist, pale, and normal or cool skin.
  C. a lack of sweating.
  D. a rapid, strong pulse.

_____ **29.** The signs and symptoms of a heat emergency in patients who have hot, dry, or moist skin include:
  A. slow, shallow breathing.   **C.** constricted pupils.
  B. seizures.   **D.** muscle cramps.

_____ **30.** When responding to a water-related emergency, you should suspect, in addition to a drowning, all of the following situations *except* that:
- **A.** substance abuse may have contributed to the incident.
- **B.** the patient may have sustained an internal injury.
- **C.** profuse perspiration is the likely cause.
- **D.** the patient may have struck his or her head or neck.

_____ **31.** The signs and symptoms of an air embolism associated with scuba diving include:
- **A.** altered mental status.
- **B.** blurred vision, paresthesia of extremities.
- **C.** seizures or stroke.
- **D.** any of the above.

_____ **32.** During a drowning submersion incident, water that hits the epiglottis causes:
- **A.** a reflex to close the mouth.
- **C.** a reflex spasm of the larynx.
- **B.** the patient to gasp for more air.
- **D.** the patient to begin hyperventilating.

_____ **33.** About 10% of drowning submersion victims die from:
- **A.** too much fluid in their lungs.
- **C.** cervical-spine injuries.
- **B.** lack of air.
- **D.** nitrogen bubble embolisms.

_____ **34.** You have been called to the river's edge, where fast moving water has a 17-year-old male pinned against a rock and some debris. If you are not an experienced swimmer, you should:
- **A.** not attempt to go into the water to do a rescue.
- **B.** don a flotation device before going into the water.
- **C.** use a boat as your first approach to conduct the rescue.
- **D.** coach the patient in floating techniques.

_____ **35.** You were called to a backyard swimming pool for a 28-year-old male who was seen diving into the shallow end of the pool. There is an abrasion on his forehead, and he is floating face up in the pool. If you suspect that this patient has a possible spine injury, you should:
- **A.** place the patient on a spine board as you pull him from the water.
- **B.** maintain inline stabilization until a backboard is used for spinal motion restriction.
- **C.** quickly remove the patient from the water to prevent hypothermia.
- **D.** encourage the patient to swim to the side of the pool.

_____ **36.** Two special medical problems that are seen in scuba diving accidents are decompression sickness and:
- **A.** carbon monoxide poisoning.
- **C.** arterial gas embolism.
- **B.** oxygen toxicity.
- **D.** arthritis.

_____ **37.** The risk of decompression sickness is increased by:
- **A.** air travel within 18 hours of a dive.
- **B.** breathing 100% oxygen immediately after the dive.
- **C.** drinking fluids before and after the dive.
- **D.** none of these.

_____ **38.** A toxin produced by some animals that is harmful to humans is:
- **A.** glycol.
- **C.** venom.
- **B.** lymph.
- **D.** an allergen.

_____ **39.** Sources of injected toxins in the United States, include _____ or insect stings.
- **A.** spider bites
- **C.** snakebites
- **B.** scorpion stings
- **D.** all of these

_____ **40.** While cleaning out the crawl space below the house, a 50-year-old female experienced blotchy skin, redness in her arm, weakness, and nausea. Her daughter has called the ambulance. After getting the history and doing an assessment, you believe it is possible that the patient:
  A. is developing heat stroke.
  B. was bitten by a poisonous spider.
  C. is having a diabetic reaction.
  D. is allergic to something in the air.

_____ **41.** A female patient was bitten by a snake while doing some yard work. Her daughter points to an area of sunny yard where a snake is, and thinks that the patient has been bitten by that snake. You should do all of the following _except_:
  A. call for medical direction.
  B. clean the injection site with soap and water.
  C. remove rings, bracelets, or other constricting items on the bitten limb.
  D. capture the snake and bring it alive in the ambulance to the emergency department.

_____ **42.** You have been called to the river's edge where a small craft will be meeting you with a patient on board. A 22-year-old female is taking lessons in scuba diving, and today was her first dive in the river. The instructor tells you that she seemed very nervous because all of her previous diving instruction has been in a swimming pool or shallow water. They were diving at an old shipwreck that is about 80–100 feet down. The patient got nervous and ascended too fast. Which of the following signs and symptoms would _not_ be likely found in this patient?
  A. Pain in the muscles and joints   **C.** Blurred vision or convulsions
  B. Extreme fatigue   **D.** Substernal pleuritic chest pain

_____ **43.** You are treating a novice diver who ascended too rapidly from a depth of 100 feet, and is now having a convulsion and lapses rapidly into unconsciousness leading to respiratory or cardiac arrest, you should suspect:
  A. decompression sickness.
  B. internal bleeding.
  C. that she was bitten by a large fish.
  D. that she may have an air embolism.

_____ **44.** If you have not been appropriately water rescue trained, methods you can use to assist a patient who has fallen into a body of water include:
  A. reach.   **C.** row.
  B. throw and tow.   **D.** all of the above.

_____ **45.** A condition that can occur when an inexperienced hiker, hiking over 8,000 feet, experiences a diffuse headache, fatigue, and dehydration would be called:
  A. HAPE.   **C.** acute mountain sickness.
  B. air embolism.   **D.** HACE.

_____ **46.** Common signs and symptoms of high altitude cerebral edema include:
  A. loss of balance and coordination.   **C.** headache that worsens over time.
  B. seizure.   **D.** any of the above.

Complete the Following

1. List six signs and symptoms that are likely in a heat emergency patient with moist, pale, normal or cool skin.

  A. _____

  B. _____

C. _____

D. _____

E. _____

F. _____

2. List seven signs and symptoms that are likely in a heat emergency patient with hot and dry or hot and moist skin.

A. _____

B. _____

C. _____

D. _____

E. _____

F. _____

G. _____

3. List thirteen signs and symptoms of injected envenomation.

A. _____

B. _____

C. _____

D. _____

E. _____

F. _____

G. _____

H. _____

I. _____

J. _____

K. _____

L. _____

M. _____

4. List eight signs and/or symptoms of a snake bite.

A. _____

B. _____

C. _____

D. _____

E. _____

F. _____

G. _____

H. _____

5. List ten signs and symptoms of hypothermia.

A. _____

B. _____

C. _____

D. _____

E. _____

F. _____

G. _____

H. _____

I. _____

J. _____

Case Study: Too Cold for Comfort

You respond to a call for a child with an altered mental status in the backyard of a private residence one early fall day. It is late in the afternoon on a windy day. On arrival, you are met by three children, ages approximately 9 to 12, who state that their little sister has been acting "funny." Their mother is grocery shopping, and they called her on her cell phone. She was the one who called 911, and she should be home any minute. Apparently, the children have been practicing diving in an unheated swimming pool for the past 4 hours. The youngest child, Robin—a very thin, frail, 7-year-old—is sitting at the edge of the pool shivering.

1. What are your primary assessment concerns with the patient?

_____

_____

2. Is it necessary for you to wait until the parent arrives to question the children?

_____

_____

3. Besides obtaining a set of baseline vital signs, what additional history may be helpful to obtain?

_____

_____

On questioning the children, you find that Robin has not been playing as part of the group for at least the last hour. When you ask the children whether they were cold, they say that they did not notice the temperature getting colder, just the wind, until a few minutes ago when the sun went down. They are able to confirm that Robin has no medical history, takes no medications, has no allergies, and has not eaten since lunchtime. When you question Robin, it is clear that she is confused. She is also shivering, cool to the touch, and breathing rapidly.

4. After ruling out trauma, you place the patient on your stretcher. What would be the best position?

_____

5. When the mother arrives on the scene, you bring her up to date on your findings. She confirms that the children gave you accurate information and is in agreement that Robin should be checked in the hospital. What do you suspect may be wrong with this child?

_____

6. Should you administer oxygen to Robin?

_____

7. If you took the patient's temperature, what do you suspect you would find?

_____

GZQ 8. Considering what you have learned, why might this the patient have been prone to hypothermia?

_____

Robin's mother tells you that the children are all very good swimmers and they are practicing for a diving competition at school. She went out for only a half-hour to go to the grocery store. The children are quick to call her on her cell phone whenever there is any kind of problem. She also says that she told them to get out of the pool before she left for the store.

GZQ 9. When she asks you how a similar incident could be prevented in the future, what should you say?

_____

Obstetrics and Gynecologic Emergencies

Core Concepts

- Anatomy and physiology of the female reproductive system
- Physiologic changes in pregnancy
- Care of the mother and baby during labor and delivery
- Care of the neonate
- Postdelivery care of the mother
- Complications of labor and delivery
- Emergencies in pregnancy
- Gynecologic emergencies

Outcomes

After reading this chapter, you should be able to:

36.1 Describe the anatomy and physiology of the female reproductive system. (pp. 1054–1059)
- Describe structures of the female reproductive system and their functions.
- Identify female reproductive organs in diagrams.
- Describe the relationship of the female reproductive cycle and potential for pregnancy.
- Identify the structures of pregnancy.
- Relate the physiologic changes of pregnancy to the risks for complications in the mother and fetus.
- Explain the characteristics of the three stages of labor.
- Recognize indications of imminent delivery of the fetus.

36.2 Summarize the management of childbirth and immediate neonatal care. (pp. 1059–1078)
- Describe the evaluation of the pregnant patient in labor.
- Describe considerations to weigh in deciding whether to transport the patient or prepare for scene-delivery.
- State the steps in preparing for delivery at the scene.
- Describe the intended use of the items in an obstetric kit.
- Describe the importance of reassuring the mother.
- Outline the steps of assisting with a delivery.
- Explain findings that may indicate the need for neonatal resuscitation.
- Outline the steps of assessing a neonate.

©2021 Pearson Education, Inc.
Emergency Care, 14th Ed.

- Outline the steps of caring for the neonate.
- Describe the procedure for clamping and cutting the umbilical cord.
- Describe the APGAR scale and Pediatric Resuscitation Triangle as they relate to decision making in the care of the neonate.
- Relate assessment findings to the specific interventions required for neonatal resuscitation.

36.3 Summarize the postdelivery care of the mother. (pp. 1078–1080)
- Describe decisions related to delivery of the placenta.
- Explain the risks of vaginal bleeding.
- Outline the steps of caring for vaginal bleeding.
- List comfort measures you can provide to the mother.
- Describe the reassessment of the mother during transport.

36.4 Summarize the approach to managing childbirth complications. (pp. 1080–1087)
- Name specific types of childbirth complications and their presentations.
- Outline the special care required for each type of childbirth complication.

36.5 Summarize the approach to managing pregnancy-related emergencies. (pp. 1087–1095)
- List specific types of pregnancy-related emergencies and their presentations.
- Outline the specific care required for each type of pregnancy-related emergency.

36.6 Summarize the approach to gynecologic emergencies. (pp. 1095–1097)
- Compare the steps in the approaches to nontraumatic vaginal bleeding and traumatic vaginal bleeding.
- Describe the special considerations required in the management of a situation in which a patient has been sexually assaulted.

Match Key Terms

Part A

A. Normal birth presentation, where the baby appears head first.

B. The lower neck of the uterus at the entrance to the birth canal.

C. When implantation of the fertilized egg is not in the body of the uterus, occurring instead in the fallopian tube (oviduct), cervix, or abdominopelvic cavity.

D. The placenta, membranes of the amniotic sac, part of the umbilical cord, and some tissues from the lining of the uterus that are delivered after the birth of the baby.

E. The baby from 8 weeks of development to birth.

F. Spontaneous abortion.

G. Expulsion of a fetus as a result of deliberate actions taken to terminate the pregnancy.

H. The sensation of the fetus moving from high in the abdomen to low in the birth canal.

I. Spontaneous (miscarriage) or induced termination of pregnancy.

J. The three stages of the delivery of a baby, which begin with the contractions of the uterus and end with the expulsion of the placenta.

K. The "bag of waters" that surrounds the developing fetus.

_____ **1.** Abortion

_____ **2.** Abruptio placentae

_____ **3.** Afterbirth

_____ **4.** Amniotic sac

_____ **5.** Breech presentation

_____ **6.** Cephalic presentation

_____ **7.** Cervix

_____ **8.** Crowning

_____ **9.** Eclampsia

_____ **10.** Ectopic pregnancy

_____ **11.** Fetus

_____ **12.** Induced abortion

_____ **13.** Labor

_____ **14.** Lightening

_____ **15.** Limb presentation

L. Amniotic fluid that is greenish or brownish-yellow rather than clear as a result of fetal defecation; an indication of possible maternal or fetal distress during labor.

M. When the baby's buttocks or legs appear first during birth.

N. When an infant's arm or leg protrudes from the vagina before the appearance of any other body part.

O. The point during childbirth when part of the baby is visible through the vaginal opening.

P. When more than one baby is born during a single delivery.

Q. A severe complication of pregnancy that produces seizures and which is very dangerous to the infant and mother.

R. A condition in which the placenta separates from the uterine wall.

S. Irregular prelabor contractions of the uterus.

_____ **16.** Meconium staining

_____ **17.** Miscarriage

_____ **18.** Multiple birth

_____ **19.** Braxton-Hicks contractions

Part B

A. When the umbilical cord presents first at the opening of the vaginal canal during birth.

B. Dizziness and a drop in blood pressure caused when the mother is in a supine position and the weight of the pregnant uterus compresses the inferior vena cava, reducing return of blood to the heart and cardiac output.

C. Any newborn weighing less than 5 1/2 pounds or born before the 37th week of pregnancy.

D. The narrow tube that connects the ovary to the uterus. Also called the oviduct.

E. Born dead.

F. The phase of the female reproductive cycle in which an egg is released from the ovary.

G. The fetal structure that contains the blood vessels that carry blood to and from the placenta.

H. The birth canal.

I. A condition in which the placenta is formed in an abnormal location (low in the uterus and close to or over the cervical opening).

J. The female reproductive organ that produces ova.

K. The muscular abdominal organ where the fetus develops.

L. When the fetus and placenta deliver before the 20th week of pregnancy; commonly called a miscarriage.

M. A complication of pregnancy in which the woman retains large amounts of fluid and has hypertension, and which may progress to eclampsia.

N. The surface area between the vagina and the anus.

O. The organ of pregnancy where exchange of oxygen, foods, and wastes occurs between mother and fetus.

_____ **1.** Ovary

_____ **2.** Ovulation

_____ **3.** Fallopian tube

_____ **4.** Perineum

_____ **5.** Placenta

_____ **6.** Placenta previa

_____ **7.** Preeclampsia

_____ **8.** Premature infant

_____ **9.** Prolapsed umbilical cord

_____ **10.** Spontaneous abortion

_____ **11.** Stillborn

_____ **12.** Supine hypotensive syndrome

_____ **13.** Umbilical cord

_____ **14.** Uterus

_____ **15.** Vagina

_____ **16.** Labia

_____ **17.** Mons pubis

_____ **18.** Embryo

_____ **19.** Neonate

P. Soft tissue that covers the pubic symphysis; area where hair grows as a woman reaches puberty.

Q. The baby from fertilization to 8 weeks of development.

R. Soft tissues that protect the entrance to the vagina.

S. A newly born infant or infant less than 1 month old.

Multiple-Choice Review

_____ **1.** The nine months of pregnancy are divided into three-month trimesters. During the second trimester, the:
  A. fetus is being formed, and there is little uterine growth.
  B. uterus grows very rapidly, while the woman's blood volume, cardiac output, and heart rate increase.
  C. uterus is often seen reaching up to the epigastrium.
  D. uterus develops to full size.

_____ **2.** The normal birth position is _____ and is called a _____ birth.
  A. headfirst; breech   **C.** feetfirst; breech
  B. headfirst; cephalic   **D.** feetfirst; cephalic

_____ **3.** You are assessing a pregnant patient who thinks that she is going into labor. The first stage of labor begins with:
  A. conception.   **C.** regular contractions of the uterus.
  B. the nine-month point.   **D.** the cervix being fully dilated.

_____ **4.** The third stage of labor begins after:
  A. the birth of the baby.   **C.** dilation of the cervix.
  B. delivery of the afterbirth. **D.** full growth of the uterus.

_____ **5.** The process by which the cervix gradually widens is called:
  A. delivery.   **C.** staining.
  B. dilation.   **D.** contraction.

_____ **6.** You are assisting in the delivery for a 26-year-old patient who is about to have her third child. She states that she has had prenatal care and is not aware of any complications. The baby is due next week. Greenish or brownish-yellow fluid is being expelled from the amniotic sac. This is called _____ and could indicate _____.
  A. a bloody show; a normal delivery
  B. vena cava syndrome; that the mother is being stressed
  C. meconium staining; potential fetal distress
  D. amniotic bile; that the infant will be a diabetic

_____ **7.** When your 22-year-old patient, who is in labor, suddenly states, "I need to go to the bathroom right now!" this most likely means that the:
  A. birth will be delayed.   **C.** delivery is nearing.
  B. uterus is almost dilated.   **D.** baby is in distress.

_____ **8.** You are treating a 21-year-old pregnant woman who is full-term and in labor. When you are timing the duration of a contraction, time it from the:
  A. start of the pain until the delivery of the infant.
  B. beginning of the contraction to when the uterus relaxes.
  C. end of a contraction to the beginning of the next one.
  D. peak of the contraction to the end of the contraction.

_____ **9.** You also need to determine the contraction interval for a women in labor. The contraction interval, or frequency, is timed from the:
  A. start of one contraction to the start of the next.
  B. beginning of the contraction to when the uterus relaxes.
  C. peak of the contraction to the end of the contraction.
  D. start of the pain until the delivery of the infant.

_____ **10.** Delivery is said to be imminent when the contractions last _____ seconds and are _____ minutes apart.
  A. 15; 5 to 8   **C.** 45; 8 to 10
  B. 30; 2 to 3   **D.** 90; 5 to 8

_____ **11.** The EMT's primary roles at a normal childbirth scene are to determine whether the delivery will occur at the scene and, if so, to:
  A. determine whether the delivery can be delayed.
  B. assist the mother as she delivers the infant.
  C. carefully deliver the infant.
  D. immobilize the patient.

_____ **12.** The sterile obstetrical kit is usually in a sealed container. It should be checked regularly, although the seal is rarely broken. The kit does *not* contain:
  A. a rubber bulb syringe for suctioning.
  B. several individually wrapped sanitary napkins.
  C. heavy, flat twine to tie the cord.
  D. cord clamps or hemostats.

_____ **13.** When you are evaluating the mother for a possible home delivery, you should check:
  A. whether pregnancy problems run in the family.
  B. the frequency and duration of contractions.
  C. whether the mother feels that she needs to urinate.
  D. the father's blood type and medical history.

_____ **14.** An important part of assessment of your 29-year-old patient, who you suspect is going to deliver soon, is to examine for crowning. It is important to ask the patient whether you can examine for crowning if she is:
  A. having an urge to push during contractions.
  B. in her ninth month of pregnancy.
  C. pregnant for the first time.
  D. It is not important to ask permission to examine the patient.

_____ **15.** You are treating a 26-year-old female who is eight months pregnant. She states that she is having contractions every 15 minutes or so that last for about 20 seconds. She is not exactly sure what labor pain is like because this is her first pregnancy. Her vital signs are pulse of 96, blood pressure of 130/70, respirations of 22, and SpO$_2$ of 98%. What should you do next?
  A. Administer oxygen and transport immediately.
  B. Prepare for a home delivery immediately.
  C. Ask whether her water broke and prepare for a quiet ride to the hospital.
  D. Tell her to call you back when the contractions are more frequent.

©2021 Pearson Education, Inc.
Emergency Care, 14th Ed.

_____ 16. If you determine that delivery is imminent because of the presence of crowning and other signs, you should:
   A. contact medical direction if local protocol requires.
   B. transport as quickly as possible.
   C. ask the mother to go to the bathroom first.
   D. ask the mother to hold her legs closed.

_____ 17. When a full-term pregnant woman lying on her back complains of dizziness and you note a drop in her blood pressure, this could be due to a condition called _____ syndrome.
   A. diabetes mellitus   **C.** Cushing reflex
   B. supine hypotensive **D.** fluid retention

_____ 18. To counteract the pressure of the uterus on the inferior vena cava, you should:
   A. raise the patient's legs.
   B. transport the patient on her left side.
   C. raise the patient's head.
   D. apply a pelvic binder.

_____ 19. You are delivering a baby in the field. Of the following, which finding would be the least likely indicator of a need for a neonatal resuscitation?
   A. The labor was induced by trauma.
   B. The patient has triplets.
   C. The infant's umbilical cord is looped around the neck.
   D. Labor was induced by drug use such as narcotics.

_____ 20. During the delivery, you should encourage the mother to:
   A. breathe rapidly and deeply.
   B. hold her breath every 2 minutes.
   C. close her mouth and breathe through her nose.
   D. breathe deeply through her mouth.

_____ 21. When supporting the baby's head during a delivery, the EMT should do all of the following _except_:
   A. pull on the baby's shoulders when they appear.
   B. apply gentle pressure to control the delivery.
   C. place one hand below the baby's head.
   D. spread the fingers evenly around the baby's head.

_____ 22. You are assisting a 23-year-old female who is about to deliver. She states that her water did not break. If the amniotic sac has not broken by the time the baby's head is delivered, you should:
   A. stop the delivery and transport immediately.
   B. use your finger to puncture the membrane.
   C. contact medical direction immediately.
   D. delay the delivery until it breaks.

_____ 23. If you cannot loosen or unwrap the umbilical cord from around the infant's neck, you should:
   A. stop the delivery and transport immediately.
   B. tell the mother to push more forcefully.
   C. clamp the cord in two places and cut between the clamps.
   D. contact medical direction for advice.

_____ 24. The normal presentation is for a baby to be born:
   A. face down and then rotate to either side.
   B. face up and then rotate to either side.
   C. feet and buttocks first and do not rotate.
   D. face up and do not rotate.

_____ 25. When suctioning a newborn:
   A. compress the bulb syringe while it is inside the baby's mouth.
   B. compress the bulb syringe before placing it in the baby's mouth.
   C. suction the nose and then the mouth.
   D. insert the syringe about 5 inches into the baby's mouth.

_____ 26. Once the baby's feet are delivered:
   A. pick the baby up by the feet using a firm grasp.
   B. lay the baby on his or her side with the head slightly lower than the torso.
   C. lay the baby on his or her side and massage the baby's back.
   D. pick the baby up by the feet and massage his or her back.

_____ 27. To assess the newborn, the EMT should do all of the following _except_:
   A. note ease of breathing.
   B. check movement in the extremities.
   C. note skin coloration.
   D. check the response to a sternal rub.

_____ 28. If assessment of the infant's breathing reveals shallow, slow, or absent respirations, the EMT should:
   A. provide oxygen by nonrebreather mask.
   B. provide a gentle but vigorous rubbing of the infant's back.
   C. provide artificial ventilations at 40–60 per minute.
   D. provide artificial ventilations at 20–30 per minute.

_____ 29. You just delivered a full-term infant who is not breathing and has a heart rate of 58. You should:
   A. provide ventilations.   C. stimulate the infant.
   B. begin chest compressions.   D. reassess vitals every five minutes.

_____ 30. The first umbilical cord clamp should be placed about _____ inches from the baby.
   A. 4   C. 8
   B. 6   D. 10

_____ 31. The second umbilical cord clamp should be placed about _____ inches from the baby.
   A. 3   C. 7
   B. 5   D. 9

_____ 32. If the placenta does not deliver within _____ minutes of the baby's birth, transport the mother and baby to a medical facility without delay.
   A. 5   C. 15
   B. 10   D. 20

_____ 33. During the delivery of a full-term newborn, the mother sustains a tear in her perineum. The EMT should:
   A. massage the uterus for at least 15 minutes.
   B. apply a sanitary napkin and gentle pressure.
   C. transport the patient on her left side immediately.
   D. contact medical direction immediately.

_____ 34. You are assisting in the delivery for a 26-year-old female who was told by her doctor that the infant is in the breech position. Which of the following is an appropriate action to take for a breech presentation?
   A. Place the mother on her left side.
   B. Provide low-concentration oxygen.
   C. Pull on the baby's legs to deliver.
   D. Initiate rapid transport upon recognition.

_____ **35.** During the examination of a 29-year-old woman with labor pains, you see the umbilical cord presenting first. You should:
   A. gently push up on the baby's head or buttocks to take pressure off of the cord.
   B. use two gloved fingers to check the cord for a pulse and keep the cord cool.
   C. raise the mother's head and lower her buttocks to lessen pressure on the birth canal.
   D. attempt to push the cord back if it is not wrapped around the baby's neck.

_____ **36.** You are about to assist in the delivery for a full-term 33-year-old female. When you check for crowning, you do not see the head, but you do see one foot. When a baby's limb presents first, you should:
   A. push gently on the extremity to prevent it from advancing.
   B. pull gently on the limb to encourage delivery.
   C. administer low-concentration oxygen to the mother.
   D. begin rapid transport of the patient immediately.

_____ **37.** You are assisting in the delivery for a 28-year-old female who is full-term; she tells you that this is her third pregnancy and that she is having twins. When you are assisting with the delivery of twins:
   A. the afterbirth will be delivered after each individual infant.
   B. clamp the cord of the first baby before the second baby is born.
   C. labor contractions will stop after the first delivery.
   D. transport the mother immediately.

_____ **38.** Newly born infants lose heat rapidly. Heat loss not only affects their comfort but also can:
   A. increase their glucose level.
   B. affect their ability to carry oxygen in their blood.
   C. cause them to develop a fever.
   D. decrease their ability to shiver.

_____ **39.** If after delivery the mother continues to bleed profusely, what should you do besides rapidly transporting?
   A. massage the uterus.
   B. encourage the mother to nurse the infant.
   C. place a sanitary napkin and treat for shock.
   D. all of the above.

_____ **40.** If you suspect meconium staining when the infant is born:
   A. contact medical direction for advice.
   B. avoid stimulating the infant before suctioning the oropharynx.
   C. suction the infant's nose, then the mouth.
   D. provide oxygen to the mother.

_____ **41.** A condition in which the placenta is formed low in the uterus and close to the cervical opening, preventing normal delivery of the fetus, is called:
   A. abruptio placentae.   **C.** placenta toxemia.
   B. stillborn birth.   **D.** placenta previa.

_____ **42.** You are treating a 22-year-old female who is eight months pregnant and just had a seizure. Which of the following is true of seizures in pregnancy?
   A. They are usually associated with low blood pressure.
   B. They tend to occur early in pregnancy.
   C. They pose a threat to the mother but not to the fetus.
   D. They are usually associated with extreme swelling of the extremities.

_____ **43.** You are assessing a 19-year old woman who is about eight months pregnant and states that she fell down the stairs. The greatest danger associated with blunt trauma to the pregnant woman's abdomen and pelvis is:
   A. cramping abdominal pains.   **C.** massive bleeding and shock.
   B. spontaneous abortion.   **D.** elevated blood pressure.

_____ **44.** Which of the following is *true* about the physiology of a pregnant woman?
  A. Her heart rate may be interpreted as suggestive of shock when it is actually normal.
  B. She has a pulse rate that is 10–15 beats per minute slower than that of the nonpregnant female.
  C. A woman in later pregnancy may have a blood volume that is up to 48% lower than what she would have in her nonpregnant state.
  D. Assessing for shock is easier in the pregnant patient than in a nonpregnant patient.

_____ **45.** You are called to the scene of a 35-year-old woman who has a complaint of abdominal pain. She tells you that she also has unexpected vaginal bleeding. Which of the following is *true* of the treatment necessary for this patient?
  A. Massage the abdomen vigorously.
  B. Assume that the woman is pregnant and transport.
  C. Treat her as if she has a potentially life-threatening condition.
  D. Determine the cause before beginning treatment.

_____ **46.** You are preparing for a neonatal resuscitation. If breathing is absent or the neonate is gasping with a heart rate less than 100, you should:
  A. begin chest compressions.
  B. stimulate the bottom of the feet.
  C. begin positive pressure ventilations.
  D. reassess the APGAR.

Complete the Following

1. List seven things you should do when evaluating a woman who is in labor and considering a transport decision.

  A. _____

  B. _____

  C. _____

  D. _____

  E. _____

  F. _____

  G. _____

2. List seven steps you should take when providing care for a woman who presents with a prolapsed cord.

  A. _____

  B. _____

  C. _____

  D. _____

  E. _____

  F. _____

  G. _____

3. Complete the following chart:

APGAR SCORE

	0	1	2
Appearance	Blue (or pale) all over	**(A)**	Pink all over
Pulse	0	Less than 100	**(B)**
Grimace (reaction to suctioning or flicking of the feet)	**(C)**	Facial grimace	Sneeze, cough, or cry
Activity	No movement	**(D)**	Moving around normally
Respiratory effort	None	Slow or irregular breathing; weak cry	**(E)**

Label the Diagrams

Fill in the name of each structure of pregnancy on the line provided.

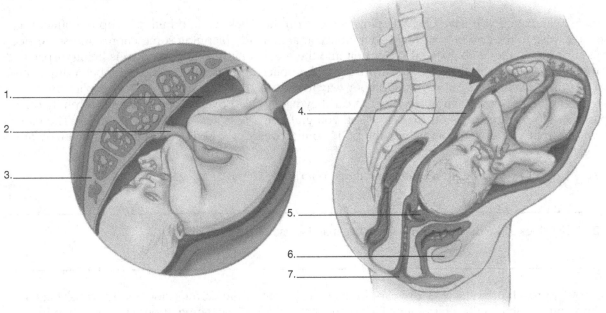

1.

2.

3.

4.

5.

6.

7.

1. _____

2. _____

3. _____

4. _____

5. _____

6. _____

7. _____

Pathophysiology: Physiologic Changes of Pregnancy

1. For the pregnant woman who has a more pink coloration to her skin, what is going on "inside" that this color relates to?

_____

2. For the pregnant woman who has nausea, vomiting, and heartburn, what is going on "inside" that these conditions relate to?

_____

3. In the woman who is in active labor when she has uterus contractions on the "inside," what would be symptoms she could tell to the EMT assisting her on the "outside"?

_____

4. If the woman who is in labor has a fetus that is not in the head-first position in the birth canal on the "inside," what might the EMT observe on the "outside" of the patient?

_____

Case Study: More Than a Speeding Ticket

It is 5:30 a.m., and you have been keeping one eye on the clock while drinking a cup of coffee. It is getting close to the end of your night shift, and you are already planning some chores and some sleep when suddenly the radio goes off. Your unit and the medic unit from across town is being dispatched to the interstate just south of Exit 6. Surprisingly, the police and rescue unit have not been dispatched, so it is most likely not a big wreck. On your way to the call, the dispatcher states the police are on the scene and there is a woman in labor in the car they have pulled over. As your partner carefully drives past the two cars and pulls off to a safe spot, you grab the assessment bag and the OB kit. The patient is in the front seat of a Toyota, which the police pulled over for speeding. It is obvious that they are all glad to see your ambulance arrive.

1. What PPE should be immediately available on a call like this?

_____

2. What does a typical OBS kit contain that may be useful on this call?

_____

As you approach the vehicle, a 25-year-old male jumps out of the driver's side and nervously starts filling you in. He identifies himself as Rafael and states that he was going about 90 mph when he got pulled over. His wife, Maria, was not due to have the baby for at least another week or two, but Rafael says that she is in labor already. They were trying to make it to the hospital on their own and did not want to bother the ambulance crews. You see that Maria, a 24-year-old woman, has the front passenger seat pushed all the way back and is trying to lie back in the seat. She is conscious and able to talk with you. He airway is open and clear, her breathing is not labored, and she has a strong radial pulse. There is no obvious external bleeding, and her skin color is a bit pale. Because she is alert (oriented to person, place, and day), you proceed to ask a few questions as your partner gets Maria's vital signs.

3. Given the urgency of the situation, what would you like to know in a history from Maria at this point?

_____

Your partner obtains Maria's vital signs, which are pulse of 100 and regular, respirations 24 and shallow, BP of 104/70 mmHg, and SpO_2 of 98%.

4. Should you administer oxygen to this patient now? If so using what device?

_____

GZQ **5.** Should your partner tell the responding medic unit to cancel or continue?

_____

Maria tells you that this is her third pregnancy and she has two healthy little ones at home, who are with a neighbor. She also tells you that she has been seeing a local OB physician who is affiliated with the hospital to which she and her husband were headed.

6. How are Maria's pregnancy history and the fact that her children are healthy relevant?

_____

7. How is the information about her physician relevant?

_____

You decide to examine for crowning before moving Maria to the ambulance on your stretcher, since she does seem to be having labor pains every few minutes. On examination, during contractions, you do not yet see crowning, but you believe that she is getting close on the basis of the history she has provided to you and the fact that she states that she is getting the urge to move her bowels, though she has not eaten in quite a while. You and your partner move Maria to the stretcher and load it into your ambulance. Within a few minutes, you are headed for the ED. Suddenly, Maria's contractions begin again. This time, they are strong enough to move the baby farther down the birth canal, and you are now seeing crowning. You lay out the parts of the OB kit and instruct your partner to pull over to a safe spot and come on back to help out. Just then, the medic unit pulls up behind you. They have been following along, and now there is plenty of help. The baby is delivered in the face-down head-first position. To everyone's relief, the delivery goes just the way it did in the movie that you saw in your EMT class.

8. What is the name for this kind of birth? If the baby had come out both feet first, what would that have been called?

_____

9. What is the third stage of the delivery? Should you wait at the side of the road?

_____

GZQ **10.** From your knowledge of emergency childbirth, what are some complications that fortunately did not occur in this case?

_____

37

Emergencies for Patients with Special Challenges

Core Concepts

- The variety of challenges that may be faced by patients with special needs
- Types of disabilities and challenges patients may have
- Special aspects of prehospital care for a patient with special challenges
- Congenital and acquired diseases and conditions
- Types of advanced medical devices patients may rely on
- How to recognize and deal with cases of abuse and neglect

Outcomes

After reading this chapter, you should be able to:

37.1 Summarize concepts related to patients who have special challenges. (pp. 1103–1107)
- Compare the characteristics of disability and of a developmental disability.
- Outline the features of selected conditions associated with special challenges.
- Analyze terminal illness, obesity, homelessness, and poverty as special challenges.

37.2 Recommend approaches of care for patients with special needs. (pp. 1108–1111)
- State the key actions the EMT can use to improve interaction with patients who have autism.
- Recognize how to obtain information to troubleshoot unfamiliar medical devices in a patient's home.
- Match specific types of medical devices with the purposes for which patients have them.

37.3 Describe general considerations in responding to patients with special challenges. (pp. 1111–1116)
- Defend the rationale for a complete history and physical in the management of a patient who has special challenges.

37.4 Recognize physical impairments and common medical devices used in the home care of patients with special challenges, including respiratory devices, cardiac devices, gastrourinary devices, and central IV catheters, and discuss EMT assessment and transport considerations for each. (pp. 1116–1128)
- Explain how to improve interaction with patients who have hearing and vision impairments that interfere with their activities of daily living.

Match Key Terms

A. A physical, emotional, behavioral, or cognitive condition that interferes with a person's ability to carry out everyday tasks such as working or caring for oneself.

B. A device that breathes for a patient.

C. A battery-powered mechanical pump that is implanted in the body to assist a failing heart in pumping blood to the body.

D. A device implanted under the skin that can detect life-threatening cardiac dysrhythmias and deliver a shock to the heart.

E. A tube used to provide delivery of nutrients to the stomach.

F. A surgical opening in the neck into the trachea.

G. A surgically created opening into the body, as with a tracheostomy, colostomy, or ileostomy.

H. A tube inserted into the bladder through the urethra to drain urine from the bladder.

I. The artificial process of filtering the blood to remove toxic or unwanted wastes and fluids.

J. A surgically inserted device used for long-term delivery of medications or fluids into the central circulation.

K. An external pouch that collects fecal matter diverted from the colon or ileum through a surgical opening in the abdominal wall.

L. A device worn by a patient that blows oxygen or air under constant low pressure through a tube and mask to keep airway passages from collapsing at the end of a breath.

M. A condition of having too much body fat, defined as a body mass index of 30 or greater.

N. A device that is implanted under the skin with wires implanted into the heart to modify the heart rate as needed to maintain an adequate heart rate.

O. Developmental disorders that affect, among other things, the ability to communicate, self-regulate behaviors, and interact with others.

P. The branch of medicine that deals with the causes of obesity as well as its prevention and treatment.

Q. An external vest worn by a patient to detect any life-threatening dysrhythmia and deliver a shock to the heart.

_____ **1.** Autism spectrum disorders (ASD)

_____ **2.** Automatic implanted cardiac defibrillator (AICD)

_____ **3.** Bariatrics

_____ **4.** Central IV catheter

_____ **5.** Continuous positive airway pressure (CPAP)

_____ **6.** Dialysis

_____ **7.** Disability

_____ **8.** Feeding tube

_____ **9.** Ventricular assist device

_____ **10.** Obesity

_____ **11.** Ostomy bag

_____ **12.** Pacemaker

_____ **13.** Stoma

_____ **14.** Tracheostomy

_____ **15.** Urinary catheter

_____ **16.** Ventilator

_____ **17.** Wearable cardioverter defibrillator (WCD)

Multiple-Choice Review

_____ **1.** To ensure proper care for the patient with special needs, the EMT must be able to _____ the patient's specific special health care needs in addition to the chief complaint.
   A. recognize
   B. understand
   C. evaluate
   D. do all of these

_____ **2.** The EMT may find patients with special care needs when responding to calls in any of the following locations _except_:
   A. the emergency department.
   B. nursing homes.
   C. specialty rehabilitation centers.
   D. specialized care facilities.

_____ **3.** One of the best resources to help you when you have a special needs patient who is on a specific device would be the:
   A. instruction manual for the device.
   B. website for the product.
   C. family member who is with the patient.
   D. medical direction physician over the radio.

_____ **4.** You are interviewing a 45-year-old female special needs patient who tells you that she has had a heart murmur since birth. A condition that is present at the birth of the patient is considered:
   A. acquired.
   B. adopted.
   C. congenital.
   D. inflamed.

_____ **5.** A device that is used by patients to help them sleep and by EMS providers in certain medical emergencies to keep the air passages from collapsing at the end of a breath and is called a(n):
   A. positive-pressure ventilator.
   B. CPAP machine.
   C. bag-mask device.
   D. endotracheal tube.

_____ **6.** You have responded to the home of a 54-year-old male patient who has a tracheostomy tube and needs to be suctioned occasionally. His wife tells you that this is especially common:
   A. during times of distress.
   B. within the first few weeks after the tube insertion.
   C. when the patient has an infection.
   D. when any of these conditions exists.

_____ **7.** You are called to the home of a 70-year-old woman who sustained a cervical spine injury about five years ago. Her caregiver tells you that she is on a device that is programmed to take over the timing and rate of her breathing. This device is called a(n):
   A. inhalator.
   B. exhalator.
   C. ventilator.
   D. CPAP device.

_____ **8.** A patient who is is attached to an artificial ventilator at home is experiencing an electrical or battery failure, so you need to begin:
   A. CPAP.
   B. using a nonrebreather mask.
   C. bag-valve-mask ventilation.
   D. attaching the AED.

_____ **9.** You are treating a 65-year-old female patient who has a long history of heart problems. She has had multiple heart attacks, and two prehospital cardiac arrests. A cardiac device was implanted in her left upper abdominal quadrant. This device is most likely a(n):
   A. LVAD.
   B. AED.
   C. heart valve.
   D. AICD.

_____ **10.** Your 52-year-old male patient is a special needs heart patient. A family member tells you that he has a cardiac device that pumps blood through the aorta to the body. This is a(n):
   A. pacemaker.
   B. bypass machine.
   C. ventricular assist device.
   D. AICD.

_____ **11.** A tube that is inserted into a patient who has lost the ability to regulate his or her urine is a(n):
- **A.** colostomy.
- **B.** urinary catheter.
- **C.** ileostomy.
- **D.** stoma.

_____ **12.** You are interviewing a 50-year-old female who has a history of hypertension and diabetes. She tells you that she needs to go for dialysis every other day in a local clinic. This procedure is done to:
- **A.** filter her blood to remove toxic waste.
- **B.** increase her blood sugar.
- **C.** remove fecal material from her bowel.
- **D.** do all of these.

_____ **13.** Devices that are commercially available under the brand names Groshong®, Hickman®, and Broviac® are:
- **A.** peripherally inserted central catheters.
- **B.** angiocaths.
- **C.** central venous lines.
- **D.** implanted port devices.

_____ **14.** A _____ is a special needle that is required to access a device implanted under the patient's skin.
- **A.** Huber.
- **B.** Port-a-Cath®.
- **C.** Mediport®.
- **D.** all of these.

_____ **15.** A major health risk that is on the rise in the United States is _____, which will ultimately increase the occurrence of _____.
- **A.** stroke; liver disease
- **B.** heart disease; sleep apnea
- **C.** obesity; type 2 diabetes
- **D.** cancer; heart failure

_____ **16.** One of the easiest ways to communicate with a patient who has hearing loss is to:
- **A.** write questions on a pad of paper.
- **B.** expect the patient to read your lips.
- **C.** find a TDD/TTY phone.
- **D.** yell your questions at the patient.

_____ **17.** A cardiac patient who has an AICD and is suddenly shocked by the device is usually instructed to call EMS for any of the following reasons *except* if:
- **A.** the patient continues to have chest pain.
- **B.** the patient becomes dizzy and does not feel well.
- **C.** the shock was momentarily painful.
- **D.** this was the second shock in a 24-hour period.

_____ **18.** In dealing with a patient who has a history of autism and who is having a meltdown, the best advice for the EMT is to:
- **A.** loudly command the patient to calm down.
- **B.** not allow the patient to express frustration.
- **C.** provide a show of force.
- **D.** remember that calm creates calm.

_____ **19.** A patient with autism is very upset. Your interaction during this crisis should be as basic as possible. This includes all of the following *except*:
- **A.** keeping your instructions simple and clear.
- **B.** asking basic questions.
- **C.** providing all treatments as quickly as possible.
- **D.** using less equipment (e.g., radios, pagers, cell phones) because they are distracting.

_____ **20.** Several serious health problems are related to homelessness. Examples include all of the following *except*:
- **A.** HIV/AIDS.
- **B.** bronchitis and pneumonia.
- **C.** wounds and skin infections.
- **D.** strokes and TIAs.

©2021 Pearson Education, Inc.
Emergency Care, 14th Ed.

Chapter 37 | Emergencies for Patients with Special Challenges 327

_____ 21. Of the following conditions, which is not considered a developmental disability?
  A. Parkinson's disease   C. Down syndrome
  B. Cerebral palsy   D. Fetal alcohol syndrome

_____ 22. Appropriate questions to ask a caregiver when there is a problem with a life-sustaining medical device would include each of the following, *except*?
  A. Has this problem occurred before?
  B. Why did you wait so long to call 911?
  C. Have you tried to fix the device?
  D. Have you been taught how to fix this problem?

_____ 23. Your patient needs an AICD installed but is waiting for insurance to authorize the surgery. He is wearing a(n) _____ designed to detect and shock a life-threatening dysrhythmia.
  A. automatic pacemaker
  B. wearable cardioverter defibrillator
  C. ventricular assist device
  D. halter monitor

_____ 24. While en route to the hospital with the patient who has a wearable cardioverter defibrillator (WCD), a siren goes off and a voice states do not touch the patient. You note the patient is unresponsive. What should you do next?
  A. Prepare for CPR but wait to see if the WCD shocks the patient.
  B. Call for an ALS unit.
  C. Remove the vest immediately.
  D. Apply defib pads to the patient's chest.

_____ 25. You are treating a 6-year-old female who shows indications that child abuse may be a contributing factor in the "accident" that occurred today. Evidence of child abuse can include all of the following *except*:
  A. repeated responses to provide care for the same child or family.
  B. poorly healing wounds or improperly healed fractures.
  C. indications of past injuries.
  D. a parent who seems concerned about the child's injuries.

_____ 26. When you respond to the home of a person who you think may be a child abuser, look for all of the following *except*:
  A. a family member who has trouble controlling anger.
  B. indications of alcohol and drug abuse.
  C. torn clothing on the child.
  D. any adult who appears in a state of depression.

_____ 27. You are treating a woman who has a broken arm and other bruises. Other signs of intimate partner violence may include:
  A. delays in seeking treatment.
  B. history that does not match injuries or injury patterns.
  C. fear of the victim of talking to EMS.
  D. all of the above.

_____ 28. When obtaining a medical history from a 19-year-old female who has sustained some suspicious injuries, you note an older woman insists on speaking for the patient and there is no available identification. You might suspect:
  A. child abuse.   C. partner violence.
  B. human trafficking.   D. the patient is disabled.

Complete the following

1. List four ways in which the concept of "basic" applies to the management of a patient with autism.

   A. _____

   B. _____

   C. _____

   D. _____

2. List ten medical conditions in which obesity increases the risk for patients.

   A. _____

   B. _____

   C. _____

   D. _____

   E. _____

   F. _____

   G. _____

   H. _____

   I. _____

   J. _____

3. List four groups of children with special challenges.

   A. _____

   B. _____

   C. _____

   D. _____

4. To address an emergency involving a home ventilator, what does the memory aid "DOPE" stand for?

   A. D - _____

   B. O - _____

   C. P - _____

   D. E - _____

38

EMS Operations

Core Concepts

- Phases of an ambulance call
- Preparation for a call
- Operating an ambulance
- Transferring and transporting the patient
- Transferring the patient to the emergency department staff
- Terminating the call, replacing and exchanging equipment, and cleaning and disinfecting the unit and equipment
- When and how to use air rescue

Outcomes

After reading this chapter, you should be able to:

38.1 Summarize the circumstances that must be attended to in order to ensure your ambulance is prepared for calls. (pp. 1144–1151)
- State the relationship between the type of ambulance and the ability to be best prepared for response.
- Recognize where to find lists of required equipment and supplies for EMT ambulances.
- Given a set of equipment and supply items, identify whether the items are required for ambulances.
- Recognize the components of the daily ambulance inspection for which EMTs are responsible.
- Describe the inspection of the patient compartment supplies and equipment.

38.2 Summarize the processes of receiving and responding to EMS calls. (pp. 1151–1152)
- Explain the information you should receive from emergency medical dispatch about a call.
- State the EMTs' process in acknowledging that they have received and are responding to the call.

38.3 Outline the concepts of professional emergency vehicle operations. (pp. 1153–1158)
- Recognize the attitudes and actions needed to safely operate an ambulance.
- Apply general concepts of emergency vehicle operations law to driving the ambulance.
- Outline the proper uses of the ambulance's warning devices.
- Identify conditions that affect the efficiency and safety of operating the ambulance.
- Compare the benefits and drawbacks of using a global positioning system (GPS) in navigation.

©2021 Pearson Education, Inc.
Emergency Care, 14th Ed.

38.4 Summarize the actions responders must take to protect the safety of themselves and the patient at a highway incident. (pp. 1158–1159)
- Explain hazards associated with highway response.
- List actions EMTs must take to improve scene safety when responding to a highway scene.

38.5 Summarize the EMT's actions in preparing patients for and transporting them to the hospital. (pp. 1159–1165)
- Evaluate characteristics of the patient and scene to select a proper means of transporting the patient to the ambulance.
- Explain what it means to package the patient for transport.
- Describe the EMT's actions while preparing the patient for transport.
- Describe the EMT's actions during transportation of the patient.

38.6 Summarize the EMT team's responsibilities in terminating the call and preparing for the next call. (pp. 1166–1171)
- Outline the steps to be taken at the hospital, including transfer of the patient to hospital staff.
- Describe steps needed to prepare the ambulance for another call.
- Outline the steps to be taken en route back to quarters to ensure your ambulance is available for another call.
- Outline the steps to be taken once you arrive back in quarters to ensure that all aspects of your ambulance are fully prepared for another response.

38.7 Summarize considerations in requesting and interacting with air rescue units. (pp. 1171–1173)
- Outline reasons for considering a call for an air rescue unit.
- State the information required to initiate an air medical response.
- Differentiate between landing zones that are correctly prepared and those that are not.
- State procedures for approaching a helicopter in the landing zone.

Match Key Terms

A. Emergency Medical Dispatcher

B. A legal term that appears in most states' driving laws and refers to the responsibility of the emergency vehicle operator to drive safely and keep the safety of all others in mind at all times

C. A call in which the driver of the emergency vehicle is excused from obeying certain traffic laws such as speed limits and stop signs because loss of life or limb is possible

D. A large, flat area without aerial obstruction in which a helicopter can land to pick up a patient

_____ **1.** Due regard

_____ **2.** EMD

_____ **3.** Landing zone (LZ)

_____ **4.** True emergency

Multiple-Choice Review

_____ **1.** The federal agency that develops specifications for ambulance vehicle designs is the:
- **A.** U.S. Department of Motor Vehicles.
- **B.** U.S. Food and Drug Administration.
- **C.** U.S. Department of Transportation.
- **D.** U.S. Department of Health, Education, and Welfare.

_____ 2. The purpose(s) for carrying an EPA-registered disinfectant solution on the ambulance is to:
   A. clean up equipment after calls.
   B. destroy mycobacterium tuberculosis.
   C. disinfect patient wounds.
   D. do all of these.

_____ 3. Each of the following on the ambulance is checked with the engine off, *except*:
   A. operation of doors and latches.
   B. dash-mounted gauges.
   C. windows for operation.
   D. fuel level.

_____ 4. When inspecting the ambulance, which is checked with the engine running?
   A. The oil level
   B. The brake pedal
   C. The mirrors
   D. The horn and emergency lights

_____ 5. On each call, you will need to take in the kit that has the equipment necessary for care of the patient's airway and ventilation. All of the following are pieces of equipment used for airway and ventilation care *except*:
   A. suction apparatus.
   B. bag-valve mask.
   C. sphygmomanometer.
   D. pulse oximeter.

_____ 6. Of the following BLS medications, which is *not* optional to carry on the ambulance?
   A. Aspirin
   B. Oxygen
   C. Nitroglycerin tablets
   D. Naloxone

_____ 7. According to federal specifications, an ambulance that is a "van type" is called a:
   A. Type I.
   B. Type II.
   C. Type III.
   D. Medium duty.

_____ 8. If you carry a toy on your ambulance, such as a teddy bear, to calm a frightened child, it should be:
   A. sanitized.
   B. soft or padded.
   C. brightly colored.
   D. all of the above.

_____ 9. Activities while at the hospital after delivering the patient include each of the following except:
   A. clean and make up the ambulance stretcher.
   B. replace airway equipment per local protocols.
   C. fill the vehicle with fuel.
   D. clean the ambulance interior.

_____ 10. Which of the following pieces of equipment carried on an ambulance or EMS vehicle for defibrillation or assisting with cardiopulmonary resuscitation is optional?
   A. Short or long spine board
   B. Mechanical CPR compressor
   C. Automated external defibrillator
   D. Kit with oral and nasal airways

_____ 11. Equipment that is carried on an ambulance or EMS vehicle for immobilization includes all of the following *except*:
   A. a traction splint.
   B. cervical collars.
   C. metal, vacuum, or wood splints.
   D. a burn sheet.

_____ 12. Supplies used for wound care should include all of the following *except*:
   A. sterile burn sheets.
   B. 4 x 4 gauze sponges.
   C. gauze roller bandages.
   D. a Hare® or Sager® traction device.

_____ 13. What is the purpose of carrying sterilized occlusive dressing on the ambulance or EMS vehicle?
A. To wrap body parts in
B. To maintain body heat
C. To make a shield over an avulsed eye
D. To seal a hole in the chest or abdomen

_____ 14. The supplies for childbirth include all the following *except*:
A. a bulb syringe.
B. a blanket.
C. large safety pins.
D. sterile gloves.

_____ 15. Of the following items checked on the ambulance or EMS vehicle, which is checked with the engine on?
A. Side to side motion of steering wheel
B. The battery and cable.
C. The vehicle's wheels and tires.
D. The vehicle's doors and latches.

_____ 16. The responsibilities of the Emergency Medical Dispatcher (EMD) include all of the following *except*:
A. dispatching and coordinating EMS resources.
B. asking questions of the caller and prioritizing the call.
C. coordinating with other public safety agencies.
D. advising the caller that an ambulance is not needed.

_____ 17. When an Emergency Medical Dispatcher (EMD) questions a patient or caller, which of the following is *not* routinely asked?
A. What is the exact location of the patient?
B. What is the problem?
C. Has the patient been in the hospital recently?
D. How old is the patient?

_____ 18. Activities to terminate the call when back at quarters include:
A. sanitize your hands.
B. clean and sanitize respiratory equipment as required.
C. remove and clean patient-care equipment as required.
D. All of the above.

_____ 19. To be a safe ambulance operator, the EMT should:
A. be tolerant of other drivers.
B. always wear glasses or contact lenses if required.
C. have a positive attitude about his or her ability as a driver.
D. do all of these.

_____ 20. Every state has statutes that regulate the operation of emergency vehicles. Under certain circumstances, vehicle operators can do all of the following *except*:
A. park the vehicle anywhere as long as it does not damage personal property.
B. proceed past red stop signals, flashing red stop signals, and stop signs.
C. exceed the posted speed limit as long as life and property are not endangered.
D. pass a school bus that has its red lights blinking.

_____ 21. You were dispatched to a priority assignment involving a motor vehicle collision. Once at the scene, you find just one patient, a 24-year-old female, and determine that she is stable. This situation is no longer a:
A. true emergency.
B. due regard.
C. cold response.
D. priority-one response.

_____ 22. Which guideline for the use of the ambulance siren is *inappropriate?*
A. Use the siren sparingly and only when you must.
B. Never assume that all motorists will hear your siren.
C. Be prepared for erratic movements of other drivers.
D. Keep the siren on until the call is completed.

_____ 23. Which of the following is *true* about the use of lights and sirens?
- **A.** Motorists are more inclined to give way to ambulances when sirens are continually sounded.
- **B.** The decision about the use of lights and sirens should be based on the patient's medical condition.
- **C.** The use of the siren has little effect on the ambulance operator.
- **D.** Four-way flashers should be used in addition to emergency lights.

_____ 24. Use of escorts or multivehicle responses is a:
- **A.** very quick and successful means of response.
- **B.** very dangerous means of response.
- **C.** means of decreasing the chance of collision.
- **D.** standard operating procedure in most communities.

_____ 25. Factors that can affect ambulance response include all of the following *except*:
- **A.** the time of day.
- **B.** the weather.
- **C.** road maintenance and construction.
- **D.** the type of emergency.

_____ 26. You are the first vehicle on the scene of an automobile collision in which one of the vehicles is on fire. You should park your vehicle _____ the wreckage until the fire apparatus arrives.
- **A.** 50 feet from
- **B.** in front (upstream) of
- **C.** behind
- **D.** downwind from

_____ 27. The sequence of operations to ready a patient for transfer is called:
- **A.** stabilization.
- **B.** packaging.
- **C.** transport.
- **D.** removal.

_____ 28. Which of the following is an action that you would *not* perform en route to the hospital?
- **A.** Recheck the patient's bandages and splints.
- **B.** Form a general impression of the patient.
- **C.** Perform reassessment and continue to monitor vital signs.
- **D.** Notify the receiving facility of your estimated time of arrival.

_____ 29. When describing the landing zone (LZ) to the air rescue service tell them:
- **A.** the terrain.
- **B.** major landmarks.
- **C.** estimated distance to nearest town.
- **D.** all of the above.

_____ 30. When delivering a patient to the hospital, the EMT should *never*:
- **A.** complete the prehospital care report (PCR) at the hospital.
- **B.** move a patient onto the hospital stretcher and just leave.
- **C.** transfer the patient's personal effects.
- **D.** obtain a release from the hospital.

_____ 31. When approaching a helicopter, first wait for the pilot or flight crew member to wave you in. Then approach from the _____ of the craft.
- **A.** rear
- **B.** uphill slope side
- **C.** front or side
- **D.** downhill slope rear

_____ 32. Which of the following patients is *least* likely to be transported in a helicopter?
- **A.** A victim of carbon monoxide poisoning
- **B.** A patient with a suspected stroke
- **C.** A cardiac arrest patient
- **D.** A patient with a critical burn

_____ 33. Some ambulance services have purchased GPS units for the dash of the ambulance to assist the vehicle operator in finding the location of the call. The EMT should remember that the benefits of GPS is all of the following *except*:
- **A.** an excellent substitute for knowledge of the response area.
- **B.** another type of distraction for the vehicle operator.
- **C.** occasionally inaccurate owing to recent road construction.
- **D.** a device for the crew chief or other front seat passenger to deal with.

©2021 Pearson Education, Inc.
Emergency Care, 14th Ed.

Complete the Following

1. List the seven questions an EMD should ask a caller who is reporting a medical emergency.

   A. _____

   B. _____

   C. _____

   D. _____

   E. _____

   F. _____

   G. _____

2. List seven factors that can affect an ambulance response.

   A. _____

   B. _____

   C. _____

   D. _____

   E. _____

   F. _____

   G. _____

3. List the four major ways in which the EMT on the scene of a collision should describe the landing zone (LZ) to the air rescue service.

   A. _____

   B. _____

   C. _____

   D. _____

4. List the five steps in terminating a call.

   A. _____

   B. _____

   C. _____

   D. _____

   E. _____

Case Study: The Ambulance Collision

You are notified by dispatch to respond to the neighboring district for a mutual aid call. You are told that an ambulance has collided with a passenger vehicle at an intersection. The ambulance, with emergency lights and siren operating, had approached the red light and had attempted to pass through it without stopping. The other vehicle's occupants are an elderly couple who were on their way to the store. As you arrive on the scene, it is obvious that there are a number of very seriously injured patients. You are assigned to look after the ambulance operator, who has minor cuts and scrapes. Fortunately, she was wearing her seat belt. Her EMT partner, who was not wearing his shoulder harness, was not as fortunate. Another ambulance has already removed him from the scene with serious head and neck injuries from being ejected through the windshield of the ambulance. Two other ambulance crews are in the process of removing the elderly man, who is in critical condition, and his wife, who has sustained leg fractures and is having a heart attack from the stress of the incident.

1. Was this a preventable collision?

_____

2. Could the serious injuries to the male EMT have been prevented?

_____

3. What should EMS service do for the patient for whom the ambulance that was involved in the accident had been responding?

_____

4. What is the first rule of medicine?

_____

The next day, a headline in the local newspaper reads: "Ambulance Kills Two en Route to an Emergency." The story reports that the patient for whom the ambulance had been responding had minor medical problems and was taken by another ambulance to the local hospital, where she was treated for flu and released. The newspaper story concludes: "The ambulance driver was suspended. The district attorney has requested that a grand jury inquiry be conducted."

GZQ **5.** Aside from the reputation of the EMT who was driving, what might this negative publicity cost the service and other EMTs who work there?

_____

6. Why might the district attorney request a grand jury for this incident?

_____

7. Is the operator of an emergency vehicle held to a higher standard than other motorists?

_____

8. Who pays for the court defense of the ambulance operator?

_____

9. Could the ambulance operator be personally sued for the injuries and deaths that occurred?

_____

GZQ **10.** How can an ambulance service prevent a collision like this from happening in its community?

_____

©2021 Pearson Education, Inc.
Emergency Care, 14th Ed.

Hazardous Materials, Multiple-Casualty Incidents, and Incident Management

Core Concepts

- How to identify and take appropriate action in a hazardous materials incident
- How to identify a multiple-casualty incident
- The Incident Command System
- Triage considerations
- Transportation and staging logistics
- Psychological aspects of multiple-casualty incidents

Outcomes

After reading this chapter, you should be able to:

39.1 Summarize concepts related to hazardous materials. (pp. 1178–1180)
- Describe the features of a hazardous material.
- Compare the federal legislation guiding the regulation of hazardous materials and the response to hazardous materials incidents.
- Explain the potential for hazardous materials incidents.
- Compare levels of hazardous materials training with the responsibilities for response at the scene of a hazardous materials incident.

39.2 Summarize the EMT's responsibilities with respect to hazardous materials incident scene management. (pp. 1180–1186)
- Recognize indications of a potential hazardous materials incident.
- Explain the process of controlling the scene.
- Identify ways an EMT can identify the substance involved in a hazardous materials incident.
- Explain the information a first-arriving EMT team at a hazardous materials incident will need to provide to a resource agency to get advice.

39.3 Summarize the EMT's roles in the treatment of others at the scene of a hazardous materials incidents. (pp. 1186–1192)
- Describe the process of rehabilitation operations.
- Describe the process of caring for injured and contaminated patients.
- Describe the processes for decontamination.

39.4 Summarize concepts related to multiple-casualty incidents. (pp. 1192–1199)
- Identify the primary feature that makes an event a multiple-casualty incident.
- Recognize the desirable characteristics of a disaster plan.
- Explain situations that have an increased likelihood of creating a mass-casualty incident.
- Identify ways for increasing the effectiveness of response to mass-casualty incidents.
- Outline the Incident Command System (ICS) structure and functions.
- Describe how to set up Incident Command if your ambulance is first on the scene at a multiple-casualty incident.
- Explain the potential psychological impacts on multiple-casualty incident (MCI) survivors and responders.

39.5 Summarize the EMS branch functions within the ICS structure. (pp. 1200–1210)
- Apply triage criteria to a variety of MCI patient portrayals.
- Outline the selection of triaged patients for secondary triage and treatment.
- Identify the relationship between the staging area and transport area at an MCI.
- Recognize the role of the staging and transportation supervisors in maintaining an organized approach to the MCI.
- Compare communication with hospitals in an MCI with routine EMS communication with hospitals.

Match Key Terms

A. A color-coded tag indicating the priority group to which a patient has been assigned.

B. The area in which secondary triage takes place at a multiple-casualty incident.

C. The process of quickly assessing patients at a multiple-casualty incident and assigning each a priority for receiving treatment.

D. The person who is responsible for overseeing triage at a multiple-casualty incident.

E. The area in which patients are treated at a multiple-casualty incident.

F. The person who is responsible for overseeing treatment of patients who have been triaged at a multiple-casualty incident.

G. The person who is responsible for communicating with sector officers and hospitals to manage transportation of patients to hospitals from a multiple-casualty incident.

H. The area where ambulances are parked and other resources are held until needed.

I. The person who is responsible for overseeing ambulances and ambulance personnel at a multiple-casualty incident.

J. Any medical or trauma incident involving multiple patients.

K. The management system used by federal, state, and local governments to manage emergencies in the United States in a consistent manner.

L. The first on the scene to establish order and initiate the Incident Command System.

_____ **1.** Cold zone

_____ **2.** Command

_____ **3.** Decontamination

_____ **4.** Disaster plan

_____ **5.** Hazardous material (HAZMAT)

_____ **6.** Hot zone

_____ **7.** Incident Command

_____ **8.** Incident Command System (ICS)

_____ **9.** Multiple-casualty incident (MCI)

_____ **10.** National Incident Management System (NIMS)

_____ **11.** Single incident command

_____ **12.** Staging area

_____ **13.** Staging supervisor

_____ **14.** Transportation supervisor

M. Any substance or material in a form that poses an unreasonable risk to health, safety, and property when transported in commerce or kept in storage.

N. Area immediately surrounding a HAZMAT incident; extends far enough to prevent adverse effects outside the zone.

O. Area where the Incident Command post and support functions are located.

P. A command organization in which a single agency controls all resources and operations.

Q. The person or persons who assume overall direction of a large-scale incident.

R. A subset of the National Incident Management System (NIMS) designed specifically for management of multiple-casualty incidents.

S. The area where personnel and equipment decontamination and hot zone support take place.

T. A command organization in which several agencies work independently but cooperatively.

U. A predefined set of instructions for a community's emergency responders.

V. A chemical and/or physical process that removes hazardous substances from employees and their equipment to the extent necessary to preclude foreseeable health effects.

W. A measurable representation of ability of a medical facility to manage a sudden influx of patients.

_____ **15.** Treatment area

_____ **16.** Treatment supervisor

_____ **17.** Triage

_____ **18.** Triage area

_____ **19.** Triage supervisor

_____ **20.** Triage tag

_____ **21.** Unified command

_____ **22.** Warm zone

_____ **23.** Surge capacity

Multiple-Choice Review

_____ **1.** On arrival at the scene of a vehicle fire involving a large truck, you observe that the large truck has placards on each of its sides. Using the *Emergency Response Guidebook*, you would find that benzene (benzol) is a chemical that:
   A. damages the eyes by eliminating moisture.
   B. has toxic vapors that can be absorbed through the skin.
   C. is used as an industrial blasting agent.
   D. is used in surgical techniques to control pain.

_____ **2.** The regulations that are meant to enhance the knowledge, skills, and safety of emergency response personnel, as well as bring about a more effective response to HAZMAT emergencies, are found in:
   A. the Ryan White CARE Act.   **C.** NFPA 1200.
   B. FEMA 1910.1030.   **D.** OSHA 29 CFR 1910.120.

_____ **3.** According to the regulations: "Those who initially respond to releases or potential releases of hazardous materials in order to protect people, property, and the environment. They stay at a safe distance, keep the incident from spreading, and protect others from any exposures." What level of training does this statement describe?
   A. First Responder Awareness
   B. First Responder Operations
   C. Hazardous Materials Technician
   D. Hazardous Materials Specialist

_____ 4. A statement in OSHA's Hazardous Waste Operations and Emergency Response standards reads, "Rescuers at this level are likely to witness or discover a hazardous substance release. They are trained only to recognize the problem and initiate a response from the proper organizations." What level of training does this describe?
   A. First Responder Awareness
   B. First Responder Operations
   C. Hazardous Materials Technician
   D. Hazardous Materials Specialist

_____ 5. The standard that deals with competencies for EMS personnel at a hazardous materials incident is:
   A. OSHA 1910.1030.
   B. NFPA #374.
   C. NFPA #473.
   D. OSHA 1910.1200.

_____ 6. You are responding to a location in your district. The dispatcher informs you that the caller has stated that there may be hazardous materials stored at the location. Which of the following is least likely to be a potential hazardous material location?
   A. A garden center
   B. A chemical plant
   C. A trucking terminal
   D. A pet store

_____ 7. Unless EMS personnel are trained to the level of _____, they must remain in the cold zone.
   A. First Responder Awareness
   B. First Responder Operations
   C. Hazardous Materials Technician
   D. Hazardous Materials Specialist

_____ 8. All victims leaving the _____ zone should be considered contaminated until proven otherwise.
   A. cold
   B. warm
   C. hot
   D. decontamination

_____ 9. The primary concern at the scene of a hazardous materials incident is
   A. the safety of the EMT and crew, patients, and the public.
   B. stabilizing the incident as fast as possible.
   C. quickly removing all exposed patients from the scene.
   D. determining the extent and cost of the damage.

_____ 10. The safe zone of a hazardous materials incident should be established in a(n) _____ location.
   A. downwind/downhill
   B. upwind/same level
   C. downwind/same level
   D. upwind/downhill

_____ 11. The role of Command at a hazardous materials incident is to delegate responsibility for all the following _except_:
   A. directing bystanders to a safe area.
   B. establishing a perimeter.
   C. immediately initiating rescue attempts.
   D. evacuating people if necessary.

_____ 12. When a contaminated victim of a HAZMAT incident comes into contact with people who are not contaminated, this is referred to as _____ contamination.
   A. secondary
   B. chemical
   C. contact
   D. clone

_____ 13. The designations on the sides of tanker trucks are called hazardous material:
   A. license plates.
   B. waybills.
   C. placards.
   D. shipping papers.

14. The commonly used placard system for fixed facilities is called the:
- **A.** SDS system.
- **B.** NFPA 704 system.
- **C.** CHEM 369 system.
- **D.** UN Classification system.

15. All employers are required to post, in an obvious spot, the information about each chemical in the workplace on a form called a(n):
- **A.** NFPA 704.
- **B.** safety data sheet (SDS).
- **C.** OSHA chemical listing.
- **D.** fair trade posting.

16. Resources that the EMT should use at a hazardous materials incident include all of the following *except*:
- **A.** copies of NFPA rules.
- **B.** the local HAZMAT team.
- **C.** the *Emergency Response Guidebook*.
- **D.** CHEM-TEL.

17. The Incident Commander at the HAZMAT incident is collecting needed information so that she can contact CHEMTREC. What is CHEMTREC?
- **A.** A twenty-four-hour service for identifying hazardous materials
- **B.** An oil refinery and manufacturer
- **C.** A national HAZMAT response team
- **D.** A round-the-clock special rescue team

18. You have been dispatched to an incident involving hazardous chemicals. EMS personnel at the scene of a hazardous materials incident are responsible for taking care of the injured and:
- **A.** identifying and controlling the substance involved.
- **B.** monitoring and rehabilitating HAZMAT team members.
- **C.** decontaminating patients exiting the hot zone.
- **D.** moving patients from the hot zone to the warm zone.

19. Which of the following is *not* a characteristic of the rehabilitation operations at a hazardous materials incident?
- **A.** They are located in the warm zone.
- **B.** They are protected from the weather.
- **C.** They are easily accessible to EMS.
- **D.** They are free from exhaust fumes.

20. As soon as possible after a HAZMAT team member exits the hot zone, the EMT in the rehab operations should:
- **A.** have the team member drink a pint of water.
- **B.** remove the team member's protective clothing.
- **C.** begin the decontamination process.
- **D.** reassess the team member's vital signs.

21. You are confronted with a patient who is at risk for causing secondary contamination in which treatment calls for irrigation with water. The HAZMAT team has not yet arrived. Which of the following actions is *not* recommended?
- **A.** Cut the patient's clothes off.
- **B.** Irrigate the patient with tepid or warmwater.
- **C.** Flush runoff water down the nearest drain.
- **D.** Use disposable equipment for treatment.

22. Which of the following is *not* a feature of a good local disaster plan?
- **A.** All emergency responders should be familiar with the plan.
- **B.** The plan must be based on the actual availability of resources.
- **C.** The plan must be rehearsed to ensure it works correctly.
- **D.** The plan should be generic and meet national standards.

23. On arrival of the first EMS unit at the scene of an MCI, the crew leader should do all of the following *except*:
- **A.** assume command.
- **B.** conduct a scene walk-through.
- **C.** call for backup.
- **D.** begin patient treatment.

_____ **24.** Which of the following is *not* a principle of good communication at an MCI?

    A. The person responsible for incident management should have a unique Command name.

    B. Responding units should be informed that a disaster plan is in effect.

    C. The majority of communications should be done via radio transmission.

    D. Communications between Command and direct subordinates should be face-to-face.

_____ **25.** Some services administer oral fluids in their rehab sectors. What fluid would be appropriate to offer the team members?

    A. Coffee that is cold or hot   **C.** Coke or diet cola

    B. Tea that is cold or hot   **D.** Watered-down sports drink

_____ **26.** You are responding to a collision between a loaded school bus and a tractor-trailer truck. You have been informed that the bus is on its side and that there are many injured children. You are quickly reviewing the roles of the management personnel at a major incident while en route. The individual at an MCI who is responsible for sorting and prioritizing patients is the _____ supervisor.

    A. triage   **C.** transportation

    B. treatment   **D.** extrication

_____ **27.** If any children at a MCI incident are assessed as having decreased mental status, they should be considered Priority:

    A. 1.   **C.** 3.

    B. 2.   **D.** 4.

_____ **28.** If any children in an MCI incident are assessed as having signs of shock, they will be considered Priority:

    A. 1.   **C.** 3.

    B. 2.   **D.** 4.

_____ **29.** If any children in an MCI incident are assessed as having multiple-bone or joint injuries but no airway problems, they will be considered Priority:

    A. 1.   **C.** 3.

    B. 2.   **D.** 4.

_____ **30.** The driver of a vehicle involved in an MCI event was assessed as having died at the MCI scene. The driver should be considered a Priority:

    A. 1.   **C.** 3.

    B. 2.   **D.** 4.

_____ **31.** The individual at an MCI incident who is responsible for maintaining a supply of vehicles and personnel at a location away from the incident site is the _____ supervisor.

    A. extrication   **C.** staging

    B. transportation   **D.** triage

_____ **32.** The individual at an MCI event who is responsible for determining patient destinations and notifying the hospitals of the incoming patients is the _____ supervisor.

    A. triage   **C.** transportation

    B. treatment   **D.** extrication

_____ **33.** Patient transport decisions at an MCI incident will be based on all of the following parameters *except*:

    A. priority.   **C.** transportation resources.

    B. destination facilities.   **D.** patient's family preferences.

©2021 Pearson Education, Inc.
Emergency Care, 14th Ed.

_____ **34.** The characteristics of the rehabilitation area must include all of the following *except* being:
   A. located in the warm zone.
   B. protected from weather as much as possible.
   C. large enough to accommodate multiple rescue crews.
   D. free from exhaust fumes.

_____ **35.** You have been assigned to the rehabilitation area at a hazardous materials incident. One of your responsibilities will be the medical monitoring of the HAZMAT team before and after working in their chemical-protective suits. One team member comes into your area and is anxious to get suited back up and go back to work. You take a set of vital signs that reveal the following: respiratory rate of 20 and regular, heart rate of 120 and bounding, blood pressure of 132/84 mmHg, and SpO$_2$ of 98%. What should you do next with this team member?
   A. Take an oral temperature.
   B. Have the team member drink some fluids, then suit back up.
   C. Have the team member sit for 15 minutes and reevaluate.
   D. Tell the team member that work is done for the day.

_____ **36.** Yours is the first unit to arrive at the scene of a multiple-casualty incident. A train car derailed in the middle of a crowded city, and there are injured people all over. Aside from confirming the incident and calling for additional help, what is one of the first steps in beginning triage using the START system?
   A. Talk to each patient and assign her or him a triage tag.
   B. Use the PA system to instruct those who can walk to go to a specific location.
   C. Locate the dead and have them removed from the scene.
   D. Evaluate the mental status of each patient.

_____ **37.** You will be using the START system during an MCI event. This system uses all of the following parameters *except*:
   A. a pulse or circulation check.
   B. a respiration assessment.
   C. the mental status of the patients.
   D. the number of broken bones each patient has.

_____ **38.** In the START system, the amount of treatment provided before tagging the patients is limited to:
   A. splinting and applying a cervical collar.
   B. opening an airway, applying pressure on a bleeding wound, or elevating an extremity.
   C. traction splinting and occlusive dressings.
   D. assisting patients in taking their own pain medications.

_____ **39.** You will be using the SALT system at future MCIs in your EMS system. In this system patients who are likely to survive with treatment are tagged as Immediate. Which one of the following patients should receive an Immediate or color red tag?
   A. A male patient without peripheral pulses.
   B. A female patient with uncontrolled external hemorrhage.
   C. A male patient who is not in respiratory distress but does have a severe injury.
   D. A female patient who makes no purposeful movements after severe head trauma.

Complete the Following

1. List eleven pieces of information that you should be prepared to give when you call for assistance from CHEMTREC.

A. _____

B. _____

C. _____

D. _____

E. _____

F. _____

G. _____

H. _____

I. _____

J. _____

K. _____

2. List six characteristics of the rehabilitation areas at a hazardous materials incident.

A. _____

B. _____

C. _____

D. _____

E. _____

F. _____

3. List seven common mechanisms for performing decontamination.

A. _____

B. _____

C. _____

D. _____

E. _____

F. _____

G. _____

Complete the Chart

Fill in the blanks to complete the chart.

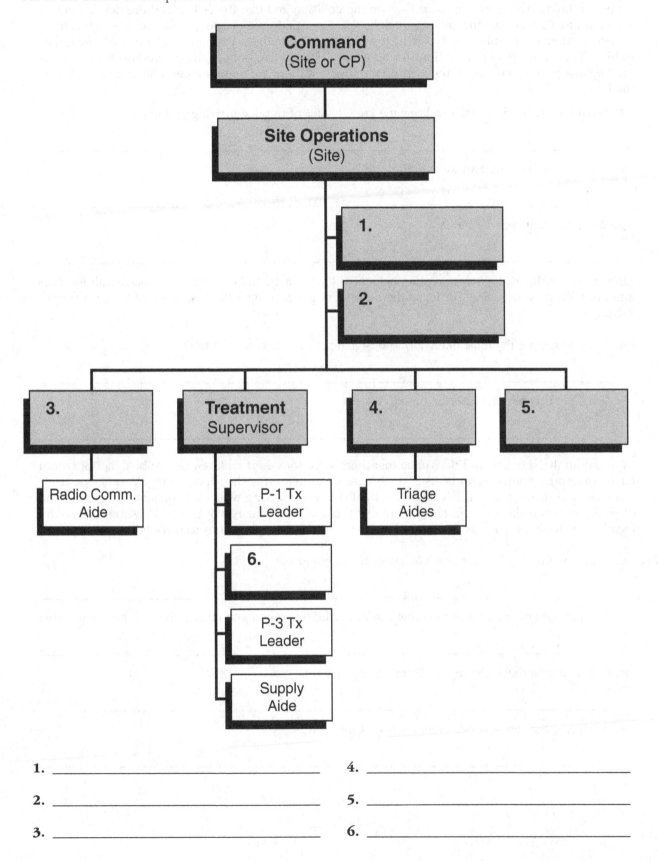

1. _____   4. _____

2. _____   5. _____

3. _____   6. _____

Case Study: School Bus MCI

You are dispatched to a school bus collision in a major intersection. The dispatcher notifies you en route that he has received numerous calls on the collision and that the police and fire department are en route. Callers state that a large truck collided at a high rate of speed with the school bus in an intersection, overturning the bus, which was full of children. As you near the center of town, the traffic is backed up in both directions for about five blocks. The police have arrived on the scene and are beginning to reroute the traffic after confirming that there are many injured children on and near the bus.

1. What would be your initial tasks as the crew leader of the first-arriving ambulance at the scene?

_____

2. Which vest from the MCI kit should you wear?

_____

3. What are your responsibilities?

_____

After declaring the MCI, confirming the incident with dispatch, and establishing contact with the police and fire officers, you begin to estimate the number of patients, with the assistance of your two crew members.

4. What would be the most likely job to designate to one of your partners?

_____

5. What are this person's specific functions?

_____

You size up the situation and determine that there were forty-four children on the bus, half of whom have numerous contusions and cuts and who are walking around the scene crying. You decide to designate a nearby store as the location for the Priority 3 "walking wounded" patients. You have one of your partners make a PA announcement that those who are injured but can walk should go to that location. In addition, you call for ten ambulances and another school bus to respond.

GZQ 6. Where would be the best place to stage the ambulances?

_____

7. What should be the role of the crew leader on the first ambulance that arrives at the staging area?

_____

8. Should any ambulances report directly to the scene?

_____

9. Are any other sector supervisors needed at this time?

_____

The fire department has cleared the bus for entry now that it has been stabilized and is no longer leaking any fuel or at risk for rolling over. Inside are fifteen patients who need to be removed from the bus. Many of them have head injuries, fractures, contusions, and glass cuts.

GZQ 10. How should these patients be removed from the bus, if it is possible?

_____

11. Once the patients have been removed from the bus, where should they be taken?

_____

Prioritize the patients described below into the following categories: Priority 1 (critical and unstable), Priority 2 (potentially unstable), Priority 3 (stable, walking wounded), and Priority 4 (or zero) (dead).

12. A 7-year-old female who complains of a swollen, deformed right lower arm and a contusion to the head with no loss of consciousness. She is alert and has vital signs that are normal for her age.

_____

13. A 9-year-old male who has a seizure disorder and who has been unconscious since the collision. He has already had two observed grand mal seizures without a lucid interval.

_____

14. A 10-year-old male who was thrown through the front window of the bus because he was standing up talking to the bus driver. He was ejected from the vehicle; was found approximately 50 feet from the bus; and has a large contusion, a depressed skull fracture, and no vital signs.

_____

15. An 8-year-old female who has a bruise on the left upper quadrant and a bruise on the forehead. She denies any loss of consciousness but is pale and clammy and has a rapid heart rate for her age.

_____

The treatment supervisor has set up a treatment area across the street from the collision in a gas station parking lot. He has set out a large yellow tarp and a large red tarp. There is also a smaller black tarp inside the gas station for the Priority 4 patients. As the incident proceeds, you are able to obtain additional assistance from the firefighters at the scene for lifting the patients who are being removed from the bus and carried on backboards to the treatment area. The area is becoming quite congested because a number of parents are arriving at the scene.

GZQ 16. What is the best thing to do with the parents of the patients?

_____

17. As a smooth flow of ambulances begins to arrive from the staging area, who should coordinate the destinations of the patient transports and communicate with the hospitals?

_____

18. What might this person want to know immediately from the local hospitals?

_____

19. Other than the bus that was ordered for the Priority 3 patients, is there any other form of transportation that should be considered for this incident?

_____

20. How should the decision be made about who rides on the bus to a hospital?

_____

21. As the incident is wrapped up, how could you, as Command, deal with the media and the emotional and physical needs of your personnel?

_____

40

Highway Safety and Vehicle Extrication

Core Concepts

- How to position emergency apparatus to create a safe work zone at a highway emergency
- How to recognize and manage hazards at the highway rescue scene
- How to stabilize a vehicle
- How to gain access to the patient in a crashed vehicle
- How to disentangle a patient from a crashed vehicle

Outcomes

After reading this chapter, you should be able to:

40.1 Summarize concepts of highway emergency operations. (pp. 1214–1219)
- Identify the hazards associated with highway emergency operations.
- Relate response to highway scenes to the incidence of line-of-duty deaths (LODD).
- Describe the actions an EMT should take at a highway scene if that EMT's ambulance is the first-arriving vehicle.
- Explain the reason for establishing Incident Command as the first-arriving unit on the scene of a highway emergency.
- Recognize the guidelines for effective placement of traffic control cones or flares.
- Outline the safety actions all EMTs should take at the scene of highway operations.

40.2 Summarize the concepts of vehicle extrication operations. (pp. 1219–1240)
- Compare the EMT's role as a team member in an extrication with that of trained rescue personnel performing the extrication procedures.
- Recognize the general steps rescuers will take in performing extrication procedures.
- Describe steps to avoid injury from damaged vehicles and structures at the scene of highway emergency operations.
- Identify safety precautions for occupants who will be inside the car during extrication procedures.
- Identify equipment that can help EMTs access a damaged vehicle while awaiting response of an extrication team.
- Describe the features of commonly used approaches to extrication.

Multiple-Choice Review

_____ **1.** One of the greatest hazards that emergency responders face on a daily basis is (are):
- **A.** high rising flood waters.
- **B.** oncoming traffic at highway incidents.
- **C.** acts of terrorism in our cities.
- **D.** routine calls involving anxious patients.

_____ **2.** The phases of extrication include all of the following _except_:
- **A.** gaining access to the patient.
- **B.** defining patient care.
- **C.** disentangling the patient.
- **D.** sizing up the situation.

_____ **3.** On arrival at the scene of a three-car motor vehicle crash, you and your crew ensure that the location is safe and begin to size up the situation. An important part of a rescue scene size-up is:
- **A.** determining the extent of entrapment.
- **B.** sweeping up all the broken glass.
- **C.** removing shattered glass from around the patient.
- **D.** informing the patient about the extent of vehicle damage.

_____ **4.** During size-up of a collision, you must be able to "read" a collision and develop an action plan based on your knowledge of rescue operations and your:
- **A.** previous experience at collision scenes.
- **B.** judgment of the extent of vehicle damage.
- **C.** estimate of the patient's condition and priority.
- **D.** evaluation of the resources available.

_____ **5.** You are on the scene of a car that crashed into a bridge overpass abutment. The patient is trapped and seriously injured. When developing an action plan for patient extrication, always keep in mind:
- **A.** the potential for observation by bystanders.
- **B.** that time is very critical to some patients' trauma management.
- **C.** the cost of further damage to the vehicle.
- **D.** the type of vehicle that is involved in the incident.

_____ **6.** If a vehicle has an airbag that deployed, the manufacturer recommends:
- **A.** airing out the car for 15 minutes before treating the patient.
- **B.** placing masks on patients before treating.
- **C.** lifting the bag and examining the steering wheel and dash.
- **D.** using HEPA masks before gaining access.

_____ **7.** The unsafe act that contributes most to injuries at collision scenes is:
- **A.** crossing over lanes of still flowing traffic on foot.
- **B.** wearing too much protective gear during rescue operations.
- **C.** not recognizing the mechanisms of injury right away.
- **D.** selecting the wrong tool for the task.

_____ **8.** Every year, EMTs and rescuers are injured at the scene of collisions. Factors that may contribute to injuries of rescuers at a collision include all of the following _except_:
- **A.** a careless attitude toward personal safety.
- **B.** a lack of skill in tool and equipment use.
- **C.** physical problems that impede strenuous effort.
- **D.** limiting the inner circle to rescuers who are in protective gear.

_____ 9. Good protective gear at the scene of a collision includes all of the following *except*:
   A. firefighter or leather gloves.
   B. fire-resistant trousers or turnout pants.
   C. steel-toed, high-top work shoes.
   D. plastic "bump caps."

_____ 10. To ensure adequate eye protection at the collision scene, the EMT should wear
   _____
   A. safety goggles with a soft vinyl frame.
   B. a hinged plastic helmet shield.
   C. a thermal mask or shield.
   D. safety glasses with small lenses.

_____ 11. During extrication, an aluminized rescue blanket may be used to:
   A. maintain the rescuer's body heat.
   B. smother a fire located in the engine compartment.
   C. protect the patient from poor weather.
   D. none of these.

_____ 12. The police have not arrived at the scene of a collision, and you have positioned
   your ambulance to temporarily block the traffic until flares have been set up.
   When using flares, the EMT should:
   A. watch for spilled fuel or other combustibles before igniting.
   B. throw them out of the moving vehicle to save time.
   C. use them as a traffic wand to divert traffic.
   D. always walk with oncoming traffic while positioning them.

_____ 13. You are just arriving on the scene of a car that crashed into a utility pole. The
   pole is broken in half, and the wires are down in the street. When there is an
   electrical hazard, the safe zone:
   A. should be established as soon as the power company arrives.
   B. does not exist because of the numerous dangers of an electrical hazard.
   C. should be far enough away to ensure that an arcing wire does not cause injury.
   D. is located at least 10 feet from the ground gradient.

_____ 14. As of 2009, federal highway standards have required that all emergency
   responders:
   A. take the incident command course.
   B. comply with NFPA 1500.
   C. wear ANSI safety vests when working in highway operations.
   D. don PPE prior to touching bleeding patients.

_____ 15. If a vehicle has been involved in a front-end collision and you notice that the
   airbag did not deploy, for safety of the crew working around the airbag, you
   should consider:
   A. immediately putting the vehicle in neutral with the parking brake on.
   B. telling all the rescuers to stay out of the vehicle until the airbag explodes.
   C. disconnecting the battery and wait 2-3 minutes, then carefully work near the bag.
   D. chaining down the steering column as soon as possible.

_____ 16. In wet weather, a phenomenon known as _____ may provide your
   first clue that a wire is down.
   A. an arc   C. lightning
   B. ground gradient   D. flash point

_____ 17. You are on the scene of a collision between a car and a utility pole. The pole is
   literally split in two and hanging by the wires. As you approach the vehicle, you
   feel a tingling sensation in your legs and lower torso. Which action should you take?
   A. Turn 180 degrees and shuffle with both feet together to safety.
   B. Turn 90 degrees and walk as quickly as possible to safety.
   C. Ask your partner for his hand and have him pull you to safety.
   D. Turn 180 degrees and crawl to safety.

_____ 18. If there is a fire in the car's engine compartment and people are trapped in the vehicle, you should do all of the following *except*:
A. quickly and carefully removing the patients.
B. ensuring that the fire department has been called.
C. donning protective gear and using your fire extinguisher.
D. applying a short spine board to the driver right away.

_____ 19. When a vehicle's hood is closed and there is an engine fire, you should do all of the following *except*:
A. using emergency moves to remove occupants.
B. letting the fire department extinguish the fire.
C. fully opening the hood to extinguish the fire.
D. letting the fire burn under the closed hood.

_____ 20. When a vehicle rolls off the roadway into a field of dried grass, a fire may be caused by the:
A. catalytic converter.
B. leaking radiator fluid.
C. ground gradient.
D. airbag deployment.

_____ 21. "Try before you pry!" is the foundation for the _____ procedure.
A. disentanglement
B. stabilization
C. simple access
D. entanglement

_____ 22. You are on the scene of a two-car, high-speed, head-on collision. The scene is safe and the traffic has been diverted by the police. Once the vehicle to which you were assigned is stabilized and an entry point has been gained, you should immediately do all of the following *except*:
A. begin the primary assessment.
B. crawl inside the vehicle.
C. provide manual spine motion restriction.
D. pull the patient out of the access hole.

_____ 23. At the scene of a 2 car frontal impact MVC, you find an unconscious 28-year-old female who is in a sitting position behind the wheel with both her legs pinned. Which is the best approach to disentanglement of this patient?
A. Displace the doors, cut the roof, and then displace the dash.
B. Pull the dash, cut the doors, and then push the seat.
C. Cut the roof, displace the doors, and then displace the dash.
D. Cut the roof, displace the dash, and then displace the doors.

_____ 24. The decision is made to remove the roof of one of the vehicles at a 2 vehicle MVC with entrapment. Which of the following is *not* a reason for removing the roof to access a patient?
A. It makes the entire interior of the vehicle accessible.
B. It creates a large exit through which to remove a patient.
C. It provides fresh air and helps cool off the patient.
D. It helps to stabilize the vehicle quickly.

Complete the Following

1. List the ten phases of the extrication or rescue process.

A. _____

B. _____

C. _____

D. _____

E. _____

F. _____

G. _____

H. _____

I. _____

J. _____

2. List six items that can be used to protect a patient from heat, cold, flying particles, and other hazards.

A. _____

B. _____

C. _____

D. _____

E. _____

F. _____

3. List the personal protective equipment that you should wear at a collision site where you will be providing patient care within the inner circle on a patient who is entrapped.

A. _____

B. _____

C. _____

D. _____

4. List eight examples of alternative fuels in vehicles on the roads today.

A. _____

B. _____

C. _____

D. _____

E. _____

F. _____

G. _____

H. _____

Case Study: Bad Wreck: Patient Pinned Under the Dash

It is about midnight, and your unit receives a call for a high speed, two-car collision on the main highway that travels east/west through your town. On your way to the call, you receive a second notice from the dispatcher requesting your estimated time of arrival, as the police are on the scene already and there are definitely two injured patients. They have also called for the fire department rescue squad, since one of the patients is trapped inside his vehicle. As you arrive, the Incident Commander tells you to drive past the collision and park off to the right of the roadway. They already have the crashed vehicles blocked by two police vehicles and are setting out flares to divert the traffic.

1. Where do you expect the fire rescue unit will be told to park their vehicle?

_____

2. What PPE should you don if you will be working in the inner circle of the crashed vehicles?

_____

You talk briefly with the police officer and are told that one patient is sitting on the lawn of a nearby house. The police officer gestures in the patient's direction. The other patient is pinned under the dash of the vehicle that has the most front-end damage. Your partner calls for another ambulance and proceeds to check on the patient who is out of his vehicle while you look into the vehicle to see what degree of entrapment there is. Both of the patient's legs are under the steering column, and the wheel and dash are crushing her. You note that the rear hatch is an access point, so you lay down a blanket. You crawl into the rear seat of the vehicle and begin to talk to the trapped patient. The patient is a 22-year old female who states that the other car came out of nowhere and slammed into the front of her car. Her name is Kayla, and she says that she might have hit her head and passed out for a few minutes, as she does not remember everything about the crash, just speeding headlights crossing the center line before the crash. You quickly determine that her mental status is a "V" (for verbally responsive) because she is talkative but confused about the day and time and exactly where she is.

3. In terms of assessment, what would be your next steps?

_____

GZQ **4.** The rescue officer asks you what you need, and you say, "We need to quickly get the vehicle off Kayla's legs so we can get her out of here." She is a high priority owing to the MOI and her mental status. You have not yet actually seen her legs. How might you assess the extent of her internal bleeding at this point?

_____

5. Will Kayla need spinal motion restriction? If so, what would be the preferred method once her legs have been freed?

_____

You note that Kayla has a very weak and fast radial pulse; she is pale, clammy and still very confused. Her breathing rate is about 26 and shallow, and she has lung sounds on both sides. She is complaining of tenderness in the left upper quadrant of her abdomen and lower left chest, and you suspect that there may be a couple of broken ribs from striking the steering wheel. The rescue officer tells you that they should have Kayla out in about 5 to 10 minutes, as they will be taking off the driver's door and removing the roof. They will then use a ram to push the dash up after making a couple of relief cuts at the rocker panel. You have worked with these firefighters before, and you know that they practice often and are good at their jobs.

©2021 Pearson Education, Inc.
Emergency Care, 14th Ed.

6. Given a few minutes more inside the vehicle as disentanglement is being accomplished, what treatment should you consider?

_____

7. Knowing that you will be taking the patient to the regional trauma center, would it be appropriate to call the emergency department and let them know her condition?

_____

Your partner lets you know that the second ambulance has arrived and is treating the other driver. Apparently, he has a few cuts, has normal vitals, and is very, very intoxicated. The roof of Kayla's car comes off and the dash is pushed up, so you are able to slide Kayla onto a long backboard and, with some help from your partner and the EMTs from the fire department, remove her from the vehicle to your stretcher, where the medic is already running through an IV line and ready to get rolling to the hospital. You look at your watch and note that the complete on-scene time has been 20 minutes including the rescue operations.

EMS Response to Terrorism

Core Concepts

- Types of terrorism and examples of tactics and doctrine
- How to identify the type of threat posed by a terrorist event
- Use of time/distance/shielding for protection at a terrorist event
- How to respond to and deal with threats from a terrorist event
- Applying strategy, tactics, and countermeasures at a terrorist event
- Self-protection and safety awareness at a terrorist event

Outcomes

After reading this chapter, you should be able to:

41.1 Summarize concepts of terrorism. (pp. 1245–1253)
- Compare the features of domestic and international terrorism.
- Describe the agents often used to create terrorism incidents.
- Relate EMT's actions in responses to incidents of terrorism to the terrorist's frequent goal of including arriving public safety personnel as targets.
- Describe EMT actions that anticipate the presence of multiple devices or terrorists.
- Identify events and structures that are at higher risk for terrorist attacks.
- Recognize the importance of specific dates in the risk for terrorist attacks.
- Give examples of on-scene indications of a potential terrorist attack.
- Describe the potential harms posed when certain agents are weaponized and disseminated.
- Name basic principles to apply during terrorist incidents.

41.2 Explain the general considerations associated with specific types of weapons used in terrorist events. (pp. 1253–1258)
- Identify the harms associated with chemical agents.
- Describe self-protection against chemical agent exposure.
- Identify the harms associated with biologic agents.
- Describe self-protection against biologic agent exposure.
- Identify the harms associated with radiologic/nuclear incidents.
- Describe self-protection measures associated with radiologic/nuclear incidents.
- Identify harms associated with explosives.
- Describe self-protective measures associated with explosives.

41.3 Explain the specific considerations associated with chemical agents of terrorism. (pp. 1258–1261)
- Give examples of the impact of each of the characteristics of a chemical agent—physical, volatility, chemical, and toxicologic—-that can impact the severity and spread of exposure.
- Describe actions of each classification of chemical agents: choking, vesicating, cyanides, nerve agents, and riot-control agents.
- Relate signs and symptoms to the possibility of nerve agent exposure.
- Relate the availability of nerve agent antidotes to the limitations in their use.
- Given a variety of hazardous material scenarios, utilize the DOT emergency guidebook to make initial decisions about establishing evacuation and work zones.

41.4 Explain the specific considerations associated with biologic agents of terrorism. (pp. 1261–1269)
- Discern between the use of living organisms and the use of toxins produced by the organisms in terms of harms caused.
- Identify the features of biologic weapons that influence their potential for use in terrorism attacks.
- Recognize specific biologic agents of concern for high potential for mass harm in terrorism attacks.
- Identify sources of information for guidance on the correct response to specific exposures.

41.5 Explain the specific considerations associated with radiologic/nuclear agents of terrorism. (pp. 1269–1270)
- Compare sources of radiation that may be used in terrorism attacks.
- Outline the progressive nature of the impact of radiation on the tissues as the dose of radiation increases.

41.6 Explain specific considerations associated with terrorism events using incendiary and explosive devices. (pp. 1270–1272)
- Identify additional risks beyond heat that may be associated with the use of incendiary devices.
- Describe the impact of blast injuries on various regions of the body.

41.7 Explain the roles of strategies and tactics in guiding the response to terrorism events. (pp. 1272–1279)
- Prioritize the outcomes desired by the use of an Incident Command System at a hazardous materials incident.
- Defend the priority of EMT protection first—before other actions.
- Size up the scene to determine the presence of clues to a possible terrorist event.

Match Key Terms

A. Terrorism directed against one's own government or population.

B. A measure of radiation dosage.

C. Spreading.

D. The dose or concentration of an agent multiplied by the time or duration.

E. The movement of a substance through a surface or, on a molecular level, through intact materials.

F. Pathways into the body, generally by absorption, ingestion, injection, or inhalation.

G. Destructive devices, such as bombs, that are placed to be activated after an initial attack and timed to injure emergency responders and others who rush in to help care for those targeted by an initial attack.

H. Terrorism that is purely foreign-based or directed.

_____ **1.** Contamination

_____ **2.** Dissemination

_____ **3.** Domestic terrorism

_____ **4.** Exposure

_____ **5.** International terrorism

_____ **6.** Permeation

_____ **7.** Rem

_____ **8.** Routes of entry

_____ **9.** Multiple devices

_____ **10.** Strategies

I. Contact with or presence of a material that is present where it does not belong and that is somehow harmful to persons, animals, or the environment.

J. Packaging or producing a material, such as a chemical, biologic, or radiologic agent, so that it can be used as a weapon.

K. The unlawful use of force or violence against persons or property to intimidate or coerce a government, the civilian population, or any segment thereof, in furtherance of political or social objectives.

L. Weapons, devices, or agents that are intended to cause widespread harm and/or fear in a population.

M. Specific operational actions to accomplish assigned tasks.

N. Able to move through the animal-human barrier: transmissible from animals to humans.

O. Broad general plans designed to achieve desired outcomes.

_____ **11.** Tactics

_____ **12.** Terrorism

_____ **13.** Weaponization

_____ **14.** Weapons of mass destruction (WMD)

_____ **15.** Zoonotic

Multiple-Choice Review

_____ **1.** In addition to armed attacks, the types of terrorism incidents may be remembered by using the mnemonic:
   A. OPQRST.
   B. CBRNE.
   C. CUPS.
   D. AVPU.

_____ **2.** Environmental terrorists, antigovernment militias, and racial-hate groups are examples of:
   A. international terrorists.
   B. state-sponsored terrorist groups.
   C. domestic terrorists.
   D. religious freedom fighters.

_____ **3.** The EMT should be alert to clues when on the scene of a suspicious incident. An acronym that was designed to help with this process is:
   A. CBRNE.
   B. TRACEM-P.
   C. SAMPLE.
   D. OTTO.

_____ **4.** Potential high-risk targets of terrorists typically include:
   A. controversial businesses.
   B. infrastructure systems.
   C. public buildings.
   D. any of these.

_____ **5.** Why is April 19 a day when the U.S. government stands at heightened security awareness for government facilities?
   A. It is the anniversary of the Pearl Harbor attack.
   B. It is the anniversary of the bombing of the Murrah building in Oklahoma City.
   C. It is the anniversary of the initial World Trade Center bombing.
   D. It is the anniversary of the Bay of Pigs incident.

_____ **6.** Responding EMTs who arrive on the scene of an incident should watch for signs that they may be dealing with a suspicious incident. Examples of unexplained patterns of illness or deaths may include all of the following *except*:
   A. car crashes involving more than two patients with serious traumatic injuries.
   B. unexplained symptoms of skin or eye irritation.
   C. unexplained vapor clouds, mists, and plumes.
   D. unexplained signs of airway irritation.

_____ **7.** The acronym TRACEM-P is designed to help rescuers understand the types of harm to which they can be exposed. The letter "E" stands for:
   A. Emergency.   **C.** Etiologic.
   B. Environmental.   **D.** Essential.

_____ **8.** Danger from alpha particles, beta particles, or gamma rays is caused by _____ harm.
   A. chemical   **C.** etiologic/biologic
   B. radiologic   **D.** mechanical

_____ **9.** The major routes through which WMD agents can enter the body include all of the following _except_:
   A. absorption.   **C.** osmosis.
   B. ingestion.   **D.** inhalation.

_____ **10.** The types of harm from radiologic or nuclear incidents include radiologic, chemical, and _____ harm.
   A. psychological   **C.** thermal
   B. mechanical   **D.** all of these

_____ **11.** The primary harm from a nuclear explosion involves _____ harm.
   A. chemical   **C.** psychological
   B. thermal   **D.** biologic

_____ **12.** The mainstays of self-protection at a radiologic incident include all of the following _except_:
   A. time.   **C.** distance.
   B. Standard Precautions.   **D.** shielding.

_____ **13.** You are on the scene where there is a suspicion that someone may have been exposed to anthrax. Which is the most lethal route of exposure to anthrax?
   A. Skin contact   **C.** Inhalation
   B. Ingestion   **D.** Injection

_____ **14.** The "OTTO" clues should arouse suspicion of terrorist involvement including:
   A. on-scene clues.   **C.** timing of the incident.
   B. type of event.   **D.** all of the above.

_____ **15.** Features that influence the potential for a biologic agent's use as a weapon include:
   A. infectivity and virulence.   **C.** transmissibility and lethality.
   B. toxicity and incubation period. **D.** all of these.

_____ **16.** When a terrorist incident is suspected at an explosion, you should do each of the following, except:
   A. wear appropriate PPE.
   B. quickly move in and evacuate patients from the scene.
   C. beware of possible multiple explosive devices.
   D. follow your Incident Command protocols.

_____ **17.** The relative ease with which an agent causes death in a susceptible population is referred to as the:
   A. stability of the product.   **C.** lethality of the agent.
   B. infectivity of the agent.   **D.** virulence of the virus.

_____ **18.** Which virus did the World Health Organization declare eradicated worldwide in 1980 through immunization efforts?
   A. Polio   **C.** Viral hemorrhagic fever
   B. Anthrax   **D.** Smallpox

_____ **19.** During an explosion, a direct consequence of the high-energy over-pressurization and most common cause of death is:
   A. abdominal injury.
   B. concussion.
   C. blast lung.
   D. tympanic membrane rupture.

_____ **20.** A virus with high human-to-human transmission would be:
   A. botulinum.
   B. smallpox.
   C. Venezuelan equine encephalitis.
   D. ricin.

_____ **21.** You have responded to a building collapse. The three-story office building is believed to have been vacant at the time of the collapse. The fire department personnel believe that there was an explosion that caused the front of the building to cave in. In addition to mechanical harm, all of the following are types of harm, that can result from an explosive incident *except*:
   A. thermal harm.
   B. asphyxiation.
   C. water damage.
   D. chemical hazards.

_____ **22.** After the scene described in question 21 is safe, you are called to the back of the building, where you find a 68-year-old man who lives in the alleyway there. He is coughing and complaining of breathing problems. It is obvious that he may have inhaled a large quantity of dust when the building collapsed. What is another danger to this patient?
   A. His skin may be very dirty or greasy.
   B. There are often toxic particles, such as asbestos, in the dust.
   C. The water he was drinking may be contaminated.
   D. He may be developing hypothermia.

_____ **23.** In recent years, investigations in the United States have uncovered groups manufacturing a chemical called _____, which is designed to interrupt the body's protein-manufacturing process at the cellular level by _____
   A. staphylococcal enterotoxin; causing extreme fat wasting.
   B. botulinum; killing off the bone marrow.
   C. ricin; altering the RNA needed for proper proteins.
   D. trichothecene mycotoxins; eliminating ascorbic acid.

_____ **24.** You were called to the scene of a 45-year-old female who is very weak and is complaining of a fever. She has a number of bruises, and the sclera of her eyes seem to be leaking blood from the tiny capillaries. She works in a lab and has been doing some top secret experiments recently. What could be the cause of this sickness?
   A. Smallpox
   B. Rabies
   C. Encephalitis
   D. A viral hemorrhagic fever

Complete the Following

1. List the four major routes of entry of poisons into the body.

A. _____

B. _____

C. _____

D. _____

©2021 Pearson Education, Inc.
Emergency Care, 14th Ed.

2. List four chemical agent properties.

A. _____

B. _____

C. _____

D. _____

3. What are the five classifications of chemical agents used as weapons?

A. _____

B. _____

C. _____

D. _____

E. _____

4. What do the letters in the mnemonic SLUDGEM stand for as a means of recalling the signs and symptoms of nerve agents?

A. S _____

B. L _____

C. U _____

D. D _____

E. G _____

F. E _____

G. M _____

5. Understand the kind of harm that can result from a terrorist incident and plan self-protective measures. The TRACEM-P harms are:

A. T _____

B. R _____

C. A _____

D. C _____

E. E _____

F. M _____

G. P _____

Interim Exam 3

Use the answer sheet on pages provided to complete this exam. It is perforated, so it can be removed easily from this workbook.

1. Your 21-year-old female trauma patient is lying across the front seat of her sports car after a head-on collision. She is making gurgling sounds as she breathes. What should you do?
   A. Ventilate her.
   B. Suction the airway.
   C. Hyperextend the neck.
   D. Apply high-concentration oxygen.

2. Sometimes a _____ can act as a full-body splint when a critical trauma patient must be carried a short distance over rough terrain.
   A. wheeled stretcher
   B. short Kendrick's extrication device
   C. warm blanket
   D. scoop stretcher

3. Compared to an adult, the pediatric patient in shock relies more on the _____ to compensate for shock.
   A. heart rate
   B. increased contractility of the heart
   C. decreased vasodilation
   D. decreased contractility of the heart

4. You are treating a 19-year-old female patient who fell from two stories and is in severe pain. Internal bleeding is not visible, so you must base the severity of blood loss on:
   A. signs and symptoms exhibited.
   B. what the patient tells you.
   C. the size of the contusion.
   D. advice from medical direction.

5. In a _____ injury, the epidermis remains intact, but cells and blood vessels in the dermis are damaged.
   A. crush   C. laceration
   B. contusion   D. bite wound

6. Blood that oozes and is dark red is most likely from a(n):
   A. vein.   C. artery.
   B. capillary.   D. contusion.

7. You are treating a 29-year-old male who slashed his wrist in an effort to end his life. The wound is spurting bright red blood, and he has decided to let you treat him. After trying direct pressure to control the bleeding, the next step would be to:
   A. apply a tourniquet at the shoulder.
   B. apply an air splint to the arm.
   C. apply a tourniquet to the lower arm.
   D. press on the brachial artery.

8. The care of an amputated finger or toe includes:
   A. placing the digit on ice to keep it cool.
   B. immersing the amputated part in salt water.
   C. sealing the digit in a plastic bag and cooling it.
   D. placing the digit on ice water.

9. You are caring for a patient that was struck by lightning. This type of injury is classified as a/an _____ burn.
   A. inhalation   C. full thickness
   B. partial thickness   D. electrical

10. In caring for a patient with an open chest wound the EMT should rapidly:
    A. prevent air from entering the chest wall injury.
    B. control the bleeding.
    C. decrease the amount of air entering the lungs.
    D. assist ventilations with high concentration oxygen.

11. You are treating a 55-year-old female patient who was assaulted. You suspect that she has some internal bleeding. The signs and symptoms of internal bleeding are:
    A. the same as those of shock.
    B. slower to present as compared to external bleeding.
    C. usually not present in elderly patients.
    D. easy to stabilize in the field.

12. Which of the following is *not* considered a type of shock?
    A. Obstructive   C. Cardiogenic
    B. Hydrophobic   D. Neurogenic

13. The point at which the body can no longer compensate for low blood volume is referred to as the _____ phase of shock.
    A. compensated   C. decompensated
    B. anaphylactic   D. terminal

14. What are the major components of the central nervous system?
    A. Cranial nerves
    B. Peripheral nerves
    C. Brain and spinal cord
    D. Brain and cranial nerves.

15. Which of the following is *not* a division of the nervous system?
   A. Central
   B. Peripheral
   C. Autonomic
   D. Voluntary

16. The skull is made up of the cranium and the facial bones. The cranium consists of the _____ of the skull.
   A. temporal, mandible, and maxilla areas
   B. frontal, parietal, and distal areas
   C. anterior, forehead, and lateral areas
   D. temporal, occipital, frontal, and parietal bones

17. The bones forming the face include all of the following *except*:
   A. vertebrae.
   B. zygomatic.
   C. mandible.
   D. maxillae.

18. The brain and spinal cord are bathed in:
   A. cerebrospinal fluid.
   B. lymphatic fluid.
   C. synovial fluid.
   D. mucosal fluid.

19. When a traumatic injury to the chest causes blood to flow into the sac surrounding the heart, the condition is called:
   A. traumatic asphyxia.
   B. cardiac tamponade.
   C. hemothorax.
   D. aortic injury.

20. A patella dislocation is associated with which joint?
   A. Elbow
   B. Hip
   C. Knee
   D. Shoulder

21. The method used most often to immobilize a dislocated shoulder is the:
   A. traction splint.
   B. air splint.
   C. padded board.
   D. sling and swathe.

22. A patient has some memory loss after a head injury. This is referred to as:
   A. bruising.
   B. amnesia.
   C. verbally responsive.
   D. "seeing stars."

23. The EMT has made the decision to apply spinal motion restriction to a small child who was involved in a significant motor vehicle collision. She could not find a pediatric cervical collar that was the right size. What should she do?
   A. Use a rolled towel to support the neck.
   B. Use the next smaller size collar.
   C. Use the next larger size collar.
   D. Skip using a collar.

24. A collection of blood within the skull or brain following a blunt head injury is called:
   A. a subdural hematoma.
   B. an epidural hematoma.
   C. an intracerebral bleed.
   D. any of these.

25. The state of shock associated with a significant spinal cord injury is:
   A. hypovolemic.
   B. autonomic.
   C. neurogenic.
   D. cardiogenic.

26. A strategy that is used to check an extremity for paralysis in a conscious patient is:
   A. checking for a proximal pulse.
   B. assessing equality of strength.
   C. checking for a distal pulse.
   D. confirming sensation is still present.

27. Which MOI is often associated with multi-system trauma?
   A. Fall < 10 feet.
   B. Fall > 20 feet.
   C. Car crash with 6 inches of intrusion.
   D. Fall off a bicycle.

28. If a patient has a significant brain injury with a skull fracture, the patient's pupils tend to be:
   A. equal.
   B. dilated.
   C. constricted.
   D. unequal.

29. Which of the following describes the blood pressure and pulse of a patient with a traumatic brain injury?
   A. Decreased BP, increased pulse
   B. Decreased BP, decreased pulse
   C. Increased BP, increased pulse
   D. Increased BP, decreased pulse

30. The spinal column is made up of _____ shaped bones.
   A. 33 regularly
   B. 33 irregularly
   C. 12 regularly
   D. 12 irregularly

31. Any blunt trauma above the clavicles may damage the _____ vertebrae.
   A. lumbar
   B. cervical
   C. sacral
   D. thoracic

32. Priapism is:
   A. a persistent erection of the penis.
   B. spasms of the hands and feet.
   C. another name for unequal pupils.
   D. uncontrolled muscle twitches of the thighs.

33. The EMT should consider that any injury of an elderly person could be a sign of:
   A. a severe fall.
   B. abuse or neglect.
   C. Alzheimer's disease.
   D. depression.

34. Obesity is defined as a condition of having a body mass index (BMI) of:
   A. 20 or more.
   B. 25 or more.
   C. 30 or more.
   D. 35 or more.

35. Your patient is a 70-year-old female. The loss of skin elasticity and shrinking of sweat glands in this woman can cause:
    A. diminished activity and tolerance of physical stress.
    B. decreased ability to clear foreign substances from the lungs.
    C. decreased energy and ability to sleep through the night.
    D. thin, dry, wrinkled skin.

36. When caring for a child with autism the EMT should remember that communication can be challenging, so consider using _____ to help the patient express their needs.
    A. sign language
    B. a white board and marker
    C. jokes and humor
    D. a picture card system

37. The EMT may be called to care for an infant with a congenital disease. This means that the patient:
    A. acquired the disease after birth.
    B. will have a coexisting chronic disease.
    C. will require advanced life support.
    D. was born with an abnormal condition.

38. An unstable foreign object impaled through the cheek wall should be:
    A. stabilized from the outside.
    B. stabilized from the inside.
    C. removed out if this can be easily done.
    D. stabilized from the inside and the outside.

39. If direct pressure and a hemostatic dressing do not control bleeding from a thigh laceration, the injury most likely involves the:
    A. carotid artery.
    B. brachial artery.
    C. subclavian vein.
    D. femoral artery.

40. A tracheostomy is a surgical opening in the neck that provides an opening:
    A. into the trachea.
    B. into the esophagus for feeding.
    C. into both the trachea and esophagus.
    D. that will always be permanent.

41. Your patient is a 55-year-old man who called EMS because he has a nosebleed that has not stopped all afternoon. The best method for control of nasal bleeding is:
    A. packing the nose with cotton.
    B. pinching the nostrils together.
    C. packing the nose with gauze.
    D. applying pressure to the facial artery.

42. The first step in caring for possible internal bleeding is:
    A. administering liquids by mouth to the patient.
    B. Keeping the SpO_2 between 90–94%.
    C. treating for shock.
    D. placing the patient in a sitting position.

43. The injury in which a flap of skin and tissue is torn loose is called a(n):
    A. laceration.
    B. amputation.
    C. incision.
    D. avulsion.

44. A 22-year-old female patient has an object impaled in her forearm. After controlling the profuse bleeding, you should:
    A. remove the object.
    B. place a pressure dressing over the site.
    C. stabilize the object.
    D. apply firm pressure to a pressure point.

45. Which of the following is a sign of shock?
    A. High BP
    B. Constricted pupils
    C. Slowed pulse rate
    D. Pale, cool, clammy skin

46. An object impaled in the eye should be:
    A. stabilized with gauze and protected with a disposable cup.
    B. removed carefully and a pressure dressing applied.
    C. shielded with a cup taped over the orbit.
    D. removed and a dressing applied with minimum pressure.

47. The EMT may be called to care for a patient with a stoma in the neck because:
    A. it caused a pneumothorax.
    B. it has become blocked.
    C. it needs to be replaced.
    D. the patient is not able to eat.

48. Before moving a supine 38-year-old male patient with a suspected spine injury onto your stretcher, you should always:
    A. align the patient's teeth and tape the jaw in place.
    B. apply a short spine board.
    C. apply a cervical collar.
    D. secure a KED to the patient.

49. The initial effort to control bleeding from a severed neck artery should include:
    A. direct pressure or pinching.
    B. applying tape.
    C. pressure points.
    D. occlusive dressing.

50. The most reliable sign of spinal-cord injury in a conscious 35-year-old female patient is:
A. pain without movement.
B. paralysis of extremities.
C. pain with movement.
D. tenderness along the spine.

51. When caring for an open abdominal wound with evisceration:
A. replace the organ but cover it with occlusive material.
B. replace the organ but cover it with a bulky dressing.
C. do not replace the organ but cover it with occlusive material.
D. do not replace the organ but cover it with a moistened dressing.

52. A 38-year-old male patient who is in acute abdominal distress denies any vomiting. He should be transported to the emergency department:
A. in the Trendelenburg position with legs straight.
B. in the coma position.
C. in the supine position with the knees bent.
D. in the recumbent position with one knee bent.

53. There is a power outage in your area of response and you are called to the home of a patient with a home ventilator. What should you be prepared to do when you arrive?
A. Bring a generator for the ventilator.
B. Transport the patient to the hospital.
C. Attempt to find a backup battery for the ventilator.
D. Assist ventilations with a bag-valve mask.

54. A fracture to the proximal end of the humerus is best cared for by immobilizing with a(n):
A. wrist sling and swathe.
B. padded board, sling, and swathe.
C. air-inflated splint.
D. sling and swathe.

55. Your 45-year-old female patient fell backward onto her left elbow and heard a loud snap. She has a distal pulse and sensation. The best way to immobilize a fractured elbow when the arm is found in the bent position and there is a distal pulse is to:
A. straighten the arm and apply an air-inflated splint.
B. keep the arm in its found position and apply a short, padded board splint.
C. keep the arm in its found position and apply an air-inflated splint.
D. straighten the arm and apply a wire-ladder splint.

56. If a severe deformity exists or distal circulation is compromised when you are splinting, you should:
A. push protruding bones back into place.
B. align to anatomical position under gentle traction.
C. immediately move the patient to a stretcher.
D. immobilize in the position found.

57. A 45-year-old male patient with a fractured pelvis should be immobilized on long spine board with:
A. legs bound together with wide cravats.
B. long padded boards secured down each side of the body.
C. stabilizing sandbags placed between the legs.
D. a pelvic wrap.

58. A fractured femur is best immobilized with a(n) _____ splint.
A. long padded
B. air-inflated
C. rigid vacuum
D. traction

59. Before immobilizing a fractured knee:
A. assess distal circulation and sensory and motor function.
B. straighten the angulation.
C. apply firm traction.
D. flex the leg at the knee.

60. A sprain is an injury in which:
A. tendons are torn.
B. ligaments are torn.
C. cartilage is crushed.
D. muscles spasm.

61. Which of the following is *not* true of open extremity injuries?
A. The skin has been broken or torn.
B. There is increased likelihood of infection.
C. Definitive care is provided in the prehospital setting.
D. Such injuries require surgery at the hospital.

62. Muscle is attached to bone by:
A. cartilage.
B. ligaments.
C. smooth muscles.
D. tendons.

63. The entire back of a 40-year-old male's right arm and his entire chest has been burned. What percentage of surface burn would you report?
A. 13.5%   C. 27%
B. 18%   D. 36%

64. Partial-thickness burns cause:
A. swelling and blistering.
B. nerve damage.
C. slight swelling.
D. scarring.

65. A 25-year-old female patient is suffering from chemical burns to the skin caused by dry lime. After you put on your PPE, your next step should be to:
A. wash the area with running water.
B. remove the lime with phenol.
C. remove the lime with alcohol.
D. brush away the lime.

66. Acid burns to the eyes should be flooded with water for at least _____ minute(s).
A. 1
B. 5
C. 10
D. 20

67. A method for estimating the extent of a burn is the:
A. rule of nines.
B. rule of percentages.
C. rule of degree.
D. burn assessment rule.

68. If a woman is having her first baby, the first stage of labor will usually last an average of _____ hours.
A. 4
B. 8
C. 12
D. 16

69. During the most active stage of labor, the uterus usually contracts every _____ minutes.
A. 1 to 2
B. 2 to 3
C. 5 to 9
D. 10 to 15

70. If the amniotic sac does not break during delivery, the EMT should:
A. do nothing; it will break after birth.
B. quickly remove it with sterile scissors.
C. puncture it with a finger.
D. transport the patient immediately.

71. To assist the mother in delivering the baby's shoulders, the EMT should gently:
A. pull at the baby's shoulders.
B. support the baby's head.
C. rotate the baby to the left or right.
D. push a gloved hand into the vagina.

72. Following delivery of a baby, if spontaneous respiration does not begin after you suction the baby's mouth and nose, you should first:
A. begin mouth-to-mouth-and-nose resuscitation.
B. apply mechanical resuscitation with 100% oxygen.

C. vigorously rub the baby's back.
D. transport immediately, administering 100% oxygen.

73. An implanted pacemaker helps the patient by:
A. regulating the time of each heartbeat.
B. squeezing the heart to improve cardiac output.
C. improving damaged cardiac muscle.
D. delivering an electrical shock to restore a normal rhythm.

74. The automated implanted cardiac defibrillator (AICD) is:
A. used for patient's needing a heart transplant.
B. carried in a special bag that the patient wears.
C. temporarily placed under the patient's skin.
D. permanently placed under the patient's skin.

75. In the following list, which is the correct order in the phases of the rescue process?
1. Sizing up the situation
2. Gaining access
3. Disentangling the patient
4. Stabilizing the vehicle

A. 1, 2, 3, 4
B. 2, 1, 4, 3
C. 1, 4, 2, 3
D. 3, 2, 1, 4

76. A battery powered mechanical pump that is implanted in the body to assist the heart in pumping blood is the:
A. wearable cardioverter defibrillator.
B. ventricular assist device.
C. automated implanted cardiac defibrillator.
D. ventricular pacemaker.

77. To minimize injuries at a collision, the EMT should:
A. use a limited number of tools.
B. deactivate the safety guards on tools.
C. wear highly visible clothing.
D. wait until the police arrive on the scene.

78. The three-step process of disentanglement described in the text includes all of the following *except*:
A. opening the trunk and cutting the battery cable.
B. creating exits by displacing doors and roof posts.
C. disentangling occupants by displacing the front end.
D. gaining access by disposing of the roof.

©2021 Pearson Education, Inc.
Emergency Care, 14th Ed.

79. Which of the following is *true* about dealing with a collision vehicle's electrical system?
   A. It should be disabled by cutting the positive battery cable.
   B. If it must be disrupted, disconnect the negative (ground) cable from the battery.
   C. Shutting off the ignition key disables the electrical systems of the car.
   D. Disconnecting the ground cable produces a spark that can ignite battery gases.

80. When positioning flares, use a formula that includes the stopping distance for the posted speed plus the:
   A. angle of the road.
   B. radius of the danger zone.
   C. reaction distance.
   D. margin of safety.

81. Once the vehicle has been stabilized, the *next* part of an extrication procedure for patient rescue is to:
   A. dispose of the vehicle's roof.
   B. displace the front end of the vehicle.
   C. displace doors and roof posts.
   D. do none of these.

82. A nasogastric tube is used to:
   A. administer medications.
   B. suction out the stomach contents.
   C. deliver nutrients.
   D. all of the above.

83. Which of the following is an *unnecessary* question for the Emergency Medical Dispatcher to ask when receiving a call for help?
   A. How old is the patient?
   B. What is the patient's gender?
   C. What is the patient's name?
   D. Is the patient conscious?

84. When operating a siren, be aware that:
   A. the continuous sound of a siren could worsen the patient's condition.
   B. all motorists will hear and honor the siren.
   C. the siren must be used continuously when the ambulance is carrying injured patients.
   D. it is necessary to pull up close to vehicles and sound the siren.

85. A common problem that the EMT will find associated with urinary catheters is:
   A. infection.
   B. hypotension.
   C. hypertension.
   D. the bag needs to be emptied.

86. When transferring a nonemergency patient to ED personnel, you should:
   A. wait for emergency staff to call for the patient.
   B. offload the patient, wheel the patient to the non-urgent treatment rooms, and leave the patient.
   C. check to see what should be done with the patient.
   D. offload the patient, wheel the patient to the designated area, and leave the patient.

87. At the hospital, as soon as you are free from patient-care activities, you should:
   A. notify dispatch that you are back in service.
   B. quickly clean the vehicle's patient compartment.
   C. prepare the prehospital care report.
   D. check on patient status with the ED.

88. The patient that requires dialysis has:
   A. diabetes.
   B. cancer.
   C. renal failure.
   D. heart failure.

89. A patient that is receiving dialysis will have a fistula that is most commonly located:
   A. in the chest.
   B. on the arm.
   C. on the back.
   D. in the abdomen.

90. You have just assisted a mother in delivering a healthy newborn. The first clamp placed on the umbilical cord should be about _____ inches from the baby.
   A. 2   C. 10
   B. 5   D. 12

91. Which of the following is the maximum amount of time the EMT should wait for the placenta to be delivered before transporting the mother and infant?
   A. 20 minutes   C. 1 hour
   B. 45 minutes   D. 2 hours

92. Delivery of the placenta is usually accompanied by the loss of no more than _____ of blood.
   A. 500 cc   C. 800 cc
   B. 600 cc   D. 1,000 cc

93. Along with physical and mental fitness, ambulance operators should be able to:
   A. move other vehicles off the roadway.
   B. perform under stress.
   C. always be up for a run.
   D. justify feelings of superiority.

94. A child with special health needs may have a ventriculoperitoneal (VP) shunt which drains fluid from the:
    A. lungs.
    B. brain.
    C. heart.
    D. abdomen.

95. If the umbilical cord presents first during birth, you should:
    A. gently push the cord back into the vagina.
    B. gently push up on the baby's head or buttocks to keep pressure off the cord.
    C. gently push on the cervix.
    D. clamp and cut the cord.

96. During a delivery, if an arm presentation without a prolapsed cord is noted, the EMT should:
    A. reach up the vagina and turn the baby.
    B. do nothing; the delivery will be normal.
    C. transport immediately and provide O_2.
    D. insert a gloved hand and push back the vaginal wall.

97. A baby is considered premature if it weighs less than 5½ pounds or is born before the _____ week of pregnancy.
    A. 35th   C. 37th
    B. 36th   D. 38th

98. The three primary ways in which elders can be abused or neglected are:
    A. financially, sexually, and physically.
    B. psychologically, sexually and emotionally.
    C. physically, psychologically, and financially.
    D. emotionally, psychologically, and physically.

99. Treatment aimed to slow the spread of venom after a snakebite may be:
    A. immobilizing or splinting the affected extremity.
    B. applying a tourniquet.
    C. cleansing the wound site.
    D. elevating the extremity above the level of the heart.

100. A 52-year-old male patient who was doing heavy garden work on a very hot day complains of severe muscle cramps in his legs and feeling faint. You should move him to a cool place and begin care by:
    A. administering oxygen.
    B. transporting him immediately.
    C. placing the patient under a fan.
    D. giving him water.

101. An emergency vehicle operator must drive with due regard:
    A. for other drivers on the road.
    B. only when there is a patient in the ambulance.
    C. only when using lights and siren.
    D. never on the way back from the hospital.

102. Which of the following might lead you to consider child abuse?
    A. Multiple skinned knees
    B. A burn from chewing an electric cord
    C. Injuries to the back, legs, and the upper arms
    D. Both ankles sprained

103. Your female Caucasian patient was outdoors on a very cold, windy day chopping wood. She did not wear gloves or a hat. You suspect that she may have early frostbite. With early frostbite, the:
    A. skin appears white and waxy.
    B. skin is commonly mottled and grayish blue.
    C. skin blisters and swells.
    D. patient may complain of burning or tingling at the site.

104. The initial sign of hypothermia is:
    A. shivering.
    B. red-colored skin.
    C. skin that is blistered and smells.
    D. white, waxy skin.

105. Extreme hypothermia is characterized by:
    A. unconsciousness and absence of discernible vital signs.
    B. shivering, numbness, and drowsiness.
    C. flaccid muscles.
    D. rapid breathing.

106. Having a police car escort an ambulance to the hospital:
    A. ensures fewer hazards than driving unescorted.
    B. means the police will drive more slowly than they normally would.
    C. means the police will drive faster than they normally would.
    D. creates additional hazards for the ambulance.

107. What agency has a system for identifying hazardous materials via placards that indicate the nature of the hazardous contents?
    A. Environmental Protection Agency.
    B. Chemical Transportation Emergency Center.
    C. National Fire Protection Association.
    D. National Highway and Traffic Safety Association.

108. The best way to stabilize a vehicle involved in a collision before gaining access to a patient is to:
   A. turn off the ignition.
   B. use three step chocks.
   C. remove the battery cables.
   D. tie ropes to the vehicle.

109. Considering blast injury patterns, the parts of the body that are especially vulnerable to injuries are the:
   A. eyes, ears, and lungs.
   B. ears, chest, and abdomen.
   C. lungs, ears, brain, and abdomen.
   D. eyes, brain, and lungs.

110. Terrorists have a history of setting traps for emergency responders that arrive on the scene to an initial attack. The term related to harming the responders in this way is:
   A. explosive devices.
   B. secondary devices.
   C. primary devices.
   D. warning signs.

111. The strong, white, fibrous material covering the bones is the:
   A. shell.
   B. perineum.
   C. marrow.
   D. periosteum.

112. The coming apart of a joint is referred to as a:
   A. fracture.
   B. sprain.
   C. dislocation.
   D. strain.

113. Overstretching or overexertion of a muscle is called a:
   A. strain.   C. dislocation.
   B. sprain.   D. fracture.

114. In a heat emergency, the patient with _____, dry skin requires rapid cooling and immediate transport.
   A. pale   C. cool
   B. hot   D. warm

115. The primary type of harm from biological incidents is:
   A. chemical.
   B. etiologic.
   C. mechanical.
   D. psychological.

116. To treat a patient with deep frostbite:
   A. immerse the limb in 105°F water and transport the patient.
   B. rub snow on the frozen area or apply cold packs if available.

   C. cover the frostbitten area, handle it as gently as possible, and transport the patient.
   D. protect the frostbitten area by keeping it cold and transport the patient.

117. Your patient fell onto his right leg. The indications for a traction splint are a painful, swollen, deformed mid-thigh with:
   A. an open fracture of the lower leg.
   B. extensive blood loss and shock.
   C. no joint or lower leg injury.
   D. either ankle or knee involvement.

118. The level of training established by OSHA for the individuals who actually plug, patch, or stop the release of a hazardous material is called:
   A. First Responder Awareness.
   B. First Responder Operations.
   C. Hazardous Materials Technician.
   D. Paramedic.

119. At a hazardous materials incident site, the safe zone should be located:
   A. downwind/downhill.
   B. downwind/same level.
   C. upwind/same level.
   D. upwind/downhill.

120. A resource that must be maintained at the work site by the employer and that must be available to all employees who work with hazardous materials is:
   A. NFPA 704.
   B. the safety data sheets.
   C. the *Emergency Response Guidebook*.
   D. a shipping manifest.

121. The responsibilities of EMS personnel at a hazmat incident include caring for the injured and:
   A. staging personnel and equipment in the warm zone.
   B. monitoring and rehabilitating the hazmat team members.
   C. decontaminating individuals exiting the hot zone.
   D. notifying medical direction about the incident.

122. You are assigning triage tags to multiple patients at a bus crash. Categorizing a patient as Priority 1 at an MCI means that the patient:
   A. is serious but does not have life-threatening injuries or illness.
   B. has minor musculoskeletal or soft-tissue injuries.
   C. is dead or fatally injured.
   D. has treatable life-threatening illness or injuries.

123. The MCI supervisor who is responsible for communicating with the treatment areas to determine the number and priority of the patients in each respective treatment area is the _____ supervisor.
   A. staging
   B. triage
   C. treatment
   D. transportation

124. A Priority 2 patient at an MCI would be color-coded as _____ to identify his or her treatment priority.
   A. black
   B. green

C. yellow
D. red

125. At an MCI, patients who are assessed as having minor injuries should be categorized as Priority:
   A. 1.
   B. 2.
   C. 3.
   D. 4.

©2021 Pearson Education, Inc.
Emergency Care, 14th Ed.

Interim Exam 3 Answer Sheet

Fill in the correct answer for each item. When scoring, note that there are 125 questions valued at 0.666 point each.

1. [ ] A   [ ] B   [ ] C   [ ] D   36. [ ] A   [ ] B   [ ] C   [ ] D
2. [ ] A   [ ] B   [ ] C   [ ] D   37. [ ] A   [ ] B   [ ] C   [ ] D
3. [ ] A   [ ] B   [ ] C   [ ] D   38. [ ] A   [ ] B   [ ] C   [ ] D
4. [ ] A   [ ] B   [ ] C   [ ] D   39. [ ] A   [ ] B   [ ] C   [ ] D
5. [ ] A   [ ] B   [ ] C   [ ] D   40. [ ] A   [ ] B   [ ] C   [ ] D
6. [ ] A   [ ] B   [ ] C   [ ] D   41. [ ] A   [ ] B   [ ] C   [ ] D
7. [ ] A   [ ] B   [ ] C   [ ] D   42. [ ] A   [ ] B   [ ] C   [ ] D
8. [ ] A   [ ] B   [ ] C   [ ] D   43. [ ] A   [ ] B   [ ] C   [ ] D
9. [ ] A   [ ] B   [ ] C   [ ] D   44. [ ] A   [ ] B   [ ] C   [ ] D
10. [ ] A   [ ] B   [ ] C   [ ] D   45. [ ] A   [ ] B   [ ] C   [ ] D
11. [ ] A   [ ] B   [ ] C   [ ] D   46. [ ] A   [ ] B   [ ] C   [ ] D
12. [ ] A   [ ] B   [ ] C   [ ] D   47. [ ] A   [ ] B   [ ] C   [ ] D
13. [ ] A   [ ] B   [ ] C   [ ] D   48. [ ] A   [ ] B   [ ] C   [ ] D
14. [ ] A   [ ] B   [ ] C   [ ] D   49. [ ] A   [ ] B   [ ] C   [ ] D
15. [ ] A   [ ] B   [ ] C   [ ] D   50. [ ] A   [ ] B   [ ] C   [ ] D
16. [ ] A   [ ] B   [ ] C   [ ] D   51. [ ] A   [ ] B   [ ] C   [ ] D
17. [ ] A   [ ] B   [ ] C   [ ] D   52. [ ] A   [ ] B   [ ] C   [ ] D
18. [ ] A   [ ] B   [ ] C   [ ] D   53. [ ] A   [ ] B   [ ] C   [ ] D
19. [ ] A   [ ] B   [ ] C   [ ] D   54. [ ] A   [ ] B   [ ] C   [ ] D
20. [ ] A   [ ] B   [ ] C   [ ] D   55. [ ] A   [ ] B   [ ] C   [ ] D
21. [ ] A   [ ] B   [ ] C   [ ] D   56. [ ] A   [ ] B   [ ] C   [ ] D
22. [ ] A   [ ] B   [ ] C   [ ] D   57. [ ] A   [ ] B   [ ] C   [ ] D
23. [ ] A   [ ] B   [ ] C   [ ] D   58. [ ] A   [ ] B   [ ] C   [ ] D
24. [ ] A   [ ] B   [ ] C   [ ] D   59. [ ] A   [ ] B   [ ] C   [ ] D
25. [ ] A   [ ] B   [ ] C   [ ] D   60. [ ] A   [ ] B   [ ] C   [ ] D
26. [ ] A   [ ] B   [ ] C   [ ] D   61. [ ] A   [ ] B   [ ] C   [ ] D
27. [ ] A   [ ] B   [ ] C   [ ] D   62. [ ] A   [ ] B   [ ] C   [ ] D
28. [ ] A   [ ] B   [ ] C   [ ] D   63. [ ] A   [ ] B   [ ] C   [ ] D
29. [ ] A   [ ] B   [ ] C   [ ] D   64. [ ] A   [ ] B   [ ] C   [ ] D
30. [ ] A   [ ] B   [ ] C   [ ] D   65. [ ] A   [ ] B   [ ] C   [ ] D
31. [ ] A   [ ] B   [ ] C   [ ] D   66. [ ] A   [ ] B   [ ] C   [ ] D
32. [ ] A   [ ] B   [ ] C   [ ] D   67. [ ] A   [ ] B   [ ] C   [ ] D
33. [ ] A   [ ] B   [ ] C   [ ] D   68. [ ] A   [ ] B   [ ] C   [ ] D
34. [ ] A   [ ] B   [ ] C   [ ] D   69. [ ] A   [ ] B   [ ] C   [ ] D
35. [ ] A   [ ] B   [ ] C   [ ] D   70. [ ] A   [ ] B   [ ] C   [ ] D

71. [ ] A   [ ] B   [ ] C   [ ] D
72. [ ] A   [ ] B   [ ] C   [ ] D
73. [ ] A   [ ] B   [ ] C   [ ] D
74. [ ] A   [ ] B   [ ] C   [ ] D
75. [ ] A   [ ] B   [ ] C   [ ] D
76. [ ] A   [ ] B   [ ] C   [ ] D
77. [ ] A   [ ] B   [ ] C   [ ] D
78. [ ] A   [ ] B   [ ] C   [ ] D
79. [ ] A   [ ] B   [ ] C   [ ] D
80. [ ] A   [ ] B   [ ] C   [ ] D
81. [ ] A   [ ] B   [ ] C   [ ] D
82. [ ] A   [ ] B   [ ] C   [ ] D
83. [ ] A   [ ] B   [ ] C   [ ] D
84. [ ] A   [ ] B   [ ] C   [ ] D
85. [ ] A   [ ] B   [ ] C   [ ] D
86. [ ] A   [ ] B   [ ] C   [ ] D
87. [ ] A   [ ] B   [ ] C   [ ] D
88. [ ] A   [ ] B   [ ] C   [ ] D
89. [ ] A   [ ] B   [ ] C   [ ] D
90. [ ] A   [ ] B   [ ] C   [ ] D
91. [ ] A   [ ] B   [ ] C   [ ] D
92. [ ] A   [ ] B   [ ] C   [ ] D
93. [ ] A   [ ] B   [ ] C   [ ] D
94. [ ] A   [ ] B   [ ] C   [ ] D
95. [ ] A   [ ] B   [ ] C   [ ] D
96. [ ] A   [ ] B   [ ] C   [ ] D
97. [ ] A   [ ] B   [ ] C   [ ] D
98. [ ] A   [ ] B   [ ] C   [ ] D

99. [ ] A   [ ] B   [ ] C   [ ] D
100. [ ] A   [ ] B   [ ] C   [ ] D
101. [ ] A   [ ] B   [ ] C   [ ] D
102. [ ] A   [ ] B   [ ] C   [ ] D
103. [ ] A   [ ] B   [ ] C   [ ] D
104. [ ] A   [ ] B   [ ] C   [ ] D
105. [ ] A   [ ] B   [ ] C   [ ] D
106. [ ] A   [ ] B   [ ] C   [ ] D
107. [ ] A   [ ] B   [ ] C   [ ] D
108. [ ] A   [ ] B   [ ] C   [ ] D
109. [ ] A   [ ] B   [ ] C   [ ] D
110. [ ] A   [ ] B   [ ] C   [ ] D
111. [ ] A   [ ] B   [ ] C   [ ] D
112. [ ] A   [ ] B   [ ] C   [ ] D
113. [ ] A   [ ] B   [ ] C   [ ] D
114. [ ] A   [ ] B   [ ] C   [ ] D
115. [ ] A   [ ] B   [ ] C   [ ] D
116. [ ] A   [ ] B   [ ] C   [ ] D
117. [ ] A   [ ] B   [ ] C   [ ] D
118. [ ] A   [ ] B   [ ] C   [ ] D
119. [ ] A   [ ] B   [ ] C   [ ] D
120. [ ] A   [ ] B   [ ] C   [ ] D
121. [ ] A   [ ] B   [ ] C   [ ] D
122. [ ] A   [ ] B   [ ] C   [ ] D
123. [ ] A   [ ] B   [ ] C   [ ] D
124. [ ] A   [ ] B   [ ] C   [ ] D
125. [ ] A   [ ] B   [ ] C   [ ] D

Appendix A

Basic Cardiac Life Support Review

Some EMT students learned cardiopulmonary resuscitation (CPR) before they began their EMT course. Others learn it in their EMT course. This section reviews the elements of CPR in accordance with the most current American Heart Association's Guidelines for Cardiopulmonary Resuscitation and Emergency Cardiovascular Care.

Multiple-Choice Review

_____ 1. Once clinical death occurs, how long does it usually take for biological death to begin to occur to your patient?
   A. 4 minutes
   B. 6 minutes
   C. 8 minutes
   D. 10 minutes

_____ 2. In the "C-A-B" sequence of cardiopulmonary resuscitation, the "A" stands for:
   A. air flow.
   B. arterial pulse.
   C. airway.
   D. aorta.

_____ 3. In the "C-A-B" sequence of cardiopulmonary resuscitation, the "C" stands for:
   A. cardiac.
   B. coronary.
   C. circulation.
   D. carotid.

_____ 4. To determine if an adult or a child (over a year old) is pulseless, the EMT should check for a pulse at the _____ artery.
   A. femoral
   B. brachial
   C. radial
   D. carotid

_____ 5. To determine pulselessness in an infant, the EMT should use the _____ artery.
   A. brachial
   B. carotid
   C. femoral
   D. apical

_____ 6. You are alone and do not have an AED. After determining unresponsiveness in an adult patient, the next thing you should do before starting CPR is:
   A. reposition the patient.
   B. activate EMS.
   C. establish an open airway.
   D. check for breathing.

_____ 7. When an unconscious patient's head flexes forward, the _____ could cause a partial airway obstruction.
   A. hypopharynx
   B. uvula
   C. tongue
   D. larynx

_____ 8. The head-tilt, chin-lift maneuver should *not* be used on a:
   A. stroke victim.
   B. diabetic patient.
   C. diving accident victim.
   D. patient who had a seizure in bed.

_____ **9.** The recommended maneuver for EMTs to open the airway of a patient with possible cervical-spine injury is the _____ maneuver.
   A. jaw-thrust   **C.** head-tilt, chin-lift
   B. mouth-to-nose   **D.** jaw-lift

_____ **10.** In an adult patient who requires rescue breathing, you should watch for chest rise as you ventilate:
   A. 12 to 20 times a minute.   **C.** with one-half of a breath.
   B. 10 to 12 times a minute.   **D.** four slow breaths.

_____ **11.** A 59-year-old female is found in bed struggling to breathe by her husband, who calls 911. When he meets you at the door, he says, frantically, that his wife has just now "passed out" and doesn't seem to be breathing at all. You rush to the patient, place her supine on the floor, and try two ventilations that do not produce chest rise. Your next step is to:
   A. continue standard mouth-to-mask ventilations.
   B. administer oxygen.
   C. perform the steps of CPR.
   D. deliver four quick breaths.

_____ **12.** A problem in the resuscitation of infants and children caused by improper head position during artificial ventilations, or, ventilations that are too quick is:
   A. spinal injury.   **C.** pulmonary trauma.
   B. gastric distention.   **D.** airway injury.

_____ **13.** Rescue breathing provided to a child should be delivered at a rate of _____ breaths per minute.
   A. 4–6   **C.** 12–20
   B. 8–10   **D.** 21–25

_____ **14.** You are ventilating an infant who was found to be not breathing. Infants should be ventilated at the rate of one breath every _____ seconds.
   A. 3–5   **C.** 8–10
   B. 5–7   **D.** 10–12

_____ **15.** When you arrived on the scene, bystanders were already performing ventilations on the patient. If a patient has a distended abdomen due to air being forced into the stomach, the EMT should:
   A. manually press on the abdomen to relieve the distention.
   B. decrease the oxygen concentration being administered to the patient.
   C. be prepared to suction should the patient vomit.
   D. increase the force of the ventilation.

_____ **16.** Why is the recovery position used?
   A. It protects the airway and allows for drainage from the mouth.
   B. It forces the mouth to remain open at all times.
   C. It protects the patient's head during a seizure.
   D. It makes oxygen administration possible in the unconscious patient.

_____ **17.** The CPR compression location for a 55-year-old male is located on the middle of the _____, centered between the nipples.
   A. clavicle   **C.** ribs
   B. substernal notch   **D.** sternum

_____ **18.** Before beginning chest compressions, the EMT can assess the patient's pulse for a maximum of _____ seconds.
   A. 10   **C.** 15
   B. 25   **D.** 20

_____ **19.** For an adult, the one-rescuer compression-to-ventilation ratio is:
   A. 5:1.   **C.** 15:2.
   B. 5:2.   **D.** 30:2.

_____ **20.** The adult CPR compressions rate in one-rescuer CPR is _____ times a minute.
   A. 60–80   **C.** 100–120
   B. 80–100   **D.** 120–140

_____ **21.** The child compression rate in one-rescuer CPR is _____ times a minute.
   A. 60–80   **C.** 100–120
   B. 80–100   **D.** 120–140

_____ **22.** The compression depth for an adult should be:
   A. at least 1 inch.
   B. at least 2 inches.
   C. one-third to one-half the depth of the chest.
   D. one-half to three-fourths the depth of the chest.

_____ **23.** The compression depth for an infant should be:
   A. 1 to 1.5 inches.
   B. at least 2 inches.
   C. at least 1/3 depth of the chest.
   D. one-half to three-quarters the depth of the chest.

_____ **24.** The compression-to-ventilation ratio for a young child or infant when there are two rescuers should be:
   A. 15:1.   **C.** 30:2.
   B. 15:2.   **D.** 5:1.

_____ **25.** The compression-to-ventilation ratio for a young child or infant when there is only one rescuer doing the CPR is:
   A. 15:1.   **C.** 30:2.
   B. 15:2.   **D.** 5:1.

_____ **26.** When opening the airway of a 9-month-old infant, use a:
   A. full head-tilt method.   **C.** slight head tilt.
   B. jaw-thrust method.   **D.** neck hyperextension method.

_____ **27.** With effective CPR, the patient's pupils may:
   A. dilate.   **C.** assume a ground-glass appearance.
   B. constrict.   **D.** begin to move.

_____ **28.** CPR compressions are delivered to children:
   A. in the same manner as they are delivered to adults.
   B. with the fingertips of the index and middle fingers.
   C. with the heel of one hand.
   D. with the fingers of two hands.

_____ **29.** With the exceptions of when defibrillation or advanced cardiac life support measures are to be initiated, CPR should not be interrupted for more than _____ seconds.
   A. a few   **C.** 15
   B. 10   **D.** 20

_____ **30.** You are treating a 45-year-old male patient with a partial airway obstruction, poor air exchange, and gray skin. You should:
   A. wait for the patient to stop breathing, then ventilate.
   B. treat the patient for a complete airway obstruction.
   C. increase the delivered oxygen concentration.
   D. do none of these.

_____ **31.** Complete airway obstruction in a conscious patient is indicated by:
   A. crowing sounds.
   B. an inability to speak.
   C. gurgling sounds.
   D. snoring sounds.

_____ **32.** When you recognize complete airway obstruction in a conscious adult or child patient, you should immediately:
A. place the patient in the supine position and check the pulse.
B. deliver four back blows in rapid succession.
C. deliver rapid abdominal thrusts until the obstruction is relieved.
D. attempt to ventilate the patient.

_____ **33.** You are treating an unresponsive 52-year-old female patient with a complete airway obstruction. You have been unsuccessful in your initial two attempts to ventilate her. Which is the correct sequence to continue your effort?
A. Finger sweeps, back blows, adominal thrusts
B. Abdominal thrusts, finger sweeps, back blows
C. Ventilations, finger sweeps, adominal thrusts
D. Chest thrusts, look in mouth, ventilations

_____ **34.** When treating a woman in her eighth month of pregnancy and who has a complete airway obstruction, the EMT should:
A. use abdominal thrusts.   C. use chest thrusts.
B. only use the back blows.   D. start rescue breathing immediately.

_____ **35.** If a patient has a partial airway (mild) obstruction and is able to speak and cough forcefully, you should:
A. perform abdominal thrusts.   C. perform the chest thrust.
B. carefully watch the patient.   D. position the patient on the floor.

_____ **36.** Which of the following is _not_ correct procedure for clearing an obstructed airway?
A. Use abdominal thrusts with conscious children.
B. Administer back slaps to infants.
C. Use blind finger sweeps with adults to remove objects you can't see.
D. Use chest thrusts with adults who are too obese for abdominal thrusts.

_____ **37.** While you are trying to clear a 52-year-old female's obstructed airway, she loses consciousness. You open her airway, look in her mouth, and attempt to ventilate. If this fails:
A. deliver CPR compressions.
B. retilt the head and again attempt to ventilate.
C. deliver four back blows.
D. attempt another finger sweep.

_____ **38.** You have been unsuccessful initially in ventilating an unconscious infant. You reposition the infant's head and attempt to ventilate again but are unsuccessful. Your next step is to perform:
A. a series of chest thrusts.
B. back blows and chest compressions.
C. abdominal thrusts.
D. a tongue-jaw lift.

_____ **39.** Which of the following is _not_ a sign of choking in an infant?
A. Ineffective cough   C. Wheezing
B. Agitation   D. Strong cry

_____ **40.** In health care provider training, in respect to the procedure of CPR, children are treated as adult patients once they have reached:
A. 8 years of age.   C. 10 years of age.
B. puberty.   D. greater than 1 year of age.

©2021 Pearson Education, Inc.
Emergency Care, 14th Ed.

Complete the Following

1. List six special circumstances in which CPR should *not* be initiated by the EMT even though the patient has no pulse.

   A. _____

   B. _____

   C. _____

   D. _____

   E. _____

   F. _____

2. Once the EMT has started CPR, list six situations in which CPR can be stopped.

   A. _____

   B. _____

   C. _____

   D. _____

   E. _____

   F. _____

3. List the information missing from the following chart.

   A. _____

   B. _____

   C. _____

   D. _____

   E. _____

   F. _____

CPR FOR ADULTS, CHILDREN, and INFANTS

Age	Adult Puberty and older	Child 1 to puberty	Infant Birth to 1 year
Compression depth	**(A)**	At least ⅓ AP diameter of chest (2 inches)	At least ⅓ AP diameter of chest (1½ inches)
Compression rate	100 to 120/min	**(B)**	100 to 120/min (newborn 120/min)
Each ventilation	1 second	**(C)**	1 second
Pulse check location	Carotid artery (throat)	**(D)**	Brachial artery (upper arm)
One-rescuer CPR compression-to-ventilation ratio	**(E)**	**(F)**	30:2 (alone) 15:2 (2 rescuers) 3:1 (newborn)
When working alone: Call 911 or emergency dispatcher.	After establishing unresponsiveness-before beginning resuscitation unless submersion, injury or overdose.	After establishing unresponsiveness and 2 minutes of resuscitation unless heart disease present.	After establishing unresponsiveness and 2 minutes of resuscitation unless heart disease present.

©2021 Pearson Education, Inc.
Emergency Care, 14th Ed.

Appendix B

Comprehensive Final Exam

Now it is time to take a practice comprehensive final examination. This format is similar to those used by a number of certifying agencies. Try timing yourself, allowing approximately 1 minute per question. That's about 1 hour and 40 minutes altogether.

The answer sheet is found at the end of the exam, and the answer key is found in the back of the book.

1. What is the level of training designed for the rescuer who is often initially on the scene and whose emphasis is on providing immediate care for life-threatening injuries as well as controlling the scene?
   A. Emergency Medical Responder
   B. Emergency Medical Technician
   C. Advanced EMT
   D. Paramedic

2. For calls at which the physician cannot be present, there should be:
   A. a detailed plan for every action of the EMT.
   B. standing orders for the patient's treatment.
   C. a chief officer present.
   D. a police officer on the scene.

3. While not directly involved as EMTs, your family may exhibit reactions because of their collateral involvement with EMS. These reactions may be due to:
   A. your unavailability to participate in certain social activities.
   B. your requirement to work some holidays and weekends.
   C. their inability to understand your emotional reactions to calls.
   D. all of the above.

4. An off-duty EMT is driving to a doctor's appointment when he passes a major vehicle collision. There are no EMRs on the scene yet. There are only Good Samaritans. The EMT is late for the appointment, so he decides not to stop and help. The driver of the vehicle dies before help arrives. One of the Good Samaritans notices the EMT license plates and writes the number down as he drives past. The Good Samaritan is angry that the EMT did not stop and help, and later tries to get the EMT fired for not assisting. Which of the following statements is true?
   A. The EMT is negligent for not stopping and helping.
   B. The EMT is negligent because the patient died.
   C. The EMT is not negligent, because he had a doctor's appointment.
   D. The EMT is not negligent, because he did not have a duty to act.

5. Positive ways of dealing with EMS work stress include all of the following except:
   A. requesting a busier work shift.
   B. exercising at least every other day.
   C. developing more healthful and positive habits.
   D. devoting time to relaxing each day.

6. The role of the EMS system is usually found in:
   A. the state's EMS enabling legislation.
   B. the state's Good Samaritan act.
   C. NFPA 423.
   D. CFR 1910.1030.

7. The set of regulations that define the extent and limits of an EMT's job are called the:
   A. advanced directive.   C. scope of practice.
   B. treatment protocol.   D. duty to act provision.

8. When informing a 45-year-old male of treatment that is needed and the associated risks, the EMT is asking for _____ consent.
   A. expressed   C. implied
   B. mutual   D. emancipated

9. In stroking the newborn's lips, the EMT is testing a nervous system reflex known as the _____ reflex.
   A. Moro   C. palmar
   B. sucking   D. rooting

10. The vessel that carries oxygen-poor blood to the right atrium is the:
    A. posterior tibia.   C. vena cava.
    B. internal jugular.   D. aorta.

11. The type of muscle that controls your legs as you walk is called:
    A. voluntary.   C. cardiac.
    B. involuntary.   D. smooth.

12. A 52-year-old man is experiencing a fight-or-flight situation, and his body is attempting to compensate by increasing his cardiac output. How does the body do this on a moment's notice?
    A. By decreasing the pulse rate   C. By increasing the heart rate
    B. By increasing the stroke volume   D. By decreasing the respiratory rate

13. The seat of the brain's respiratory control is a section called the:
    A. medulla oblongata.   C. cerebellum.
    B. foramen magnum.   D. cerebrum.

14. A 19-year-old female is reported to have taken too many narcotic pain pills that were prescribed for her recent elbow surgery. She is extremely sleepy with very shallow breathing. Her color is pale, and her SpO2 is 84 percent. Her body is probably attempting to compensate for her poor level of ventilatory effort by stimulating the respiratory system to increase rate and tidal volume. Normally, respiratory drive is triggered by changing levels of:
    A. carbon dioxide.   C. pH.
    B. oxygen.   D. glucose.

15. A powder prepared from charred wood administered by some EMS systems to conscious poisoning patients is called:
    A. Zofran.   C. activated charcoal.
    B. naloxone.   D. ipecac.

16. Your patient is a 68-year-old female with a long history of emphysema. She is sitting up in the tripod position and complaining of severe shortness of breath. You should:
    A. suction the airway with a rigid suction catheter.
    B. administer 4 lpm of oxygen via nasal cannula.
    C. insert a nasal airway and ventilate.
    D. apply a nonrebreather mask to administer 15 lpm of oxygen.

17. Your 79-year-old male patient appears to show all the signs and symptoms of a stroke. His mental status has rapidly deteriorated, he is now unconscious, and he can no longer control his own airway. While you intervene to manage his airway, the best position in which to keep fluid or vomitus from occluding his airway would be the _____ position.
    A. supine
    B. Fowler's
    C. recovery
    D. prone

18. Your 70-year-old male patient is having trouble breathing. When you auscultate his lungs, you hear crackles (rales), and you are concerned that he may have pulmonary edema. His SpO2 is 92 percent, so you place him on 100 percent oxygen via nonrebreather mask. His breathing gets a little easier with the oxygen. Later, as you are completing your reassessment, you see that his respirations have slowed to 8 times per minute and he is barely staying awake. What should you do next?
    A. Ask your partner to pull over and wait for an ALS backup.
    B. Assist the patient with using his metered-dose inhaler (MDI).
    C. Shake the patient to keep him awake.
    D. Begin ventilating the patient with a BVM.

19. You are responding to a 54-year-old female patient in respiratory distress. She is on home oxygen by nasal cannula at 2 lpm. She has diminished lung sounds bilaterally with wheezes. She appears malnourished and has a barrel chest. Which condition do you suspect?
    A. Pulmonary embolism
    B. Asthma
    C. Chronic obstructive pulmonary disease
    D. Congestive heart failure

20. A 17-year-old male is having an asthma attack after participating in some strenuous activity at school. He has taken several doses of his own bronchodilator with little relief. Your partner immediately administers oxygen. Providing supplemental oxygen will increase the amount of oxygen molecules carried by the _____ in the patient's blood, helping oxygenate critical organs such as the brain.
    A. plasma
    B. hemoglobin
    C. white blood cells
    D. albumin

21. Which of the following questions will most likely elicit your patient's chief complaint?
    A. What made you call 911 this evening?
    B. Do you have any medical problems?
    C. How have you been feeling lately?
    D. Have you been drinking today?

22. When should you assess the scene for safety?
    A. Only at the beginning of the call
    B. At the beginning and throughout the entire call
    C. Only when needed
    D. After the patient has been treated for life-threatening injuries

23. Of the following scenarios, which presents the *greatest immediate* danger for an EMT's safety?
    A. Two women shouting at each other
    B. A college student who has overdosed on "angel dust"
    C. A longtime street alcoholic who is verbally abusive
    D. A young man who appears to be intoxicated

24. You arrive on the scene of a car crash. The MOI suggests a rear-end collision. Which of the following injury patterns should you most likely suspect in the unrestrained driver of the vehicle that was struck from the rear?
    A. Neck injury
    B. Chest injury
    C. Leg injury
    D. Arm injury

25. In assessing the respirations of an infant, it is important to remember that the infant's respiratory rate:
    A. is basically the same as that of the adult.
    B. is usually slower than that of an adult.
    C. is usually faster than that of an adult.
    D. does not tell you much about the patient's condition.

26. You are treating a 52-year-old female for chest pain. You have gathered all pertinent history of present illness, completed two sets of vital signs, talked with medical control, and assisted the patient with two doses of her nitroglycerin. Determination of whether the nitroglycerin was effective is made during the:
    A. primary assessment.
    B. secondary assessment.
    C. reassessment.
    D. primary and secondary assessment.

27. You are caring for a 48-year-old female who sustained a head injury as a result of a domestic dispute. You suspect that she has a closed head injury. You have been monitoring her vital signs every 5 minutes, and you see that her BP is rising and her pulse is dropping. This part of the assessment is called:
    A. modified secondary assessment.
    B. crisis management.
    C. trending.
    D. intervention check.

28. The MOI is evaluated during the:
    A. scene size-up and primary assessment.
    B. reassessment.
    C. detailed focused exam.
    D. All of the above

29. You are assessing a 28-year-old male trauma patient who has no significant MOI. After the primary assessment, you should:
    A. assess the areas that the patient tells you are painful.
    B. continue to assess every body part from head to toe.
    C. focus on just the patient's airway and cervical spine.
    D. complete only the reassessment.

30. After arriving in the ED you should introduce the patient by name, summarize what was in your radio report, and:
    A. provide history that was not given previously.
    B. discuss additional treatment given en route.
    C. update the vital signs.
    D. All of the above

31. A 65-year-old female patient complains of abdominal pain. While you are completing a SAMPLE history, she tells you that she is not currently being treated by a physician and takes no medications. You should:
    A. transport the patient to the hospital immediately.
    B. reassess the patient's complaint and redo the primary assessment.
    C. palpate the abdomen to assess for tenderness.
    D. do a physical examination of the body systems involved.

32. You arrive on the scene of a 53-year-old male patient. The ambulance was called because he has had chest pain for the past hour. The chest pain in this situation is referred to as the:
    A. major past illness.
    B. chief complaint.
    C. presenting diagnosis.
    D. call type.

33. A 75-year-old female is unresponsive but still breathing. You should obtain pertinent patient history information from:
   A. bystanders or family members.
   B. the family physician by telephone.
   C. the responding ALS unit.
   D. all of the above.

34. A secondary assessment is appropriate for:
   A. the trauma patient who is unresponsive en route to the hospital.
   B. the medical patient who is responsive.
   C. the trauma patient without a significant MOI.
   D. all of the above.

35. You respond to the scene of a 48-year-old male complaining of heartburn. He says that it's just his "acid reflux," but his partner panicked and called 911 anyway. What information would lead you to suspect that something more serious is occurring?
   A. The patient had a stroke 10 years ago.
   B. The patient has a history of gastric reflux.
   C. The patient is flushed and diaphoretic.
   D. The patient is hypotensive.

36. Your adult patient has a heart rate of 82, a respiratory rate of 16, and a BP of 120/80, and does not appear to be in any distress. You should repeat vital sign measurements at least every _____ minutes.
   A. 5   **C.** 15
   B. 10   **D.** 20

37. If you receive an order from on-line medical direction for 10 times the normal dose of a medicine (e.g., 1,500 mg of ASA instead of 150 mg) you should:
   A. switch to another radio frequency to find another physician.
   B. question the physician about the order.
   C. follow the physician's order as stated.
   D. ignore the order and do what you believe is correct.

38. You are on the scene of a 74-year-old female patient who is complaining of posterior chest pain that she states feels "like someone is tearing out my back." What condition do you suspect?
   A. Myocardial infarction
   B. Congestive heart failure
   C. Aortic aneurysm
   D. Angina pectoris

39. You are called to the home of a 54-year-old male who is complaining of difficulty breathing. He is alert and presents with hives over his chest, stridor, a swollen tongue, and wheezing in the upper fields. His breathing rate is 32 times per minute and shallow. He is speaking in two- to three-word sentences. What is the best treatment for this patient?
   A. Administering epinephrine with consent from medical control
   B. Administering oxygen at 15 liters per minute by nonrebreather mask
   C. Administering oxygen at 15 liters per minute by bag-valve mask
   D. Rapid transport to the nearest facility

40. Albuterol and epinephrine both have bronchodilation properties that improve the amount of oxygen that a person can inhale and absorb. However, albuterol is administrated only for asthma, whereas epinephrine is administered for both asthma and anaphylaxis. Why is epinephrine, not albuterol, the first choice for anaphylaxis?
   A. Albuterol makes the heart rate increase too much.
   B. Albuterol slows down the heart rate too much.
   C. Albuterol drops the blood pressure too low.
   D. Albuterol is not a vasoconstrictor.

41. An elderly female patient who is experiencing a myocardial infarction is more likely to complain of which of the following symptoms than would be a younger male patient?
    A. Shortness of breath without chest pain
    B. Shortness of breath with chest pain
    C. Chest pain without shortness of breath
    D. No chest pain or shortness of breath

42. In dealing with a person experiencing a psychiatric emergency, why is it important to gather a detailed medical history?
    A. It is not. You want to get the call resolved as quickly as possible, and this will delay it.
    B. It will alert you to past issues as well as medications.
    C. It will help you to determine whether the police are needed.
    D. It will help you to determine whether you need to restrain the patient.

43. Suctioning in pediatric patients is not very different than suctioning adult patients. Both rigid and flexible suction catheters have appropriate pediatric sizes. The difference is:
    A. Time stimulating the hypopharynx should be minimized.
    B. Infants are very sensitive to vagal stimulation.
    C. Bulb syringes are used in the emergency childbirth setting.
    D. All of the above are true.

44. You are about to apply a BP cuff to an unconscious female when you notice that she appears to have a tube under the skin of her arm. The tube feels as though it has fluid going through it. You should:
    A. move the cuff down to the forearm and inflate.
    B. continue to take the BP in the arm.
    C. use the other arm to measure the BP.
    D. use an automatic BP cuff instead.

45. Compared with an adult's airway structures, the pediatric patient's respiratory system includes:
    A. a narrower trachea.
    B. a softer and more flexible trachea.
    C. a smaller mouth and nose.
    D. all of the above.

46. Epinephrine is a _____ drug name.
    A. brand   C. generic
    B. trade   D. marketing

47. Which of the following substances most effectively prevents the patient from digesting an ingested poison?
    A. Salt   C. Activated charcoal
    B. Milk   D. Narcan

48. Why could a prescribed inhaler be helpful for a patient who is suffering from asthma, emphysema, or chronic bronchitis?
    A. Inhalers slow the patient's heart rate.
    B. Inhalers enlarge constricted bronchial tubes.
    C. Inhalers reduce pain.
    D. Inhalers constrict bronchial tubes.

49. Your patient is a child who is having difficulty breathing. The structure of an infant or child's airway is different from an adult's in all of the following ways except that:
    A. All airway structures are smaller and more easily obstructed in the infant or child.
    B. Their tongues are proportionately larger than an adult's.
    C. The trachea is softer and more flexible.
    D. The cricoid cartilage is more rigid.

50. The relationship of glucose to insulin is often described as:
    A. oppositional.   C. a lock-and-key mechanism.
    B. synergistic.   D. antagonistic.

51. You transported a 58-year-old female who presented with a number of the signs and symptoms of a stroke to the emergency department yesterday. You are talking with your Medical Director about the call, and he tells you that the signs and symptoms were completely resolved within the past 24 hours. This patient was most likely suffering from a(n):
    A. altered mental status.
    B. transient ischemic attack.
    C. acute myocardial infarction.
    D. hypoglycemic incident.

52. Which of the following is a generic name for a prescribed inhaler?
    A. Procainamide   C. Albuterol
    B. Furosemide   D. Tolbutamide

53. A substance secreted by plants, animals, or bacteria that is poisonous to humans is called a:
    A. chemical.   C. narcotic.
    B. toxin.   D. drug.

54. _____ is an infection in the lungs that may lead to sepsis in elderly patients.
    A. Hepatitis B   C. Croup
    B. Mumps   D. Pneumonia

55. You are interviewing a 38-year-old male who is experiencing "severe and sudden epigastric pain" that radiates to his shoulder. He says that it got worse when he ate. Which of the following is the most likely cause?
    A. Ectopic pregnancy   C. A hernia
    B. Cholecystitis   D. Renal colic

56. You are treating a 68-year-old male who states that he has not been feeling well since returning home from his dialysis appointment. All of the following are common complications of dialysis except:
    A. development of an aortic aneurysm.
    B. bleeding from the site of the A-V fistula.
    C. clotting and loss of function of the A-V fistula.
    D. a bacterial infection of the blood.

57. Which of the following is a contraindication for the use of nitroglycerin?
    A. The patient has a history of respiratory problems.
    B. The patient complains of chest pain.
    C. The patient has previously had a heart bypass.
    D. The patient's systolic BP is less than 90.

58. Treatment of a conscious 12-year-old female with a history of diabetes may include:
    A. providing cardiac compressions.
    B. giving oral glucose.
    C. administering the patient's prescribed insulin.
    D. giving low-concentration oxygen by nasal cannula.

59. You are not sure whether your conscious 38-year-old female diabetic patient has too much or too little sugar in her blood. What should you do if she has an altered mental status?
    A. Treat only after determining the glucose level.
    B. Give nothing by mouth.
    C. Give glucose if she is able to swallow.
    D. Transport, since no other field treatment is indicated.

60. In what medication form does oral glucose come?
    A. Gel   C. Fine powder
    B. Oral suspension   D. Slurry

61. A 12-year-old female patient complains of an "itchy feeling" in her throat. She also complains of difficulty breathing. She tells that you she was just stung by a bee. You suspect that she is suffering from:
    A. high BP.
    B. low blood sugar.
    C. an allergic reaction.
    D. an impending seizure.

62. Why do patients suffering from allergic reactions have difficulty breathing?
    A. Allergens use up oxygen molecules.
    B. Allergens destroy the respiratory drive in the brain.
    C. Tissues swell in the respiratory system.
    D. The cardiac rhythm is disturbed.

63. Your 32-year-old male patient is experiencing an allergic reaction after eating shellfish. He denies breathing difficulty, and his vital signs are within normal ranges. You should:
    A. continue with your physical examination.
    B. assist the patient in using his epinephrine auto-injector.
    C. give oxygen by nasal cannula.
    D. All of the above

64. The most important part of the treatment of your patient with an absorbed poison is to:
    A. neutralize the poison with vinegar.
    B. remove the poison from the skin.
    C. neutralize the poison with baking soda in water.
    D. administer activated charcoal.

65. You suspect that your nearly unconscious 33-year-old female patient has ingested sleeping pills and alcohol. She is breathing inadequately. You should be prepared to immediately:
    A. give her oxygen by nasal cannula.
    B. administer activated charcoal.
    C. administer syrup of ipecac.
    D. assist her ventilations with a BVM device.

66. Which of the following infectious diseases is often considered a childhood disease, but can return in adults in a different form?
    A. Meningococcal meningitis
    B. Croup
    C. Varicella zoster
    D. Measles

67. To prevent fatigue while performing CPR, how often should you switch positions with your partner?
    A. Every five cycles of CPR   C. Each time you deliver a shock
    B. Every minute   D. Each time you ventilate

68. Do not perform finger sweeps on an unresponsive infant with a foreign body airway obstruction:
    A. because the patient may bite.   C. because the patient may cough.
    B. unless your gloves are sterile.   D. unless the object is visible.

69. The depth of compressions in performing CPR on a 55-year-old male is:
    A. 1 to 1 ½ inches.   C. 2 to 2.4 inches.
    B. ½ to ¾ inch.   D. ¾ to 1 inch.

70. What is the ventilation rate in performing rescue breathing for a 6-year-old female?
    A. 10–12 breaths per minute   C. 15–30 breaths per minute
    B. 12–20 breaths per minute   D. 25–30 breaths per minute

©2021 Pearson Education, Inc.
Emergency Care, 14th Ed.

71. A 16-year-old male has ingested hallucinogenic mushrooms. He is vomiting excessively. He agrees to treatment but does not want to be transported. Your next action should be to:
   A. contact medical direction and the patient's parent.
   B. leave after advising the family physician of the situation.
   C. request that the patient sign a release form, after which you return to the station.
   D. stay with the patient until he has recovered.

72. Which of the following characteristics may lead you to believe that the patient could become hostile?
   A. The patient complains of a severe headache.
   B. The patient displays slow physical movement and slurred speech.
   C. The patient displays rapid speech and physical movement.
   D. The patient complains of chest pain.

73. In performing CPR, what is the rate of chest compressions per minute for a 58-year-old female?
   A. At least 80
   B. At least 90
   C. 100–120
   D. 120 or more

74. To minimize the delay in beginning compressions for a 62-year-old male in cardiac arrest, the EMT should:
   A. open the airway while determining unresponsiveness.
   B. look, listen, and feel for breathing.
   C. check for a pulse at least 20 seconds.
   D. immediately begin chest compressions.

75. The ratio of compressions to ventilations for single-rescuer CPR for adult, child, and infant patients is:
   A. 1 compression:6 ventilations.
   B. 2 compressions:15 ventilations.
   C. 15 compressions:2 ventilations.
   D. 30 compressions:2 ventilations.

76. A blood vessel with thick, muscular walls that carries blood away from the heart is called a(n):
   A. artery.
   B. capillary.
   C. vein.
   D. venule.

77. Your care for a 52-year-old male patient taking blood thinners, who you suspect has internal bleeding, should include all of the following except:
   A. maintaining ABCs.
   B. fluids by mouth.
   C. control of any external bleeding.
   D. immediate transport to the appropriate facility.

78. Despite your best efforts to help, a 7-year-old child with a known airway obstruction has become unresponsive. You should next:
   A. perform abdominal thrusts till dislodged.
   B. open the airway and attempt to ventilate.
   C. perform chest compressions.
   D. ventilate the patient for 2 minutes.

79. When force is transmitted to the body's internal structures, causing internal organs to rupture or bleed internally, the injury is called a(n):
   A. crushing.
   B. concussion.
   C. contusion.
   D. avulsion.

80. A bruise may be an indication of internal injuries and internal bleeding. It is important for you to monitor your patient for any signs and symptoms of:
   A. low blood sugar.
   B. shock.
   C. infection.
   D. hypothermia.

81. You respond to a burn patient at a house fire. On your arrival, one of the firefighters is assisting a 36-year-old female into your ambulance. She is conscious and alert with full-thickness burns to both hands and forearms. She also has partial-thickness burns to her chest. Your treatment should include:
   A. soaking the burned areas in saline and wrapping them with a sterile dressing.
   B. carefully wrapping the burned areas with a dry sterile dressing.
   C. applying an antiseptic ointment to the burns to prevent infection.
   D. applying ice to the burned areas to cool them down.

82. If you apply a leg splint too loosely to your 22-year-old male patient, complications may include all of the following except:
   A. further soft tissue injury.
   B. an open fracture.
   C. excessive movement.
   D. immobilization of the adjacent joints.

83. Use of a traction splint is contraindicated if your adult patient has:
   A. a knee injury.
   B. a back injury.
   C. a femur injury.
   D. no distal pulse in the injured extremity.

84. You should consider using a SAM splint for splinting an injury to:
   A. the neck.   C. the elbow.
   B. the femur.   D. all of the above.

85. The major components of the nervous system are the:
   A. cranium and vertebrae.   C. brain and spinal cord.
   B. muscles and tendons.   D. arteries and veins.

86. Your 21-year-old female patient is taking a drug that was prescribed to help regulate her emotional activity and keep neurotransmitter levels from dropping too low. This type of drug is an:
   A. analgesic.
   B. antidepressant.
   C. antidysrhythmic.
   D. anticonvulsant.

87. A KED is appropriate to use in spinal motion restriction of a patient with signs of spine injury who is:
   A. standing.   C. lying on a soft surface.
   B. lying on a hard surface.   D. seated in a vehicle.

88. For the purposes of CPR, a child is defined as a patient who is:
   A. less than 1 year of age.
   B. age 1 year to puberty.
   C. age 1–8 years.
   D. age 1–17 years.

89. A 21-year-old male has a serious open wound to the neck. You are concerned about the possibility of an air embolism. An air embolism can occur because of:
   A. the higher pressure in the vessels of the neck.
   B. the high pressure in the chest.
   C. vessel pressure that is lower than atmospheric pressure.
   D. damage to the trachea.

90. You are approaching a 47-year-old female who has bright red blood spurting from her right leg. She is screaming, and she begs you to help. You should:
   A. ask her to calm down.
   B. control the bleeding.
   C. assess her airway.
   D. apply oxygen.

91. You are caring for an 18-month-old male with a fever. He experiences a seizure. Your treatment should include all of the following except:

    A. obtaining a good history of previous seizure activity.

    B. applying rubbing alcohol to lower the patient's fever.

    C. providing blow-by oxygen.

    D. positioning the patient on his side after the convulsion ends.

92. If the heart's electrical system fails completely and no electricity is created, this would show _____ on a cardiac monitor.

    A. PEA

    B. ventricular fibrillation

    C. asystole

    D. ventricular tachycardia

93. Experiencing a strong emotional response after caring for a critical pediatric patient is a normal reaction. If this occurs, you should consider all of the following except:

    A. talking to other EMTs about your feelings.

    B. talking with a professional counselor.

    C. contacting your area CISM team.

    D. working through the stress alone with a few beers.

94. The supplies in your ambulance for childbirth include all of the following, except:

    A. a bulb syringe.

    B. sanitary napkins.

    C. large safety pins.

    D. sterile surgical gloves.

95. You respond to a 15-year-old female in labor. Which of the following findings may indicate the need for neonatal resuscitation?

    A. A patient with a blood pressure of 130/82 mmHg

    B. A mother who has had three previous births

    C. A young mother who has not had prenatal care

    D. A patient whose water has already broken

96. You are called to a nursing home for an 82-year-old male complaining of abdominal pain. The patient has a history of dementia and cannot describe the pain to you. The nurse states that the patient has been vomiting dark coffee ground emesis for about an hour. His blood pressure is 90/40 mmHg, his pulse is 100 regular, and his respiratory rate is 24. Aside from the airway, what is your greatest concern?

    A. The patient will go into hypovolemic shock.

    B. The patient will have a myocardial infarction.

    C. The patient will have a stroke.

    D. The patient will become combative.

97. The key elements of quality CPR in an adult patient include:

    A. hand placement on lower third of the sternum.

    B. compression depth of 2 inches allowing full chest recoil.

    C. compression rate of 100–120 per minute.

    D. all of the above.

98. According to typical state vehicle and traffic laws, when in an emergency vehicle on an emergency operation, the driver may do any of the following, while displaying a red beacon 360 degrees and sounding an audible device, except:

    A. exceed the posted speed limit.

    B. pass a school bus that has its red light blinking.

    C. travel opposite the direction of travel.

    D. proceed through a red light with caution.

99. The national HAZMAT standard written specifically for first responders to a hazardous materials incident is:

    A. OSHA 1910.1030.

    B. NFPA 473.

    C. EPA 472.

    D. OSHA 1910.120.

100. According to START triage guidelines, a patient on the scene of an MCI who is alert and has a capillary refill time of less than 2 seconds is deemed a _____ patient.

    A. Priority 0

    B. Priority 1

    C. Priority 2

    D. Priority 3

Comprehensive Final Exam Answer Sheet

Fill in the correct answer for each item. When scoring, note that there are 100 questions valued at 1 point each.

1. [ ] A	[ ] B	[ ] C	[ ] D	**34.** [ ] A	[ ] B	[ ] C	[ ] D
2. [ ] A	[ ] B	[ ] C	[ ] D	**35.** [ ] A	[ ] B	[ ] C	[ ] D
3. [ ] A	[ ] B	[ ] C	[ ] D	**36.** [ ] A	[ ] B	[ ] C	[ ] D
4. [ ] A	[ ] B	[ ] C	[ ] D	**37.** [ ] A	[ ] B	[ ] C	[ ] D
5. [ ] A	[ ] B	[ ] C	[ ] D	**38.** [ ] A	[ ] B	[ ] C	[ ] D
6. [ ] A	[ ] B	[ ] C	[ ] D	**39.** [ ] A	[ ] B	[ ] C	[ ] D
7. [ ] A	[ ] B	[ ] C	[ ] D	**40.** [ ] A	[ ] B	[ ] C	[ ] D
8. [ ] A	[ ] B	[ ] C	[ ] D	**41.** [ ] A	[ ] B	[ ] C	[ ] D
9. [ ] A	[ ] B	[ ] C	[ ] D	**42.** [ ] A	[ ] B	[ ] C	[ ] D
10. [ ] A	[ ] B	[ ] C	[ ] D	**43.** [ ] A	[ ] B	[ ] C	[ ] D
11. [ ] A	[ ] B	[ ] C	[ ] D	**44.** [ ] A	[ ] B	[ ] C	[ ] D
12. [ ] A	[ ] B	[ ] C	[ ] D	**45.** [ ] A	[ ] B	[ ] C	[ ] D
13. [ ] A	[ ] B	[ ] C	[ ] D	**46.** [ ] A	[ ] B	[ ] C	[ ] D
14. [ ] A	[ ] B	[ ] C	[ ] D	**47.** [ ] A	[ ] B	[ ] C	[ ] D
15. [ ] A	[ ] B	[ ] C	[ ] D	**48.** [ ] A	[ ] B	[ ] C	[ ] D
16. [ ] A	[ ] B	[ ] C	[ ] D	**49.** [ ] A	[ ] B	[ ] C	[ ] D
17. [ ] A	[ ] B	[ ] C	[ ] D	**50.** [ ] A	[ ] B	[ ] C	[ ] D
18. [ ] A	[ ] B	[ ] C	[ ] D	**51.** [ ] A	[ ] B	[ ] C	[ ] D
19. [ ] A	[ ] B	[ ] C	[ ] D	**52.** [ ] A	[ ] B	[ ] C	[ ] D
20. [ ] A	[ ] B	[ ] C	[ ] D	**53.** [ ] A	[ ] B	[ ] C	[ ] D
21. [ ] A	[ ] B	[ ] C	[ ] D	**54.** [ ] A	[ ] B	[ ] C	[ ] D
22. [ ] A	[ ] B	[ ] C	[ ] D	**55.** [ ] A	[ ] B	[ ] C	[ ] D
23. [ ] A	[ ] B	[ ] C	[ ] D	**56.** [ ] A	[ ] B	[ ] C	[ ] D
24. [ ] A	[ ] B	[ ] C	[ ] D	**57.** [ ] A	[ ] B	[ ] C	[ ] D
25. [ ] A	[ ] B	[ ] C	[ ] D	**58.** [ ] A	[ ] B	[ ] C	[ ] D
26. [ ] A	[ ] B	[ ] C	[ ] D	**59.** [ ] A	[ ] B	[ ] C	[ ] D
27. [ ] A	[ ] B	[ ] C	[ ] D	**60.** [ ] A	[ ] B	[ ] C	[ ] D
28. [ ] A	[ ] B	[ ] C	[ ] D	**61.** [ ] A	[ ] B	[ ] C	[ ] D
29. [ ] A	[ ] B	[ ] C	[ ] D	**62.** [ ] A	[ ] B	[ ] C	[ ] D
30. [ ] A	[ ] B	[ ] C	[ ] D	**63.** [ ] A	[ ] B	[ ] C	[ ] D
31. [ ] A	[ ] B	[ ] C	[ ] D	**64.** [ ] A	[ ] B	[ ] C	[ ] D
32. [ ] A	[ ] B	[ ] C	[ ] D	**65.** [ ] A	[ ] B	[ ] C	[ ] D
33. [ ] A	[ ] B	[ ] C	[ ] D	**66.** [ ] A	[ ] B	[ ] C	[ ] D

©2021 Pearson Education, Inc.
Emergency Care, 14th Ed.

67.	[ ] A	[ ] B	[ ] C	[ ] D
68.	[ ] A	[ ] B	[ ] C	[ ] D
69.	[ ] A	[ ] B	[ ] C	[ ] D
70.	[ ] A	[ ] B	[ ] C	[ ] D
71.	[ ] A	[ ] B	[ ] C	[ ] D
72.	[ ] A	[ ] B	[ ] C	[ ] D
73.	[ ] A	[ ] B	[ ] C	[ ] D
74.	[ ] A	[ ] B	[ ] C	[ ] D
75.	[ ] A	[ ] B	[ ] C	[ ] D
76.	[ ] A	[ ] B	[ ] C	[ ] D
77.	[ ] A	[ ] B	[ ] C	[ ] D
78.	[ ] A	[ ] B	[ ] C	[ ] D
79.	[ ] A	[ ] B	[ ] C	[ ] D
80.	[ ] A	[ ] B	[ ] C	[ ] D
81.	[ ] A	[ ] B	[ ] C	[ ] D
82.	[ ] A	[ ] B	[ ] C	[ ] D
83.	[ ] A	[ ] B	[ ] C	[ ] D

84.	[ ] A	[ ] B	[ ] C	[ ] D
85.	[ ] A	[ ] B	[ ] C	[ ] D
86.	[ ] A	[ ] B	[ ] C	[ ] D
87.	[ ] A	[ ] B	[ ] C	[ ] D
88.	[ ] A	[ ] B	[ ] C	[ ] D
89.	[ ] A	[ ] B	[ ] C	[ ] D
90.	[ ] A	[ ] B	[ ] C	[ ] D
91.	[ ] A	[ ] B	[ ] C	[ ] D
92.	[ ] A	[ ] B	[ ] C	[ ] D
93.	[ ] A	[ ] B	[ ] C	[ ] D
94.	[ ] A	[ ] B	[ ] C	[ ] D
95.	[ ] A	[ ] B	[ ] C	[ ] D
96.	[ ] A	[ ] B	[ ] C	[ ] D
97.	[ ] A	[ ] B	[ ] C	[ ] D
98.	[ ] A	[ ] B	[ ] C	[ ] D
99.	[ ] A	[ ] B	[ ] C	[ ] D
100.	[ ] A	[ ] B	[ ] C	[ ] D

Answer Key

CHAPTER 1: Introduction to Emergency Medical Services

Match Key Terms

1. (K) Evidence-based techniques: Techniques of practices that are supported by scientific evidence of their safety and efficacy, rather than merely supposition and tradition. (p. 20)

2. (E) Off-line medical direction: Consists of standing orders issued by the Medical Director that allow EMT's to give certain medications or perform certain procedures without speaking to the Medical Director or another physician at that moment. (p. 20)

3. (H) On-line medical direction: Orders from the on-duty physician given directly to an EMT in the field by radio or telephone. (p. 20)

4. (A) 911 system: A system for telephone access to report emergencies. (p. 20)

5. (C) Medical direction: Oversight of the patient-care aspects of an EMS system by the Medical Director. (p. 20)

6. (D) Medical director: A physician who assumes ultimate responsibility for the patient-care aspects of the EMS system. (p. 20)

7. (B) Quality improvement: A process of continuous self-review with the purpose of identifying and correcting aspects of the system that require improvement. (p. 20)

8. (F) Protocols: Lists of steps, such as assessments and interventions, to be taken in different situations. (p. 20)

9. (G) Standing order: Policies or protocols issued by a Medical Director that authorize EMTs and others to perform particular skills in certain situations. (p. 20)

10. (J) Patient outcomes: The long-term survival of patients. (p. 20)

11. (I) Peer reviewed: Submitted to a professional journal and reviewed by several of the researcher's peers. (p. 20)

Multiple-Choice Review

1. (B) The earliest documented emergency medical service was in France in the 1790s. (p. 3)

2. (C) In 1966, the National Highway Safety Act charged the U.S. Department of Transportation with developing EMS standards and helping the states to upgrade the quality of their prehospital emergency care. (p. 4)

3. (B) Computerization is not a major component in the NHTSA's EMS system assessment. (pp. 4–5)

4. (C) A trauma center is an example of a specialty hospital in an EMS system. (p. 6)

5. (A) The NREMT provides certification after successful completion of examinations for national levels of EMS training in EMR, EMT, AEMT, and paramedic. (p. 12)

6. (C) The major emphasis of EMT education deals with basic-level assessment and care of the ill or injured patient in the prehospital setting. (p. 7)

7. (B) Patient care provided by the EMT should be based on assessment findings. (p. 9)

8. (A) Providing pertinent patient information to the hospital staff helps ensure continuity during the transfer of care of the patient. (p. 9)

9. (D) Patient advocacy is speaking up for your patient. (p. 9)

10. (A) Good personality traits are very important to the EMT. You should be cooperative and resourceful. (p. 10)

11. (D) An EMT who is not in control of personal habits might be disrespectful or condescending, make inappropriate decisions, and render improper care. (pp. 10–11)

12. (C) To prevent violating patient confidentiality, the EMT should avoid inappropriate conversation about the patient. (p. 11)

13. (C) An EMT may maintain up-to-date knowledge and skills through continuing education such as attending EMS conferences. (p. 12)

14. (C) A process of continuous self-review of all aspects of an EMS system for the purpose of identifying and correcting aspects of the system that require change is called quality improvement. (p. 13)

15. (B) In some states the role of the EMT has been expanded to assist local public health departments with seasonal flu vaccinations. (p. 16)

16. (C) Participation in continuing education and keeping carefully written documentation are examples of the EMT's role in quality improvement. (p. 13)

17. (D) Every EMS service or agency must have a Medical Director. (p. 14)

18. (C) It is important that each EMT know his or her Medical Director. An EMT is operating as the Medical Director's eyes and ears in the field. (p. 14)

19. (D) The difference between on-line and off-line medical direction is that on-line orders are given by the on-duty physician, usually over the radio or phone. (p. 15)

20. (D) An example of a pharmaceutical carried by EMTs that may require a physician consultation to administer is aspirin. (p. 15)

CHAPTER 1: (continued)

21. (B) As a new EMT, you will witness many changes in the EMS system and patient care, moving from practices that have been based on tradition to those that are based on research. (p. 17)

22. (C) The EMT has many jobs to do. It is the responsibility of the EMT to treat patients in a nonjudgmental and fair manner. (p. 11)

23. (D) Your Medical Director has stated that EMS is moving closer to science-based guidelines. A general procedure involved in making evidence-based patient care decisions is reviewing the literature, an evaluation of evidence, and forming a hypothesis. (p. 17)

24. (B) Your service has been seeing an increase in injuries to the aging population, and your leadership is planning to do something about it. Injury prevention for geriatric patients are examples of an EMT's role in public health. (p. 16)

25. (B) In a process developed by Galileo almost 400 years ago, called the scientific method, general observations are turned into a hypothesis. (p. 18)

26. (C) Which of the following is *not* a challenge when EMTs conduct research in the field: lengthy patient encounters. A lengthy patient encounter would be a benefit for research. Most often, though, the patient encounter is brief and it is difficult to conduct a research interview. (p. 18)

Complete the Following

1. The categories and standards of an EMS system established by NHTSA may include any six of the following: (pp. 4–5)
   - Regulation and policy
   - Resource management
   - Human resources and training
   - Transportation
   - Facilities
   - Communications
   - Public information and education
   - Medical direction
   - Trauma systems
   - Evaluation

2. Five types of specialty hospitals are: (p. 7)
   - Trauma centers
   - Burn center
   - Pediatric centers
   - Cardiac centers
   - Stroke centers

3. The four levels of EMS certifications are: (pp. 7–8)
   - EMR
   - EMT
   - AEMT
   - Paramedic

4. The responsibilities of the EMT may include any six of the following: (p. 9)
   - Personal safety
   - Safety of the crew, patient, and bystanders
   - Working with other public safety professionals
   - Patient assessment
   - Patient care
   - Lifting and moving
   - Transport
   - Transfer of care
   - Patient advocacy

Case Study: Introduction to the Gray-Zone

1. The Paramedic is an advanced life support provider who performs all of the skills of the EMT and AEMT plus additional advanced-level assessment, decision making, and treatment.

In most states, this is the highest level of prehospital provider and can be registered by the NREMT. (p. 8)

2. The Medical Director is a physician who assumes ultimate responsibility for the patient-care aspects of the EMS system. (p. 14)

3. Treatment protocols are lists of steps, such as assessments and interventions, to be taken in different situations. Protocols are developed by the Medical Director of an EMS system. (pp. 14–15)

CHAPTER 2: The Well-Being of the EMT

Match Key Terms

1. (C) Contamination: The introduction of dangerous chemicals, disease, or infectious materials. (p. 52)

2. (E) Pathogens: The organisms that cause infection, for example, viruses and bacteria. (p. 52)

3. (F) Multiple-casualty incident (MCI): An emergency involving multiple patients. (p. 52)

4. (A) Standard Precautions: A strict form on infection control that is based on the assumption that all blood and other body fluids are infectious; also known as body substance isolation (BSI). (p. 52)

5. (B) Critical incident stress management (CISM): A comprehensive system that includes education and resources to both prevent stress and deal with stress appropriately when it occurs. (p. 52)

6. (G) Decontamination: The removal or cleansing of dangerous chemicals and other dangerous or infectious materials. (p. 52)

7. (H) Hazardous material incident: The release of a harmful substance into the environment. (p. 52)

8. (J) Stress: A state of physical and/or psychological arousal to a stimulus. (p. 52)

9. (D) Personal protective equipment (PPE): Equipment that protects the EMS worker from infection and/or exposure to the dangers of rescue operations. (p. 52)

10. (I) Resilience: Toughness; an ability to recover quickly from difficult situations. (p. 52)

Multiple-Choice Review

1. (D) Fever of an unknown origin is likely caused by an organism called a pathogen. (p. 25)

2. (C) Procedures that protect you from blood and body fluids are called Standard Precautions. (p. 25)

3. (C) To provide the appropriate level of precautions to protect from infectious diseases in the field, the EMT may need to use disposable gloves and eye protection. (pp. 26–27)

4. (A) When covering the patient's mouth and nose to prevent the spread of an airborne disease the EMT should monitor the patient's respirations and airway closely. (p. 30)

5. (B) Preplanning safety precautions include vaccinations but does not involve keeping lists of patients with certain diseases in your district. (p. 38)

6. (C) All EMTs should be immunized for tetanus, hepatitis B, and influenza. The TST is not a vaccine, just a tuberculin skin test. (p. 38)

©2021 Pearson Education, Inc.
Emergency Care, 14th Ed.

7. (C) The federal agency that issues guidelines for employee safety around biohazards is OSHA. (p. 25)

8. (C) Employers of EMTs must provide all employees the hepatitis B vaccination. (p. 35)

9. (B) The federal act that establishes procedures by which emergency responders can find out if they have been exposed to a life-threatening infectious disease is the Ryan White CARE Act. (p. 35)

10. (C) After contact with the blood or body fluids of a patient, an EMT should submit a request for a determination of exposure to his or her designated officer. (pp. 35–36)

11. (B) Sometimes the EMT does not have the complete patient history for every patient when deciding which level of Standard precautions to utilize. Always assume that any person with a productive cough has TB. (p. 32)

12. (C) The diseases chicken pox, German measles, and whooping cough are all spread by airborne droplets. (p. 32)

13. (D) The EMT can safeguard his or her well-being by understanding and dealing with job stress, ensuring scene safety, and practicing Standard Precautions. (pp. 24–25)

14. (B) Examples of calls that have a high potential for causing acute stress reactions on the EMT would include trauma to multiple children, a plane crash with many victims, or a death or serious injury of a coworker. (p. 41)

15. (C) Some warning signs that an EMT is being affected by stress include indecisiveness and guilt. (p. 42)

16. (D) Avoiding a discussion about feelings is not a beneficial way to deal with stress. Lifestyle changes that may benefit an EMT in preventing and dealing with job stress include developing more healthful and positive dietary habits, devoting time to relaxing, and exercising. (pp. 42–43)

17. (C) A meeting held by a team of peer counselors and mental health professionals within 24 to 72 hours after a major incident is called a critical incident stress debriefing. (p. 44)

18. (A) A smaller meeting conducted within a few hours of a major incident with a few rescuers who were directly involved in the most stressful aspects of the call is called a defusing session. (p. 44)

19. (A) Most medical professionals and EMS leaders agree that the best course of action for an EMT who is experiencing significant stress from a serious call that involved multiple deaths is to seek help from a mental health professional who is experienced in these issues. (p. 44)

20. (C) A person who finds out that he or she is dying may go through the emotional stages of depression and acceptance. (p. 45)

21. (B) The emotional stages typically occur in this order: denial, anger, bargaining, depression, and then acceptance. (p. 45)

22. (B) Telling the patient that everything will be fine is false reassurance. When assisting the patient with a terminal illness, experts suggest listening empathetically to the patient, being tolerant of angry reactions from the patient or family members, and trying to recognize the patient's needs. (p. 45)

23. (C) Running is not a correct response to danger because you might put yourself more in harm's way. The words that sum up the actions required to respond to danger when a call gets violent include plan, observe, and react. (p. 48)

24. (C) The body's response to stress was studied by Hans Selye who found there is a general adaptation syndrome. (p. 39)

25. (C) The phases of adaptation to stress include alarm, resistance and exhaustion. (pp. 39–40)

26. (B) A stress reaction that involves either physical or psychological behavior manifested days or weeks after an incident is called posttraumatic stress disorder. (p. 40)

27. (D) If you suspect your patient may have active TB when transporting it is appropriate to wear disposable gloves, eye shield, and an N-95 or HEPA mask. (p. 38)

28. (C) The normal mode of transmission of chicken pox is through airborne droplets. (p. 32)

29. (A) Hepatitis is a bloodborne spread disease. Bacterial meningitis, pneumonia, and influenza are spread by respiratory secretions or oral or nasal secretions. (p. 32)

30. (B) A disease that mothers are thought to be able to pass to their unborn child is AIDS. (p. 32)

31. (B) The incubation period for Ebola is 2 to 21 days. (p. 32)

32. (C) Late signs of an Ebola patient would include extensive bruising. (p. 33)

33. (B) The Emergency Response Guidebook is helpful in estimating safe perimeters and evacuation distances at the scene of a hazardous materials incident. (p. 46)

34. (B) If you suspect danger or violence at a call it is best to call for a police backup to secure the scene. (p. 49)

35. (D) The "A" in eSCAPEe curriculum stands for Anticipate what happens next. (p. 43)

Complete the Following

1. Five types of calls with high potential stress for EMS personnel would include: (p. 41)
   - Multiple-casualty incidents
   - Calls involving infants and children
   - Severe injuries
   - Abuse and neglect
   - Death of a coworker

2. List five signs or symptoms of stress: (p. 42)
   - Irritability with family, friends, and coworkers
   - Inability to concentrate
   - Changes in daily activities such as difficulty sleeping or nightmares
   - Loss of appetite
   - Loss of interest in sexual activity
   - Anxiety
   - Indecisiveness
   - Guilt
   - Isolation
   - Loss of interest in work

3. List five critical elements of the standard Title 29 Code of Federal Regulations 1910.1030. (pp. 34–35)
   - Infection exposure control plan
   - Adequate education and training
   - Hepatitis B vaccination
   - Personal protective equipment
   - Methods of control
   - Housekeeping
   - Labeling
   - Post exposure evaluation and follow-up

4. List four factors to address in planning for a potentially violent call. (p. 49)
   - Wear safe clothing
   - Prepare your equipment so it is not cumbersome
   - Carry a portable radio whenever possible
   - Decide on safety roles

CHAPTER 2: (continued)

Case Study: Just a Fall in the Kitchen

1. What Standard Precautions would be appropriate in this situation? Gloves, eye shield, mask, and a gown to prevent soiling your uniform. (pp. 26–32)

2. Would it be appropriate to remove the patient's clothing and clean her up in the house? This depends on her condition and would take into consideration your best clinical judgement. It may be best to clean her up in her home, which is private and indoors. On the other hand, you need to take the physical findings, vital signs, and her overall condition into consideration. Since an altered level of consciousness is considered a critical finding, she would be considered unstable—hence time on scene should be minimized.

3. Once you determine that the patient is breathing, has an open airway, and has a pulse, what exam should you conduct on her? It would be appropriate to do a rapid trauma assessment (secondary survey) head to foot.

4. What medical history would be appropriate to obtain from the patient's son? Get the patient's history. Find out what prior medical problems the patient has had and any medications she should be taking (which were missed on the days she was lying on the floor). Although she has not been traveling, he has recently traveled. Consequently, knowing the location may be helpful if you are suspecting a regional infectious disease. (p. 33)

5. Based on the potential for exposure to body fluids, how should you handle this patient? Dress appropriately, and follow the guideline, "If it is wet and not yours, don't touch it without appropriate protection." (pp. 27–32)

6. If you noticed that your glove was ripped, what should you do to maintain your own personal protection? Take off the glove, wash your hands, and put on another glove. (p. 31)

7. Does the updated information that you were given in the ED change how you should have managed the hazards in this situation for your own protection? If you were following the advice in answer 5 above and wore PPE, this should not be a problem at all. You should have a hepatitis B series of shots, and equipment from your agency. If for any reason you believe you may have had an exposure, call your agency's supervisor and follow the established policies. If you have any questions, call your Medical Director. (p. 35)

CHAPTER 3: Lifting and Moving Patients

Match Key Terms

1. (C) Power grip: Gripping with as much hand surface as possible in contact with the object being lifted, all fingers bent at the same angle and hands at least 10 inches apart. (p. 77)

2. (E) Body mechanics: The proper use of the body to facilitate lifting and moving and preventing injury. (p. 77)

3. (D) Direct carry: A method of transferring a patient from bed to stretcher, in which two or more rescuers curl the patient to their chests, then reverse the process to lower the patient to the stretcher. (p. 77)

4. (B) Direct ground lift: A method of lifting and carrying a patient from ground level to a stretcher in which two or more rescuers kneel, curl the patient to their chests, stand, then reverse the process to lower the patient to the stretcher. (p. 77)

5. (H) Draw-sheet method: A method of transferring a patient from bed to stretcher by grasping and pulling the loosened bottom sheet of the bed. (p. 77)

6. (A) Bariatric: Having to do with patients who are significantly overweight or obese. (p. 77)

7. (F) Extremity lift: A method of lifting and carrying a patient during which one rescuer slips hands under the patient's armpits and grasps the wrists, while another rescuer grasps the patient's knees. (p. 77)

8. (G) Power lift: A lift from a squatting position with weight to be lifted close to the body, feet apart and flat on the ground, body weight on or just behind balls of feet, and the back locked in. The upper body is raised before the hips. (p. 77)

Multiple-Choice Review

1. (C) To ensure your personal safety when lifting an adult patient, it is important to use your legs, not your back, to lift. (p. 56)

2. (B) Do not twist while you are lifting as it can injure your back. (p. 56)

3. (A) When lifting the cot you should use four rescuers if on rough or uneven terrain. (p. 67)

4. (A) When you place all fingers and the palm in contact with the stretcher as you prepare to lift, you are using the technique known as the power grip. (p. 57)

5. (A) When you must pull an object, you should keep the line of pull through the center of your body by bending your knees. (p. 58)

6. (D) An emergency move would not be used in the situation where the dispatcher is holding another EMS call. (p. 58)

7. (C) The patient on the floor who needs an emergency move can be moved by pulling on her clothing in the neck and shoulder area. (p. 60)

8. (B) If your 55-year-old male patient has an altered mental status, you should consider an urgent move. (p. 59)

9. (C) When doing a log roll, you should lean from your hips and use your shoulder muscles to help with the roll. (p. 62)

10. (A) The final step in packaging a patient for transport on a wheeled stretcher involves securing the stretcher to the ambulance. (p. 66)

11. (D) If you and your partner are going to be carrying this patient down the stairway, you should use a stair chair instead of a stretcher. (p. 68)

12. (D) It would be helpful to have your partner call for powered loading equipment, a bariatric stretcher, and additional crew members. (p. 67)

13. (A) The patient being lowered by the Fire Department will lower down a ladder bed should be placed in the plastic basket stretcher prior to movement. (p. 70)

14. (B) The long spine board would be most appropriate for this transfer of a confirmed spinal injured patient. (pp. 68, 70)

15. (A) The pack strap carry is an example of an emergency move for a patient who has no spine injury. (p. 61)

16. (B) Another name for the squat-lift used by weight lifters and EMTs is the power lift. (p. 57)

17. (D) The EMT's feet should be positioned at a comfortable distance apart, flat on the ground, and weight on the balls of the feet when lifting. (p. 57)

©2021 Pearson Education, Inc.
Emergency Care, 14th Ed.

18. (B) The EMT who has to lift with one hand, as in a litter carry, must be careful not to compensate by leaning. (p. 56)

19. (C) A comfortable device that can be used to transport a patient in the supine position who has sustained a spinal injury is a vacuum mattress. (p. 70)

20. (B) When a vacuum mattress is used, the patient is placed on the device and the air is withdrawn by a pump. Then the mattress will form a rigid and conforming surface around the patient. (p. 70)

Complete the Following

1. List five patient-carrying devices illustrated in the chapter. (pp. 63–64, 70)
   - Wheeled stretcher or Power stretcher
   - Portable stretcher
   - Scoop (orthopedic) stretcher
   - Basket (Stokes) stretcher
   - Flexible (Reeves) stretcher
   - Stair chair

2. List four general principles that will help you prevent injury when reaching for a patient. (p. 57)
   - Keep your back in a locked-in position.
   - Avoid twisting while reaching.
   - Avoid reaching more than 20 inches in front of your body.
   - Avoid prolonged reaching when strenuous effort is required.
   - Avoid reaching overhead.

3. List five general principles that will help you prevent injury when pushing or pulling a patient. (p. 58)
   - Push, rather than pull, whenever possible.
   - Keep your back locked in.
   - Keep the line of pull through the center of your body by bending your knees.
   - Keep the weight close to your body.
   - If the weight is below your waist level, push or pull from a kneeling position.
   - Avoid pushing or pulling overhead.
   - Keep your elbows bent and arms close to your sides.

4. List three situations that may require an emergency move. (p. 58)
   - The scene is hazardous.
   - Care of life-threatening conditions requires repositioning.
   - You must move a closer patient in order to reach other patients who are more critically injured.

Label the Photographs (pp. 60–62)

1. Shoulder drag

2. Incline drag

3. Foot drag

4. Clothes drag

5. Firefighter's drag

6. Blanket drag

7. One Rescuer assist

8. Cradle carry

9. Pack strap carry

10. Piggy back carry

11. Firefighter's carry

12. Two Rescuer assist

Case Study: More Than the Average Patient

1. Normally, a stair chair is used to remove patients on the second floor. However, considering the size he would unlikely fit in a stair chair. Additionally, the fact that his back is hurting him, it makes sense to keep him in the supine position. (p. 64)

2. A direct ground lift with such a heavy patient would be dangerous to the EMT. A draw-sheet method lift would be more appropriate, especially if the sheet could be replaced with blankets and several sheets for added strength while lifting. (p. 75)

3. The decision to call the fire department to obtain more rescuers was a wise decision because this is a very heavy patient.

4. A bariatric unit is designed to transport obese patients. These units have special stretchers rated for more weight and larger patients as well as lifts and ramps to prevent the need for the EMTs to lift the stretcher into the ambulance. (p. 67)

5. A scoop stretcher has points to hold onto and is designed for smaller patients. It could be used with a larger patient, but you would need a lot of lifting assistance, so it would be difficult to get everyone on the side and also go down the stairs. The Reeves stretcher can be placed under an obese patient and has many hand-holds for carrying. With a large patient, these would come in handy. The Reeves stretcher can also slide on the floor or stairs if needed. Each situation may be different, so this could be a case in that gray zone where you should use your best judgement, taking into consideration the environment and the number of personnel you have. (p. 70)

6. If the Reeves stretcher did not work, another option would be a plastic Stokes basket, provided that is rated for the size and weight of the patient. (p. 70)

7. The highest priority for the EMS providers should always be the safety of the EMTs. For the patient, being able to maintain an open airway would certainly be a high priority. When a large patient has an altered mental status and is in a supine position, it can be difficult to keep the airway open. Having a lot of help in this instance was a good thing so that no rescuer goes home with a back injury. (p. 67)

CHAPTER 4: Medical, Legal, and Ethical Issues

Match Key Terms

Part A

1. (M) Abandonment: Leaving a patient after care has been initiated and before the patient has been transferred to someone with equal or greater medical training. (pp. 99–100)

2. (P) Slander: False, injurious information stated verbally. (pp. 99–100)

3. (L) Confidentiality: The obligation not to reveal information obtained about a patient except to other health care professionals involved in the patient's care, or under subpoena, or in a court of law, or when the patient has signed a release of confidentiality. (pp. 99–100)

4. (F) Consent: Permission from the patient for care or other action by the EMT. (pp. 99–100)

5. (I) Safe haven law: A law that permits a person to drop off an infant or child off at a police, fire, or EMS station or to deliver the infant or child to any available public safety personnel. (pp. 99–100)

6. (K) Do not resuscitate (DNR) order: A legal document, usually signed by the patient and physician which states that the patient has a terminal illness and does not wish to prolong life through resuscitative efforts. (pp. 99–100)

7. (D) Duty to act: An obligation to provide care to a patient. (pp. 99–100)

8. (E) Expressed consent: Consent given by adults who are of legal age and mentally competent to make a rational decision with regard to their medical well-being. (pp. 99–100)

CHAPTER 4: (continued)

9. (G) Good Samaritan laws: A series of laws, varying by state, designed to provide limited legal protection for citizens and some health care personnel when they are administering emergency care. (pp. 99–100)

10. (O) HIPAA: The Health Insurance Portability and Accountability Act, a federal law protecting the privacy of patient-specific health care information and providing the patient with control over how this information is used and distributed. (pp. 99–100)

11. (A) Implied consent: The consent that is presumed a patient or patient's parent or guardian would give if they could, such as for an unconscious patient or a child whose parents cannot be contacted when care is needed. (pp. 99–100)

12. (C) Liability: Being held legally responsible. (pp. 99–100)

13. (J) Negligence: A finding that there was failure to act properly in a situation in which there was a duty to act that needed care as would reasonably be expected of the EMT was not provided, and that harm was caused to the patient as a result. (pp. 99–100)

14. (N) Organ donor: A person who has completed a legal document that allows for donation of organs and tissues in the event of death. (pp. 99–100)

15. (H) Scope of practice: A set of regulations that define the scope, or extent and limits, of the EMT's job. (pp. 99–100)

16. (B) POLST: Physician orders that state not only the patient's wishes regarding resuscitation attempts but also the patient's wishes regarding artificial feeding, antibiotics, and other life-sustaining care if the person is unable to state the person's desires later. (pp. 99–100)

Part B

1. (F) *In loco parentis*: Literally "in place of a parent," indicating a person who may give consent for care of a child when the parents are not present or able to give consent. (pp. 99–100)

2. (E) Assault: Placing a person in fear of bodily harm. (pp. 99–100)

3. (G) Battery: Causing bodily harm or restraining a person. (pp. 99–100)

4. (A) Tort: A civil, not a criminal, offense; an action or injury caused by negligence from which a lawsuit may arise. (pp. 99–100)

5. (H) *Res ipsa loquitur*: A Latin term meaning "the thing speaks for itself." (pp. 99–100)

6. (B) Moral: Regarding personnel standards or principles of right and wrong. (pp. 99–100)

7. (I) Ethical: Regarding a social system or social or professional expectations for applying principles of right and wrong. (pp. 99–100)

8. (C) Libel: False, injurious information in written form. (pp. 99–100)

9. (K) Advance directive: A DNR order; instructions written in advance of an event. (pp. 99–100)

10. (J) Crime scene: The location where a crime has been committed or any place where evidence relating to a crime may be found. (pp. 99–100)

11. (D) Standard of care: For an EMT providing care for a specific patient in a specific situation, the care that would be expected to be provided by an EMT with similar training when caring for a patient in a similar situation. (pp. 99–100)

Multiple-Choice Review

1. (B) The collective set of regulations governing the EMT is called the EMT's scope of practice. (p. 81)

2. (B) Laws that govern the skills and treatments that an EMT may perform are different from state to state. (p. 81)

3. (C) When the EMT advocates for the physical/emotional needs of the, this is considering an ethical responsibility. (p. 98)

4. (C) Applied consent is not a type of consent by the EMT. (p. 83)

5. (A) When you inform the adult patient of a procedure you are about to perform and its associated risks, you are asking for the patient's expressed consent. (p. 83)

6. (C) You are assessing a 28-year-old male patient who was found unconscious at the bottom of a stairwell. Consent that is based on the assumption that this patient would approve your life-saving care is called implied consent. (p. 83)

7. (C) You are treating a 22-year-old female who decides that she does not want a cervical collar and definitely does not want to be transported to the hospital. The record of her refusal of medical care and/or transport should include informing the patient of the risks and consequences of refusal, documenting the steps you took, and obtaining a release form with the patient's witnessed signature. Signing of the form by the Medical Director would not be included in the record of her refusal of medical care. (pp. 84–85)

8. (B) It is clear that your 24-year-old competent male patient does not want to go to the hospital. Forcing him to go to the hospital against his will may result in assault charges against the EMT. (p. 85)

9. (C) If a 36-year-old female refuses care, the EMT should not tell the patient to call her family physician if the problem reoccurs, rather she should be instructed to call 911 again. (p. 85)

10. (D) Another name for a DNR order is an advance directive. (p. 87)

11. (A) There may be varying degrees of DNR orders in your state, which may be expressed through a variety of detailed instructions that may be part of the order, such as allowing CPR only if cardiac or respiratory arrest was observed. (p. 90)

12. (B) In a hospital, long-term life-support and comfort-care measures would consist of intravenous feeding and the use of a respirator. (p. 90)

13. (B) If an EMT with a duty to act fails to provide the standard of care and if this failure causes harm or injury to the patient, the EMT may be accused of negligence. (p. 90)

14. (C) Leaving your 82-year-old male patient on the hallway stretcher in a busy ED and leaving without giving a report to a health care professional is an example of abandonment. (p. 92)

15. (D) The EMT should not discuss information about a patient except to relay pertinent information to the physician at the ED. Information that is considered confidential includes patient history gained through interview, assessment findings, and treatments rendered. (p. 92)

16. (A) The EMT should not release confidential patient information. The exception to this rule would be to inform other health care professionals who need to know information to continue care. (p. 92)

17. (D) Patches would not be a form of medical identification. Medical identification devices worn to indicate serious medical conditions are available in bracelets, necklaces, and cards. (p. 94)

©2021 Pearson Education, Inc.
Emergency Care, 14th Ed.

18. (B) When treating a patient with a severe head injury who happens to be an organ donor you should treat the patient the same as any other patient and inform the ED physician. (p. 95)

19. (A) At the crime scene the EMT should avoid disturbing any evidence at the scene unless emergency care requires. (pp. 95–97)

20. (B) Crimes in public places are not commonly a required reporting situation. Commonly required reporting situations in most states include child and elder abuse, sexual assault, and suspected human trafficking. (p. 98)

21. (C) The extent of limits of an EMT's occupation is referred to as the scope of practice. (p. 81)

22. (B) The patient who admits to drinking "half a dozen beers" in the last 90 minutes may not be mentally competent to sign a refusal. (p. 84)

23. (C) The federal law designed to protect the patient's private medical information is called HIPAA. (p. 93)

24. (A) Your highest priority in transporting the patient to the local ED is to monitor the patient's mental status and vital signs. (p. 83)

25. (B) Examples of microscopic evidence at a crime scene would be any dirt and carpet fibers. (p. 97)

26. (B) You are on the scene where a 46-year-old female who is refusing to go to the hospital. After arguing for 20 minutes you decide to just restrain her and remove to the ED as her family wishes so they can get a break from her complaining. If the patient is of sound mind you could be charged with a battery. (p. 85)

27. (C) The concept use in tort law is *res ipsa loquitur* which is Latin for "the thing speaks for itself." (p. 91)

28. (C) When conducting a physical exam of an unconscious adult patient with a suspected medical problem, you remember that there was a "Vial of Life" sticker on the front door of the residence. This is important because it may reveal that additional medical identification is in the refrigerator. (p. 87)

Complete the Following

1. List four conditions that must be fulfilled for a patient to refuse care or transport. (p. 84)
   • Patients must be legally able to consent.
   • Patients must be awake and oriented.
   • Patients must be fully informed.
   • Patients will be asked to sign a "release" form.

2. A finding of negligence, or failure to act properly, requires that all of the following circumstances be proven. (p. 90)
   • The EMT had a duty to the patient.
   • The EMT did not provide the standard of care (committed a breach of duty).
   • There was proximate causation (the concept that the damages to the patient were the result of action or inaction by the EMT).

3. Four medical conditions that may be listed on a medical identification device (such as a necklace, bracelet, or card) are: (p. 94)
   • Heart conditions   • Diabetes
   • Allergies   • Epilepsy

4. Describe the purpose of the typical state "safe haven" law and how it may affect your EMS agency. (p. 95)

   Most states have implemented come sort of "safe haven" law. Under such a law, a person may drop an infant or child off at any police, fire, or EMS station or deliver the child to any public safety personnel.

Case Study: A Witnessed Collision: First on the Scene

1. No, unless your state law requires you to stop. If you do stop you should not leave the patient except in the hands of another EMT or advanced EMT. Leaving a patient is abandonment which is an example of gross negligence. (p. 92)

2. Yes and no. Anyone can be sued. Most states do have a Good Samaritan law or some law dealing specifically with EMS personnel that have limited protections in this situation as long as your treatment is not grossly negligent. (p. 92)

3. Yes, in most states. (p. 92)

4. 9-1-1 is the universal emergency number in the USA.

5. Questions such as:
   • What is the exact location of the sick or injured person?
   • What is your call-back number?
   • How old is the patient?
   • What is the problem?
   • What is the patient's sex?
   • Is the patient breathing?

6. The police, the fire department and the ambulance service.

7. Assign them to perform manual cervical spine motion restriction of the head and neck and to help with lifting the patient once the ambulance arrives.

8. The patient could have additional broken bones, internal bleeding, or a head or neck injury to name a few.

9. No permission is needed since consent is implied with the unconscious patient.

10. A ruptured spleen, fractured ribs, and back and neck injuries, in addition to the obvious leg injury.

11. Assign someone to lift the patient's injured leg and hold it as still as possible.

12. Yes, he is conscious and must give expressed consent.

13. Not until you check with the EMT or paramedic in charge to be sure that your assistance is no longer needed and you have provided any pertinent patient information to them. Additionally, you may have to make statements to the police as you witnessed the accident itself.

14. Usually, this is an example of gross negligence due to abandonment. If you say you are going to assist and then leave before additional help arrives, the patient might not get access to life-saving assistance. Additionally, you may have to give a statement to the police as you witnessed an MVC in which there was a fatality.

CHAPTER 5: Medical Terminology

Match Key Terms

Part A

1. (E) Compound: A word formed from two or more whole words. (pp. 112–113)

2. (F) Root: Foundation of a word that is not a word that can stand on its own. (pp. 112–113)

3. (A) Combining form: A word root with an added vowel that can be joined with other words, roots, or suffixes to form a new word. (pp. 112–113)

4. (D) Prefix: A word part added to the beginning of a root or word to modify or qualify its meaning. (pp. 112–113)

CHAPTER 5: (continued)

5. (C) Suffix: A word part added to the end of a root or word to complete its meaning. (pp. 112–113)

6. (B) Anatomy: The study of body structure. (pp. 112–113)

7. (G) Physiology: The study of body function. (pp. 112–113)

8. (Q) Anatomic position: The standard reference position for the body in the study of anatomy. In this position, the body is standing erect, facing the observer, with arms down at the sides and the palms of the hands forward. (pp. 112–113)

9. (J) Plane: A flat surface formed when slicing through a solid object. (pp. 112–113)

10. (I) Midline: An imaginary line drawn down the center of the body, dividing it into right and left halves. (pp. 112–113)

11. (H) Medial: Toward the midline of the body. (pp. 112–113)

12. (K) Lateral: To the side, away from the midline of the body. (pp. 112–113)

13. (P) Bilateral: On both sides. (pp. 112–113)

14. (O) Unilateral: Limited to one side. (pp. 112–113)

15. (M) Midaxillary: A line drawn vertically from the middle of the armpit to the ankle. (pp. 112–113)

16. (N) Anterior: The front of the body or body part. (pp. 112–113)

17. (L) Posterior: The back of the body or body part. (pp. 112–113)

Part B

1. (C) Ventral: Referring to the front of the body. (pp. 112–113)

2. (E) Dorsal: Referring to the back of the body or the back of the hand or foot. (112–113)

3. (B) Superior: Toward the head. (pp. 112–113)

4. (A) Inferior: Away from the head; usually compared with another structure that is closer to the head. (pp. 112–113)

5. (D) Proximal: Closer to the torso. (pp. 112–113)

6. (J) Distal: Further away from the torso. (pp. 112–113)

7. (H) Torso: The trunk of the body; without the head and extremities. (pp. 112–113)

8. (G) Palmar: Referring to the palm of the hand. (pp. 112–113)

9. (F) Plantar: Referring to the sole of the foot. (pp. 112–113)

10. (I) Midclavicular: The line through the center of each clavicle. (pp. 112–113)

11. (L) Abdominal quadrants: Four divisions of the abdomen used to pinpoint the location of a pain or injury: the right upper quadrant (RUQ), the left upper quadrant (LUQ), the right lower quadrant (RLQ), and the left lower quadrant (LLQ). (pp. 112–113)

12. (K) Supine: Lying on the back. (pp. 112–113)

13. (N) Prone: Lying facedown. (pp. 112–113)

14. (O) Recovery position: Lying on the side. (pp. 112–113)

15. (M) Fowler position: A sitting position. (pp. 112–113)

Multiple-Choice Review

1. (A) The word electrocardiogram is actually a combination of three roots. (p. 104)

2. (B) If a patient is lying on his or her side, the patient is said to be in the recovery position. (p. 111)

3. (C) When a patient who has been having difficulty breathing is placed in a sitting position on a stretcher, this is called Fowler. (p. 111)

4. (B) A patient lying flat on her back would be in the supine position. (p. 111)

5. (A) Your patient is being treated for heart disease and was referred to a specialist for further treatment. The type of physician she is going to see is most likely a cardiologist. (p. 104)

6. (C) When you see the suffix "itis" in a patient's chart, it means inflammation. (p. 104)

7. (B) Your service encourages the use of abbreviations and acronyms on the prehospital care report to save time. The downside of this is that they can lead to communication errors. (p. 106)

8. (D) The universal reference position of the body used when discussing human anatomy is called the anatomic position. (p. 107)

9. (C) A patient who has absent lung sounds in both the right and left upper lobes is said to have bilateral findings. (p. 109)

10. (B) Your patient was stabbed in the front of the chest on the left side, and you suspect that his heart may have been injured due to the wound location at the left nipple level in the mid-clavicular line. (p. 110)

Complete the Following

1. Describe each of the following planes or directional terms: (pp. 109–110)
- Midline – down the center of body, dividing into right and left.
- Medial – toward the midline of the body.
- Lateral – to the side, away from midline.
- Midaxillary line – a line drawn vertically from the middle of armpit to ankle.
- Anterior – the front of the body or body part.
- Posterior – the back of the body or body part.
- Superior – toward the head.
- Inferior – away from the head.
- Midclavicular line – the line through the center of each clavicle.

2. Name the organ(s) or body system that is the specialty of each of the following doctors: (p. 105)
- Pulmonologist – lungs
- Gastroenterologist – digestive system
- Cardiologist – heart
- Neurologist – nervous system

3. Define the following medical prefixes: (p. 105)
- Ante – before
- Brady – slow
- Contra – against
- Dys – difficult or painful
- Hyper – above normal/high
- Inter – between
- Peri – around
- Poly – many
- Super/supra – above or in excess
- Uni – one

Pathophysiology: Dissecting a Compound Word

1. If you break the medical term cholecystitis down into three parts, they are chol/e, cyst, and itis. (p. 106)

2. The parts mean: bile (chol/e), sac (cyst), and inflammation (-itis). (p. 106)

3. The patient should not be eating greasy fried food because she cannot digest it since the inflamed gallbladder is unable to secret the bile into the GI system to help emulsify fat in the digestive process. (p. 106)

Label the Diagrams

Anatomic Postures (p. 111)

1. Supine
2. Prone
3. Lateral recumbent (recovery)

Anatomical Positions (pp. 108–110)

1. distal
2. proximal
3. midline
4. midclavicular line
5. medial
6. lateral
7. palmar
8. left
9. dorsal
10. right
11. anterior (ventral)
12. posterior (dorsal)
13. superior
14. midaxillary
15. inferior

CHAPTER 6: Anatomy and Physiology

Match Key Terms

Part A (pp. 150–152)

1. (H) Anatomy: The study of body structure.
2. (P) Physiology: The study of body function.
3. (G) Thyroid cartilage: The wing-shaped plate of cartilage that sits anterior to the larynx and forms the Adam's apple.
4. (O) Musculoskeletal system: The system of bones and skeletal muscles that support and protect the body and permit movement.
5. (F) Skeleton: The bones of the body.
6. (N) Muscle: Tissue that can contract to allow movement of a body part.
7. (E) Ligament: Tissue that connects bone to bone.
8. (I) Tendon: Tissue that connects muscle to bone.
9. (A) Skull: The bony structure of the head.
10. (J) Cranium: The top, back, and sides of the skull.
11. (B) Mandible: The lower jaw.
12. (K) Maxillae: The two fused bones forming the upper jaw.
13. (C) Nasal bones: Bones that comprise the nasal cavity.
14. (Q) Orbits: The bony structures around the eyes.
15. (D) Zygomatic arches: Bones that form the structure of the cheeks.
16. (M) Vertebrae: The bones of the spinal column.
17. (L) Buffer system: A system that helps manage the pH of the blood.

Part B (pp. 150–152)

1. (H) Thorax: The chest.
2. (P) Sternum: The breastbone.
3. (G) Manubrium: The superior portion of the pelvis.
4. (O) Xiphoid process: The inferior portion of the sternum.
5. (F) Pelvis: The basin-shaped bony structure that supports the spine and is the point of attachment for the lower extremities.
6. (N) Ilium: The superior and widest portion of the pelvis.
7. (E) Ischium: The lower, posterior portions of the pelvis.
8. (I) Pubis: The medial anterior portion of the pelvis.
9. (A) Acetabulum: The pelvic socket into which the ball at the proximal end of the femur fits to form the hip joint.
10. (J) Femur: The large bone of the thigh.
11. (B) Patella: The kneecap.
12. (K) Tibia: The medial and larger bone of the lower leg.
13. (C) Fibula: The lateral and smaller bone of the lower leg.
14. (L) Malleolus: Bony protrusions seen on either side of the ankle joint.
15. (D) Tarsals: The ankle bones.
16. (Q) Metatarsals: The foot bones.
17. (M) Lymphatic system: Composed of organs, tissues, and vessels, these help to maintain the fluid balance of the body and contributes to the body's immune system.

Part C (pp. 150–152)

1. (H) Calcaneus: The heel bone.
2. (P) Phalanges: The bones of the fingers and toes.
3. (G) Clavicle: The collarbone.
4. (O) Scapula: The shoulder blade.
5. (F) Acromion process: The highest portion of the shoulder.
6. (N) Acromioclavicular joint: The joint where the acromion and the clavicle meet.
7. (E) Humerus: The bone of the upper arm, between the shoulder and the elbow.
8. (I) Radius: The lateral bone of the forearm.
9. (A) Ulna: The medial bone of the forearm.
10. (Q) Carpals: The wrist bones.
11. (B) Metacarpals: The hand bones.
12. (K) Joint: The point where two bones come together.
13. (C) Voluntary muscle: Muscle that can be consciously controlled.
14. (L) Involuntary muscle: Muscle that responds automatically to brain signals but cannot be consciously controlled.
15. (D) Cardiac muscle: Specialized involuntary muscle found only in the heart.
16. (M) Automaticity: The ability of the heart to generate and conduct electrical impulses on its own.
17. (J) Radial artery: Artery of the lower arm; the artery felt when taking the pulse at the thumb side of the wrist.

CHAPTER 6: (continued)

Part D (pp. 150–152)

1. (K) Respiratory system

2. (P) Oropharynx: The area directly posterior to the mouth.

3. (G) Nasopharynx: The area directly posterior to the nose.

4. (N) Pharynx: The area directly posterior to the mouth and nose. It is made up of the oropharynx and the nasopharynx.

5. (C) Epiglottis: A leaf-shaped structure that prevents food and foreign matter from entering the trachea.

6. (O) Larynx: The voice box.

7. (E) Cricoid cartilage: The ring-shaped structure that forms the lower portion of the larynx.

8. (M) Trachea: The "windpipe"; the structure that connects the pharynx to the lungs.

9. (A) Lungs: The organs where the exchange of atmospheric oxygen and waste carbon dioxide takes place.

10. (J) Mainstem bronchi: The two large sets of branches that come off the trachea and enter the lungs. There are right and left bronchi.

11. (B) Alveoli: The microscopic sacs of the lungs where gas exchange with the bloodstream take place.

12. (H) Diaphragm: The muscular structure that divides the chest cavity from the abdominal cavity; a major muscle of respiration.

13. (F) Inhalation: An active process in which the intercostal (rib) muscles and the diaphragm contract, increasing the size of the chest cavity and causing air to flow into the lungs.

14. (L) Exhalation: A passive process in which the intercostal (rib) muscles and the diaphragm relax, causing the chest cavity to decrease in size and air to flow out of the lungs.

15. (D) Ventilation: The mechanical process of moving gases to and from the alveoli.

16. (I) Respiration: The process of moving oxygen and carbon dioxide between circulating blood and the cells.

Part E (pp. 150–152)

1. (K) Cardiovascular system: The system made up of the heart and the blood vessels.

2. (P) Atria: The two upper chambers of the heart.

3. (G) Ventricles: The two lower chambers of the heart.

4. (N) Venae cava: This is the major venous structure that returns blood from the body to the right atrium.

5. (C) Valve: A structure that opens and closes to permit the flow of a fluid in only one direction.

6. (O) Cardiac conduction system: A system of specialized muscle tissues that conducts electrical impulses that stimulate the heart to beat.

7. (E) Artery: Any blood vessel carrying blood away from the heart.

8. (M) Coronary arteries: The blood vessels that supply the muscle of the heart (myocardium).

9. (A) Aorta: The largest artery in the body. It transports blood from the left ventricle to begin systemic circulation.

10. (J) Pulmonary arteries: The vessels that carry deoxygenated blood from the right ventricle of the heart to the lungs.

11. (B) Carotid arteries: The large neck arteries, one on each side of the neck, that carry blood from the heart to the head.

12. (H) Femoral artery: The major artery supplying the leg.

13. (F) Brachial artery: Major artery of the upper arm.

14. (L) Posterior tibial artery: Artery supplying the foot, behind the medial ankle.

15. (D) Dorsalis pedis artery: Artery supplying the foot, lateral to the large tendon of the big toe.

16. (I) Arteriole: The smallest kind of artery.

Part F (pp. 150–152)

1. (K) Capillary: A thin-walled, microscopic blood vessel where the oxygen/carbon dioxide and nutrient/waste exchange with the body's cells takes place.

2. (P) Venule: The smallest kind of vein.

3. (G) Vein: Any blood vessel returning blood to the heart.

4. (N) Pulmonary veins: The vessels that carry oxygenated blood from the lungs to the left atrium of the heart.

5. (C) Plasma: The fluid portion of the blood.

6. (O) Red blood cells: Components of the blood. They transport oxygen and carbon dioxide.

7. (E) White blood cells: Components of the blood. They help the body fight infection.

8. (M) Platelets: Components of the blood. These participate in the clotting of blood.

9. (A) Pulse: The rhythmic beats caused as waves of blood move through and expand arteries.

10. (J) Peripheral pulses: The radial, brachial, posterior tibial, and dorsalis pedis pulses are all examples of these.

11. (B) Central pulses: The carotid and femoral pulses, which can be felt in the central part of the body.

12. (H) Blood pressure: The pressure remaining in the arteries when the left ventricle contracts and forces blood into circulation.

13. (F) Systolic blood pressure: The pressure created in the arteries when the left ventricle contracts and forces blood into circulation.

14. (L) Diastolic blood pressure: The pressure created in the arteries when the left ventricle is refilling.

15. (D) Perfusion: The supply of oxygen to and removal of wastes from, the cells and tissue of the body as a result of the flow of blood through the capillaries.

16. (I) Hypoperfusion: Inability of the body to adequately circulate blood to the body's cells to supply them with oxygen and nutrients.

Part G (pp. 150–152)

1. (J) Nervous system: The system of brain, spinal cord, and nerves that governs sensation, movement, and thought.

2. (C) Central nervous system: The brain and spinal cord.

3. (G) Peripheral nervous system: The nerves that enter and leave the spinal cord and travel between the brain and organs without passing through the spinal cord.

©2021 Pearson Education, Inc.
Emergency Care, 14th Ed.

4. (N) Autonomic nervous system: The division of the peripheral nervous system that controls involuntary motor functions.

5. (P) Digestive system: The system by which food travels through the body and is digested, or broken down into absorbable forms.

6. (O) Stomach: The muscular sac between the esophagus and the small intestine where digestion of food begins.

7. (L) Small intestine: The muscular tube between the stomach and the large intestine, divided into the duodenum, the jejunum, and the ileum, which receives partially digested food from the stomach and continues digestion. Nutrients are absorbed by the body through its walls.

8. (M) Large intestine: The muscular tube that removes water from waste products received from the small intestine and moves anything not absorbed by the body toward excretion from the body.

9. (D) Liver: The largest internal organ of the body, which produces bile to assist in breakdown of fats and assists in the metabolism of various substances in the body.

10. (K) Gallbladder: A sac on the underside of the liver that stores bile produced by the liver.

11. (B) Pancreas: A gland located behind the stomach that produces insulin and juices that assist in digestion of food in the duodenum of the small intestine.

12. (H) Spleen: An organ located in the left upper quadrant of the abdomen that acts as a blood filtration system and a reservoir for blood.

13. (F) Appendix: A small tube located near the junction of the small and large intestines in the right quadrant of the abdomen.

14. (E) Skin: The layer of tissue between the body and the external environment.

15. (A) Epidermis: The outer layer of the skin.

16. (I) Dermis: The inner (second) layer of the skin, rich in blood vessels and nerves, found beneath the epidermis.

Part H (pp. 150–152)

1. (J) Subcutaneous layers: The layers of fat and soft tissues found below the dermis.

2. (C) Endocrine system: A system of glands that produce chemicals called hormones that help to regulate many body activities and functions.

3. (G) insulin: A hormone produced by the pancreas to help with glucose transport into cells.

4. (N) Epinephrine: A hormone produced by the body. As a medication, dilates respiratory passages and is used to relieve severe allergic reactions.

5. (I) Renal system: The body system that regulates fluid balance and the filtration of blood.

6. (O) Kidneys: Organs of the renal system that filter blood and regulate fluid levels in the body.

7. (L) Bladder: The round saclike organ of the renal system used as a reservoir for urine.

8. (M) Ureters: The tubes connecting the kidneys to the bladder.

9. (D) Urethra: The tube connecting the bladder to the vagina or penis for excretion of urine.

10. (K) Reproductive system: The body system that is responsible for human reproduction.

11. (B) Testes: The male organs of reproduction used for the production of sperm.

12. (H) Penis: The organ of male reproduction responsible for sexual intercourse and the transfer of sperm.

13. (F) Ovaries: Egg-producing organs within the female reproductive system.

14. (E) Uterus: The female organ of reproduction that is used to house the developing fetus.

15. (A) Vagina: The female organ of reproduction used for both sexual intercourse and as an exit from the uterus for the fetus.

Multiple-Choice Review

1. (C) The abdominal is not a body system. (pp. 119–122)

2. (B) The musculoskeletal system has four functions. It supports and protects the body, and forms blood cells and stores minerals. (p. 118)

3. (C) The name of the bone for the upper jaw is the maxillae. (p. 124)

4. (A) The spinal column includes the thoracic and coccyx vertebrae. (p. 124)

5. (C) An injury to the spinal cord at the cervical level may be fatal because control of the muscles of breathing arise from the spinal cord at this level. (p. 125)

6. (A) The bones in the lower extremities that he may have broken include the femur, calcaneus, and phalanges. (p. 126)

7. (A) The bones in the upper extremities include the humerus and radius. (p. 126)

8. (D) The types of muscle tissue include voluntary, involuntary, and cardiac. (p. 126)

9. (A) A patient who is walking is using voluntary muscle. (p. 126)

10. (B) involuntary (smooth) muscle is found in the blood vessels. (p. 126)

11. (B) The structure in the throat that is described as the voice box is called the larynx. (p. 127)

12. (B) A leaf-shaped valve that prevents food and foreign objects from entering the trachea during swallowing is called the epiglottis. (p. 127)

13. (C) Oxygen passes from the environment to the lungs in this order; mouth, pharynx, trachea, bronchi, alveoli. (p. 127, 129)

14. (C) When the diaphragm and intercostal muscles relax, the size of the chest cavity decreased, causing exhalation. (p. 129)

15. (D) The difference between the adult airway and the pediatric airway is that all structures are smaller and more easily obstructed in a child. (p. 129)

16. (B) The body system that is responsible for the breakdown of food into absorbable forms is called the digestive system. (p. 142)

17. (C) A hollow organ containing acidic gastric juices that begin the breakdown of food into components that the body will be able to convert to energy is the stomach. (p. 142)

18. (B) The major artery in the thigh is called the femoral. (p. 133)

19. (C) The vessel that caries oxygen-poor blood from the portions of the body below the heart and back to the right atrium is called the inferior vena cava. (p. 131, 134)

CHAPTER 6: (continued)

20. (B) The heart has a right and left side as well as upper and lower chambers. The left atrium receives blood from the pulmonary veins. (p. 131)

21. (C) The formed fluid that carries the blood cells and nutrients is called plasma. (p. 135)

22. (B) The blood component that is essential to the formation of blood clots is called platelets. (p. 135)

23. (B) The components of the blood involved in destroying microorganisms (germs) and producing antibodies are the leukocytes. (p. 135)

24. (A) The two main divisions of the nervous system are central and peripheral. (pp. 139,142)

25. (D) The nerves that carry information from throughout the body to the spinal cord and brain are sensory nerves. (p. 142)

26. (C) One of the functions of the integumentary system is to aid in temperature regulation. (p. 121, 143)

27. (C) The system that secretes hormones, such as insulin and epinephrine, and that is responsible for regulating many body activities is called the endocrine system. (p. 121, 144)

28. (C) The kidneys and ureters are structures of the renal/urinary system. (p. 122, 144)

29. (D) Fluid balance of the body and a contribution to the body's immune system are functions of the lymphatic system. (p. 120, 139)

30. (B) The organs which are part of the lymphatic system include the thymus adenoids and the spleen. (p. 139)

31. (D) As food is digested, water is removed from waste products prior to their elimination from the body by the large intestine. (p. 142)

32. (D) When epinephrine and norepinephrine are released by the adrenal gland they can cause; increased cardiac force of contraction, increased heart rate, and bronchiole dilation. (p. 144)

Complete the Following

1. List the names of nine arteries in the body. (pp. 133–134)
   - Coronary arteries
   - Aorta
   - Pulmonary artery
   - Carotid arteries
   - Femoral artery
   - Brachial artery
   - Radial artery
   - Posterior tibial artery
   - Dorsalis pedis artery

2. Four structures found in the integumentary system. (p. 121)
   - Skin
   - Hair
   - Nails
   - Sweat glands

3. List five structures in the heart's conduction system. (p. 132)
   - Sinoatrial node
   - Atrioventricular node
   - Atrioventricular bundle (bundle of His)
   - Bundle branches
   - Purkinje fibers

Pathophysiology: Recognizing Sympathetic Nervous System Response. (p. 142, 144, 130)

1. Elderly patients, females, and diabetics often have silent MIs.

2. During a stress reaction or compensation from blood loss, the brain tells the adrenal glands to secrete epinephrine and norepinephrine. The epinephrine causes increased heart rate, and the norepinephrine causes vasoconstriction in the periphery, causing an increase in blood pressure.

3. The endocrine system.

4. The cardiovascular system.

Label the Diagrams

1. Skeletal system: A. nasal bone, B. mandible, C. radius, D. patella, E. fibula, F. tibia, G. metatarsals, H. cervical vertebra, I. clavicle, J. scapula, K. humerus, L. lumbar vertebra, M. pelvis, N. phalanges, O. femur

2. Respiratory system: A. nasal cavity, N. nostrils or nares, C. epiglottis, D. larynx, E. right lung, F. pharynx, G. esophagus, H. trachea, I. rib, J. diaphragm

3. Digestive system: A. mouth, B. tongue, C. teeth, D. epiglottis, E. liver, F. gallbladder, G. appendix, H. hypopharynx/esophagus, I. stomach, J. large intestine

CHAPTER 7: Principles of Pathophysiology

Match Key Terms

1. (J) Pathophysiology: The study of how disease processes affect the function of the body. (p. 182)

2. (C) Electrolyte: A substance that, when dissolved in water, separates into charged particles. (p. 182)

3. (R) Metabolism: The cellular function of converting nutrients into energy. (p. 182)

4. (P) Aerobic metabolism: The cellular process in which oxygen is used to metabolize glucose. (p. 182)

5. (T) Anaerobic metabolism: The cellular process in which glucose is metabolized into energy without oxygen. (p. 182)

6. (O) Patent: Open and clear: free from obstruction. (p. 182)

7. (N) Tidal volume: The volume of air moved in one cycle of breathing. (p. 182)

8. (Q) Dead air space: Air that occupies the space between the mouth and alveoli but does not actually reach the area of gas exchange. (p. 182)

9. (S) Chemoreceptors: Chemical sensors in the brain and blood vessels that identify changing levels of oxygen and carbon dioxide. (p. 182)

10. (U) Plasma oncotic pressure: The pull exerted by large proteins in the plasma portion of blood that tends to pull water from the tissues into the bloodstream. (p. 182)

11. (K) Hydrostatic pressure: The pressure within a blood vessel that tends to push water out of a vessel. (p. 182)

©2021 Pearson Education, Inc.
Emergency Care, 14th Ed.

12. (B) Cardiac output: The amount of blood ejected from the heart in one minute (HR × SV). (p. 182)

13. (M) Systemic vascular resistance (SVR): The pressure in the peripheral blood vessels that the heart must overcome to pump blood in the system. (p. 182)

14. (V) V/Q match: This implies that the alveoli are supplied with enough air and that the air in the alveoli is matched with sufficient blood in the pulmonary capillaries to permit optimum exchange of oxygen and carbon dioxide. (p. 182)

15. (I) Perfusion: The supply of oxygen to and removal of wastes from the cells and tissues of the body as a result of the flow of blood through the capillaries. (p. 182)

16. (G) Dehydration: An abnormally low amount of water in the body. (p. 182)

17. (F) Edema: Swelling associated with the movement of water into the interstitial space. (p. 182)

18. (H) Hypersensitivity: An exaggerated response by the immune system to a particular substance. (p. 182)

19. (L) Stretch receptors: Sensors in the blood vessels designed to identify internal pressure. (p. 182)

20. (D) FiO_2: Fraction of inspired oxygen; the concentration of oxygen in the air we breathe. (p. 182)

21. (E) Minute volume: The amount of air breathed in during each respiration multiplied by the number of breaths per minute. (p. 182)

22. (A) Stroke volume: The amount of blood ejected from the heart in one contraction. (p. 182)

23. (Y) Hypoperfusion: The inability of the body to adequately circulate blood to the body's cells to supply them with oxygen and nutrients. (p. 182)

24. (X) Shock: The non-medical term referring to hypoperfusion. (p. 175)

25. (W) Diaphoresis: Sweating: condition of cool, pale, and moist/sweaty skin. (p. 182)

Multiple-Choice Review

1. (C) The study of how disease processes affect the function of the body is called pathophysiology. (p. 157)

2. (B) The cell structure that contains the DNA is called the nucleus. (p. 158)

3. (D) Water management by the cells of the body is important because: it influences the concentrations of electrolytes, interrupts basic cellular functions, and causes cells to dehydrate and die. (p. 159)

4. (B) When the legs are crushed under a slab of concrete, the blood supply is diminished to the cells in the legs. The condition may result in lactic acid being produced. (p. 159)

5. (A) Movement of air into and out of the chest requires a patent airway. (p. 163)

6. (C) You are assessing the ventilations of a 35-year-old female who appears to be having an asthma attack. The best assessment of the amount of air that gets into and out of the lungs each minute is the minute volume. (p. 164)

7. (D) An example of a patient whose minute volume is likely to have diminished considerably would be each of the examples listed. (p. 164)

8. (A) The respiratory control center of the brain is the medulla oblongata. (p. 165)

9. (B) Respiration is activated by changing pressure within the thorax. Inhalation is an active process, and exhalation is a passive process. (p. 165)

10. (C) The sensory information provided to the respiratory system to increase the rate and/or tidal volume originates with the chemoreceptors in the brain and vascular system. (p. 165)

11. (B) Energy for the cell is produced largely by the mitochondria, which are responsible for conversation of glucose and nutrients into ATP. (p. 158)

12. (D) Your patient is dehydrated yet also has massive edema. This is not due to hyperventilating under stress. (p. 177)

13. (B) When a patient's blood vessels constrict because of external blood loss, this process was originated by the brain because of messages received from the stretch receptors in certain blood vessels. (p. 170)

14. (B) Anaerobic metabolism is inefficient because it causes the body to expend more energy to eliminate CO_2. (p. 159)

15. (C) Patients who develop sepsis are prone to problems that affect blood vessel constriction. (p. 175)

16. (D) The average person ejects approximately 70 mL of blood per contraction of the heart. This is known as stroke volume. (p. 173)

17. (B) The more forceful the squeezing of the heart, the greater the stroke volume. This concept refers to the contractility of the heart. (p. 173)

18. (D) The patient's stroke volume depends on afterload, contractility, and preload. (p. 173)

19. (C) A 60-year-old female patient is experiencing a fight-or-flight situation, and her body is attempting to compensate by increasing her cardiac output by increasing the heart rate. (p. 173)

20. (C) When a cardiac patient has a repeat heart attack and his cardiac output drops, this is often due to a decrease in the strength of contractions. (p. 173)

21. (D) Fluid distribution is determined by the brain and kidneys regulating thirst and eliminating excess fluid, the large proteins in blood plasma pulling fluid into the bloodstream, and the permeability of both cell membranes and the walls of the capillaries helping to determine how much water can be held in and pushed out of cells and blood vessels. (p. 177)

22. (B) You are treating a 50-year-old male patient who has had severe vomiting and diarrhea for the past day. You suspect that he may have a condition called dehydration. (p. 178)

23. (D) You are assessing a patient who you suspect may be having a stroke. He has signs of neurological impairment, including inability to speak or difficulty speaking, visual or hearing disturbance, and weakness (sometimes limited to one side). (p. 179)

24. (A) An example of a condition in which glands of the body are producing too much of a hormone is Graves' disease. (p. 180)

25. (B) The most common disorder of the digestive system are diarrhea and nausea and vomiting. (p. 180)

26. (B) When the brain cells are significantly deprived of glucose a patient will develop, signs and symptoms that mimic the signs and symptoms of stroke. (p. 179)

27. (D) A 42-year-old female with a history of blood clots in her left leg suddenly developed difficulty breathing as a result of a clot moving to the lung. (p. 175)

28. (A) When a patient develops an infection that reaches the brain and spinal cord the body system most affected is the nervous system. (p. 179)

29. (B) A patient with severe nausea and vomiting due to a digestive problem can quickly become dehydrated. (p. 180)

30. (C) Endocrine disorders most commonly occur due to illness. (p. 180)

31. (D) A patient who is experiencing a new stroke might exhibit which sign? Visual disturbance (p. 179)

32. (C) When a pediatric patient experiences vasoconstriction it is a very powerful response. It can be sustained thru massive volume loss and therefore the EMT should not wait for hypotension to recognize shock. (p. 171)

33. (D) Infants and young children rely a great deal on heart rate to compensate for poor perfusion. This is because they have less contractile heart muscle cells than an adult. (p. 173)

34. (B) A clinical finding that EMTs can use to indicate poor perfusion, considered helpful in children but less reliable in adults, is capillary refill time. (p. 171)

35. (A) When assessing a pediatric patient who has fallen off a skateboard, the EMT should be especially concerned in finding an increased heartrate, which may be the earliest indicator of compensation in a young child. (p. 173)

Complete the Following

1. For the "air to go in and to go out and blood to go round and round," the system must be working. List what needs to be functioning properly. (pp. 162–163, 168)
   A. In the respiratory system: must be able to move oxygen into the lungs and carbon dioxide out of the lungs.
   B. In the cardiovascular system: must be able to move oxygenated blood to all the cells and remove deoxygenated blood from the cells.

2. A ventilation/perfusion (V/Q) match involves: (p. 174)
   A. Alveoli that are supplied with enough air
   B. Pulmonary capillaries that have sufficient blood to permit optimum exchange of oxygen and carbon dioxide.

3. Shock is commonly defined as: Inadequate perfusion. (p. 174)

4. Four groupings of shock are: (p. 175)
   • Hypovolemic shock
   • Distributive shock
   • Cardiogenic shock
   • Obstructive shock

5. Water comprises approximately 60 percent of the body's weight. How much water is in each of these three spaces? (p. 176)
   • Intracellular fluid (70 percent)—This is water that is inside the cells.
   • Intravascular fluid (5 percent)—This is water that is in the bloodstream.
   Interstitial fluid (25 percent)—This is water that can be found between cells and blood vessels.

Pathophysiology: Recognizing Compensation

On the basis of the discussion of recognizing compensation in the text, list five things that happen to the body during a fight-or-flight situation: (p. 175)

• Slight mental status changes, including anxiety and feeling of impending doom
• Increased heart rate
• Increased respiratory rate
• Delayed capillary refill time
• Pale skin that is cool
• Sweating, or diaphoretic skin that is moist to the touch

Case Study: Major Life-Threatening Bleeding Injury

1. Injured spleen due to the ULQ pain from a major high-speed collision leads you to suspect spleen injury.

2. Hypovolemic shock due to bleeding externally from the leg injury and internally from the possible ruptured spleen.

3. Nonrebreather mask, since this is major trauma and SpO_2 is 94% (or less). In the past, most patients would automatically get high-concentration oxygen. In this case, good clinical judgment suggests that it would be appropriate to give the patient high concentration oxygen due to the extensive blood loss, evolving shock, and SpO_2.

4. Ten minutes or less on the scene because of the major bleeding.

5. A slight mental status changes, increased heart rate, increased respiratory rate, delayed capillary refill, pale clammy skin, and sweating.

6. Calling ahead to the ED so that they can be ready to move the patient to surgery would be one way of getting them prepared to assess and manage and move the patient along. Good clinical judgment comes into play here and can be life-saving. Can you think of other ways of saving time with this patient? Perhaps you should discuss this with your Medical Director.

7. The blood pressure is dropping.

CHAPTER 8: Life Span Development

Match Key Terms

1. (H) Infancy: Stage of life from birth to 1 year of age. (p. 197)

2. (P) Moro reflex: A response to being startled in which the infant throws out both arms, spreads the fingers, then grabs with the fingers and arms. (p. 197)

3. (I) Palmar reflex: A grasping reflex in which an infant grabs onto a finger placed in the infant's palm. (p. 197)

4. (B) Rooting reflex: A reflex response in which a hungry infant automatically turns toward the stimulus when the cheek or one side of the mouth is touched. (p. 197)

©2021 Pearson Education, Inc.
Emergency Care, 14th Ed.

5. (A) Sucking reflex: A reflex in which stroking a hungry infant's lips causes the infant to start sucking. (p. 197)

6. (O) Bonding: The sense that needs will be met. (p. 197)

7. (J) Trust versus mistrust: Concept developed from an orderly, predictable environment versus a disorderly, irregular environment. (p. 197)

8. (M) Scaffolding: Building on what one already knows. (p. 197)

9. (C) Temperament: The infant's reaction to the infant's environment. (p. 197)

10. (D) Toddler phase: Stage of life from 12 to 36 months. (p. 197)

11. (N) Preschool age: Stage of life from 3 to 5 years. (p. 197)

12. (K) School age: Stage of life from 6 to 12 years. (p. 197)

13. (E) Adolescence: Stage of life from 13 to 18 years. (p. 197)

14. (F) Early adulthood: Stage of life from 19 to 40 years. (p. 197)

15. (L) Middle adulthood: Stage of life from 41 to 60 years. (p. 197)

16. (G) Late adulthood: Stage of life from 61 years and older. (p. 197)

Multiple-Choice Review

1. (B) Your patient is primarily a nose breather, and her head is equal to 25 percent of her total body weight. She is in the infancy age group. (p. 186)

2. (C) You are assessing an infant who is very congested. Why can nasal congestion be a major problem in the first few months of life? Because children of this age are primarily nasal breathers. (p. 186)

3. (D) Infants get their immunity and antibodies from: breastfeeding from their mother, the vaccinations they receive, and producing their own antibodies from exposure to diseases. (p. 186)

4. (A) You are evaluating an infant whose mother states that the infant "has been very sleepy all day." The Cushing reflex is a nervous system reflex that is not normally found in an infant. (pp. 186–187)

5. (B) When the mother strokes the infant's lips and the baby starts sucking, this is a nervous system reflex known as the sucking reflex. (p. 187)

6. (B) A mother states that her baby daughter is developing her reactions to the environment. This is also known as the psychosocial characteristic of temperament. (p. 188)

7. (A) When an infant develops anxiety and insecurity, this is often due to the psychosocial characteristic of trust versus mistrust. (p. 188)

8. (C) A toddler has continuing developments and changes from infancy. Examples include each of the following except that the toddler is less susceptible to illness. The toddler is actually *more* susceptible because of no longer having immunity from the mother. (p. 189)

9. (A) The adolescent years often include the beginning of self-destructive behaviors. (p. 193)

10. (B) The peak physical condition occurs between the ages of 19 and 26. (p. 193)

11. (D) According to your understanding of typical activities of different age groups, her most likely age group is middle adulthood. (p. 194)

12. (D) Some examples of the psychosocial challenges that a person in late adulthood face include financial burdens, self-worth, and living environment. (p. 196)

13. (D) How might the age of a patient affect your assessment? The parent or caregiver will need to help you when you assess an infant. The patient who is in late adulthood is likely to have cardiovascular disorders, and the adolescent often experiments with alcohol and tobacco. (pp. 187–197)

14. (C) An EMT's ability to communicate with a patient can be complicated by each of the following except separation anxiety. (p. 192)

15. (B) During the adolescent years of development, both males and females reach reproductive maturity. (p. 193)

16. (B) Girls are usually finished growing by the age of 16. (p. 193)

17. (C) Boys are usually finished growing by the age of 18. (p. 193)

18. (B) Serious family conflicts occur in some adolescents as the child strives for independence and the parents strive for control. (p. 193)

19. (C) The leading cause of death in the early adulthood age group is/are accidents. (p. 193)

20. (D) The highest levels of job stress occur in the early adult age group. (p. 193)

Complete the Following

1. List the eight stages of life discussed in the textbook. (p. 185)
- Infancy
- Toddler phase
- Preschool age
- School age
- Adolescence
- Early adulthood
- Middle adulthood
- Late adulthood

2. Many changes occur during the first months of life. List a developmental characteristic for each of the following month in the child's first year: (p. 188)
- 2 months – tracks objects with eyes & recognizes familiar faces.
- 3 months – moves objects to mouth with hands & distinct facial expressions.
- 4 months – drools without swallowing & begins to reach out to people.
- 5 months – sleeps through the night without waking for feeding & discriminates between family and strangers.
- 6 months – sits upright in high chair & begins making one syllable sounds.
- 7 months – exhibits fear of strangers & moods shift quickly.
- 8 months – begins responding to the word no & can sit alone & can play peek-a-boo.
- 9 months – responds to adult anger & pulls self up to standing position & explores objects by mouthing, sucking, chewing, and biting.
- 10 months – pays attention to own name & crawls well.
- 11 months – attempts to walk without assistance & begins to show frustration about restrictions.
- 12 months – walks with help & knows own name.

3. What would the normal pulse rate be for each of the following age groups?
   - Newborn: 100–170 (p. 187)
   - Infant: 90–160 (p. 187)
   - Toddler: 80–140 (p. 189)
   - Preschooler: 70–120 (p. 191)
   - School age: 65–120 (p. 192)
   - Adolescence: 60–100 (p. 193)
   - Early adulthood: 60–100 (p. 193)

4. List four psychosocial changes in the early adulthood years: (p. 193)
   - Highest levels of job stress
   - Love develops, both romantic and affectionate
   - Childbirth is most common in this group
   - Accidents are leading cause of death

CHAPTER 9: Airway Management

Match Key Terms

1. (E) Airway: The passageway by which air enters or leaves the body. The structures of the airway are the nose, mouth, pharynx, larynx, trachea, bronchi and lungs. (p. 234)

2. (C) Patent airway: An airway that is open and clear to the passage of air into and out of the body. (p. 234)

3. (F) A means of correcting blockage of the airway by the tongue by tilting the head back and lifting the chin. Used when no trauma, or injury, is suspected. (p. 234)

4. (A) Jaw-thrust maneuver: A means of correcting blockage of the airway by moving the jaw forward without tilting the head or neck used when trauma, or injury, is suspected. To open the airway without causing further injury to the spinal cord in the neck. (p. 234)

5. (B) Oropharyngeal airway: A curved device inserted through the patient's mouth into the pharynx to help maintain an open airway. (p. 234)

6. (H) Nasopharyngeal airway: A flexible device inserted through the patient's nostril into the pharynx to help maintain an open airway. (p. 234)

7. (D) Gag reflex: Vomiting or retching that results when something is placed in the back of the pharynx. This is tied to the swallow reflex. (p. 234)

8. (G) Suctioning: Use of a vacuum device to remove blood, vomitus, and other secretions or foreign materials from the airway. (p. 234)

9. (K) Bronchoconstriction: The contraction of smooth muscle that lines the bronchial passages that result in a decreased internal diameter of the airway and increased resistance to flow. (p. 234)

10. (J) Stridor: A high-pitched inspiratory sound generated from partially obstructed airflow in the upper airway. (p. 234)

11. (I) Glottic opening: the space between the vocal cords that defines the boundary between the upper and lower airways.

Multiple-Choice Review

1. (C) The movement of air into and out of the lungs requires that airflow is unobstructed and moving freely. (p. 203)

2. (C) When a patient inhales, air enters the body and finally travels through the laryngopharynx prior to entering the trachea. (p. 203)

3. (B) The hypopharynx is also called the laryngopharynx. (p. 203)

4. (C) The large leaflike structure that protects the opening to the trachea is called the epiglottis. (p. 203)

5. (B) When we say that a patient is experiencing lower airway obstruction, it is likely that the patient's bronchial passages or alveoli are congested. (p. 205)

6. (B) You believe that your patient is exhibiting signs of an inadequate airway. These signs will include all of the following except air that can be felt at the nose or mouth on expiration. (p. 209)

7. (D) When inserting an OPA into a pediatric patient insert it straight in, do not rotate or flip over the tongue, and consider using a tongue depressor. (p. 220)

8. (C) If the choking infant becomes unconscious you should begin CPR. (p. 216)

9. (B) if a conscious infant is choking severely, you must intervene with backslaps and chest thrusts. (p. 215)

10. (C) One indication that a child is experiencing labored breathing is that she has nasal flaring when she breathes. (p. 208)

11. (C) The optimal airway position in unresponsive infants and children can be achieved by aligning the patient's ear to the level of the suprasternal notch. (p. 212)

12. (B) You are about to manage the airway of a 22-year-old male who fell face down a flight of stairs. What is the importance of mechanism of injury to airway care? The procedure for opening the patient's airway is different in trauma. Trauma victims may require the jaw-thrust maneuver instead of the head-elevated, sniffing position to open the airway safely and prevent potential spinal cord injury. (pp. 210–212)

13. (A) Your patient has sustained a high-energy impact to the head and neck. To open the airway of a patient with a suspected head, neck, or spine injury, the EMT should use a jaw-thrust maneuver. (p. 213)

14. (B) You are deciding which airway adjunct to use to assist in keeping open the airway of a 30-year-old female who you suspect has sustained a basilar skull fracture. You note clear fluid running out of her ears. It is best to choose an OPA if she has no gag reflex. (p. 217)

15. (D) When performing the jaw-thrust maneuver, the EMT should do each one of the following except tilting the head by applying gentle pressure to the patient's forehead. (p. 214)

16. (B) The main purpose of the jaw-thrust maneuver is to open the airway without moving the head or neck. (pp. 213–214)

17. (C) An oral or nasal airway should be used to help keep an airway open. (p. 217)

18. (C) it is always important to be careful when inserting an OPA. If something is placed in the patient's throat, the gag reflex may cause the patient to vomit or retch. (p. 217)

19. (A) An OPA of proper size extends from the corner of the patient's mouth to the tip of the earlobe. (p. 217)

20. (A) In an adult patient an OPA should be inserted upside down, with the tip toward the roof of the mouth, then flipped 180 degrees over the tongue. (p. 218)

21. (B) A nasopharyngeal airway should be measured from the patient's nostril to the tip of the earlobe or angle of the jaw. (p. 221)

22. (D) To assist in airway maintenance, you have decided to use a nasopharyngeal airway. When inserting an NPA, lubricate the outside of the tube with a water-based lubricant. Petroleum-based lubricants can damage tissue and increase risk of infection. (p. 221)

23. (C) Your service requires that you bring the suction unit on all priority calls where you might need to use it. The purposes of suctioning may include removal of blood, vomitus, and other secretions. (p. 227)

24. (A) When a patient begins to vomit or produce a gurgling sound, it is essential that you have a suction unit ready to go at the patient's side. (p. 227)

25. (C) Which is not true of the Yankauer suction tip? It is not true that the Yankauer is used most successfully with responsive patients. (p. 230)

26. (D) Compared to an adult's airway structures, the pediatric patient's respiratory system includes a narrower trachea, a softer and more flexible trachea, and a smaller mouth and nose. (p. 205)

27. (B) Why is nasal obstruction a more urgent problem in an infant as opposed to an adult? Infants and newborns typically breathe through their noses. (p. 205)

28. (B) Lying a small child, with altered mental status, flat can be problematic because flexion of the neck can cause airway obstruction. (p. 212)

29. (D) Suctioning in pediatric patients is not very different than suctioning in adults. Both rigid and flexible suction catheters have appropriate pediatric sizes. The difference is time stimulating the hypopharynx should be minimized, and infants are very sensitive to vagal stimulation, and bulb syringes are used in the emergency childbirth setting. (p. 230)

30. (D) Some patients will benefit from a supraglottic airway. They should be considered when proper positioning will not work, the patient does not have a gag reflex, and basic airway management measures have failed. (p. 223)

31. (C) In the supine position an optimal airway position can be achieved by creating a head elevated, sniffing position. (p. 211)

32. (B) The slowing of the pulse is most-likely due to vagal stimulation caused by the catheter contacting the hypopharynx of the child. (p. 230)

33. (D) Compared to an adult's airway physiology, the pediatric airway includes more dependency on the diaphragm for breathing, a chest wall that is softer, and a tongue that takes up more space proportionally in the child's mouth than in the adult's. (p. 205)

Pathophysiology: Sounds of a Partially Obstructed Airway (p. 207)

1. Stridor

2. Hoarseness

3. Snoring

4. Gurgling

Complete the Following

1. List eight signs of an inadequate airway in adults and/or pediatric patients. (p. 209)
   • There are no signs of breathing or air movement.

• There is evidence of foreign bodies in the airway, including blood, vomit, or objects such as broken teeth.
• No air can be felt or heard at the nose or mouth, or the amount of air exchanged is below normal.
• The patient is unable to speak or has great difficulty speaking.
• The patient's voice has an unusual hoarse or raspy quality.
• Chest movements are absent, minimal, or uneven (be aware, however, that patients can have chest movement even with an obstructed airway.)
• Movement associated with breathing is limited to the abdomen (abdominal breathing).
• Breath sounds are diminished or absent.
• Noises such as wheezing, stridor, snoring, gurgling, or gasping are heard during breathing.
• In children, there may be retractions (a pulling in of the muscles) above the clavicles and between and below the ribs.
• Nasal flaring (widening of the nostrils of the nose with respirations) may be present, especially in infants and children.

2. List six general rules for the use of OPAs and NPAs. (p. 217)
   • Use an OPA only on patients who do not exhibit a gag reflex. A patient with a gag reflex who cannot tolerate an OPA may be able to tolerate an NPA.
   • Open the patient's airway manually before using an adjunct device.
   • When inserting the airway, take care not to push the patient's tongue into the pharynx.
   • Have suction ready prior to inserting any airway.
   • Do not continue inserting the airway if the patient begins to gag.
   • When an airway adjunct is in place, you must maintain the head-tilt, chin-lift maneuver or jaw-thrust maneuver and monitor the airway.
   • After an airway adjunct is in place, continue to be ready to provide suction if fluid such as vomitus or blood obstructs the airway.
   • If the patient regains consciousness or develops a gag reflex, remove the airway immediately.
   • Use infection-control practices while maintaining the airway. Wear disposable gloves, a mask and goggles or other protective eyewear to prevent body fluid contact.

3. Complete this chart. (p. 208)
   Look.
   • Visually, inspect the airway to ensure it is free from foreign bodies and obvious trauma.
   • Look for visual clues of potential airway dangers such as facial burns, external neck trauma, and bleeding in and around the mouth and nose.
   • Look for visual signs of breathing such as the chest rising.
   • Look at the patient's position. Does the patient need to sit bolt upright to keep breathing?

   Listen.
   • Listen for the sound of breathing.
   • Listen for sounds of obstructed air movement such as stridor, gurgling, and gasping.

   Feel.
   • Feel for air movement at the mouth.
   • Feel the chest for rise and fall.

Will the airway stay open?
- Are there immediate correctable threats?
- If no airway, then open it.
- Consider how you might keep an unstable airway open.
- Consider ALS for more definitive airway care.

Are there potential threats that may develop later?
- Reassess, reassess, reassess.
- Assess for signs of impending collapse such as stridor or voice changes.
- Consider conditions that may later threaten the airway (such as anaphylaxis).
- Consider the patient's mental status. Can the patient maintain and protect the airway? Will that mental status likely change over time?

Case Study: Rapidly Changing Airway

1. The patient most likely has a partial lower airway obstruction. At this point, you do not have a lot of information, but your clinical instincts tell you that it is likely lower airway. Do not put the blinders on; continue to evaluate for upper airway too (i.e. swelling in airway or an obstruction). The patient is still moving air, but the wheezing is caused by air being forced through her narrowed bronchioles.

2. The short, choppy sentences are an indication of severe shortness of breath or respiratory distress.

3. If she loses consciousness, insert an OPA as long as she does not have a gag reflex.

4. This is a medical patient, and you have no evidence of head or neck trauma, so use the head-tilt, chin-lift to position the airway.

5. The most common reason patients make a snoring noise is partial obstruction of the tongue in the back of the throat. Reposition her airway so that it is open all the way, and the snoring should cease.

6. Gurgling sounds in the airway are usually due to fluid. Roll her to the side, scoop out any large particles, and then remove the fluid by suctioning out her airway.

7. The fact that the wheezing is getting quieter without the assistance of a bronchodilator treatment is not a good sign. It is likely that the patient is not moving enough air to create the wheezing sound. Use your clinical judgment here to make the decision that you will need to take over ventilations for this patient. Discuss this case and how to handle it with your Medical Director.

CHAPTER 10: Respiration and Artificial Ventilation

Match Key Terms

Part A

1. (I) Ventilation: Breathing in and out (inhalation and exhalation), or artificial provision of breaths). (p. 286)

2. (J) Alveolar ventilation: The amount of air that reaches the alveoli during inhalation. (p. 286)

3. (B) Diffusion: A process by which molecules move from an area of high concentration to an area of low concentration. (p. 286)

4. (N) Pulmonary respiration: The exchange of oxygen and carbon dioxide between the alveoli and circulating blood in the pulmonary capillaries. (p. 286)

5. (G) Cellular respiration: The exchange of oxygen and carbon dioxide between cells and circulating blood. (p. 286)

6. (K) Respiration: The diffusion of oxygen and carbon dioxide between the alveoli and the blood and between the blood and the cells. (p. 286)

7. (M) Hypoxia: An insufficiency of oxygen in the body's tissues. (p. 286)

8. (D) Respiratory distress: Increased work of breathing: a sensation of shortness of breath. (p. 286)

9. (L) Respiratory failure: The reduction of breathing to the point at which oxygen intake is not sufficient to support life. (p. 286)

10. (E) Respiratory arrest: When breathing completely stops. (p. 286)

11. (H) Cyanosis: A blue or gray color resulting from lack of oxygen in the body. (p. 286)

12. (F) Artificial ventilation: Forcing air or oxygen into the lungs when a patient has stopped breathing or has inadequate breathing. (p. 286)

13. (C) Positive pressure ventilation: The process of forcing air and/or oxygen into the lungs when breathing has stopped. (p. 286)

14. (A) Pocket face mask: A device, usually with a one-way valve, to aid in artificial ventilation. It also acts as a barrier to prevent contact with a patient's breath or body fluids. (p. 286)

Part B

1. (I) Bag-valve mask (BVM): A handheld device with a face mask and self-filling bag that can be squeezed to provide artificial ventilations to a patient. (p. 286)

2. (C) Venturi mask: A face mask that delivers very specific concentrations of oxygen by mixing oxygen with inhaled air. (p. 286)

3. (B) Stoma: A permanent surgical opening in the neck through which the patient breathes. (p. 286)

4. (A) Tracheostomy mask: A device designed to be placed over a stoma or tracheostomy tube to provide supplemental oxygen. (p. 286)

5. (G) Automatic transport ventilator (ATV): A device that provides positive pressure ventilations. It includes settings designed to adjust ventilation rate and volume, is portable, and is easily carried on an ambulance. (p. 286)

6. (J) Oxygen cylinder: A cylinder filled with oxygen under pressure. (p. 286)

7. (L) Pressure regulator: A device connected to an oxygen cylinder to reduce cylinder pressure so that it is safe for delivery of oxygen to a patient. (p. 286)

8. (D) Flowmeter: A valve that indicates the flow of oxygen in liters per minute. (p. 286)

9. (K) Humidifier: A device connected to the flowmeter to add moisture to the dry oxygen coming from an oxygen cylinder. (p. 286)

10. (E) Nonrebreather (NRB) mask: A face mask and reservoir bag device that delivers high concentrations of oxygen. The patient's exhaled air escapes through a valve and is not rebreathed. (p. 286)

©2021 Pearson Education, Inc.
Emergency Care, 14th Ed.

11. (H) Nasal cannula: A device that delivers low concentrations of oxygen through two prongs that rest in the patient's nostrils. (p. 286)

12. (F) Partial rebreather mask: A face mask and reservoir oxygen bag with no flutter valves on the mask, allowing the patient to breath in atmospheric air along with oxygen. (p. 286)

Multiple-Choice Review

1. (D) During the process of ventilation the diaphragm and chest muscles contract and relax to change the pressure in the chest. (p. 239)

2. (B) Respiratory failure is inadequacy of breathing with insufficient oxygen intake. (p. 243)

3. (C) You are assessing a 45-year-old female who called the ambulance because she was having difficulty breathing. Severely diminished breath sounds upon auscultation of the lungs. (p. 245)

4. (D) You are assessing a 6-year-old male who is having difficulty breathing. Signs of inadequate breathing may include cyanotic skin, lips, tongue, or earlobes, retractions between and below the ribs, and nasal flaring. (p. 249)

5. (B) Each of the following is a sign of labored breathing in an adult patient except breathing rate in an adult of 14 to 18 breaths per minute. (p. 245)

6. (B) You are treating a patient who has signs of inadequate breathing. These signs could include all of the following except air that can be felt at the nose or mouth on exhalation. (p. 245)

7. (D) Inadequate breathing in a child (4 years old) is defined as: fewer than 12 per minute, more than 36 per minute, or cyanosis of the lips and earlobes. (pp. 248–249)

8. (A) Which of the following is a difference in signs between respiratory distress and respiratory failure? A patient with respiratory failure has cyanotic or gray skin color. (p. 245)

9. (D) Your patient may be becoming cyanotic. You check for cyanosis by observing the patient's lips and tongue, nail beds, and earlobes. (p. 249)

10. (C) One indication that a patient is experiencing inadequate breathing is that she talks in short, choppy sentences. (p. 249)

11. (B) When the diffusion of oxygen and carbon dioxide takes place between the cells and circulating blood this accomplishes cellular respiration. (p. 241)

12. (B) This medicine has been known to depress respirations and lead to hypoxia. (p. 250)

13. (B) The normal, or adequate, breathing rate for a 50-year-old adult should be 12 to 20 breaths per minute. (p. 248)

14. (D) When the EMT determines that the patient is not breathing or that breathing is inadequate, it is necessary to provide positive pressure ventilation, artificial ventilation, or assistance with a BVM device. (p. 245, 251)

15. (A) The negative side effects of positive pressure ventilation include each of the following except hypothermia. (p. 251)

16. (B) Your partner states that you should be careful not to hyperventilate the patient because is causes vasoconstriction and limited blood flow to the brain. (p. 251)

17. (A) Given plenty of trained helpers, which would be least effective? One rescuer using a bag-valve mask. (p. 252, 260)

18. (A) Which of the following indicates you are ventilating the patient adequately? The patient's chest rises and falls with each ventilation. (p. 252)

19. (C) If an adult has a tidal volume of 500 mL and is breathing 12 times a minute, what would be the alveolar ventilation per minute? (500 – 150 dead space = 350 × 12 = 4,200 mL per minute). (p. 239)

20. (B) The adult sized bag-valve mask on your EMS unit should have a non-jam valve with an oxygen inlet. (p. 259)

21. (A) The bag-valve mask should be capable of withstanding cold temperatures. (p. 259)

22. (D) In ventilating a 35-year-old male head trauma patient with a bag-valve mask, it is most effective to do all of the following except maintain the head-tilt, chin-lift maneuver. (p. 260)

23. (D) In ventilating a 22-year-old unconscious female, a bag-valve mask should be used with a reservoir bag, an oral airway, and an oxygen tank and liter flow regulator. (p. 259)

24. (D) If the patient's chest does not rise and fall during ventilation using a bag-valve mask, the EMT should do all of the following except increase the rate at which the bag is squeezed. (p. 262)

25. (C) If the patient has a stoma and needs ventilatory assistance, the best device to use is a bag-valve mask. (p. 262)

26. (D) When you question an elderly woman with a respiratory complaint, she speaks in short, two- or three-word sentences. Is this significant? Yes, she is probably very short of breath. (p. 249)

27. (B) A prehospital modality of therapy for treating patients with inadequate breathing and respiratory distress that assists with ventilations of a breathing patient is a BVM device. (p. 278)

28. (B) When prolonged ventilations need to be done on a patient and there is only one EMT on the airway, you should consider using a/an automatic transport ventilator. (p. 264)

29. (C) A fully pressurized portable oxygen tankshould have approximately 2,000 psi. (p. 265)

30. (B) Which portable oxygen cylinder, when full, lasts the longest when delivering oxygen? The "E" tank. (pp. 265–266)

31. (B) Before connecting a regulator to an oxygen supply cylinder, the EMT should crack the main valve for one second. (p. 271)

32. (C) Humidified oxygen is not needed in adult patients who are being transported for short distances. (p. 269)

33. (A) Concerns about the dangers of giving too much oxygen to patients with chronic COPD are invalid in the out-of-hospital setting when clinically appropriate to administer. (p. 270)

34. (D) Your patient may be having a heart attack. He is in moderate distress and his SpO_2 is 92%. The best method for you to use when giving a high concentration of oxygen to this breathing patient is a nonrebreather mask. (p. 275)

35. (D) The oxygen concentration of a nonrebreather mask is between 80% and 90%. (p. 275)

36. (B) The flow rate of a nonrebreather mask should be 12 to 15 liters per minute. (p. 275)

37. (C) The oxygen concentration of a nasal cannula is between 24% and 44%. (p. 275)

38. (B) You are treating a 68-year-old female who fell and injured her ribs. She was found breathing at a rate of 44 and shallowly, yet she is starting to turn cyanotic. Why is this a serious threat to her life? Her minute volume may be diminished. (p. 244)

39. (D) What is meant by anatomical dead space? The area in the lungs that does not participate in gas exchange. (p. 239, 240)

40. (B) What is the most important consideration in assessing and managing the breathing of a child? Children consume oxygen at a higher rate than adults do. (p. 280)

Complete the Following

1. To determine the signs of adequate breathing, the EMT should: (p. 248)
- Look for adequate and equal expansion of both sides of the chest when the patient inhales.
- Listen for air entering and leaving the nose, mouth, and chest.
- Feel for air moving out of the nose or mouth.
- Check for typical skin coloration.
- Note the rate, rhythm, quality, and depth of breathing typical for a person at rest.

2. The signs of inadequate breathing include the following: (pp. 248–249)
- Altered mental status
- Chest movements are absent, minimal, or uneven.
- Slow pulse rate in infants and children.
- Movement associated with breathing is limited to the abdomen or, especially in children, is exaggerated in alternating rise and fall of the chest and the abdomen.
- No air can be felt or heard at the nose or mouth, or the amount of air exchanged is below normal.
- Breath sounds are diminished or absent.
- Noises such as wheezing, crowing, stridor, snoring, gurgling, or gasping are heard during breathing.
- Rate of breathing is too rapid or too slow.
- Breathing is very shallow, very deep, or appears labored.
- The patient's skin, lips, tongue, ear lobes, or nail beds are blue or gray.
- Inspirations are prolonged or expirations are prolonged.
- Patient is unable to speak, or the patient cannot speak full sentences because of shortness of breath.
- In children, there may be retractions above the clavicles and between and below the ribs.
- Nasal flaring may be present, especially in pediatrics.
- Low oxygen saturation reading (<95%).
- Body position changes such as tripod position.

3. List three mechanical failures of the cardiopulmonary system and two examples of each: (pp. 241–242)
- Mechanics of breathing disrupted – patient stabbed in the chest, a patient loses nervous system control of respiration, a patient sustains chest wall injuries, a patient has airway problems such as bronchoconstriction.
- Gas exchange interrupted – low oxygen levels in the outside air, diffusion problems.
- Circulation issues – not enough blood, hemoglobin problems

Pathophysiology: Respiratory Distress to Respiratory Failure (pp. 244, 247–248)

1. The respiratory rate will increase.

2. The blood vessels in the arms and legs will constrict.

3. The wheezes are due to bronchoconstriction and air being forced through narrowed passageways.

4. The patient often becomes anxious because of hypoxia of the brain.

5. When the patient gets tired, the chest muscles might no longer support the effort of breathing and this may be pre-respiratory arrest. This is never a good sign.

Case Study: Complicated Airway: The Self-Inflicted Shooting

1. Open the airway by jutting the jaw and pulling the tongue forward out of the throat. This is easy to say but may be difficult to do depending on how much of the jaw is intact. Use your best clinical judgment here. You need to be aggressive to make sure this patient can breathe and does not drown in his own blood. This is a good example of a situation to discuss with your Medical Director!

2. Yes, the patient needs to be suctioned.

3. Yes, an oral airway would be helpful to this patient.

4. A bag-valve mask should be used to assist this patient's ventilations. Of course, you should use your best clinical judgment, as he needs adequate oxygenation and ventilation but you do not want to cause him to aspirate on his own blood. This would be a good situation to discuss with your Medical Director.

5. Use 12 to 15 liters per minute. CPAP would not be appropriate for this patient, owing to poor seal, side effects of hypotension in an already bleeding patient, and potential for vomiting.

6. A full D tank contains about 350 liters and has a pressure of 2,000 to 2,200 pounds per square inch (psi).

7. It takes about 19 to 20 minutes to run the tank down to 200 psi (which is 10 percent left in the tank). Let's say that the full tank contains 350 liters. By subtracting 10 percent (350 − 35 = 315) and then dividing 315 by 15 liters per minute, you are left with 21. To be on the safe side, round down 1 minute because you never know for sure that the tank actually had every bit of the 2,200 psi when you began.

8. Do not exceed 15 seconds. You are removing oxygen when you suction the patient. A rigid Yankauer suction tip is most appropriate in this patient.

9. This patient is a high priority. His complicated airway is the major problem, making him a priority patient. He should be transported right away to a trauma center if there is one in your region.

10. ALS may be helpful for fluid infusion en route to the hospital, advanced airway procedures, and more trained hands to manage the patient.

11. If you heard bubbling around the mask, suction and reassess your mask seal.

Interim Exam 1

1. (C) Most EMT training programs today are based on standards developed by the National Highway Traffic Safety Administration (NHTSA). The American Red Cross (ARC)

©2021 Pearson Education, Inc.
Emergency Care, 14th Ed.

is involved in disaster relief and in basic first aid and CPR training. The American Heart Association (AHA) is involved in basic and advanced life support training as well as cardiovascular research. The National Institutes of Health (NIH) provides grants for health research. (p. 4)

2. (D) Being pleasant, cooperative, sincere, and a good listener. Do not put patient safety above your own, and do not lie to the patient by saying that everything is all right when it is not. (pp. 10–11)

3. (C) Negligence is (1) a failure to act properly in a situation in which there was a duty to act, (2) needed care as would reasonably be expected of the EMT was not provided, and (3) harm was caused to the patient as a result. Abandonment means that you left the patient in no one's care. (p. 90)

4. (D) To refuse care or transport, a patient must be mentally competent, oriented fully, and informed of potential consequences of refusing care. Document the refusal on a release form. (p. 84)

5. (B) In the case of an unconscious patient, consent may be assumed. This is known as implied consent. *Triage* is a French word that means "to sort." Immunity is a protection from liability. (p. 83)

6. (D) Even though the child's injury is not described as life threatening, parental consent is still required. A minor cannot give expressed consent. Only life-threatening situations involve implied consent. (p. 83)

7. (C) Good Samaritan laws, which many states have, grant immunity from liability to off-duty rescuers who act in good faith to provide care to the level of their training. (p. 92)

8. (B) The form of infection control based on the presumption that all body fluids are infectious is called Standard Precautions. (p. 25)

9. (C) Shoulder drags and fireman's carries are urgent moves. A nonurgent move should be used on patients without immediate life threats. (p. 59)

10. (C) Use the leg muscles. Do not twist or use your back muscles while lifting; both actions may cause injury. Keep communicating with your partner. (p. 56)

11. (C) Keep your arms bent, not fully straight, when pushing or pulling objects. (p. 58)

12. (D) The preferred carrying device to move patients out of vehicles is a long spine board. (p. 68)

13. (B) This is an extremity lift. The draw-sheet method involves a sheet. The direct ground lift requires lifting the patient from a supine position onto the rescuer's knees and then to the stretcher. The direct carry involves two rescuers lifting and curling the patient into their chests, returning to a standing position, and then walking together with the patient. (p. 71)

14. (B) When managing the airway of an infant padding should be placed under the shoulders to achieve a neutral airway. (p. 212)

15. (A) The vena cava returns blood to the right atrium of the heart. (p. 130)

16. (A) The coronary arteries supply the heart with blood. (p. 133)

17. (B) To control the patient's airway and bleeding, use an urgent move, the rapid extrication procedure. Taking time to apply a short backboard may cause a deadly delay in removing the patient. (p. 59)

18. (B) The red blood cells carry oxygen to the body cells and carry carbon dioxide away from the body cells. (p. 135)

19. (C) Inadequate circulation of blood through the body is shock (hypoperfusion). (p. 136)

20. (D) The lymphatic system helps to maintain the body's immune system and fluid balance. (p. 139)

21. (B) The liver is a large solid organ located in the upper right and left quadrants. (p. 110)

22. (D) Proper personal protective equipment can prevent injuries to you and your crew, and an injured EMT is of little help to the patient. (p. 25)

23. (A) When a threat presents itself, retreat to a safe area. (p. 50)

24. (B) Eustress is positive stress. Distress is negative, can be cumulative, and may require a critical incident debriefing. (p. 42)

25. (C) In responding to a violent situation, observation begins when you enter the neighborhood or immediate area of the scene. (p. 49)

26. (B) Crew members should always carry a portable radio to enable them to call for police assistance if necessary. (p. 49)

27. (B) Quickly control bleeding. Then have the dog secured in another room so that it doesn't try to protect its owner by attacking you or just get in the way of your work. (p. 50)

28. (B) An advance directive is the expressed wishes of the patient in writing. If one of these documents is signed and at the patient's side, it can simplify resuscitation situations. (p. 87)

29. (D) Providing care within the scope of your practice, using proper documentation, and being courteous and respectful can prevent lawsuits. (p. 81, 91, 99)

30. (D) The skin in conjunction with the nervous and vascular system, not the musculoskeletal system, regulates body temperature. The musculoskeletal system gives the body shape, protects internal organs, and provides for body movement. (p. 118)

31. (C) The superior portion of the sternum is called the manubrium. (p. 125)

32. (B) The protrusion on the inside of the ankle is called the medial malleolus. The lateral malleolus is on the outside of the ankle. (pp. 125–126)

33. (B) Automaticity is the ability of the heart to generate and conduct electrical impulses on its own. (p. 126)

34. (A) The autonomic nervous system, a division of the peripheral nervous system, controls involuntary motor functions. (p. 142)

35. (B) The anatomic position is a standard reference position for the body in which the body is standing erect, facing the observer. The arms are down at the sides, and the palms of the hands are facing forward. (p. 107)

36. (D) Plantar refers to the sole of the foot. (p. 110)

37. (C) The zygomatic bones are the cheekbones. (p. 124)

38. (B) Knees are proximal, or closer to the torso, compared to the toes. The toes are distal, or farther away from the torso, compared to the knees. (p. 109)

CHAPTER 10: (continued)

39. (C) Supine means lying on the back. Prone means lying face down. (p. 111)

40. (C) The abdomen is divided into four parts, or quadrants. (p. 110)

41. (A) The torso consists of the abdomen, pelvis, and thorax. (p. 108)

42. (C) The structure that divides the chest from the abdominal cavity is the diaphragm. (p. 129)

43. (C) The kneecap is the patella. The ilium is a pelvic bone, the malleolus is in the ankle, and the phalanges are fingers and toes. (p. 123)

44. (C) The cranium is the skull minus the facial bones, that is, the top, back and sides. (p. 118)

45. (A) The acromion process of the scapula is the highest portion of the shoulder. (p. 126)

46. (B) Unconsciousness in adults or children allows implied consent, thus allowing for care to begin. (p. 83)

47. (C) For negligence, three actions must be proved: The EMT had a duty to act, the EMT breached that duty, and this breach of duty caused physical or psychological harm to the patient. (p. 90)

48. (C) Patients who are dying over a period of time go through the following stages, though not necessarily in this order: denial, anger, bargaining, depression, and then acceptance. (p. 45)

49. (B) The National Registry of EMTs was founded in 1970 to establish professional standards. (p. 4)

50. (B) Quality improvement is a continuous self-review of the EMS system or service. (p. 13)

51. (B) The Medical Director assumes the ultimate responsibility for the patient-care aspects of the EMS system. (p. 5)

52. (A) A common cause of lawsuits against EMS agencies is patients who refuse care. (p. 84)

53. (D) The scope of practice defines the legal limits of the EMT's job skills. (p. 81)

54. (A) Decisiveness is not a sign of stress. (p. 42)

55. (D) Most motor vehicle collisions do not result in excessive stress reactions. (p. 41)

56. (B) Increasing consumption of fatty foods is the wrong reaction to stress. (p. 24)

57. (D) The integumentary system protects the body from the environment, bacteria, and other organisms. (p. 143)

58. (C) After a major EMS incident, stress is normal and expected. (p. 40)

59. (B) The five stages of grief include a stage in which the patient may retreat to a world of his or her own. This stage is called depression. (p. 45)

60. (B) A crushing injury causes anaerobic metabolism and will increase the production of lactic acids at the cellular level. (pp. 159–160)

61. (C) A disease that is spread by exposure to an open wound or sore of an infected individual may be caused by a bloodborne pathogen. (p. 25)

62. (D) Hepatitis is an infection that causes inflammation of the liver. (p. 31)

63. (C) Airborne diseases are spread by inhaling or absorbing droplets from the air through the eyes, nose, or mouth. (p. 31)

64. (D) The hepatitis B virus kills approximately 200 health workers every year in the United States. (p. 31)

65. (B) For safety, assume that a patient with a productive cough has tuberculosis and take the necessary precautions. (p. 32)

66. (D) HIV is not an airborne disease; it is spread by blood, semen, and other body fluids. (p. 32)

67. (A) There is less than a 0.5% (less than half of one percent) chance of contracting HIV from an infected needle. (p. 32)

68. (C) To protect yourself from TB, take Standard Precautions and wear a HEPA or N-95 respirator. A surgeon's mask will not protect you from this airborne disease. (p. 30)

69. (A) Use a pocket mask with one-way valve when you are confronted with a nonbreathing patient and you are alone. The bag-valve mask needs two rescuers to be used effectively. (p. 261)

70. (B) The Ryan White CARE Act establishes procedures for emergency response workers to find out whether they have been exposed to life-threatening infectious diseases. OSHA does not require this. There is no such thing as the AIDS protection act. (pp. 34–35)

71. (A) OSHA 1910.1030 requires an exposure control plan and annual training. (p. 34)

72. (A) The suffix -*itis* means inflammation. (p. 105)

73. (C) Homeostasis is the body's ability to maintain stability within cells and the body using nervous system feedback and messaging. (p. 161)

74. (B) When a choking victim becomes unresponsive the EMT should begin CPR. (p. 216)

75. (B) High-risk locations for TB do not include daycare centers because children are not prone to having TB. (p. 32)

76. (A) Notify police immediately if there may be any weapons at the scene. The police are responsible for weapons control; your responsibility is patient care. (p. 50)

77. (A) Respiratory failure is the reduction of breathing to the point at which oxygen intake is not sufficient to support life. Anoxic (or anaerobic) metabolism occurs in the absence of oxygen from not breathing. Respiratory support is what the EMT provides. Respiratory arrest occurs when breathing stops. (p. 243)

78. (C) Cyanosis, or blue or gray skin, is not a sign of adequate breathing. (p. 248)

79. (B) Widening of the nostrils with respirations is called nasal flaring. Increased breathing rate is hyperventilation. Wheezes are a musical tone caused by spasms of the small airways. (p. 209)

80. (B) Blue or gray skin is called cyanosis. Stridor is a harsh sound during respiration caused by airway obstruction. Pallor is pale skin. Anemia is a disease in which the patient has too few red blood cells. (p. 249)

81. (C) Inability to speak in full sentences is a sign of shortness of breath. Snoring is a noise made from a partial airway obstruction caused by the tongue. (p. 249)

82. (B) EMTs do not routinely insert endotracheal tubes. All other answers listed are principal procedures used by the EMT to treat life-threatening respiratory problems. (pp. 250–253)

83. (A) The tongue is involved in most airway problems. (p. 206)

84. (D) If the unconscious patient is found at the bottom of a stairwell, you will need to assume a neck or spine injury and use the jaw-thrust maneuver. (p. 213)

85. (C) Artificial ventilation may be inadequate if the rate of ventilation is too fast or too slow. (p. 245, 263)

©2021 Pearson Education, Inc.
Emergency Care, 14th Ed.

86. (D) The pediatric airway is very small so the OPA must be inserted straight in to prevent injury to the soft palate, with the aid of a tongue depressor to displace the tongue. (p. 220)

87. (B) The proper airway adjunct to use on a patient with clenched teeth is a nasopharyngeal airway. (p. 220)

88. (C) The proper bag-valve mask oxygen flow rate is 15 liters per minute. (p. 259)

89. (B) The most recent American Heart Association guidelines now state that ventilation (i.e., mouth-to-mask, bag-valve mask, or other forms of ventilation with or without supplementary oxygen) should involve sufficient ventilation volume to achieve visible chest rise. (p. 259)

90. (C) The first step in artificial ventilation of a stoma breather is to clear any mucus or secretions that may be obstructing the stoma. (p. 262)

91. (A) Suctioning an airway can cause a vagal stimulation that slows the heart rate. The infant is very sensitive to vagal stimulation. (p. 230)

92. (B) The oropharyngeal and nasopharyngeal airways are the most common airway adjuncts. (p. 217)

93. (D) Use an oropharyngeal airway on unconscious patients with no gag reflex. Airway usage is not restricted to only medical or only trauma patients. (p. 217)

94. (C) When suctioning a patient, never suction for longer than 10 seconds. You do not *hypo*ventilate but do *hyper*ventilate the patient before and after suctioning. Always wear eye protection and a mask when suctioning. Suction on the way out. (p. 232)

95. (A) The EMT is authorized to use the supraglottic airway in some states where they are properly trained. (p. 222)

96. (C) Insufficiency in the supply of oxygen to the body's tissues is called hypoxia. Anoxia means no oxygen is being supplied to the cells. Cyanosis is a result of hypoxia. There is no such thing as no-oxia. (p. 250)

97. (A) Change the oxygen cylinder before the pressure gauge reads 200 psi at the lowest; otherwise, you may damage the inside of the tank. (p. 266)

98. (C) Store cylinders in a cool, dry area, not in a warm, humid one. (p. 267)

99. (A) Use a nonrebreather mask for high-concentration oxygen delivery to the breathing patient. EMTs do not use partial rebreather masks in the field. A nasal cannula is a low-concentration device. A bag-valve mask is used on patients who are not breathing. (p. 275)

100. (B) The concentration of oxygen administered by a nasal cannula is between 24% and 44%. (p. 275)

101. (B) Do not remove the dentures unless they are loose. Dentures allow for an improved seal between the patient's face and mask. (p. 234)

102. (A) A child's mouth and nose are smaller and more easily obstructed than an adult's. The child's chest wall is softer. The child's trachea is narrower, so it is more easily obstructed. (p. 205)

103. (A) Respiratory arrest is complete breathing stoppage. (p. 243)

104. (D) If positive pressure ventilations are not performed with good technique the stomach can fill with air. (p. 251)

105. (A) A flowmeter allows the control of oxygen in liters per minute. A humidifier helps to keep the oxygen from being too dry. A reservoir is used on the BVM to increase the oxygen concentration. (p. 268)

106. (C) Hyperventilation (ventilating too quickly) causes too much carbon dioxide to be blown off, which causes vasoconstriction of blood vessels, which causes decreased blood flow to the brain. (p. 251)

107. (A) Some EMS systems use oxygen humidification to prevent drying out the patient's mucous membranes. Humidifiers are usually not used in systems with short transports and, unless they are disposable, may increase the potential for infection spread. (p. 269)

108. (C) The ATV has settings to adjust the ventilation rate and tidal volume. (p. 264)

109. (A) The child's metabolism consumes oxygen at a higher rate than an adult. (p. 280)

110. (D) With an air mattress, the patient is placed on the device, and the air is withdrawn by the pump. The mattress then forms a rigid and conforming surface around the patient. (p. 70)

111. (C) The digestive system is responsible for the breakdown of food into absorbable forms. The nervous system is the body's communication system and controls almost all body systems, the urinary system eliminates the liquid wastes from the bladder, and the integumentary system covers the surface of the body. (p. 180)

112. (B) Gastric distension, or air in the stomach, pushes against the diaphragm leaving little room for the lungs to expand. (p. 280)

113. (D) Twelve breaths per minute times 500 milliliters of air per breath = 6,000 milliliters per minute in the adult patient. (p. 240)

114. (C) Dehydration can be caused by loss of fluids for multiple days, which can occur with severe diarrhea and vomiting. (p. 180)

115. (A) A patient who is short of breath often speaks in short, choppy sentences. (p. 249)

116. (B) Young infants breathe primarily through their noses, and they are unable to blow their noses on their own, so nasal congestion can be a major problem. (p. 205)

117. (B) When the mother strokes the infant's lips and the baby starts sucking, this nervous system reflex is known as the sucking reflex. (p. 187)

118. (C) The adolescent years are the beginning of self-destructive behaviors. (p. 193)

119. (D) Pediatric circulation is commonly assessed using the capillary refill test. (p. 171)

120. (D) The family conflict of control versus independence becomes an issue with adolescents in some cases. (p. 193)

121. (B) Girls are usually finished growing by the age of 16. (p. 193)

122. (B) A patient who sits upright and leans forward with their hands on their knees to improve breathing is called the tripod position. (p. 249)

123. (B) The proper way to open the airway of a patient who you do not suspect has neck trauma is to use the head-tilt, chin-lift maneuver. The modified jaw-thrust and the head-tilt, neck-lift maneuvers have not been taught since early 2000. (p. 213)

124. (C) Measure the nasopharyngeal airway from the tip of the nose to the earlobe. Insert the airway in the right nostril with the open side of the bevel facing the nasal septum. (p. 221)

125. (C) Respiratory distress leads to respiratory failure, which in turn leads to respiratory arrest if it is not treated appropriately. (p. 243)

CHAPTER 11: Scene Size-Up

Match Key Terms

1. (G) Scene size-up: Steps taken when approaching the scene of an emergency call. (p. 310)

2. (D) Danger zone: The area around the wreckage of a vehicle collision or other incident within which special safety precautions should be taken. (p. 310)

3. (C) Mechanism of injury: A force or forces that may have caused injury. (p. 310)

4. (A) Penetrating trauma: Injury caused by an object that passes into or through the skin or other body tissues. (p. 310)

5. (B) Blunt-force trauma: Injury caused by a blow that does not penetrate the skin or other body tissues. (p. 310)

6. (E) Index of suspicion: Awareness that there may be injuries based on the mechanism of injury. (p. 310)

7. (F) Nature of the illness: What is medically wrong with a patient. (p. 310)

Multiple-Choice Review

1. (A) It begins as you approach the scene, surveying it to determine whether there are any threats to your own safety. (p. 290)

2. (C) If there is active shooting going on, it will be too risky to get to the patient for EMTs, so of the choices listed this would be the one where retreat would be most appropriate. Retreat means moving to a safer position and returning with the police! (p. 298)

3. (B) If you arrive at a multiple-vehicle collision scene where police, fire vehicles, and other ambulances are already present, you should conduct your own scene size-up. (p. 291)

4. (D) Which of the following is not an appropriate action when you near the scene of a traffic collision? Attempt to park your vehicle downhill from the scene. Generally EMS should park uphill and upwind from any scene if possible. (p. 292)

5. (A) When you are in sight of the collision scene, you should watch for the signals of police officers and other emergency service personnel because they may have information about hazards or the location of injured persons. (p. 293)

6. (B) When there are no apparent hazards, consider the danger zone to extend at least 50 feet in all directions from the wreckage. (p. 294)

7. (C) When a collision vehicle is on fire, consider the danger zone to extend at least 100 feet in all directions, even if the fire appears small and limited to the engine compartment. (p. 294)

8. (A) Your scene size-up should identify the potential for a violent or dangerous situation. (p. 290)

9. (D) The EMT's equipment/supplies for Standard Precautions during the scene size-up may include all of the following except nonrebreather mask. (p. 299)

10. (B) Standard Precautions should be taken with all patients. The key element of Standard Precautions is to always have personal protective equipment readily available. (p. 299)

11. (B) Certain injuries are common to particular situations. Injuries to bones and joints are usually associated with falls and vehicle collisions. (p. 299)

12. (D) Some idea of potential forces involved in the mechanism of injury (MOI) assists the EMT in predicting various injury patterns, deciding if spine motion restriction precautions may be warranted, and predicting various injury patterns. (p. 299)

13. (C) One of those laws, the law of inertia, states that a body in motion will remain in motion unless acted upon by an outside force. (p. 301)

14. (A) To which part of her body was she most likely to have sustained injuries? Skull. (p. 302)

15. (C) Which of the following is least likely to be considered a mechanism of injury (MOI) for an unrestrained patient who was in a head-on crash and followed the "up-and-over" pathway? Brake pedal because the body would likely be moving away from it in an "up and over" trajectory. (p. 302)

16. (C) Your patient has stable vital signs and is complaining of knee, leg, and hip pain. He also states that he was in the front passenger seat of the vehicle and was not wearing his seat belt. What type of collision did he most likely experience? Head-on, down-and-under. (p. 302)

17. (D) Which type of collision is most serious when the occupant is not restrained because it has the potential for multiple impacts? Roll-over. (p. 303)

18. (D) All of the following are indications of mechanisms of injury except a flat tire. (pp. 302–303)

19. (A) According to the CDC, a severe fall for an adult is over 20 feet. (p. 306)

20. (A) You are evaluating a patient who sustained a penetrating injury. In a low-velocity injury, the injury is usually limited to the penetrated area. (p. 306)

21. (C) The pressure wave around a bullet's track through the body is called cavitation. (p. 306)

22. (C) This type of injury is called a blunt-force trauma. (p. 306)

23. (B) In which of the following situations would it be necessary for you and your partner to call for additional assistance? Your patient is a 450-pound male who fell down the stairs and has a broken leg. (p. 308)

24. (A) Three members of the same family have the same symptoms. You should immediately evacuate all people from the building. (p. 308)

25. (B) If the number of patients is more than the responding units can effectively handle, the EMT should call for additional EMS resources immediately. (p. 308)

26. (B) When arriving at the scene of a collision, the EMT should don an ANSI approved reflective vest. (p. 294)

27. (C) What should you do next? Retreat to a safe location and ask for the police to respond to secure the scene. (p. 296)

28. (A) You arrive on the scene of a large fire. If the personnel at the scene are using the incident command/management system, you should follow the instructions of the Incident Commander. (p. 294)

29. (C) A fall over 10 feet for a child under 15-years-old is considered a severe fall by the CDC. (p. 306)

30. (D) Vehicles with airbags should still require the occupants to use passenger restraint systems properly because they only deploy once during the collision, the airbags may cause injury themselves, and airbags may damage the windshield. (p. 300)

©2021 Pearson Education, Inc.
Emergency Care, 14th Ed.

Complete the Following

1. List five signals that violence may be a danger on your call. (pp. 296–297)
   - Fighting or loud voices.
   - Weapons visible or in use.
   - Signs of alcohol or other drug use.
   - Unusual silence.
   - Knowledge of prior violence.

2. List the guidelines for establishing a danger zone around the wreckage of a vehicle collision. (p. 294)
   - When there are no apparent hazards: at least 50 feet (152 meters) in all directions from the wreckages.
   - When fuel has been spilled: a minimum of 100 feet (30.4 meters) in all directions from the wreckage.
   - When a vehicle is on fire: at least 100 feet (30.4 meters) in all directions, even if the fire seems small and limited to the engine compartment.
   - When wires are down: the area in which people or vehicles might be in contact with energized wires. Park the ambulance at least one full span of wires away from the poles to which broken wires are attached.
   - When a hazardous material is involved: Check the *Emergency Response Guidebook* or ask the Incident Commander to seek advice about where to park. Depending on circumstances you may be able to park 50 feet (15.2 meters) from the wreckage when no hazardous material has been released or as much as 2000 feet (609.6 meters) from the wreckage when high explosives may detonate. Always park upwind if a hazardous material is present or on the same level if gases or fumes may rise. Park behind a natural barrier if possibe.

3. List five types of motor vehicle collisions and the common injury patterns for each. (pp. 302–303)
   - Head-on collision: up and over- head/neck, chest/abdomen.
   - Head-on collision: down and under – knees/legs and hips injuries.
   - Rear-end collision: neck and head injuries.
   - Side-impact collision: neck injury and head, chest, and abdomen/pelvis injury.
   - Rollover collision: possibility of multiple impacts and ejections causing any type of serious injury pattern.
   - Rotational collision: possibility of multiple impacts causing multiple injury patterns.

4. When you are determining the nature of the illness this information can be obtained from: (p. 307)
   - The family members or bystanders.
   - The patient.
   - The scene.

Label the Diagram (p. 300)

1. Forced flexion or hyperextension
2. Twisting
3. Indirect
4. Direct blow (lateral)
5. Direct blow (lateral)
6. Direct blow (downward)

CHAPTER 12: Primary Assessment

Match Key Terms

1. (C) A-B-Cs: Airway, breathing, and circulation. (p. 335)
2. (F) AVPU: A memory aid for classifying a patient's level of responsiveness, or mental status. The letters stand for alert, verbal response, painful response, unresponsive. (p. 335)
3. (D) Chief complaint: In emergency medicine, the reason EMS was called, usually in the patient's own words. (p. 335)
4. (A) General impression: Impression of the patient's condition that is formed on first approaching the patient, based on the patient's environment, chief complaint, and appearance. (p. 335)
5. (G) Interventions: Actions taken to correct or manage a patient's problem. (p. 335)
6. (B) Mental status: Level of responsiveness. (p. 335)
7. (E) Primary assessment: The first element in a patient's assessment: steps taken for the purpose of discovering and dealing with any life-threatening problems. The six parts are: forming a general impression, assessing mental status, assessing airway, assessing breathing, assessing circulation, and determining the priority of the patient for treatment and transport to the hospital. (p. 335)
8. (H) Priority: The decision regarding the need for immediate transport of the patient versus further assessment and care at the scene. (p. 335)
9. (J) Manual stabilization: Using one's hands to prevent movement of a patient's head and neck until a cervical collar can be applied. (p. 335)
10. (I) Spinal motion restriction: The use of specific procedures and equipment for limiting movement of the head, neck, and spine when spinal injury is possible or likely. (p. 335)

Multiple-Choice Review

1. (D) Which of the following steps is not a part of the primary assessment for this patient? Obtain the patient's blood pressure. (p. 314)
2. (D) The general impression is based on an evaluation of all of the following except the past medical history. (p. 318)
3. (B) Finding drug-use paraphernalia at the scene of an emergency is an example of the environment part of the general impression. (p. 318)
4. (B) When a 45-year-old female tells you, in her own words, why she requested an ambulance, this is called the chief complaint. (p. 321)
5. (B) If your patient is not alert and breathing is inadequate due to an insufficient minute volume you should provide positive pressure ventilations. (p. 322)
6. (D) What does the "A" in AVPU stand for? Alert. (p. 321)
7. (C) What does the "V" in AVPU stand for? Verbal response. (p. 321)
8. (B) One major difference between the primary assessment of a responsive trauma patient and the primary assessment of an unresponsive trauma patient is the unresponsive patient is a higher priority for immediate transport. (pp. 327–328)

CHAPTER 12: (continued)

9. (D) She is not alert, and her breathing rate is less than 8 per minute and shallow. As an EMT in charge, you should provide positive pressure ventilations with 100% oxygen. (p. 322)

10. (B) During your primary assessment of a 42-year-old female patient who is alert and has a breathing rate that is greater than 24 with signs of respiratory distress and SPO_2 of 93%, you should provide her with high-concentration oxygen via nonrebreather mask. (p. 331)

11. (D) In the primary assessment of a 53-year-old male patient, the circulation assessment includes evaluating the pulse, skin characteristics, and bleeding severity. (p. 327)

12. (D) You are evaluating a 22-year-old male patient. If his skin is warm, dry, and a normal color, it would indicate good circulation. (p. 327)

13. (C) Your 38-year-old male patient has no life-threatening external hemorrhage, but his skin is cool, pale, and moist. This could indicate poor circulation. (p. 327)

14. (A) To evaluate skin color in a dark-skinned patient, the EMT should also evaluate the tissues of the lips or nail beds. (p. 327)

15. (C) When assessing the circulation during the primary assessment, the EMT should check for and control severe bleeding. This is important to do because a patient can bleed to death in minutes. (p. 327)

16. (B) When a life threat is observed in the primary assessment, the EMT should treat it immediately. (p. 327)

17. (D) On completion of your primary assessment, you decide that your patient is a high priority. High-priority conditions include poor general impression, unresponsive, and shock. (p. 328)

18. (C) All of the following would be considered high-priority conditions except an uncomplicated childbirth. (p. 328)

19. (A) During the primary assessment of a 55-year-old female with a chief complaint of chest pain, you note that her breathing rate is 24 and SPO_2 is 95%. You should consider providing oxygen to the patient. (p. 329)

20. (B) When doing an assessment on a patient who appears lifeless, the approach is adapted to include the C-A-B approach per AHA Guidelines. (p. 316, 323)

21. (B) For a patient to be considered stable he/she needs to have vital signs that are in the normal or just slightly abnormal range. (p. 327)

22. (D) When assessing a child who is responsive and appears stable on general impression, it is helpful to take a moment to kneel at her level, establish a rapport with the child, and check the capillary refill. (p. 332)

23. (C) In the early part of your patient assessment of a trauma patient your primary concern is to treat the patient's life-threatening conditions while providing spinal motion restriction. (p. 318)

24. (A) If an infant is not initially alert you should shout a verbal stimulus to stimulate responsiveness or crying. (p. 334)

Complete the Following

1. The primary assessment is the first element in the total assessment of the patient. List the six steps of the primary assessment. (p. 315)
   - Forming a general impression
   - Assessing the patient's mental status (and manually stabilizing the head and neck, when appropriate)
   - Assessing the patient's airway
   - Assessing the patient's breathing
   - Assessing the patient's circulation
   - Determining the patient's priority

2. State what the letters in AVPU stand for. (p. 321)
   - A = alert
   - V = verbal response
   - P = painful response
   - U = unresponsive

3. List five examples of patients who may be critical. (pp. 319–320)

   Any of these:
   - Appears lifeless.
   - Has an obviously altered mental status.
   - Is unusually anxious
   - Appears pale and sweaty.
   - Has obvious trauma to head, chest, abdomen, or pelvis.
   - Has assumed any specific position that indicates distress.
   - Has uncontrolled bleeding.
   - Is breathing inadequately.
   - Displays an occluded or partially occluded airway.

4. List the basic three possible results of a pulse-rate check during the primary assessment. (p. 327)
   - Within normal limits.
   - Abnormally slow.
   - Abnormally fast.

5. List six high-priority conditions. (p. 328)

   Any of these:
   - Poor general impression.
   - Unresponsive.
   - Responsive, but not following commands.
   - Difficulty breathing.
   - Shock (hypoperfusion).
   - Complicated childbirth.
   - Chest pain consistent with cardiac problems.
   - Uncontrolled bleeding.
   - Severe pain anywhere.

Case Study: Car Versus Bike Crash

1. Attend to the scene size-up and other safety issues.

2. Primary assessment.

3. The mechanism of injury or MOI.

4. You were not there to see what happened, so the bystander's information is very helpful in determining the MOI, which is a major clue to the patient's possible injuries.

5. To assess the patient's mental status.

6. Alert ("A" on the AVPU scale) because Tony knows his name, where he is, and the day of the week (is oriented to person, place, and time).

7. The primary assessment is always done in order so that essential steps are not missed. If a life threat is identified, the EMT should manage it and move on to the next step. Since Tony's mental status is alert, having him take a deep breath helps assess his airway and breathing and, if that is painful, whether he may have an injury involving his thorax or lungs. As always, use your best clinical judgment.

8. The C step ("circulation") includes assessment of the pulse (present and/or within normal range); the external bleeding; and the skin's color, temperature, and condition.

9. To be safe, it would be best to make Tony a priority patient because he might have some internal bleeding in addition to the possibly fractured clavicle because he was moving

©2021 Pearson Education, Inc.
Emergency Care, 14th Ed.

along at some speed when he crashed. Rapid movement before crashing into something (in this case the car door and then the pavement), can be a significant mechanism of injury, and good clinical judgement should lead you to consider this a high priority.

CHAPTER 13: Vital Signs and Monitoring Devices

Match Key Terms

Part A

1. (L) Auscultation: The act of listening with a stethoscope is used to auscultate for characteristic sounds.

2. (C) Blood Pressure: The force of blood against the walls of the blood vessels. (p. 366)

3. (J) Brachial artery: The major artery of the upper arm. (p. 366)

4. (B) Bradycardia: A slow pulse; any pulse rate below 60 beats per minute. (p. 366)

5. (D) Carotid pulse: The pulse felt along the large artery on either side of the neck. (p. 366)

6. (N) Constrict: Get smaller in diameter. (p. 366)

7. (M) Dilate: Get larger in diameter. (p. 366)

8. (A) Diastole blood pressure: The pressure remaining in the arteries when the left ventricle of the heart is relaxed and refilling. (p. 366)

9. (E) Palpation: Assessing the patient through touch or feeling with the hands. (p. 366)

10. (H) Pulse: The rhythmic beats as the heart pumps blood through the arteries. (p. 366)

11. (I) Pulse quality: The rhythm (regular or irregular) and force (strong or weak) of the pulse. (p. 366)

12. (F) Pulse rate: The number of pulse beats per minute. (p. 366)

13. (K) Pupil: The black center of the eye. (p. 366)

14. (O) Radial pulse: The pulse felt at the wrist. (p. 366)

15. (G) Reactivity: The changing size of the pupils when light is shown into them. (p. 366)

Part B

1. (B) Respiratory quality: The normal or abnormal (shallow, labored or noisy) character of breathing. (p. 366)

2. (A) Respiratory rate: The number of breaths taken in one minute. (p. 366)

3. (E) Respiratory rhythm: The regular or irregular spacing of breaths. (p. 366)

4. (F) Oxygen saturation: The ratio of the amount of oxygen present in the blood to the amount that could be carried, expressed in a percentage. (p. 366)

5. (G) Respiration: The act of breathing in and breathing out. (p. 366)

6. (H) Sphygmomanometer: The cuff and gauge used to measure blood pressure. (p. 366)

7. (D) Systolic blood pressure: The pressure created when the heart contracts and forces blood out into the arteries. (p. 366)

8. (C) Tachycardia: A rapid pulse; any pulse rate above 100 beats per minute. (p. 366)

9. (L) Blood pressure monitor: A machine that automatically inflates a blood pressure cuff and measures blood pressure. (p. 366)

10. (K) Pulse oximeter: An electronic device for determining the amount of oxygen carried in the blood, known as the oxygen saturation or SpO_2. (p. 366)

11. (I) Vital signs: Outward signs of what is going on inside the body, including respiration; pulse, skin color, temperature, and condition (plus capillary refill in infants and young children); pupils; and blood pressure. (p. 366)

12. (J) Brachial pulse: The pulse felt in the upper arm. (p. 366)

Multiple-Choice Review

1. (D) The components of the vital signs you will be measuring include all of the following except blood sugar level. (p. 340)

2. (B) A sign that gives important information about the patient's condition but is not considered a vital sign is mental status. (p. 340)

3. (B) Why is it essential that vital signs be recorded as they are obtained? To prevent forgetting them and to note trends in the condition. (p. 340)

4. (D) You take her pulse, and the rate exceeds 100 beats per minute. This is called tachycardia. (p. 341)

5. (D) On the basis of the pulse alone, a sign that something may be seriously wrong with a patient could be a sustained rate below 48 beats per minute, a sustained rate above 126 beats per minute, or a rate above 150 beats per minute. (p. 341)

6. (B) In addition to the answer to multiple-choice question 5, another serious indicator found in the pulse may be an irregular rhythm. (p. 341)

7. (C) Assessing the quality of the pulse includes determining the rhythm and force. (p. 344)

8. (C) A 50-year-old male patient who sustained serious trauma from an ATV crash is described as having a "thready" pulse. This patient most likely has a weak pulse. (p. 344)

9. (C) The normal pulse rate for a school-age child (6–10 years) is 65 to 120. (p. 341)

10. (A) When assessing the pulse rate of a typical adult who is not in distress, you would expect to obtain a rate of 60 to 100. (p. 341)

11. (B) The pulse at the thumb side of the wrist is referred to as the radial pulse. (p. 344)

12. (C) When assessing the carotid pulse, the EMT should be aware that excessive pressure can slow the heart. (p. 344)

13. (C) The number of breaths a patient takes in one minute is called the respiratory rate. (p. 345)

14. (A) The respiratory rate is classified as normal, slow, or rapid. (p. 345)

15. (D) If the EMT is treating a patient with a sustained respiratory rate above 24 or below 10 breaths per minute, this is serious and high-concentration oxygen should be considered. (p. 346)

16. (B) your partner obtains a set of vitals and tells you that the 45-year-old male patient has a normal respiratory rate. The patient's rate at rest should be 12 to 20. (p. 346)

17. (D) The normal respiration rate for a toddler (1–3 years) is 24 to 40. (p. 346)

CHAPTER 13: (continued)

18. (A) Shallow breathing occurs when there is only slight movement of the chest or abdomen. (p. 346)

19. (B) Many resting people breathe more with their diaphragm than with their chest muscles. (p. 346)

20. (D) Signs of labored breathing include all of the following except delayed capillary refill. (p. 346)

21. (B) A high-pitched harsh sound when the patient inhales is called stridor. (p. 346)

22. (C) When the quality of a patient's respirations is abnormal because something is blocking the flow of air, this is referred to as noisy breathing. (p. 346)

23. (A) During your primary assessment, you hear an airway sound that usually indicates the need for suction. This sound is called gurgling. (p. 346)

24. (B) Two of the best places to assess circulation by skin color in adults are the inside of the cheek and the nail beds. (p. 347)

25. (C) Your patient sustained a significant blood loss from an injury. This condition may result in skin that is pale. (p. 347)

26. (D) A patient with a lack of oxygen in the red blood cells resulting from inadequate breathing or inadequate heart function will exhibit a bluish discoloration known as cyanotic skin. (p. 347)

27. (D) Your patient's liver abnormality may help explain why his skin appears jaundiced. (p. 347)

28. (B) Your patient was found lying in a parking lot. You note that he has cold, dry skin, which is frequently associated with exposure to cold. (p. 348)

29. (A) Hot, dry skin is frequently associated with high fever and heat exposure. (p. 348)

30. (B) A sudden increase in end-tidal CO_2 on capnography during CPR is a signal that you should stop compressions and check for a pulse. (p. 365)

31. (C) The reading on the device to test blood sugar level is reported in milligrams of glucose per deciliter of blood. (p. 362)

32. (B) When you assess her pupils, you should cover the patient's eyes for a few moments, then uncover one eye at a time. (p. 350)

33. (D) The pupils may be unequal as a result of any of the following conditions except shock. (p. 350)

34. (B) Fright, blood loss, drugs, and treatment with eye drops may cause the patient's pupils to become dilated. (p. 350)

35. (A) When the left ventricle of the heart is in the relaxation and refilling phase, the pressure in the arteries is called the diastolic pressure. (p. 350)

36. (B) The pulse oximeter should be used routinely with patients who complain of respiratory problems. (p. 360)

37. (A) The pulse oximeter is helpful because it helps the EMT properly titrate oxygen therapy. (p. 360)

38. (C) Your partner reminds you that the pulse oximeter produces falsely high readings in patients with carbon monoxide poisoning. (p. 361)

39. (B) Chronic smokers may have a pulse oximeter reading that is higher than the actual oxygen saturation. (p. 361)

40. (C) In a healthy person, one would expect the oximeter reading to be 96% and above. (p. 360)

41. (C) To determine a patient's skin temperature, the EMT often feels the patient's skin with the back of the hand. (p. 348)

42. (C) The normal blood glucose meter reading is usually at least 70 to 100 mg/dL. (p. 364)

43. (A) The systolic blood pressure is created when the heart contracts. (p. 350)

44. (C) In a situation like this (a noisy atmosphere), it makes sense to take the patient's BP by palpation, revealing only the systolic pressure. (pp. 352–353)

45. (C) Serious hypotension in an adult patient is normally defined as a systolic below 90 mmHg. (p. 352)

46. (D) In assessing a patient who has an altered mental status, it is not uncommon for the EMT to utilize a glucose meter, a BP cuff and stethoscope, and/or a pulse oximeter. (pp. 340, 359–364)

47. (D) When a child is under 3 years-old the BP may be difficult to assess in the field. More useful information about the condition can be obtained by observing for respiratory distress, sick appearance, or unconsciousness. (p. 356)

48. (B) When assessing the skin of a child under the age of 6 you should also evaluate capillary refill. (p. 348)

Complete the Following

1. List the six vital signs assessed by the EMT. (pp. 342–343)
- Pulse
- Blood pressure
- Skin (color, temperature, condition)
- Respirations
- Pupils
- Pulse oximetry

2. List some potential causes of the following: (pp. 347–348, 350–351)
- **A.** High BP: medical condition, exertion, fright, emotional distress, stimulant drug overdose or excitement.
- **B.** Low BP: athlete or other person with normally low BP, blood loss, late sign of shock, depressant drug overdose.
- **C.** Cool, clammy skin: sign of shock, anxiety.
- **D.** Cold, moist skin: body is losing heat.
- **E.** Cold, dry skin: exposure to cold.
- **F.** Hot, dry skin: high fever, heat exposure.
- **G.** Hot, moist skin: high fever, heat exposure.
- **H.** Dilated pupil: fright, blood loss, drugs, prescription eye drops.
- **I.** Unequal pupils: stroke, head injury, eye injury, artificial eye, prescription eye drops.

3. List three different methods used to measure blood pressure. (p. 352)
- Auscultation
- Palpation
- Blood pressure monitor

4. List three methods of measuring temperature. (p. 356, 359)
- Tympanic membrane.
- Oral.
- Rectal.

Label the Diagram

TABLE 13–1 Pulse (p. 341)

1. 60–100

2. Preschoolers

3. 80–140 (awake: slightly lower when asleep)

4. 90–160 (awake: slightly lower when asleep)

©2021 Pearson Education, Inc.
Emergency Care, 14th Ed.

5. 100–170 (awake: slightly lower when asleep)

6. Abnormal electrical activity in the heart

7. Cardiac arrest. Note: if a patient is awake and talking to you, but has no carotid pulses, ask if he has a ventricular assist device.

Case Study: "Man Down" in the Alley

1. In the primary assessment, the EMT determines the mental status and checks the airway, breathing, and circulation, then prioritizes the patient.

2. Gurgling means that there is fluid in the upper airway, so you should have your suction unit and rigid-tip Yankauer ready to go.

3. The patient can talk to you and answer questions but he is not oriented to person, place, and time, so he is "V" for "verbal."

4. Normal vitals for a young adult male would be a respiration of 12 to 20 and regular, a pulse rate of 60 to 100 and regular, and a BP of around 120/80 mmHg. (p. 341, 346, 351)

5. If the patient is a diabetic with an altered mental status, check the blood sugar level with a glucometer. Use your best clinical judgment, and follow your regional protocols in assessing and managing this patient. (pp. 361–364)

6. Yes, in most EMS systems.

7. Every five minutes because an altered mental status is unstable. If the patient becomes alert, every 15 minutes would be fine. (p 356)

CHAPTER 14: Principles of Assessment

Match Key Terms

1. (G) Chief complaint: The patient's statement that describes the symptom or concern associated with the primary problem the patient is having. (p. 401)

2. (A) Crepitation: The grating sound or feeling of broken bones rubbing together. (p. 401)

3. (D) Diagnosis: A description or label for a patient's condition that assists a clinician in further evaluation and treatment. (p. 401)

4. (I) Past medical history (PMH): Information gathered regarding the patient's health problems in the past. (p. 401)

5. (C) Closed-ended question: A question requiring only a "yes" or "no" answer. (p. 401)

6. (H) Differential diagnosis: A list of potential diagnoses compiled early in the assessment of the patient. (p. 401)

7. (E) SAMPLE: A memory aid in which the letters stand for elements of the past medical history: signs and symptoms, allergies, medications, pertinent past history, last oral intake, and events leading to the injury or illness. (p. 401)

8. (B) Jugular vein distention: Bulging of the neck veins. (p. 401)

9. (K) Open-ended questions: A question requiring more than just a "yes" or "no" answer. (p. 401)

10. (J) History of the present illness (HPI): Information gathered regarding the symptoms and nature of the patient's current concern. (p. 401)

11. (F) OPQRST: A memory aid in which the letters stand for questions asked to get a description of the present illness: onset, provokes, quality, radiation, severity, and time. (p. 401)

Multiple-Choice Review

1. (B) When obtaining a history it is best to begin with an open-ended question such as "What can you tell me about your chest pain?" (p. 371)

2. (D) In the field we seek to answer the question, What does this patient need? (p. 371)

3. (C) An example of a closed-ended question would be Do you feel like you are going to pass out? (p. 371)

4. (B) From a general perspective, preschoolers can usually be interviewed if you take your time and keep your language simple. (p. 374)

5. (C) When evaluating a patient during the physician exam, the EMT will observe, auscultate, and palpate each body part. (p. 377)

6. (B) When a patient tells you that he called because he cut his wrist with a razor, this is called the chief complaint. (p. 372)

7. (B) The history of the present illness and PMH includes interviewing bystanders to ask about each of the following except how the patient could have prevented the illness from occurring. (pp. 370–371)

8. (B) The "M" in the memory aid SAMPLE refers to medications. (p. 373)

9. (A) The "P" in the mnemonic OPQRST refers to provocation (what provokes the pain or causes it to flare up). (p. 372)

10. (A) All of the following are key questions to answer in taking a patient history, regardless of the type of medical or traumatic complaint, except Does the patient walk down this street often? (pp. 373–374)

11. (A) In obtaining history during the secondary assessment of a patient with a respiratory complaint, which of the following questions would the EMT least likely ask? Has the patient checked his or her blood glucose recently? (p. 379)

12. (C) The mental status assessment is key to the physical examination of patients with respiratory and neurological system complaints. (pp. 382–384)

13. (B) When a patient with a respiratory complaint states that she has breathing difficulty when lying down, this is called orthopnea. (p. 379)

14. (A) When assessing the abdomen of an adult male trauma patient, the EMT should observe and palpate for pain in addition to wounds and deformities. (pp. 387–388)

15. (A) The cardiovascular assessment includes checking for a narrowing pulse pressure. This is defined as the difference between the systolic and diastolic pulse pressure. (p. 384)

16. (D) The components of the secondary assessment for a medical patient with a cardiovascular system complaint include all of the following except performing the Cincinnati Prehospital Stroke Scale. (pp. 383–384)

17. (B) Many memory aids are used during the secondary assessment process. OPQRST is a memory aid to help the EMT remember the questions that expand on the history of the present illness. (p. 372)

18. (B) When you ask a male patient with back pain, "How bad is the pain?" you are questioning him about severity. (p. 372)

19. (C) Why is it important for the EMT to determine the "T" in OPQRST when questioning a 58-year-old male with a chief complaint of chest pain? It is helpful to determine the time when the pain began. (p. 372)

CHAPTER 14: (continued)

20. (A) The 58-year-old male continues to discuss his condition with you. His chief complaint is chest pain. When you ask, "Do you have nausea or have you been vomiting?" you are questioning him about his signs and symptoms. (p. 373)

21. (B) The alert 58-year-old male who is complaining of chest pain goes on to describe other recent hospitalizations and the medical condition for which his doctor is treating him. In the SAMPLE history, this information is considered pertinent past history. (p. 374)

22. (C) When you ask an elderly female patient, "How have you been feeling today?" you are asking her about her about the events leading to the current illness. (p. 374)

23. (C) When interviewing a patient who has a neurologic system complaint, during your assessment you should examine the patient's mental status and assess movement and sensation of the extremities. (p. 385)

24. (B) In conducting a body system examination of the patient with a GI system complaint, which of the following questions would be appropriate to ask in the secondary assessment? Have you had a bowel movement recently? (p. 388)

25. (C) When assessing a 28-year-old female patient who has a medical complaint involving the endocrine system, be sure to ask whether the patient is currently sick. (p. 387)

26. (C) When conducting a physical exam on the unconscious patient you see a medical bracelet on the patient's wrist. This is important because it may reveal the patient's medical condition. (p. 387)

27. (D) Your patient is a young child who was injured. During the physical exam which of the following should you do and why? Use a reassuring voice to help calm the patient. (p. 378)

28. (C) When conducting an assessment on a child the EMT should do each of the following except use the same terms you do for adults. (p. 376)

29. (D) If you must expose the small child to conduct a physical exam, remember to protect the child from stares of onlookers, quickly cover the child after the exam, and do not rush the child into accepting all that is happening. (p. 378)

30. (C) Which is not considered a part of the body system exam of a patient with a cardiac complaint? The breath odors. (p. 380)

31. (C) The analytical process that assists the EMT in reaching a field diagnosis is referred to as critical thinking. (p. 392)

32. (B) The basic approach that clinicians use to arrive at a diagnosis includes each of the following except administering lab tests. (p. 392)

33. (C) When a clinician draws up a list of conditions that may be the cause of the patient's condition today, this is referred to as the differential diagnosis. (p. 393)

34. (D) A highly experienced physician who reaches an incorrect diagnosis while using heuristics (shortcuts) may have been subject to any of the listed failings except lack of confidence. (In fact the list of shortcuts that can lead to biases includes *over*confidence as well as search satisfying, representativeness, and confirmation bias.) (pp. 397–398)

35. (A) The traditional approach to diagnosis involves narrowing down a long list of possible diagnoses. (p. 393)

36. (B) A clinician who is specifically looking for evidence that supports the diagnosis he or she already has in mind is committing a confirmation bias. (p. 398)

37. (B) When a patient does not fit the classic pattern, such as a cardiac patient without crushing chest pain, the EMT has to be careful not to make a representativeness error or bias (that is, concluding that the patient is not having a heart attack because he or she doesn't fit the classic pattern). (p. 397)

38. (D) You recently had a patient with heat stroke. The next time you have a patient in a warm environment, you are more likely to think of a diagnosis of heat stroke instead of more common problems such as dehydration. This bias is referred to as availability. (p. 397)

39. (D) The EMT should be skeptical about one condition being the actual cause of another condition a patient presents with. Drawing quick conclusions about the cause of a diagnosis can lead to anchoring, illusory correlation, or search satisfying bias. (p. 398)

40. (D) if you stop the search for a diagnosis as soon as you come up with a likely cause of an obvious problem, this can lead to missing out on a secondary diagnosis, overconfidence and misdiagnosis, or confirmation bias. (pp. 397–398)

41. (B) During your body system exam of a patient, checking the blood glucose is likely associated with a(n) endocrine system chief complaint. (p. 381)

Complete the Following

1. List questions that are usually asked when using the OPQRST to elaborate on the chief complaint. (p. 372)
- O – What were you doing when the pain or problem began?
- P – Does anything seem to trigger the pain or problem? Does anything make it feel better?
- Q – Can you describe the pain or problem for me?
- R – Where is the pain? Will you please point toward it? Does it seem to shoot or spread anywhere?
- S – How bad is the pain or problem? If zero is no pain or problem and ten is the worst you can imagine, what number would you say your pain or problem is right now?
- T – When did the pain or problem start? Has it changed at all since it started?

2. List questions you might ask when using the SAMPLE history acronym. (pp. 373–374)
- S – What's wrong?
- A – Are you allergic to medications or foods, or do you have environmental allergies?
- M – What medications are you currently taking or are you supposed to be taking (prescription, over-the-counter, or recreational)?
- P – Have you been experiencing any medical problems?
- L – When did you last eat or drink? What did you eat or drink?
- E – What sequence of events led to today's problem?

3. List six questions you would ask in gathering your history of a patient with a respiratory complaint. (p. 379)
- Determine the onset. How long have you had this shortness of breath?
- Dyspnea on exertion. Is it increasingly difficult for patients to catch their breath after they have exerted themselves?

©2021 Pearson Education, Inc.
Emergency Care, 14th Ed.

- Weight gain. Does the patient report recent, rapid weight gain or that their clothes are tight?
- Orthopnea. Does the patient have difficulty breathing when lying down?
- Does the patient sleep on pillows?
- Does the patient have a cough? Has the cough been productive? If so what does the patient cough up?
- Has the patient had any respiratory conditions recently?
- Does the patient have a chronic illness that affects the respiratory system?

4. List four questions you would consider or ask the patient or bystander in gathering the history of a patient with a neurologic complaint. (p. 385)
   - What is the patient's current mental status?
   - What is the patient's normal state of mental functioning?
   - Does the patient have a history of neurologic conditions?
   - Does the patient's speech sound normal?

5. List four questions you would ask in gathering your history of a patient with a gastrointestinal complaint. (pp. 387–388)
   - Does the patient complain of any abdominal pain?
   - Has the patient had any recent oral intake?
   - Does the patient have a history of any gastrointestinal issues?
   - Has the patient vomited? How much and how frequently? What did the vomit look like?
   - Has the patient had bowel movements recently? If so, how frequently? How does this compare with normal? What did the stool look like?

6. List eight ways in which an EMT can learn to think like a highly experienced physician. (pp. 398–400)
   - Learn to love ambiguity.
   - Understand the limitations of technology and people.
   - Realize that no one strategy works for everything.
   - Form a strong foundation of knowledge.
   - Organize the data in your head.
   - Change the way you think.
   - Learn from others.
   - Reflect on what you have learned.

Case Study; A Motorcycle Mishap

1. Standard Precautions: Protect yourself from blood and other body fluids found on the patient.
2. Scene safety: most notably the traffic
3. Mechanism of injury: a two-vehicle collision
4. The number of patients
5. Forming a general impression helps you to determine how serious the patient's condition is, which helps you set priorities for care and transport. The general impression is based on an immediate assessment of the environment and the patient's chief complaint and appearance. It gives you an idea of the sex and age of the patient, what happened and why EMS was called, whether the patient is injured or ill, and the severity of the patient's condition.
6. Using good clinical judgment, based on the MOI and the situation, you should consider the potential for a neck injury. One of your partners should be holding manual in-line stabilization of the patient's head and neck. The situations in which we immobilize patients may be changing, but according to what we know so far, the immobilization is appropriate. This is a good case for discussion with your Medical Director.

7. The patient appears to be alert, or "A" on the AVPU scale.
8. His broken legs might not be the worst problem, and you must assess him for life-threatening injuries first. Use your best assessment skills and clinical judgment here, and do not let the patient tell you how to do the assessment!
9. The primary assessment for Jesse should consist of forming a general impression, assessing mental status (both of which you have already done), assessing his ABC (airway, breathing, and circulation), and determining priority.
10. Signs of developing shock make Jesse a high-priority patient.
11. Call for ALS right away. If they are not there by the time Jesse is packaged, try to arrange a quick meeting en route to the hospital. But do not delay transport waiting for an ALS unit to arrive.
12. Wounds, deformities, and tenderness
13. In addition to the SAMPLE History (Signs and symptoms, Allergies, Medications, Pertinent past medical history, Last oral intake, Events leading up to incident), consider asking Jesse the following:
    - Whether he has had prior injuries in the area where you suspect injury
    - Whether he takes blood-thinning medications or medications that delay clotting. This may help to predict bleeding that can be severe and difficult to control.
    - Use the history to determine whether a medical problem caused the traumatic injury. (p. 373)
14. Assess respirations, pulse, blood pressure, skin (color, condition, temperature), and pupils.
15. A physical examination of Jesse would include an assessment of everything that was examined in the rapid trauma assessment plus the face, ears, eyes, nose, and mouth.

CHAPTER 15: Secondary Assessment

Match Key Terms

1. (N) Medical patient: A patient with one or more medical diseases or conditions. (p. 451)
2. (F) Reassessment: A procedure for detecting changes in a patient's condition after assessment and care has started. (p. 451)
3. (I) Past medical history (PMH): Information gathered regarding the patient's health problems in the past. (p. 451)
4. (L) Detailed physical exam: An assessment of the head, neck, chest, abdomen, pelvis, extremities, and posterior of the body to detect signs and symptoms of injury. (p. 451)
5. (K) Distension: A condition of being stretched, inflated, or larger than normal. (p. 451)
6. (J) History of present illness (HPI): Information gathered regarding the symptoms and nature of the patient's current concern. (p. 451)
7. (E) Symptom: Something regarding the patient's condition that the patient tells you. (p. 451)
8. (H) Sign: Evidence of the patient's condition that you can see. (p. 451)

9. (B) Paradoxical motion: Movement of part of the chest in the opposite direction to that of the rest of the chest during breathing. (p. 451)

10. (C) Priapism: Persistent erection of the penis that can result from spinal injury and some medical problems. (p. 451)

11. (D) Rapid trauma assessment: An assessment of the head, neck, chest, abdomen, pelvis, extremities, and posterior of the body in an injured patient who is unresponsive. (p. 451)

12. (G) Stoma: A permanent surgical opening in the neck through which the patient breathes. (p. 451)

13. (A) Tracheostomy: A surgical incision into the trachea that is held open by a metal or plastic tube. (p. 451)

14. (M) Trauma patient: A patient suffering from one or more physical injuries. (p. 451)

Multiple-Choice Review

1. (D) Why is the secondary assessment performed after the scene size-up and the primary assessment? Before the secondary assessment, you need to be sure there are no immediate life threats requiring intervention, you must be sure you are functioning at a safe scene, and you need to have called for all the resources you need. (p. 405)

2. (B) A patient suffering from one or more physical injuries is which type of patient? Trauma patient. (p. 406)

3. (D) When performing a secondary assessment, you will generally complete the: physical exam, patient history, and vital signs. (p. 406)

4. (D) Which statement is correct about a "sign" and/or a "symptom"? The patient tells you about a symptom. (pp. 406–407)

5. (B) When gathering a history from a child kneel or find another way to get on the level of the child. (p. 412)

6. (C) An alternative to using the mnemonic DCAP-BTLS suggested by the authors would be to remember wounds, tenderness and deformities. (p. 424)

7. (C) In reference to pediatrics the Guidelines for Field Triage of Injured Patients state: "< 15 years: Fall > 10 feet (3 meters)," should transport to a trauma ED. (p. 429)

8. (B) Listen to infant's lung sounds in the midaxillary position to ensure the sounds are not referred from the opposite lung. (p. 446)

9. (C) In the secondary assessment, you will be checking the patient for pain and tenderness. The difference between pain and tenderness is that tenderness may not hurt unless the area is palpated, whereas pain is evident without palpation. (p. 424)

10. (D) When assessing the responsive medical patient the steps include obtaining vital signs and: gathering the chief complaint and HPI, gathering a PMH from the patient, and conducting a physical exam. (p. 408)

11. (A) You are treating a baseball player who was hit in the face by a pitch. You remember from your EMT training that any blow above the clavicles may damage the cervical spine. (p. 425)

12. (A) If a cervical collar is the wrong size, it may cause additional injury to the spine. (p. 425)

13. (B) What is the correct statement about the typical order of the steps of secondary assessment of the responsive or the unresponsive medical patient? The chief complaint and the HPI come first in the responsive patient. (p. 408)

14. (C) When assessing and interviewing a patient, we ask about and look for signs and symptoms. What is a sign? An objective finding that you can see, hear, or feel when examining the patient. (p. 406)

15. (D) When a patient has shortness of breath additional history should include: fever or chills, cough, and dyspnea on exertion. (p. 411)

16. (B) You are treating a patient who was in the front seat of an automobile involved in a collision. You observe a spiderweb crack in the windshield and the facial lacerations on the patient. Most-likely the patient did not wear a seat belt or three-point harness. (p. 421)

17. (C) When asking about additional history items such as fever, nausea and vomiting, diarrhea, or constipation, you are most-likely gathering a history for a medical patient with abdominal pain. (p. 411)

18. (C) When assessing the head of an adult male critical trauma patient, the EMT should inspect and palpate for crepitation in addition to wounds, tenderness, and deformities. (p. 430)

19. (A) When assessing the neck of an adult female critical trauma patient, the EMT should inspect and palpate for jugular vein distention in addition to wounds and deformities. (p. 431)

20. (B) When assessing the pelvis of an adult male critical trauma patient, the EMT should inspect and palpate for distended areas in addition to wounds, deformities, and tenderness. (p. 432)

21. (B) If you are treating a severely injured trauma patient, it may be appropriate to skip the detailed physical exam. (p. 448)

22. (B) A difference between the detailed physical examination and the rapid trauma assessment is the detailed examination is usually done en route to the ED. (p. 423)

23. (D) The final step of the detailed physical examination is to roll the patient to examine the posterior of the body. (p. 433)

24. (C) You are examining a patient who was struck on the head last night. His mental status is altered, and he has a bruise behind one ear. This is referred to as Battle sign. (p. 435)

25. (C) When performing a rapid assessment of the head in a trauma patient, you note blood in the anterior chamber of the eyes. This tells you that the eye sustained significant force and is bleeding inside. (p. 435)

26. (B) Clear fluid that is draining from the ears and nose is cerebrospinal fluid. (p. 436)

27. (D) In addition to looking for deformities, you should look for all of the following except crepitation when examining the mouth. (p. 431)

28. (D) You will be conducting a rapid physical examination on an unresponsive 54-year-old female medical patient. You should include all of the following steps except asking the SAMPLE history questions. (p. 416)

29. (D) All of the following are high-risk patients (per CDC Guidelines) except intrusion > 6 inches into the occupant side of car. (p. 429)

©2021 Pearson Education, Inc.
Emergency Care, 14th Ed.

30. (D) It is important to realize that even people who were wearing seat belts may sustain injury to the neck arteries, the bowel, and abdominal organs. (p. 433)

31. (B) Flat neck veins in a patient who is lying down may be a sign of blood loss. (p. 437)

32. (B) When conducting the rapid trauma exam of the chest you note the patient has a number of rib fractures broken at both ends. This condition can lead to paradoxical motion during breathing. (p. 438)

33. (B) When examining an infant who sustained trauma you should do each of the following except apply pressure to the soft spots on the head to feel for swelling. (p. 444)

34. (C) The best position to maintain for the injured child's airway is the neutral position. (p. 447)

35. (B) The neck veins are usually not visible when the patient is sitting up. (p. 437)

Complete the Following

1. List four steps of secondary assessment in their usual order for a responsive medical patient. (p. 408)
 A. Gather the chief complaint and history of the present illness.
 B. Gather past medical history and SAMPLE information.
 C. Conduct a physical exam (per body system).
 D. Obtain baseline vital signs.

2. List four steps of secondary assessment in their usual order for an unresponsive medical patient. (p. 408)
 A. Conduct rapid physical exam.
 B. Obtain baseline vital signs.
 C. Gather HPI and OPQRST.
 D. Gather PMH and SAMPLE.

3. List five significant injuries and signs of significant injuries. (p. 434)
 A. Unresponsive or AMS.
 B. Penetrating wound of the head, neck, chest, or abdomen.
 C. Airway that is not patent.
 D. Respiratory compromise.
 E. Pallor, tachycardia, and other signs of shock.

4. When conducting a physical exam/trauma assessment in addition to examining for wounds, tenderness and deformities, what else should be checked for: (p. 435)
 • Head – crepitation, trachea.
 • Neck – JVD, crepitation.
 • Chest – paradoxical motion, crepitation, breath sounds.
 • Abdomen – firmness, softness, distention.
 • Pelvis – pain, tenderness, motion.
 • Extremities – distal circulation, sensation, motor function.

5. List four general principles to remember when examining a patient. (443)
 A. Tell the patient what you are going to do.
 B. Expose any injured area before examining it.
 C. Try to maintain eye contact.
 D. Consider spine motion restriction protocols.

Case Study: Just a Bit Dizzy

1. Mental status, airway, breathing, circulation, and determining patient priority

2. Physical examination, patient history, and vital signs

3. Examples of questions include the following:
 • S—Signs and symptoms: What's wrong?
 • A—Allergies: Are you allergic to medications or foods or to anything in the environment?

 • M—Medications: What medications are you currently taking or are you supposed to be taking?
 • P—Pertinent past history: Do you have any medical problems? Have you been feeling ill? Have you recently had any surgery or injuries? Have you been seeing a doctor? What is your doctor's name?
 • L—Last oral intake: When did you last eat or drink? What did you eat or drink? (Also if a patient will need to go to surgery, the hospital staff must know when he or she last had anything to eat or drink.)
 • E—Events leading to the injury or illness: What sequence of event led up to today's problem?

4. Endocrine

5. Seven specific questions are as follows (others may also be appropriate):
 A. What is the patient's history of endocrine conditions?
 B. Does the patient takes medications and, if so, when were they last taken?
 C. Has the patient eaten?
 D. Has the patient been exerting herself at an unusual level?
 E. Is the patient currently sick?
 F. Has the patient checked her blood glucose recently?
 G. Does the patient have an insulin pump?

6. Linda, a diabetic, has been at the mall all day, missed lunch, and probably got hypoglycemic. The candy bar was a little too late, and she is lucky that she is still alert. But she needs to have more sugar to bring her blood glucose level back to her normal level.

CHAPTER 16: Reassessment

Match Key Terms

1. (B) Trending: Changes in a patient's condition over time, such as slowing respirations or rising pulse rate, that may show improvement. (p. 459)

2. (A) Reassessment: A procedure for detecting changes in a patient's condition. It involves four steps: repeating the primary assessment, repeating and recording vital signs, repeating the physical exam, and checking interventions. (p. 459)

Multiple-Choice Review

1. (D) Which of the following most accurately describes the purpose of performing a reassessment on your patient? To repeat key elements of assessment procedures already performed to detect changes in patient condition. (p. 454)

2. (D) Your patient is a young child who was suddenly injured. During the reassessment, which of the following should you do and why? (p. 454)

3. (C) You are treating a 45-year-old male who sustained multiple injuries in a fall. En route to the hospital, you will be conducting a reassessment, which includes all the following steps except repeating the detailed physical exam. (p. 454)

4. (D) Which is not something you should do when performing the reassessment of the 25-year-old male with a rib fracture? Apply a cervical collar. (p. 455)

5. (D) During your reassessment of a 22-year-old female who is complaining of abdominal cramps, you note that her pulse is rapid and her skin is cool, pale, and clammy. This may indicate the onset of shock. (p. 455)

CHAPTER 16: (continued)

6. (B) If the patient has normal vital signs, you would consider his condition to be stable, and the recommended interval for reassessment is every 15 minutes. (p. 457)

7. (D) Examples of subtle changes you should pick up on during reassessment would include anxiety, restlessness, and sweating. (p. 454)

8. (A) You are transporting an unstable 30-year-old male trauma patient directly to the Regional Trauma Center. How often should you be doing your reassessment? Every 5 minutes. (p. 457)

9. (A) Her only medical history is a past stroke and taking blood thinner medication. On reassessment her pulse jumped up 20 points. Your next reassessment should be in 5 minutes. (p. 458)

Complete the Following

1. List three things you should always evaluate when checking interventions during your patient reassessment. (p. 457)
   A. Ensure adequacy of oxygen delivery and artificial ventilation.
   B. Ensure the management of any bleeding is effective.
   C. Ensure adequacy of other interventions.

2. When reassessing your patient, you need to repeat the primary assessment. List the six key steps to re-check: (p. 455)
   A. Reassess the mental status.
   B. Maintain open airway.
   C. Monitor breathing for rate and quality.
   D. Reassess the pulse for rate and quality.
   E. Monitor skin color and temperature.
   F. Reestablish patient priorities.

3. How would the mental status of an unresponsive child or infant be reassessed? (p. 456)
   A. Check by speaking loudly (verbal stimuli) or flicking the feet (painful stimuli).

4. List three tips to consider when reassessing a pediatric patient. (p. 454)
   A. Maintain eye contact with a conscious child.
   B. Stay on the child's level as much as possible.
   C. Explain what you are doing in a quiet and reassuring voice.

CHAPTER 17: Communication and Documentation

Match Key Terms

1. (E) Base station: A two-way radio at a fixed site such as a hospital or dispatch center. (p. 491)

2. (C) Cell phone: A phone that transmits through the air instead of over wires so that the phone can be transported and used over a wide area. (p. 491)

3. (D) Mobile radio: A two-way radio that is used or affixed in a vehicle. (p. 491)

4. (F) Portable radio: A handheld two-way radio. (p. 491)

5. (B) Repeater: A device that picks up signals from lower-power radio units, such as mobile and portable radios, and retransmits them at a higher power. It allows low-power radio signals to be transmitted over longer distances. (p. 491)

6. (H) Watt: The unit of measurement of the output of a radio. (p. 491)

7. (A) Drop report (or transfer report): An abbreviated form of the PCR that an EMS crew can leave at the hospital when there is not enough time to complete the PCR before leaving. (p. 491)

8. (G) Telemetry: The process of sending and receiving data wirelessly. (p. 491)

Multiple-Choice Review

1. (D) After arriving in the ED you should introduce the patient by name, summarize what was in your radio report, and provide history that was not given previously, discuss additional treatment given en route, and update the vital signs taken en route. (p. 469)

2. (D) The components of an EMS communications system include base stations, mobile radios, and portable radios. (pp. 464–465)

3. (C) This device, which boosts up the power and retransmits it, is called a repeater. (p. 465)

4. (A) The U.S. government agency that is responsible for maintaining order on the airwaves is the FCC. (p. 466)

5. (C) The reason for always closely following the general principles of radio transmission is to allow everyone to use the frequencies and to prevent delays. (p. 466)

6. (C) The correct order, of those listed, would be: unit identification and level of provider, chief complaint, major past illness, and emergency medical care given. (p. 468)

7. (B) You arrive at the office of a 52-year-old male. Your unit was alerted because he has had chest pain for the past 45 minutes. The chest pain is referred to as the chief complaint. (p. 481)

8. (D) During your radio report, you state, "The patient's abdomen feels rigid." You are advising the ED of pertinent findings of the physical examination. (p. 469)

9. (C) During your radio report you state. "The patient's mental status has not changed during our care." You are attempting to advise the ED of the response of the patient to the emergency medical care you have provided. (p. 469)

10. (A) Whenever you request an order for medical direction over the radio, it is good practice to repeat the physician's order word for word back to the physician. (p. 469)

11. (B) If you receive an order from the on-line physician for ten times the normal dose of a medication, what should you do? Question the physician about the order. (p. 469)

12. (B) You notice that your partner is standing with arms crossed looking down at the patient. What nonverbal message is your partner sending to the patient? "I am not really interested." (p. 472)

13. (D) The most appropriate response would be "Yes it is, and I will be as gentle as possible in splinting it." (p. 472)

14. (A) In treating a 2-year-old who is sitting on the couch crying and complaining of "tummy" pain, the best approach would be to kneel down so that you are at the child's level. (p. 474)

15. (C) The PCR has many functions. It serves as a legal document as well as an aid to research, education, and administrative efforts. (p. 476)

©2021 Pearson Education, Inc.
Emergency Care, 14th Ed.

16. (B) Why is it necessary to complete a PCR/drop report if, on each call, you give the ED staff a good oral report? It provides a means for the ED staff to review the patient's prehospital care. (p. 476)

17. (C) The copy of the PCR that is provided to the hospital becomes part of the patient's permanent hospital record. (p. 476)

18. (C) Which of the following will best help you recall the events of the call? A complete and accurate PCR. (p. 476)

19. (D) The person who completed the PCR may be called to a court of law to testify about the call in a criminal proceeding, care provided to the patient, and call in a civil proceeding. (p. 476)

20. (B) The routine review of PCRs for conformity to current medical and organizational standards is part of a process called quality improvement. (p. 478)

21. (B) Each individual box on a PCR, either paper or electronic, is called a data element. (p. 478)

22. (C) According to the NHTSA, in addition to the data elements, the minimum data set on a PCR should include all of the following except the patient's Social Security number. (p. 479)

23. (B) The time of incident is an example of run data on the PCR. (p. 479)

24. (A) The PCR serves a number of purposes for the EMS system and EMTs. An example of patient information on a PCR would be the date of birth and age of the patient. (p. 480)

25. (C) EMTs should consider a good PCR to be one that paints a picture of the patient. (p. 480)

26. (B) A statement such as "The patient has a swollen, deformed extremity" on the narrative portion of the PCR is an example of objective information. (p. 481)

27. (C) All the following are examples of information that should be put in quotation marks on the PCR except objective information. (p. 481)

28. (B) In the narrative section of a PCR, the EMT should include pertinent negatives. (p. 481)

29. (C) Medical abbreviations should be used on a PCR only if they are standardized. (p. 481)

30. (D) Before leaving the scene, you should document assessment findings and care given, try again to persuade the patient to go to a hospital, and ensure that the patient is able to make a rational, informed decision. (p. 483)

31. (D) When completing a PCR involving a patient refusal, the EMT should document all of the following except the patient's definitive diagnosis. (p. 484)

32. (A) An EMT who forgot to administer a treatment that is required by the state or regional treatment protocols should document on the PCR only treatment that was actually given. (p. 486)

33. (A) Falsification of information on a PCR may lead to suspension or revocation of your license or certification. (p. 486)

34. (B) To correct an error that is discovered while writing the PCR, you should draw a line through the error, initial it, and write the correct information. (p. 487)

35. (C) If information was omitted by mistake, you should add a note with the correct information, date it, and initial it. (p. 487)

36. (A) An example of an instance in which it would not be unusual for the EMT to obtain only a limited amount of information is during a multiple-casualty incident (MCI). (p. 487)

37. (A) Special situation reports document events that should be reported to local regulatory authorities. (p. 488)

38. (B) Ambulance services and EMS personnel are required by HIPAA to take steps to safeguard patient confidentiality. (p. 482)

39. (A) An example of a method that an ambulance service would use to safeguard patient confidentiality is requiring employees to place completed PCRs in a locked box. (p. 482)

40. (D) The policy that an ambulance service develops concerning patient rights and confidentially must take into consideration state regulations, local regulations, and HIPAA. (p. 482)

Complete the Following

1. List six examples of components of a communications system. (pp. 464–465)
   A. Base station
   B. Mobile radios
   C. Portable radios
   D. Repeaters
   E. Cell phone
   F. Telemetry

2. List six interpersonal communications guidelines to use when dealing with patients, families, friends, and bystanders. (pp. 471–473)
   A. Use eye contact.
   B. Be aware of your position and body.
   C. Use language the patient can understand.
   D. Be honest.
   E. Use the patient's proper name.
   F. Listen.

3. List five examples of patient information on a PCR. (p. 480)
   A. Patient's name, address and phone number
   B. Patient's sex, age, and date of birth
   C. Patient's weight
   D. Patient's race and/or ethnicity
   E. Billing and insurance information

4. List five examples of situations that may require the use of a special incident report. (p. 488)
   A. Exposure to infectious disease
   B. Injury to yourself or another EMT
   C. Hazardous or unsafe scenes to which other crews should be alerted
   D. Referrals to social service agencies for elderly or other patients in need of home care
   E. Mandatory reports for child or elder abuse

5. List six principles of radio communication. (p. 466)

   (Any six of the following)
   - Make sure that your radio is on and the volume is adjusted properly.
   - Reduce background noise by closing the vehicle window when possible.
   - Listen to the frequency and ensure that it is clear before beginning a transmission.
   - Press the "press to talk" (PTT) button on the radio, then wait one second before speaking.
   - Speak with your lips about 2–3 inches from the microphone.
   - When calling another unit or base station, use their unit number or name, followed by yours.
   - If the unit you are calling tells you to "Stand by," wait until they tell you they are ready to take your transmission.

- Speak slowly and clearly.
- Keep the transmissions brief.
- Use plain English. Avoid codes.
- Do not use phrases such as "be advised." These are implied and serve no purpose.
- Courtesy is assumed, so there is no need to say "Please," "Thank you."
- When transmitting a number that might be unclear give the number and then repeat the individual digits.
- Anything said over the radio can be heard by the public on a scanner. Do not use the patient's name over the radio.
- Use "we" instead of "I." As an EMT you will rarely be acting alone.
- "Affirmative" and "Negative" are preferred over "Yes" and "No."
- Give assessment information about your patient but avoid offering a field diagnosis of the patient's problem.
- Avoid slang or abbreviations that are not authorized.
- Use EMS frequencies only for authorized EMS communications.

Case Study: Asleep at the Wheel

1. You may have already used a mobile radio and a portable radio.

2. The reason why the ambulance was called in this case—the chief complaint in the patient's own words—was for a car crash.

3. Initially, your partner or another EMS provider should consider the need for spinal motion restriction.

4. No. This should not be a gray zone decision. This should be black and white, so use your clinical judgment to get out of the gray zone and realize that on the basis of the MOI and situation, this patient should not be allowed to sign off. If you are not sure, discuss this case with your Medical Director.

5. On the basis of the MOI, frontal striking a tree with lots of damage to the vehicle and the fact that the patient did strike his head and wants to sleep now, you should make every effort to talk him into being seen in the ED.

6. If you cannot convince the patient to be seen in the ED and your partner can't convince him, try getting your supervisor or your Medical Director on the radio or cell phone or a police officer to talk with the patient.

7. On the basis of the information we have, the medical radio report would at least say:

This is unit number XXX.

This is EMT XXX.

I have an ETA of XXX.

En route to your facility with a 28-year-old male.

He was involved in a single car crash with significant damage to the front of his vehicle.

He is alert and states, "I was tired and may have fallen asleep at the wheel." He denies any loss of consciousness but does have a laceration on his forehead, which has stopped bleeding. He also states that he wants to sleep now.

He denies any major illness or other medical history.

We have his head bandaged; he has received spinal motion restriction precautions; and we have no requests for orders.

He is resting comfortably at this point.

8. Additional information you have found out since the radio report and any changes in the patient's condition as well as more detailed information you might not want to take the time to transmit over the radio.

CHAPTER 18: General Pharmacology

Match Key Terms

1. (H) Atomizer: A device attached to the end of a syringe that turns medicine into fine droplets upon administration. (p. 515)

2. (E) Aspirin: A medication used to reduce the clotting ability of blood to prevent and treat clots associated with myocardial infarction. (p. 515)

3. (L) Contraindication: Specific circumstances under which it is not appropriate and may be harmful to administer a drug to a patient. (p. 515)

4. (F) Epinephrine: A drug that helps to constrict the blood vessels and relax passages of the airway. It may be used to counter a severe allergic reaction. (p. 515)

5. (A) Indications: Specific signs or circumstances under which it is appropriate to administer a drug to a patient. (p. 515)

6. (B) Inhaler: A device with a mouthpiece that contains a dry aerosolized form of a medication that a patient can spray into their mouth while they breathe in. (p. 515)

7. (M) Nitroglycerin: A drug that helps to dilate the coronary vessels that supply the heart muscle with blood. (p. 515)

8. (D) Oral glucose: A medication given by mouth to treat an awake patient (who is able to swallow) with an altered mental status and a history of diabetes. (p. 515)

9. (G) Oxygen: A gas commonly found in the atmosphere, that is also a medication that can be used to treat patients with respiratory distress and hypoxia. Pure oxygen is used as a drug to treat any patient whose medical or traumatic condition may cause hypoxia, or low oxygen. (p. 515)

10. (C) Pharmacology: The study of drugs, their sources, their characteristics, and their effects. (p. 515)

11. (I) Pharmacodynamics: The study of the effects of medications on the body. (p. 515)

12. (K) Side effect: Any action of a drug other than the desired action. (p. 515)

13. (J) Untoward effect: An unexpected effect of a medication in addition to its desired effect that may be potentially harmful to the patient. (p. 504)

14. (O) Parenteral: Referring to a route of medication administration that does not use the gastrointestinal tract, such as an intravenous medication. (p. 515)

15. (P) Enteral: Referring to a route of medication administration that uses the gastrointestinal tract, such as swallowing a pill. (p. 515)

16. (N) Naloxone: An antidote for narcotic overdoses. (p. 515)

Multiple-Choice Review

1. (D) The study of drugs, their sources, and their effects is referred to as pharmacology. (p. 496)

2. (D) Medications that EMTs can routinely administer or assist with in the field include aspirin, oral glucose, naloxone, nitroglycerin, epinephrine, and prescribed inhalers. (p. 496)

3. (C) According to treatment protocols, an EMT in the field would administer aspirin to help prevent clot formation. (p. 497)

4. (B) When would aspirin administration be contraindicated? If the patient has a history of GI bleeding. (p. 497)

5. (B) Poorly managed diabetes can cause altered mental status. (p. 497)

6. (A) Oral glucose is given between the patient's cheek and gum, using a tongue depressor, because this method promotes fast absorption into the bloodstream and easy swallowing. (p. 497)

7. (C) Examples of medications he may have in his possession that you may assist him in taking, under the appropriate circumstances are epinephrine auto-injector, a bronchodilator inhaler, nitroglycerin, and aspirin. (pp. 499–501)

8. (C) Your 52-year-old female patient states that she has a long history of asthma and chronic bronchitis. It would be expected that she carry a bronchodilator in her purse. (p. 499)

9. (C) Your 62-year-old male patient has a history of cardiac problems and states that he takes nitroglycerin when he gets chest pain. Nitroglycerin is used to dilate the coronary vessels. (p. 501)

10. (C) The comprehensive U.S. government publication that lists all drugs is called the *U.S. Pharmacopoeia (USP)*. (p. 503)

11. (B) The name that the manufacturer uses in marketing a drug is called the trade name. (p. 503)

12. (D) A circumstance in which a drug should not be used because it may cause harm to the patient is called a contraindication. (p. 504)

13. (A) An action of a drug that is other than the desired action is called a side effect. (p. 504)

14. (D) Before administering the medication, you must know all of the following except both the generic and chemical names. (p. 505)

15. (B) Drugs prescribed for pain relief are called analgesics. (p. 509)

16. (D) Drugs that are prescribed to reduce high blood pressure are called antihypertensives. (p. 509)

17. (C) Drugs that are prescribed for heart rhythm disorders are called antidysrhythmics. (p. 509)

18. (B) Medications that are prescribed to relax the smooth muscles of the bronchial tubes are called bronchodilators. (p. 509)

19. (C) Drugs that are prescribed for prevention and control of seizures are called anticonvulsants. (p. 509)

20. (A) This type of drug is called an antidepressant. (p. 509)

21. (C) When a patient is administered tiny aerosolized particles of medicine to treat a disease such as asthma, this is considered the inhaled route of administration. (p 506)

22. (B) An example of an understanding of the pharmacodynamics of a specific medication is knowing that medications may have a longer effect in geriatric patients. (p. 507)

23. (B) Your patient may have taken an OD of an opiate/narcotic and is unresponsive and having very slow and very shallow respirations. While assisting ventilations with a BVM you should consider administering naloxone by the intranasal route. (p. 499)

24. (C) A powder prepared from charred wood administered by some EMS Systems to theconscious poisoning patient is called activated charcoal. (p. 498)

25. (D) When assisting an ALS provider in starting an IV on a patient, you notice that the fluid is not flowing thru the drip chamber of the administration set. What could be the problem? The clamp may be closed on the tubing, the constricting band was left on the arm, and the tubing may be kinked. (p. 513)

26. (C) The antidote used in medicine when an overdose of a narcotic has caused a slow respiratory drive is naloxone. (p. 499)

Pathophysiology: How Medications for Asthma and Anaphylaxis Work

1. Air does not move in and out easily, and you will likely hear wheezes as well as a prolonged expiratory phase.

2. The small airways are becoming reactive and constricted.

3. Exercise, allergens, respiratory viruses, and even aspirin and NSAIDs can trigger this reaction.

4. Albuterol is commonly administered by inhaler or small-volume nebulizer. Its role is to dilate the small airways, making it much easier for the patient to breathe.

5. An allergic reaction is a life-threatening condition that can have severe effects on the airway, respiratory system, the cardiovascular system, and other systems of the body. The major concerns are airway closure, shock, and decreased blood pressure, an altered mental status, and severe respiratory distress. This patient could also wheeze, so remember that wheezes occur not just with asthma.

6. Histamines and other substances cause the cells to leak, causing vasodilatation and shock as well as bronchoconstriction.

7. An Epi-Pen® or other epinephrine self-injector

8. Epinephrine causes vasoconstriction, which reverses the shock. It also reduces vascular permeability and the edema found in the face and airways. It also causes bronchodilation, opening up the constricted airways.

Complete the Following

1. List seven medications that an EMT can administer or assist a patient in taking.
   A. Bronchodilator (albuterol). (p. 496)
   B. Nitroglycerin.
   C. Epinephrine auto-injector.
   D. Aspirin.
   E. Oral glucose.
   F. Oxygen.
   G. Naloxone.

2. List the five questions to ask yourself to assure you are addressing the five "rights" when administering a medication. (p. 505)
   A. Do I have the right patient?
   B. It is the right time to administer this medication?
   C. Is this the right medication?
   D. Is this the right dose?
   E. Am I giving this medication by the right route of administration?

3. List eight routes of administration of medications. (pp. 506–507)
   A. Oral, or swallowed.
   B. Sublingual, or dissolved under the tongue.

    C. Inhaled, or breathed into the lungs.
    D. Intranasal, or sprayed into the nostrils.
    E. Intravenous, or injected into a vein.
    F. Intramuscular, or injected into a muscle.
    G. Subcutaneous, or injected under the skin.
    H. Intraosseous, or injected into the bone marrow cavity.
    I. Endotracheal, or sprayed directly into a tube inserted into the trachea.

4. List what the following herbal agents are used for. (p. 510)
    A. Gingko – dementia, poor circulation to the legs, ringing in the ears.
    B. Garlic – high cholesterol.
    C. Ginger root – nausea and vomiting.
    D. Evening primrose oil – premenstrual syndrome.
    E. Kava kava – anxiety.

Case Study: Altered Mental Status

1. Respiratory distress turns into respiratory failure and then respiratory arrest.

2. Assist the patient's ventilations with a BVM and oxygen.

3. Yes, you should definitely continue to have them respond for more help and more assistance with altered mental status as well as airway management.

4. Hypoxia, head injury, hyperthermia, hypothermia, shock, hypoglycemia, stroke, and drug overdose are some potential causes of altered mental state.

5. Bring them along to the emergency department.

6. When you have a moment en route to the hospital, you could check your resources in the ambulance or on your smart phone.

7. The patient should become more alert, and his respiratory rate and depth should improve. If given too much of a dose too fast, he could wake up in withdrawal and be violent, so be careful.

8. Give him another dose according to your regional protocol, and of course check his blood sugar with your glucometer.

9. (A) Prozac is an antidepressant, (B) Topamax is an antiseizure medication, and (C) OxyContin is a narcotic analgesic

CHAPTER 19: Respiratory Emergencies

Match Key Terms

1. (C) Bronchoconstriction: Abnormal narrowing of the smaller airways of the lungs from conditions such as allergies or pulmonary conditions. (p. 546)

2. (D) Exhalation: Another term for expiration. (p. 552)

3. (F) Expiration: A passive process in which the intercostal (rib) muscles and the diaphragm relax, causing the chest cavity to decrease in size and force air from the lungs. (p. 552)

4. (B) Inhalation: Another term for inspiration. (p. 552)

5. (A) Inspiration: An active process in which the intercostal (rib) muscles and the diaphragm contract, expanding the size of the chest cavity and causing air to flow into the lungs. (p. 552)

6. (E) Continuous positive airway pressure (CPAP): A form of noninvasive positive pressure ventilation (BPPV) consisting of a mask and a means of blowing oxygen or air into the mask to prevent airway collapse or to help alleviate difficulty breathing. (p. 552)

Multiple-Choice Review

1. (C) The thin, umbrella-shaped muscle that divides the chest cavity from the abdominal cavity is called the diaphragm muscle. (p. 521)

2. (B) In the mechanical process of breathing, expiration is a passive process that involves the relaxation of the intercostal muscles and the diaphragm. (p. 521)

3. (D) To determine the quality of breathing in an asthma patient, you should check for all of the following except breathing rhythm. (p. 524)

4. (C) Aside from quickly checking his pulse, your treatment of this patient should involve immediate ventilation with supplemental oxygen. (p. 526)

5. (B) He is using the muscles in his neck and abdomen to assist his breathing. These muscles are referred to as the accessory muscles of breathing. (p. 523)

6. (D) Oxygenation of the body's tissue is reduced in a patient with inadequate breathing, so the skin may be blue in color and feel clammy and cool. (p. 524)

7. (A) You are treating an unresponsive 38-year-old female. If she is making snoring or gurgling sounds, she may have a serious problem requiring your immediate intervention. (p. 526)

8. (C) Of the following causes of death, statistically, the leading killer of infants and children is respiratory conditions. (p. 525)

9. (D) You need to recall that the structure of an infant's or child's airway is different from an adult's in each of the following way except the cricoid cartilage is more rigid. (p. 525)

10. (B) Because the chest wall is softer in infants and children, they depend more heavily on the diaphragm for breathing. (p. 525)

11. (D) In infants and children, signs of inadequate breathing include all of the following except lip quivering. (p. 525)

12. (B) To move air, the respiratory system changes pressure within the chest cavity. Negative pressure is used to move air in and positive pressure is used to move air out. (p. 520)

13. (B) The appropriate rate of artificial ventilations for a nonbreathing adult patient who still has a pulse is 10 to 12 breaths per minute. (p. 527)

14. (C) The appropriate rate of artificial ventilations for the nonbreathing infant or child who has a palpable pulse is 12 to 20 breaths per minute. (p. 527)

15. (C) If an infant or a child has a slow pulse in the setting of a respiratory emergency, this usually indicates trouble. (p. 525)

16. (B) A respiratory rate of 18 to 30 would be considered adequate for a school-age child. (p. 522)

17. (B) In observing the breathing of a 45-year-old female, all of the following are important observations for you to make except the lung sounds. (pp. 529–530)

18. (B) In neonates and infants the rib cage flares outward at the bottom as compared to an adult's rib cage which flares inward. What is the problem posed by this difference in

©2021 Pearson Education, Inc.
Emergency Care, 14th Ed.

anatomy? A flatter diaphragm makes it more difficult for infant to generate negative pressure. (p. 522)

19. (C) You are talking to a 62-year-old female who is speaking in short, choppy sentences. This could be an indication that she is experiencing breathing difficulty. (p. 523)

20. (B) Your patient is seated in the tripod position. This means that she is leaning forward with hands resting on knees. (p. 529)

21. (D) Which pair of signs/symptoms is not commonly associated with breathing difficulty? Vomiting/headache. (p. 530)

22. (B) During your assessment, you decide that he is breathing adequately. If oxygen is administered, it should be given via nonrebreather mask. (p. 526)

23. (C) If a 62-year-old male is experiencing breathing difficulty and is breathing adequately, it is usually best to place him in the sitting-up position on your stretcher. (p. 534)

24. (B) Infants and children are subject to respiratory infections that may cause swelling of airway passages. The care of these patients includes all of the following except check the airway with a tongue depressor. (p. 528)

25. (C) Once you receive permission from medical direction to assist a patient with an inhaler, make sure that you have all of the following except a large enough syringe. (p. 549)

26. (A) Before coaching the patient from question 25 in the use of the inhaler, you should shake the inhaler vigorously. (p. 549)

27. (B) To ensure that the most medication is absorbed in using an inhaler, encourage the patient to hold the breath as long as possible. (p. 547)

28. (A) Using CPAP on a patient with respiratory distress is a means of preventing the alveoli from collapsing at the end of inhalation. (p. 535)

29. (C) To help improve the volume of the medication that the patient is able to self-administer when in distress, the physician may prescribe a spacer device. (p. 546)

30. (B) Of the prescribed inhalers listed below, which is not considered a medication that would be used in an emergency to reverse airway constriction because its use in intended to prevent attacks by reducing inflammation? Advair. (p. 547)

31. (D) This sound, caused by fluid in the alveoli, is called crackles. (p. 531)

32. (D) Although CPAP is frequently effective in relieving a patient's difficulty with breathing, it can have a side effect to: producing hypotension, pneumothorax, and gastric distension. (p. 536–537)

33. (B) If a patient who has been treated with CPAP for the past 10 minutes starts to experience a decrease in mental status, the EMT should remove CPAP and ventilate with a BVM. (p. 537)

34. (B) Your 58-year-old female patient has a chronic respiratory disease that has episodic exacerbations or flares. She is most likely suffering from asthma. (p. 540)

35. (A) He is 30 years old, is very thin and tall, and complains of a sudden sharp unilateral chest pain with each breath. What is his most likely respiratory condition? Spontaneous pneumothorax. (p. 542)

36. (C) The use of CPAP may be indicated if the patient whom you suspect has acute pulmonary edema also has stable vital signs. (p. 535)

37. (D) A respiratory condition that may be caused by a deep vein thrombosis (DVT) after sitting for a very long flight is called pulmonary embolism. (p. 543)

38. (A) A respiratory condition that used to be prominent with children but has been virtually eliminated by vaccination of infants is epiglottitis. (p. 543)

39. (D) For a child with a suspected respiratory infection you should transport quickly if they have: wheezing, stridor or grunting, flared nostrils or retracted muscles of breathing, and pale or cyanotic lips or mouth. (p. 528)

40. (C) By inhaling and exhaling against the flow of air created by CPAP, patients increase their PEEP. (p. 535)

41. (B) Of the following signs of respiratory distress in a child, which is not an early sign? Decreased heart rate. (pp. 532–534)

42. (B) Your patient has a respiratory disease in which the walls of the alveoli break down, reducing surface area for respiratory exchange. What condition is most likely? Emphysema. (p. 539)

43. (C) A condition common in children where small airways become inflamed because of viral infections is most likely bronchiolitis. (p. 544)

Complete the Following

1. List eight observations during your primary and secondary assessment of the patient with breathing difficulty and inadequate breathing. (p. 524)
   A. Fast respiratory rate.
   B. Slowing or irregular respirations.
   C. Inability to speak.
   D. Silent chest.
   E. Low oxygen saturation despite supplemental oxygen.
   F. Agonal respirations.
   G. Uneven rhythm.
   H. Poor quality.

2. List three of the prehospital indications for CPAP. (p. 536)
   A. Pulmonary edema.
   B. Drowning.
   C. Pulmonary conditions such as asthma and COPD.
   D. Impending respiratory failure.

3. List and describe four of the common abnormal lung sounds. (p. 531)
   A. Wheezes - musical or tone-like sounds.
   B. Crackles - fine popping or crackling sounds.
   C. Rhonchi - loud course sounds heard in the larger airways.
   D. Stridor - high pitched airway sound, most commonly heard during inspiration.

4. Oxygen should be administered to all patients with severe respiratory distress, regardless of their oxygen saturation readings. The oximeter reading in a normal, healthy person is typically (A) greater than 95%. An oximeter reading below (B) 94% often indicates hypoxia. (p. 534)

5. List the indications and contraindications and side effects for albuterol.
   A. Indications:
      • Patient exhibits signs and symptoms of respiratory emergency.
      • Patient has physician-prescribed handheld inhaler.
      • Medical direction gives specific authorization to use.
   B. Contraindications:
      • Patient is unable to use the device.
      • Inhaler is not prescribed for the patient.
      • No permission has been given by medical direction.
      • Patient has already taken the maximum prescribed dose prior to the EMT's arrival.

CHAPTER 19: (continued)

C. Side effects:
- Increased pulse rate.
- Tremors.
- Nervousness. (p. 549)

Label the Diagrams

1. relaxation
2. muscle contraction
3. inspiration
4. muscle relaxation (p. 521)

Case Study: The Three A.M. Call: "Mom Simply Cannot Breathe"

1. As you approach the patient, your Standard Precautions should include disposable gloves and a surgical mask at a minimum.

2. An N-95 mask should be used if there is a possibility that the patient may have active TB.

3. Awake and alert patients who have breathing difficulty usually find the Fowler or semi-Fowler position (sitting up) most comfortable.

4. Patients who talk in short, choppy sentences usually have respiratory distress.

5. The initial oxygen administration should be given via a nonrebreather mask.

6. If the patient's breathing were too fast, too slow, or too shallow, the bag-mask device or pocket face mask would be more appropriate. Use your clinical judgment on this, and assess the SpO$_2$. Also call for ALS on this call.

7. Albuterol is given, with medical direction approval, by inhaling two puffs through the patient's MDI.

8. No, the patient's family member's medicine cannot be used for the patient. Use only the patient's prescribed medicine(s). If in your clinical judgment, you feel strongly that the patient needs this medication, consult with Medical Direction, stating clearly that the medication you have available is not actually the patient's.

9. A spacer can be used, and some patients are more comfortable with the spacer device attached to their MDI.

10. Expect to see tachycardia, slight tremors, and some anxiety from the medication.

CHAPTER 20: Cardiac Emergencies

Match Key Terms

Part A

1. (D) Acute coronary syndrome (ACS): A blanket term used to represent any symptoms related to lack of oxygen (ischemia) in the heart muscle. Also called cardiac compromise. (p. 587)

2. (G) Acute myocardial infarction (AMI): The condition in which a portion of the heart muscle dies as a result of occlusion; often called a heart attack by laypersons. (p. 578)

3. (F) Angina pectoris: Pain in the chest occurring when blood supply to the heart is reduced and a portion of the heart muscle is not receiving enough oxygen. (p. 578)

4. (E) Aneurysm: The dilation, or ballooning, of a weakened section of the wall of an artery. (p. 587)

5. (H) Bradycardia: When the heart rate is slow, usually below 60 beats per minute. (p. 578)

6. (I) Cardiovascular system: The heart and the blood vessels. (p. 578)

7. (A) Cardiac compromise: Another term for acute coronary syndrome. (p. 578)

8. (C) Coronary artery disease (CAD): Diseases that affect the blood vessels of the heart. (p. 578)

9. (B) Dyspnea: Shortness of breath; labored breathing or difficult breathing. (p. 578)

10. (J) Dysrhythmia: A disturbance in the heart rate and/or rhythm. (p. 578)

Part B

1. (H) Embolism: Blockage of a vessel by a clot or foreign material brought to the site by the blood current. (p. 578)

2. (C) Nitroglycerin: A medication that dilates the blood vessels. (p. 578)

3. (G) Occlusion: Blockage, as of an artery by fatty deposits. (p. 578)

4. (D) Pedal edema: Accumulation of fluid in the feet or ankles. (p. 578)

5. (B) Pulmonary edema: Accumulation of fluid in the lungs. (p. 578)

6. (A) Heart failure (HF): The failure of the heart to pump efficiently, leading to excessive blood or fluids in the lungs, the body, or both; previously known as congestive heart failure (CHF). (p. 578)

7. (F) Tachycardia: A heart rate of more than 100 beats per minute. (p. 578)

8. (E) Thrombus: A clot formed of blood and plaque attached to the inner wall of an artery or vein. (p. 578)

Multiple-Choice Review

1. (C) Your 58-year-old male patient is going to be admitted to the hospital for ACS. ACS is a blanket term that refers to any time the heart may not be getting enough oxygen. (p. 558)

2. (C) Chest discomfort from the heart is typically described by the patient as a "squeezing sensation." It is also often described as any of the following except tearing. (p. 559)

3. (A) When it is due to a heart problem, pain commonly radiates to the arms and jaw. (p. 559)

4. (C) In addition to chest pain or discomfort, the patient with ACS may also complain of dyspnea. (p. 559)

5. (C) Patients with heart problems may complain of any of the following except sudden onset of sharp abdominal pain. (p. 559)

6. (B) This is a very important vital sign because if the heart is beating too fast or too slow, the patient with ACS may also lose consciousness. (pp. 559–560)

7. (C) Her signs and symptoms may include any of the following except sharp lower abdominal pain and a fever. (p. 559)

8. (C) The EMT management of the patient with suspected ACS should include all of the following except administering CPAP. (pp. 565–567)

9. (B) An interruption to the heart's supply of oxygenated blood can result in significant problems. This is because, having no reserve of oxygen, heart muscle needs a constant supply of oxygenated blood. (p. 558)

10. (B) You should consider using nitroglycerin when a 65-year-old female patient has her own nitroglycerin and has crushing chest pain. (p. 568)

11. (C) Which of the following is the best description of the role of medical direction in the treatment of a 55-year-old male who you suspect has ACS? Authorizing the EMT to assist the patient in taking his prescribed nitroglycerin. (p. 567)

12. (C) For the EMT to administer nitroglycerin, all of following conditions must be met except that the patient's BP must be at least 80 mmHg systolic. (p. 568)

13. (C) The maximum number of doses of nitroglycerin routinely given by the EMT with medical control permission or taken by the patient at the advice of his or her physician is three. (p. 568)

14. (A) Nitroglycerin is contraindicated for a patient who has an obvious head injury and AMS. (p. 568)

15. (B) Of the following considerations, which would not be pertinent to administering this medication? The patient has a history of emphysema. (p. 567)

16. (C) After administering the nitroglycerin, it is important for you to reassess the BP. (p. 569)

17. (D) When conducting a physical exam of a suspected ACS patient you should look for findings such as: Levine's sign, sweating, and pale or gray skin. (p. 560)

18. (D) When managing a pediatric patient who appears to be suffering from an unknown or unclear cardiac condition you should transport to a facility capable of managing the patient's condition, ask caregivers how this condition differs from normal (baseline) for the child, and manage primary assessment issues in the same way you would for other children. (p. 577)

19. (B) A condition that is often the result of the buildup of fatty deposits on the inner walls of the arteries is called coronary artery disease. (p. 570)

20. (D) Factors that put a person at risk for developing CAD include: age, cigarette smoking, and obesity. (p. 570)

21. (C) Which of the following risk factors can be modified to reduce the risk of CAD? Hypertension. (p. 570)

22. (A) Most cardiac-related medical emergencies result from changes in the inner walls of the arteries. (p. 570)

23. (B) Angina pectoris means, literally: a pain in the chest. (p. 570)

24. (B) Why is nitroglycerin administered to the patient with chest pain? It dilates the blood vessels and decreases the work of the heart. (pp. 570–571)

25. (B) A condition in which a portion of the myocardium dies as a result of oxygen starvation is known as acute myocardial infarction. (p. 572)

26. (C) A cardiac arrest that occurs within 2 hours of the onset of cardiac symptoms is referred to as sudden death. (p. 573)

27. (B) These weak spots begin to dilate to form a condition that is known as an aneurysm. (p. 576)

28. (B) Because of his difficulty breathing and normally sedentary lifestyle, you suspect that he may be experiencing heart failure (HF). HF is failure of the heart to pump blood with normal efficiency. (p. 574)

29. (B) Damage to the left ventricle causes blood to back up into the lungs. Fluid shifting into the lungs is referred to as pulmonary edema. (p. 575)

30. (D) If your patient has HF and presents with acute pulmonary edema the prehospital management should include contacting ALS immediately, CPAP if the patient is alert, and nitroglycerin if your protocol allows. (p. 575)

31. (C) You are treating a 59-year-old male patient whose wife called EMS because he had difficulty breathing and was acting anxious and confused. He is diaphoretic and cyanotic, and his vitals are rapid respirations, tachycardia, and hypertension. He has swollen ankles and is coughing up pink sputum. What do you suspect is wrong with this patient? He has HF affecting both the right and left heart. (p. 574)

32. (C) A patient with pulmonary edema is likely to have each of the following in the field except flat neck veins. (p. 575)

33. (B) If a young child has a cardiac history it is likely to be congenital, due to a birth defect. (p. 569)

Complete the Following

1. List the nine signs and symptoms that are often associated with ACS: (p. 560)
   A. Pain, pressure, or discomfort in the chest, jaw, neck, arms or upper abdomen.
   B. Difficulty breathing.
   C. Palpitations.
   D. Sudden onset of sweating and nausea or vomiting.
   E. Syncope.
   F. Anxiety.
   G. Unusual generalized weakness.
   H. Abnormal pulse.
   I. Abnormal BP.

2. List the four steps recommended for 12-lead ECG Placement: (pp. 561–562)
   A. Step 1 – Place the limb leads.
   B. Step 2 – Place V1 and V2 leads.
   C. Step 3 – Place V4 and V3 leads.
   D. Step 4 – Place V5 and V6 leads.

Case Study: The patient was "Just Stacking Wood."

1. As you approach the patient, what are your immediate concerns? The breathing difficulty as well as the chest pain. Important to determine this patient's history and get an ALS unit to the scene.

2. When would you consider administering oxygen to the patient and with which device? As soon as you note he is short of breath consider oxygen and listen to his lung sounds right away.

3. If the patient with a chief complaint of chest pain is awake and alert, in what position would it be best for him to assess and manage him? The position of comfort which is usually sitting up. If he is dizzy he may want to lie down but that could make it more difficult to breathe.

4. What line of questioning would help to elaborate on the chief complaint? Use the OPQRST to elaborate on the chief complaint and get a SAMPLE history.

CHAPTER 20: (continued)

5. What oxygen device is most appropriate for the initial oxygen administration to this patient? With mild shortness of breath a nasal cannula would be appropriate to start with.

6. **GZQ:** If the patient is believed to have cardiac "ischemic" chest pain which equipment should be available at your side? Your oxygen, your AED, and the monitor to acquire a 12-Lead ECG if your protocols allow.

7. If Bill has his own nitroglycerin prescribed to him and you have a standing order protocol to assist him, how is this administered and what is the usual dose? The nitro is given sublingually by a pill or single spray. The dose is 0.4 mg. This patient may have taken aspirin already today but it would be appropriate to consider chewing four baby aspirins (dose of 324 mg).

8. **GZQ:** Your protocol is to acquire a quick 12-Lead ECG to assist in the transport/hospital destination decision. Why is this an important procedure that should be done quickly? The 12-Lead could indicate the patient is having an ST segment elevated acute myocardial infarction (STEMI). If this is occurring, the mantra is "time is muscle," so transportation to the appropriate cardiac hospital destination should not be delayed.

9. If Bill's vitals are still similar to the initial set will the medic consider another nitroglycerin? Yes, it is likely another dose of nitroglycerin would be appropriate and the medic may choose an even stronger pain reliever as well.

10. The medic reviews the ECG and states the patient is having a ST-elevation myocardial infarction (STEMI). How does this affect the hospital destination? This confirmation underscores the need to transport this patient to the nearest appropriate hospital that is equipped to handle cardiac emergencies.

CHAPTER 21: Resuscitation

Match Key Terms

1. (E) Agonal breathing: Irregular, gasping breaths that precede apnea or death. (p. 617)

2. (G) Apnea: No breathing. (p. 617)

3. (I) Asphyxial cardiac arrest: A cardiac arrest caused by systemic hypoxia, typically due to a respiratory disorder, airway occlusion, or significant impedance of the bellows action of the chest. (p. 617)

4. (K) Asystole: A condition in which the heart has ceased generating electrical impulses. Commonly called flatline. (p. 617)

5. (M) Cardiac arrest: A state in which the heart is no longer pumping blood. (p. 617)

6. (O) Cardiopulmonary resuscitation (CPR): Actions taken to revive a person by keeping the person's heart and lungs working artificially. (p. 617)

7. (P) Chain of survival: A metaphor that describes the key elements of cardiac arrest management. A representation of different but interconnected interventions that optimize care for cardiac arrest patients. (p. 617)

8. (B) Commotio cordis: A cardiac arrest dysrhythmia caused by acute blunt force trauma to the chest. (p. 617)

9. (A) Compression fraction: The amount of time chest compressions are being performed compared with the total time of patient contact. (p. 617)

10. (N) Defibrillation: Delivery of an electrical shock to stop the fibrillation of heart muscles and restore a normal heart rhythm. (p. 617)

11. (L) Dysrhythmia: An electrical disturbance in heart rate and/or rhythm. (p. 617)

12. (C) Pulseless electrical activity (PEA): A condition in which the heart's electrical rhythm remains relatively normal, yet the mechanical pumping activity of the heart fails, causing cardiac arrest. (p. 617)

13. (J) Return of spontaneous circulation (ROSC): The heart beating again after successful resuscitation. (p. 617)

14. (H) Sudden cardiac arrest: A cardiac arrest occurring due to the abrupt onset of a dysrhythmia. (p. 617)

15. (F) Ventricular fibrillation (VF): A condition in which the heart's electrical impulses are disorganized, preventing the heart muscle from contracting normally. (p. 617)

16. (D) Ventricular tachycardia (VT): A cardiac dysrhythmia originating in the larger chambers of the heart, that if rapid enough, will not allow for sufficient pumping of blood to meet the body's needs. (p. 617)

Multiple-Choice Review

1. (B) The most common mechanical reason the heart ceases to function correctly is loss of normal heart muscle structure. (p. 583)

2. (B) When a patient is in cardiac arrest and the monitor shows an organized ECG rhythm this is referred to as pulseless electrical activity (PEA). (p. 584)

3. (C) If the heart's electrical system fails completely and no electricity is created, this would show as asystole on the cardiac monitor. (p. 584)

4. (D) The five elements of the chain of survival include early activation and immediate high-quality CPR, rapid defibrillation, and basic and advanced emergency medical care. (p. 582)

5. (C) Poor blood supply to a portion of the heart muscle can lead to irritability causing a dysrhythmia which in turn can lead to life-threatening ECG rhythms including ventricular fibrillation (VF). (p. 584)

6. (B) Which of the following steps is not necessary to ensure that CPR can be delivered earlier to cardiac arrest victims? Ensure that heart specialists are involved in CPR training. (p. 590)

7. (A) This condition was most-likely caused by commotio cordis. (p. 585)

8. (D) When the heart stops pumping due to issues related to systemic hypoxia this is referred to as asphyxial cardiac arrest. (p. 585)

9. (C) This reflex is not always present but called agonal breathing and should be treated with CPR. (p. 585)

10. (D) When providing a notification to the family that your resuscitation efforts have been terminated, per medical direction, you should use straightforward language and no vague terms, allow the family some time with the deceased, do not suggest you know how they feel. (p. 612)

11. (D) The key elements of quality CPR in an adult patient include: hand placement on lower third of the sternum, compression depth of 2 inches (5 cm), allowing full chest

©2021 Pearson Education, Inc.
Emergency Care, 14th Ed.

recoil, and compression rate of 100–120 per minute. (pp. 591–592)

12. (A) When doing compressions on an infant and there are two rescuers, the preferred method is the two thumb encircling hands technique. (p. 591)

13. (A) The shockable rhythms include all of the following except asystole and PEA. (p. 596)

14. (A) A nonshockable but electrically organized rhythm that can be the result of a heart muscle with mechanical problems or severe blood loss is called pulseless electrical activity. (p. 597)

15. (C) A nonshockable rhythm that is commonly called flatline is named asystole. (p. 584, 597)

16. (B) When the AED is analyzing the patient's heart rhythm, the EMT must avoid touching the patient. (p. 606)

17. (C) High-quality CPR includes a minimum of pauses in compressions. All efforts should be made to provide a compression fraction of 90 percent during a resuscitation. (p. 593)

18. (C) After the first shock, the patient seems to move, and you assess a strong carotid pulse. The patient is also breathing adequately. You should use a pulse oximeter to titrate oxygen to at least 95% saturation. (p. 600)

19. (C) When a cardiac arrest patient has ROSC you should prepare to transport to the most appropriate receiving hospital. (p. 600)

20. (A) Which of the following is not a general principle of AED use? Hook up oxygen before beginning defibrillation. (p. 608–09, 611)

21. (D) Of the cardiac arrest patients listed, assuming they are in ventricular fibrillation, assuming they are in ventricular fibrillation, which should be defibrillated immediately? The patient with an implanted defibrillator. (p. 615)

22. (A) If a patient is wearing a nitroglycerin or other medication patch, you should carefully remove it before defibrillation because the patch's adhesive can burn and may impede defibrillation. (p. 613)

23. (C) If a 55-year-old patient with an implanted cardiac pacemaker needs to be defibrillated, the EMT should position the pad several inches away from the pacemaker battery. (p. 614)

24. (C) What does this patient likely have? A left ventricular assist device (LVAD). (p. 615)

25. (B) When assessing the pulse of an infant use the brachial pulse. (p. 587)

26. (D) The causes of a sudden unexplained infant death syndrome (SUIDS) include each of the following except trauma to the head. (p. 588)

27. (C) If you suspect a SUIDS you should attempt a resuscitation unless there is rigor mortis or lividity. (p. 588)

28. (D) Often the public is trained in hands only CPR. Once EMS arrives ventilations should play a role in the resuscitation especially in suspected asphyxia arrest (patient is hypoxic), pediatric patients, and suspected opiate arrests (respirations are depressed). (p. 594)

29. (D) When using an AED on a pediatric patient under 8 years old, you can: place pads in anterior-posterior configuration, use pediatric pads, or use adult pads if they are only ones available. (p. 609)

30. (D) Resuscitation is a team effort and the likelihood of success is increased when high-quality CPR is performed, rescuers are rotated to minimize fatigue, and the team is well-practiced. (p. 601)

31. (D) When assessing a 2-year-old child who is unconscious and has a heart rate of 56 and is hypotensive your priorities are to begin assisting ventilations with oxygen, start CPR compressions if the pulse does not increase, and alert ALS and prepare for transport. (p. 587)

32. (B) If you are the lone rescuer and find a pulseless child, the first priority is to immediately begin chest compressions and ventilations for two minutes then apply the AED. (p. 604)

Complete the Following

1. Once you have started resuscitation, you must continue to provide resuscitation (CPR, defibrillation) until: (p. 612)
   A. Spontaneous circulation occurs.
   B. Another trained rescuer can take over for you.
   C. You turn care of the patient over to a person with a higher level of training.
   D. You are too exhausted to continue.
   E. You receive a "cease resuscitation" order from a physician or other authority per local protocols.

2. List the five links in the adult chain of survival: (p. 582)
   A. Recognition and activation of the emergency response system (and prevention strategies, especially for children)
   B. Immediate high-quality CPR.
   C. Rapid defibrillation.
   D. Basic and advanced emergency medical services.
   E. Advanced life support and post arrest care.

3. List five suggestions to consider when making a death notification to family members after an unsuccessful resuscitation. (p. 612)
   A. Be straightforward and use direct language.
   B. When possible, allow the family time with the deceased patient.
   C. Take time and be patient.
   D. Do not suggest that you "know how they feel."
   E. Be yourself. If you are sad, it is okay to be sad. Do not fake emotions. Your deception will be obvious.

CHAPTER 22: Diabetic Emergencies and Altered Mental Status

Match Key Terms

1. (B) Diabetes mellitus: The medical condition brought about by decreased insulin production or the inability of the body cells to use insulin properly. (p. 648)

2. (G) Epilepsy: A medical condition that causes seizures. (p. 648)

3. (A) Glucose: A form of sugar, the body's basic source of energy. (p. 648)

4. (H) Hyperglycemia: High blood sugar. (p. 648)

5. (F) Hypoglycemia: Low blood sugar. (p. 648)

6. (C) Insulin: A hormone produced by the pancreas that facilitates the transfer of glucose into the body's cells. (p. 648)

CHAPTER 22: (continued)

7. (I) Seizure: A sudden change in sensation, behavior, or movement. Capable of producing violent muscle contractions called convulsions. (p. 648)

8. (E) Status epilepticus: A prolonged seizure or the situation in which a person suffers two or more convulsive seizures without regaining full consciousness. (p. 648)

9. (J) Stroke: A condition of altered function caused when an artery in the brain is blocked or ruptured, disrupting the supply of oxygenated blood or causing bleeding into the brain. (p. 648)

10. (D) Syncope: Fainting. (p. 648)

11. (K) Aura: A sensation experienced by a seizure patient right before the seizure that might be a smell, sound or general feeling. (p. 648)

12. (L) Diabetic ketoacidosis (DKA): A condition that occurs as the result of high blood sugar (hyperglycemia), characterized by dehydration, altered mental status, and shock. (p. 648)

13. (M) Generalized seizure: A seizure that affects both sides of the brain. (p. 648)

14. (N) Partial seizure: A seizure that affects only one part or one side of the brain. (p. 648)

15. (O) Postictal phase: The period of time immediately following a tonic-clonic seizure in which the patient goes from full loss of consciousness back to a normal mental status. (p. 648)

16. (P) Reticular activating system: A series of neurologic circuits in the brain that control the functions of staying awake, paying attention, and sleeping. (p. 648)

17. (Q) Tonic-clonic seizure: A generalized seizure in which the patient loses consciousness and has jerking movements of paired muscle groups. (p. 648)

Multiple-Choice Review

1. (C) The relationship between glucose and insulin if often described as a lock-and-key mechanism. (p. 624)

2. (A) This condition is known as diabetes mellitus. (p. 624)

3. (C) The most common medical emergency related to diabetes is hypoglycemia. (p. 625)

4. (A) She is a little confused about where she is and the day of the week. She has most likely developed hypoglycemia. (p. 625)

5. (B) Eating candy too fast is not a cause of hypoglycemia. (p. 625)

6. (A) If sugar is not replenished quickly for the patient described in question 4, she may sustain permanent brain damage. (p. 625)

7. (C) The clues that he may be a diabetic may include all the described findings except non-lactose ice cream in the freezer. (p. 626)

8. (D) In the patient found with an altered mental status, you should always consider scene safety from a potentially agitated/violent patient. (p. 626)

9. (B) Diabetics can present with all of the described signs and symptoms except decreased heart rate. (p. 628)

10. (A) Typically prehospital protocols state that for an EMT to administer oral glucose, the patient must have an altered mental status and have a history of diabetes and be awake enough to swallow. (p. 629)

11. (C) What action should you take? Consult medical direction about whether to administer more glucose. (p. 631)

12. (C) Which statement about children with the disease diabetes is most accurate? Children are more at risk than adults for developing hypoglycemia. (p. 630)

13. (C) Which of the following would most likely indicate an alteration in the patient's blood sugar level? Change in mental status. (p. 631)

14. (B) Before and after administering the medication, you should make sure to document the patient's mental status. (p. 623, 632)

15. (D) A trade name for the medication oral glucose is Insta-glucose. (p. 632)

16. (D) Before deciding that he has a behavioral problem, you should consider all the described conditions/findings except glucose allergy. (p. 634)

17. (B) People with diabetes routinely test the level of sugar in their blood using a glucose meter. (p. 630)

18. (D) Complications of diabetes can include kidney failure, heart disease, and blindness. (p. 630)

19. (C) The reading on a glucometer is reported in milligrams of glucose per deciliter of blood. (p. 631)

20. (D) A diabetic who is symptomatic and has a sugar level below 60 mg/dL is considered hypoglycemic. (p. 630)

21. (A) A diabetic who is symptomatic and has a sugar level above 140 mg/dL is considered hyperglycemic. (p. 631)

22. (C) The most common cause of seizures in adults is not taking prescribed antiseizure medication. (p. 635)

23. (A) Seizures are commonly caused by all of the following except exposure to cold. (p. 635)

24. (A) Seizures lasting longer than 10 minutes is not a characteristic of idiopathic seizures. (p. 635)

25. (A) Convulsive seizures may be seen with epilepsy or hypoglycemia. (p. 635)

26. (B) The most common condition that results in seizures is epilepsy. (p. 635)

27. (C) The reticular activating system is a part of the brain responsible for staying awake, paying attention, and sleeping. (p. 622)

28. (D) In obtaining the medical history from a seizure patient, also interview the bystanders to find out each of the following except what the family's reaction was to the seizure. (p. 636)

29. (C) As the convulsions end, what action should you take? Provide artificial ventilations with supplemental oxygen. (p. 637)

30. (B) The most common cause of seizures in infants and toddlers is a high fever. (p. 635)

31. (A) A seizure will normally last no more than 2 to 3 minutes. (p. 638)

32. (B) This is a serious condition called status epilepticus and the treatment will include possible ALS intercept. (p. 638)

33. (D) If you suspect that a conscious 49-year-old female has had a stroke, you should transport her in the semisitting position and pay close attention to her airway. (p. 643)

34. (B) When assessing your 53-year-old male patient, you determine that he is having difficulty saying what he is thinking, even though he clearly understands you. This is called expressive aphasia. (p. 639)

35. (C) When assessing your 42-year-old female patient, you determine that she can speak clearly but cannot understand what you are saying. This is called receptive aphasia. (p. 639)

36. (D) A symptom that you would expect her to exhibit is headache. (p. 639)

37. (D) The signs and symptoms of stroke might include: vomiting, seizures, loss of bladder control. (p. 641)

38. (B) This patient is most likely suffering a(n) transient ischemic attack (TIA). (p. 639)

39. (C) When a patient faints, the medical terms to describe this is usually syncope or a syncopal episode, and the treatment would involve oxygen administration. (p. 647)

40. (B) Lightheadedness or dizziness is a symptom that is often due to poor perfusion to the brain. (p. 644)

41. (C) If a patient demonstrates one of the three findings of the Cincinnati Prehospital Stroke Scale, that patient will have a 70 percent chance of having an acute stroke. (p. 642)

42. (C) If you can determine the time last seen normal in your stroke patient you may have up to 3 hours for them to be administered thrombolytic drugs if they are a candidate. (p. 643)

Pathophysiology: Hypoglycemia (p. 625)

1. Blood vessels constrict, the heart pumps faster and harder, and breathing accelerates.

2. Confusion, stupor, unconsciousness, vital sign changes, and seizures are common.

Pathophysiology: Hyperglycemia (pp. 625–626)

1. Systemic dehydration and potential hypovolemic shock develop.

2. The production of ketones can result in the fruity or acetone smell on the breath of the diabetic patient.

Pathophysiology: Tonic-Clonic Seizure (p. 635)

1. The tonic phase causes the body to become rigid, stiffening for about 30 seconds. Breathing may stop, and the patient might bite his or her tongue and become incontinent.

2. The clonic phase involves the body jerking about violently for about 1 to 2 minutes. The patient may foam at the mouth and drool. His or her face and lips may become cyanotic.

3. The postictal phase occurs when the convulsions stop. The patient may be drowsy and very tired during this period.

Complete the Following

1. List nine signs and symptoms associated with a diabetic emergency. (p. 628)
  A. Rapid onset of altered mental status.
  B. Intoxicated appearance, staggering, slurred speech, and unconsciousness.
  C. Elevated heart rate.
  D. Cold, clammy skin.

  E. Hunger.
  F. Seizures.
  G. Uncharacteristic behavior.
  H. Anxiety.
  I. Combativeness.

2. Give four reasons why a diabetic may develop hyperglycemia. (p. 625)
  A. The patient has not taken enough insulin to make up for the deficiency in natural insulin.
  B. The patient has forgotten to take his or her insulin.
  C. The patient has overeaten.
  D. An infection has upset the patient's insulin–glucose balance.

3. List ten causes of seizures. (p. 635)
  A. Hypoxia.
  B. Stroke.
  C. Traumatic brain injury.
  D. Toxins.
  E. Hypoglycemia.
  F. Brain tumor.
  G. Congenital brain defects.
  H. Infection.
  I. Metabolic.
  J. Idiopathic.

4. List the four categories of causes of dizziness and syncope. (pp. 644–646)
  A. Hypovolemic causes.
  B. Metabolic and structural causes.
  C. Environmental/toxicological causes.
  D. Cardiovascular causes.

5. List ten signs or symptoms of a stroke. (p. 641)

May include any ten of these:
  • Confusion.
  • Dizziness.
  • Numbness, weakness, or paralysis (usually on one side of the body).
  • Loss of bowel or bladder control.
  • Impaired vision.
  • High blood pressure.
  • Difficulty respiration or snoring.
  • Nausea or vomiting.
  • Seizures.
  • Unequal pupils.
  • Headache.
  • Loss of vision in one eye.
  • Unconsciousness (uncommon).

Case Study: Call for a "Man Down"

1. Use the head-tilt, chin-lift maneuver.

2. Use the BVM, and assist ventilations with 100 percent oxygen.

3. It could have been the result of a seizure, no access to a bathroom, or intoxication.

4. Seizure patients take Dilantin, so the patient could have a history of seizures.

5. No, that would be jumping to a conclusion. Seizure is a likely cause, but you need to investigate further.

6. The oxygen is for potential hypoxia. The vitals are a baseline to compare the next set to and may help to determine whether there is internal bleeding. The blood sugar test helps to determine whether the altered mental status is due to hypoglycemia. Use your best clinical judgment here, and be careful not to just jump to a quick conclusion. There are, as you have learned in this chapter, many reasons for an altered level of consciousness.

7. A glucometer reading of 60 indicates hypoglycemia. This could be in the Gray Zone, since the normal glucose level is a range of 70–100, and not all state or regional protocols allow for EMTs to begin treatment until a patient with a history of diabetes and an altered mental status has a blood sugar level below a specific point. The bottom line here is that the EMT should consider the patient's mental status and the clinical picture. Calling for an ALS unit is a wise decision, since they often have more aggressive treatment protocols.

8. Type 2 diabetes often develops in later life when the pancreas is no longer able to supply enough insulin or the body is unable to use the insulin effectively. Only some type 2 diabetics take insulin injections. Many can control their diet and take oral medications to properly regulate their glucose levels.

CHAPTER 23: Allergic Reaction

Match Key Terms

1. (C) Allergen: Something that causes an allergic reaction. (p. 667)

2. (F) Allergic reaction: An exaggerated immune response. (p. 667)

3. (B) Anaphylaxis: A severe or life-threatening allergic reaction in which the blood vessels dilate, causing a drop in blood pressure, and the tissues lining the respiratory system swell, interfering with the airway. (p. 667)

4. (E) Auto-injector: A syringe preloaded with medication that has a spring-loaded device and pushes the needle through the skin to deploy the medication when the tip of the device is pressed firmly against the body. (p. 667)

5. (D) Epinephrine: A hormone produced by the body. As a medication, it constricts blood vessels and dilates respiratory passages, and is used to relieve severe allergic reactions. (p. 667)

6. (A) Hives: Red, itchy, raised blotches on the skin that often result from an allergic reaction. (p. 667)

Multiple-Choice Review

1. (C) A 27-year-old male's exaggerated response of his body's immune system to any substance is called an allergic reaction. (p. 651)

2. (D) Why would an anaphylactic reaction sometimes be treated as a high-priority patient? An anaphylactic reaction can cause airway obstruction. (p. 652)

3. (C) The first time a person is exposed to an allergen, the person's immune system forms antibodies. (p. 653)

4. (A) The second time a person is exposed to the same allergen, the body reactions may include all of the following except destruction of antibodies; the reaction causes an increase in antibodies. (p. 653)

5. (D) When interviewing a 23-year-old male, you should consider the common causes of allergic reactions, which include all of the following except red fruits and vegetables. (p. 652)

6. (C) It is possible for a patient to be allergic to peanuts and not to walnuts or almonds because peanuts are legumes and not nuts. (p. 652)

7. (B) He was stung by a few bees when mowing the lawn. The respiratory signs and symptoms of anaphylactic shock include all of the following except hives. (p. 654)

8. (D) The effects on the cardiac system of an allergic reaction for a 35-year-old male could described in question 7 include increased heart rate and decreased blood pressure. (p. 655)

9. (C) For an immune response to be considered a severe allergic reaction, the patient must have signs and symptoms of shock or respiratory distress. (p. 655)

10. (A) After you administer epinephrine by an auto-injector, you should prepare to administer another dose if condition worsens. (p. 659)

11. (B) When capillaries become leaky, fluid moves into the tissue and appears as swelling, called angioedema, especially around the site of an injection (or sting) and to the face—including eyes, lips, ears, and tongue—and to the airway.(p. 653)

12. (A) Your 22-year-old male patient has an epinephrine auto-injector in his backpack. Besides helping him take his medication, you should always ask the patient whether he has any spare auto-injectors for the trip to the hospital. (p. 663)

13. (B) The recommended location for injection with an epinephrine auto-injector is the lateral mid-thigh. (p. 661)

14. (B) The child size epinephrine auto-injector (for children weighing less than 66 pounds) contains 0.15 mg. (p. 661)

15. (B) Which statement is true regarding anaphylactic reactions in infants and children? Many children outgrow allergies as they mature. (p. 662)

16. (B) Which of the following is a sign of a patient experiencing a minor allergic reaction? The allergic reaction has local swelling. (p. 656)

Pathophysiology: Allergic Reactions or Anaphylactic Reactions (p. 656)

1. List the signs and symptoms in allergic reaction which are not life-threatening below:
   A. Respiratory complaints – sneezing, cough.
   B. Respiratory sounds – normal.
   C. Skin findings – local hives, local redness.
   D. Swelling – local swelling.
   E. Vital signs – normal or nearly normal vital signs.
   F. Mental status – normal, may be anxious.

2. List the signs and symptoms in anaphylaxis which are life-threatening below:
   A. Respiratory complaints – dyspnea, tightness in chest.
   B. Respiratory sounds – wheezing, muffled voice, stridor.
   C. Skin findings – widespread hives, pallor, diffuse redness.
   D. Swelling – swelling of face, lips, eyes, tongue, mouth, injection site.
   E. Vital signs – tachycardia, hypotension, tachypnea, decreased oxygen saturation.
   F. Mental status – syncope, altered mental status, feeling of impending doom.

Complete the Following

1. List 14 signs and symptoms of allergic reaction or anaphylactic shock. (pp. 654–655)

May include any 14 of these:
- Skin – itching, hives, flushing, swelling of face, neck, hands, feet, or tongue, warm, tingling feeling in the face, mouth, chest, feet, and hands.

- Respiratory – tightness in the throat or chest, cough, rapid breathing, labored, noisy breathing, hoarseness, muffled voice, loss of voice entirely, stridor, wheezing.
- Cardiac – increased heart rate, decreased BP.
- Generalized findings – itchy, watery eyes, headache, runny nose, patient-expressed sense of impending doom.
- Signs and symptoms of shock – AMS, flushed, dry skin or pale, cool, clammy skin, nausea or vomiting, changes in vital signs: increased pulse, increased respirations, decreased BP.

2. List 8 side effects of Epinephrine Auto-Injector. (p. 661)
   A. Increased heart rate.
   B. Pallor.
   C. Dizziness.
   D. Chest pain.
   E. Headache.
   F. Nausea.
   G. Vomiting.
   H. Excitability, anxiety.

3. During your secondary assessment of a patient with a chief complaint of allergic reaction. What six factors should you inquire about? (p. 655)
   A. History of allergies
   B. What the patient was exposed to (what triggered the reaction)
   C. How the patient was exposed (contact, ingestion, and so on)
   D. What signs and symptoms the patient is having
   E. Progression (What happened first? Next? How rapidly?)
   F. Interventions (Has any care been provided? Has the patient taken any medication?)

Label the Diagrams (p. 652)

1. insect bites
2. food products
3. plants
4. medications

Case Study: The Lakefront Emergency

1. No, because there is only one patient.

2. Yes, you should have an ALS unit sent to the scene or at least to intercept you en route to the hospital because of the breathing difficulty

3. She likely has breathing difficulty and cannot inhale deeply enough to speak for normal time periods.

4. She is alert and oriented.

5. The sound is most likely a wheeze, which can be caused by asthma, upper airway obstruction, anaphylaxis, left heart failure.

6. Additional signs of breathing difficulty could be her posture or position, such as an upright tripod position; intercostal separation or retractions; accessory muscle use; cyanosis; and others

7. This patient should be given oxygen by a nonrebreather mask at 15 liters per minute. Use your best clinical judgment, and you can also use the pulse oximetry reading and the vital signs to guide your therapy.

8. This is a high-priority patient because of her breathing difficulty, and she should be transported rapidly.

9. The position of comfort is generally best. But if she is able to breathe adequately, lay her down to relieve her dizziness.

10. SAMPLE (signs and symptoms, allergies, medications, past medical history, last intake, and events leading up to illness)

11. Epinephrine is the medication contained within bee-sting kit (auto-injector). It would be appropriate to assist her with her epinephrine auto-injector. Of course, you need to use good clinical judgment and follow your state or regional protocols. If you have questions on this case, discuss them with your medical director.

12. You must call medical direction for permission to administer epinephrine to the patient. Make sure the epinephrine auto-injector is prescribed to the patient, has not expired, and is clear.

13. You would report that the chief complaint is breathing difficulty with chest pain, and that you suspect the patient is having an allergic reaction. You would also report OPQRST findings, vital signs, SAMPLE findings, and treatment given thus far (e.g., oxygen, positioning, epinephrine auto-injector per medical direction).

14. The paramedic would establish an IV, administer intravenous fluids, evaluate the need for airway or breathing management, and assess the need for additional epinephrine or other medications.

CHAPTER 24: Infectious Diseases and Sepsis

Match Key Terms

1. (C) Infectious diseases: Diseases that can be spread by bacteria, viruses, and other microbes. (p. 692)

2. (A) Communicable diseases: Diseases that can be passed from one individual to another, through either direct contact or contact with secretions from an infected person. (p. 692)

3. (B) Sepsis: A life-threatening condition resulting from an abnormal and counterproductive response by the body that causes damage to tissues and organs after the body is invaded by a pathogen. (p. 675)

Multiple-Choice Review

1. (B) Viruses are not a cell and have a protein coat or shell that encloses what they need to reproduce. In order for them to survive and replicate, they must be in a host cell to do so. (p. 671)

2. (A) People who have an infection have a microbe inside their body, but they are not necessarily sick, although they may become sick over time. (p. 674)

3. (D) When an infection worsens, it can spread to the blood stream or certain other organs and cause lift-threatening changes in the body. (p. 674)

4. (D) Pneumonia is one of the most common respiratory infections that may lead to sepsis. (p. 675)

5. (C) Meningitis in an infection that causes inflammation of the tissues surrounding the brain and cord. (p. 676)

6. (A) Dried scabs do not spread the disease, hence the patient should be isolated until that time. (p. 676)

7. (A) Some people who had chicken pox (varicella zoster) as children, later experience herpes zoster, also known as shingles (herpes zoster) as an adult, if and when the virus reactivates years later. (p. 673, 678)

CHAPTER 24: (continued)

8. (D) Mumps (the condition the listed symptoms indicate) is spread through droplets and direct contact with a patient's saliva. (p. 672, 681)

9. (B) When the EMT suspects sepsis he/she should alert the emergency department with a "sepsis alert" to give advance warning which can lead to earlier treatment. (pp. 675–677)

10. (A) Any infectious disease that is spread by contact with airborne droplets puts the EMT as risk for exposure. The EMT should take standard precautions immediately upon hearing or seeing coughing and sneezing. (p. 672)

11. (A) EMTs must consider what risks (if any) that patients with infectious diseases pose to them and must know how to reduce those risks. (p. 671)

12. (C) Many patients display a rash within a week that looks like bull's-eye target. The rash fades, and months to years later, the patient can develop complications of the disease, including neurologic problems. (p. 690)

13. (C) Tuberculosis can be pulmonary (in the lungs), and it also can infect many other organs and tissues. (p. 688)

14. (A) Hepatitis A is spread from person to person by the fecal-oral root. Hepatitis E is spread by the same route but by a different strain of virus. (p. 682)

15. (D) Rubeola (or measles), is a highly infectious viral diseases that starts with a fever, cough, and eye irritation. (p. 679)

16. (C) There are several safe and effective medication regimens for eradicating the hepatitis C virus from a patient, but there is no vaccination. (p. 684)

17. (B) Antiviral medications are used to reduce and suppress a patient's viral load. (p. 684)

18. (D) The risk for exposure to EMTs comes from contact with blood or other body fluids, such as a needle stick or contact on an open wound. (p. 672)

19. (B) More than two dozen viruses can cause influenza. (p. 685)

20. (B) Pertussis or whooping cough begins like a typical upper respiratory infection, then worsens with "fits" of coughing and lasts 1–2 months. (p. 686)

Complete the Following

1. List ten communicable diseases and their mode of transmission. (p. 672)

   Any ten of these.
   - Chicken pox – airborne droplets and open sores.
   - Measles – airborne droplets and direct contact with nasal and throat secretions.
   - Mumps – droplets of saliva or contact with objects contaminated by saliva.
   - Hepatitis A – fecal-oral route.
   - Hepatitis B – blood, semen, CSF, amniotic fluid, vaginal secretions.
   - Hepatitis C – blood semen, CSF, amniotic fluid, vaginal secretions.
   - HIV/AIDS – blood, semen, CSF, amniotic fluid, vaginal secretions, breast milk.

- Influenza – airborne droplets and direct contact.
- Croup – airborne droplets and direct contact.
- Pertussis – airborne droplets.
- Pneumococcal pneumonia – droplets.
- Tuberculosis – airborne droplets.
- Meningococcal meningitis – direct contact.

2. In an adult with suspected infection, what are the assessment criteria used to determine if the patient may also have sepsis? (p. 676)
   A. Temperature lower than 96.8°F or higher than 101°F.
   B. Heart rate over 90.
   C. Respiratory rate greater than 20.
   D. Systolic blood pressure lower than 90 mmHg.
   E. New onset altered mental status or worsened mental status.

3. List eight examples of emerging new infectious diseases: (p. 691)
   A. MRSA.
   B. VRE.
   C. C. diff.
   D. MDR-TB.
   E. SARS.
   F. Ebola.
   G. MERS-CoV.
   H. Zika.

Case Study: "Just Another Rash"

1. As you approach the patient, what Standard Precautions should you take? Strongly suggest gloves, mask and eyeshield at this point.

2. With this rash expanding over time from the face to the chest could this be serious? Yes. Might want to make sure there are no threats to airway, breathing, and circulation right away.

3. Why would it make sense to inquire who else lives in the home? There could be others who may also have similar signs and symptoms.

4. Should you inquire as to what the school nurse's concerns have been about Tommy? Yes. Obviously, this is a sensitive topic but just make sure it is relevant to today's complaint.

5. The mother tells you that her husband has very strong opinions about no vaccinations for their children. Could this information be relevant to the secondary assessment? Yes. The mother is likely fighting with the school nurse over state and or local policy preventing student who are not vaccinated against childhood diseases from attending school.

6. What disease do you suspect Tommy might have? Rubeola or the measles. Based on the initial fever, cough and itchy eyes which has moved to a rash on the face and then trunk and/or rest of the body.

7. Who might be at high-risk of contracting this disease? Anyone who is immune deficient, non-vaccinated, infants less than 1 year, and pregnant woman.

8. Is any special notification needed before arriving at the ED? They may want to isolate the patient from other patients so best to give them a heads up prior to wheeling him into the ED.

©2021 Pearson Education, Inc.
Emergency Care, 14th Ed.

CHAPTER 25: Poisoning and Overdose Emergencies

Match Key Terms

1. (D) Absorbed poisons: Poisons that are taken into the body through unbroken skin. (p. 723)

2. (H) Activated charcoal: A substance that adsorbs many poisons and prevents them from being absorbed by the body. (p. 723)

3. (P) Antidote: A substance that will neutralize the poison or its effects. (p. 723)

4. (K) Delirium tremens (DTs): A severe reaction that can be part of alcohol withdrawal, characterized by sweating, trembling, anxiety, and hallucinations. Severe alcohol withdrawal with the DTs can lead to death if untreated. (p. 723)

5. (I) Dilution: Thinning down or weakening a poison by mixing with something else. Ingested poisons are sometimes diluted by drinking water or milk. (p. 723)

6. (E) Downers: Depressants, such as benzodiazepines, that depress the central nervous system, often bring on a more relaxed state of mind. (p. 723)

7. (M) Hallucinogens: Mind-affecting or mind-altering drugs that act on the central nervous system to produce excitement and distortion of perceptions. (p. 723)

8. (F) Ingested poisons: Poisons that are swallowed and which are often used. (p. 723)

9. (L) Inhaled poisons: Poisons that are breathed in. (p. 723)

10. (J) Injected poisons: Poisons that are inserted through the skin, for example, by needle, snake fangs, or insect stinger. (p. 723)

11. (G) Narcotics: A class of drugs that affects the nervous system and changes many normal body activities. Their legal use is for relief of pain. Illicit use is to produce an intense state of relaxation. (p. 723)

12. (A) Poison: Any substance that can harm the body by altering cell structure or functions. (p. 723)

13. (N) Toxin: A poisonous substance secreted by bacteria, plants, or animals. (p. 723)

14. (B) Uppers: Stimulants, such as cocaine and methamphetamine that affect the central nervous system to excite the user. (p. 723)

15. (O) Volatile chemicals: Vaporized compounds, such as cleaning fluid, that are breathed in by an abuser to produce a "high." (p. 723)

16. (C) Withdrawal: Referring to alcohol or drug withdrawal in which the patient's body reacts severely when deprived of the abused substance. (p. 723)

Multiple-Choice Review

1. (B) Which of the following is an environmental clue at the scene that can be used to help you determine whether she has been poisoned? There is an empty pill bottle on her night table. (p. 697)

2. (A) The most accurate definition of a poison would be that it is any substance that can potentially harm the body (sometimes seriously enough to create a medical emergency). (p. 697)

3. (C) Most of the more than two million poisonings in the United States each year are due to accidents involving young children. (p. 697)

4. (B) Any substance secreted by plants, animals, or bacteria that is poisonous to humans is called a toxin. (p. 697)

5. (D) Because of the poisons they produce, mistletoe, mushrooms, and rubber plants can be dangerous to humans. (p. 697)

6. (B) Bacteria may produce toxins that cause deadly diseases such as botulism. While bacteria is known to cause diseases such as tuberculosis, it is not due to the "toxins" they create. HIV and covid-19 are caused by viruses. (p. 697)

7. (B) The body's reaction to most poisonous substances is often most severe in the elderly and the ill. (p. 697)

8. (D) Poisons may enter the body through any of the following routes except excretion. (pp. 698–699)

9. (C) Carbon monoxide, chlorine, and sulfur are examples of inhaled poisons. (p. 698)

10. (A) Examples of absorbed poisons include insecticides and agricultural chemicals. (p. 698)

11. (B) The venom of a bite from a rattlesnake is an example of an injected poison. (p. 699)

12. (A) You are treating a 32-year-old female who was found unconscious by her roommate when the roommate got home late at night. If it is being assumed that she was poisoned, why is it important to determine when the ingestion of a poison occurred? Different poisons act on the body at different rates. (p. 700)

13. (B) The most common findings of ingesting a poison are nausea and vomiting. (p. 700)

14. (C) You are having a discussion with medical direction about an order to use activated charcoal for a conscious patient who ingested a poison. Activated charcoal is used to reduce the amount of poison absorbed by the body. (p. 702)

15. (C) The decision on when to use activated charcoal is best made with medical direction or consultation with the poison control center. (p. 702)

16. (D) Activated charcoal is not routinely used with ingestion of caustic substances, strong acids, and strong alkalis. (p. 703)

17. (B) Examples of caustic substances include all of the listed substances except venom. (p. 703)

18. (A) The appropriate treatment for this patient should not include activated charcoal. (p. 703)

19. (C) When a physician orders dilution of an ingested substance, in most cases you can use either water or milk. (p. 704)

20. (C) The most common inhaled substance at poisonous levels is carbon monoxide. (p. 709)

21. (A) What should you do? Stand back and attempt to learn more about the chemical involved. (p. 708)

22. (B) The principal prehospital treatment of a 40-year-old female patient who has inhaled poison is administering high-concentration oxygen. (p. 709)

23. (C) Besides motor vehicle exhaust, where else might you find carbon monoxide? Around an improperly vented wood-burning stove. (p. 709)

24. (B) How does carbon monoxide affect the body? It impairs the normal carrying of oxygen by the red blood cells. (p. 709)

25. (D) The least likely finding of those described associated with carbon monoxide poisoning is cherry-red lips. (p. 709)

26. (A) After ensuring you own safety with PPE, you should brush off as much of the powder as possible, then irrigate. (p. 713)

27. (B) There is a strong smell of rotten eggs. What would you suspect? The mixture may have produced hydrogen sulfide, which can be deadly. (p. 712)

28. (A) Which of the following signs and symptoms is not seen with alcohol abuse but is seen in a diabetic emergency? Acetone breath. (p. 716)

29. (C) The sweating, trembling, anxiety, and hallucinations that are found in the patient experiencing alcohol withdrawal are called delirium tremens. (p. 716)

30. (B) It is important to determine an infant or child's weight and estimated amount of substance ingested in cases of pediatric poisonings. (p. 705)

31. (A) These drugs are called uppers. (p. 718)

32. (B) These pills are examples of downers. (p. 719)

33. (B) These types of drugs are called downers. (p. 719)

34. (C) These types of medications are called narcotics. (p. 718)

35. (D) This drug was most likely a hallucinogen. (p. 719)

36. (B) Cleaning fluid, glue, and model cement are examples of volatile chemicals. (p. 719)

37. (A) A 21-year-old female who has overdosed on an upper may have signs and symptoms such as excitement, increased pulse and breathing rates, dilated pupils, and rapid speech. (p. 720)

38. (B) You can expect to observe signs and symptoms such as sluggishness, sleepiness, and lack of coordination of body and speech. (p. 720)

39. (C) A 32-year-old female patient who has overdosed on psilocybin (magic mushrooms) may have signs and symptoms such as fast pulse rate, dilated pupils, flushed face, and seeing or hearing things. (p. 720)

40. (D) If he has overdosed on the narcotic he takes, he might have signs and symptoms such as reduced pulse rate and rate and depth of breathing, pinpoint pupils, and sweating. (p. 720)

41. (D) The patient who took ipecac before your arrival should be monitored closely for: vomiting, potential for airway obstruction, and potential for aspiration. (p. 703)

42. (D) Which of the following would not indicate an airway that was injured by smoke inhalation? Pinpoint pupils. (p. 711)

Pathophysiology: Acetaminophen Overdose (p. 705)

1. The patient who overdoses on acetaminophen is likely to have what type of internal organ damage?
   • Toxic effects do not appear right away, but over time the liver becomes overwhelmed and unable to detoxify the substance away, but over time the liver sustains irreparable damage if nothing is done.

2. What are some common signs and symptoms of an acetaminophen overdose?
   • Signs and symptoms are often delayed and not specific, however during first 4–12 hours patient may experience loss of appetite, nausea, and vomiting. A day or two later, when it's too late for antidote, the patient experiences URQ pain, liver failure, and jaundice.

Complete the Following

1. What are the steps in the care of the patient who has ingested a poison? (p. 704)
   A. Detect and treat immediately life-threatening problems in the primary assessment. Evaluate the need for prompt transport for critical patients.
   B. Perform secondary assessment.
   C. Assess baseline vital signs.
   D. Consult medical direction or poison control.
   E. Transport the patient with all containers, bottles, and labels from the substance if it is safe to do so.
   F. Perform reassessment en route.

2. List at least eight signs and symptoms of alcohol abuse. (p. 716)

   Any eight of these:
   • Odor of alcohol on the patient's breath or clothing.
   • Swaying and unsteadiness of movement.
   • Slurred speech, rambling through patterns, or incoherent words or phrases.
   • A flushed appearance to the face, often with the patient sweating and complaining of being warm.
   • Nausea or vomiting.
   • Poor coordination.
   • Slowed reaction time.
   • Blurred vision.
   • Confusion.
   • Hallucinations, visual or auditory.
   • Lack of memory
   • Altered mental status.

3. What is the phone number for the poison control center? (p. 714)
   • 1-800-222-1222

Label the Diagrams (p. 699)

1. inhalation
2. injection
3. ingestion
4. absorption

Complete the Chart (720)

• 1, 8, 9, – Uppers
• 3, 4, 11, 12, 13, 16, 22 – Mind Altering
• 5, 15, 24 – Volatile Chemicals
• 6, 7, 10, 19, 21 – Downers
• 2, 14, 17, 18, 20, 23 – Narcotics

Case Study: Not a Fun Party for Everyone

1. The first assessment and treatment priority is to make sure the patient's airway is open and clear.

2. The raspy cough and gurgling may indicate fluid in the airway, and the patient needs to be suctioned. Airway management may turn out to be not just your highest priority but your *only priority* in such a patient. Use your best clinical judgment in caring for this patient, and consider ALS as soon as possible to help manage the airway.

3. If ALS is available, they should be called.

4. This is a high-priority call.

5. Rule out aspiration of a foreign substance, alcohol intoxication, drug abuse.

©2021 Pearson Education, Inc.
Emergency Care, 14th Ed.

6. This is a critical patient given her suspected overdoses and airway concerns. She should be transported to the ED as rapidly as possible. Using your best clinical judgment, you should recognize that this patient has a problem that can be life-threatening and is not easily resolved in the field. Consult your medical director to discuss this case further.

7. Activated charcoal would not be indicated because of the patient's depressed mental status. The patient could regurgitate and possibly aspirate the stomach contents.

CHAPTER 26: Abdominal Emergencies

Match Key Terms

1. (D) Parietal pain: A localized, intense pain that arises from the outer layer (parietal peritoneum), of the lining of the abdominal cavity. (p. 743)

2. (E) Peritoneum: The two thin membranes that lines the abdominal cavity (the parietal peritoneum) and covers the organs within it (the visceral peritoneum). (p. 743)

3. (A) Referred pain: Pain that is felt in a location other than where the pain originates. (p. 743)

4. (B) Tearing pain: Sharp pain that feels as if body tissues are being ripped apart. (p. 743)

5. (C) Visceral pain: A poorly localized, dull, or diffuse pain that arises from the abdominal organs, or viscera. (p. 743)

6. (F) Retroperitoneal space: The area posterior to the peritoneum, between the peritoneum and the back. (p. 743)

Multiple-Choice Review

1. (B) The membrane that covers the abdominal organs is called the visceral peritoneum. (p. 728)

2. (C) The organs outside the peritoneum that are found between the abdomen and the back are in the retroperitoneal space. (p. 728)

3. (C) Pain felt in a location other than where it originates is called referred. (p. 730)

4. (D) The pain is often described as intermittent and dull, diffuse, and achy. (730)

5. (C) Colicky pain is often visceral pain from a hollow organ in the abdomen. (p. 730)

6. (B) Why might the pain in his right shoulder blade be a symptom of gallbladder problems? Nerve pathways from the gallbladder return to the spinal cord by way of shared pathways with the shoulder; this type of pain is called referred pain. (p. 730)

7. (A) Why is last oral intake an important part of your SAMPLE history for this patient? The food may have been spoiled or related to current complaint. (p. 738)

8. (B) It would be appropriate to ask her where she is in her menstrual cycle to begin to focus on the possibility of an ectopic pregnancy. (p. 734)

9. (A) When you palpate the abdomen, be sure to palpate the area with the pain last. (p. 739)

10. (B) He denies any difficulty breathing yet has a pulse of 110 regular, a BP of 98/68 mmHg, and an SpO_2 of 91%. You should administer 10–15 lpm oxygen by nonrebreather mask because signs are consistent with a patient in shock and hypoxia. (p. 741)

11. (C) When a 61-year-old male patient tells you that he has a tearing sensation in his lower back and denies any recent injury, you should suspect an abdominal aortic aneurysm. (p. 732)

12. (B) Of the following choices, which is the most likely cause? Cholecystitis or inflammation of the gallbladder. (p. 731)

13. (D) What would you suspect is his most likely problem? Renal colic. (p. 733)

14. (B) Because this came on suddenly during exercising, you suspect that it could be a hernia. (p. 733)

15. (C) What do you suspect is the most likely problem? A bleeding ulcer. (p. 732)

16. (B) When assessing a geriatric patient you may find difficulty obtaining a history of pain from the abdomen due to decreased ability to perceive pain. (p. 738)

17. (B) When a patient has a hole in the muscle layers of the abdominal wall that allows intestine to protrude, this is called a hernia. (p. 732)

18. (D) Common abdominal conditions in the pediatric patient include gastroenteritis, appendicitis, and constipation. (p. 731)

19. (C) A serious condition that can involve pain in the epigastric area radiating to the back and made worse by chronic alcohol use is pancreatitis. (p. 732)

20. (B) When a patient with abdominal pain is found with the knees drawn up and arms across the abdomen, this is called the guarding position. (p. 736)

Complete the Following

1. List four solid structures (organs) found in the abdomen. Any four of the following. (p. 727)
   A. Spleen
   B. Liver
   C. Pancreas
   D. Kidney
   E. Overies

2. List six hollow structures (organs) found in the abdomen. (p. 727)
   A. Stomach
   B. Gallbladder
   C. Duodenum
   D. Large intestine
   E. Small intestine
   F. Bladder

3. In doing an assessment on a female patient with a chief complaint of abdominal pain, what are six important questions to ask? (p. 737)
   A. Where are you in your menstrual cycle?
   B. Is your period late?
   C. Do you have bleeding from the vagina now that is not menstrual bleeding?
   D. If you are menstruating, is the flow normal?
   E. Have you had this pain before?
   F. If you had this pain before, when did it happen and what was it like?

Label the Diagrams

Solid Organs (p. 727)

   A. Spleen
   B. Liver
   C. Pancreas
   D. Kidneys

Hollow Organs (p. 727)

A. Stomach

B. Gallbladder

C. Duodenum

D. Large intestine

E. Small intestine

F. Urinary bladder

Case Study: Just a Belly Ache

1. As you approached the patient, he was in fetal position on the couch, and when he sat up, he was guarding the painful abdomen with his forearm. Also there is evidence that he was vomiting.

2. If he saw blood (i.e., frank red or coffee ground color), it could indicate GI bleeding.

3. There is a good indication of appendicitis based on the periumbilical pain migrating to the lower right quadrant.

4. If his appendix ruptured, it would have released chemicals into the abdomen which can cause irritation and infection. Since he may already be infected, and his body could be fighting the infection with a fever and mobilizing his white blood cells. It might be good to check his temperature.

5. On the basis of your clinical judgment, you suspect that an abdominal organ is causing the pain. Of course, you still might suspect GI or cardiac causes too. It is not highly likely that the patient would be given pain relievers in the field, although this is a question the paramedic should answer. In either instance, summoning ALS would be a good idea given the intensity of his pain.

6. No, of the source of his pain is a ruptured appendix, he is likely going to surgery, so it is good that he has an empty stomach.

CHAPTER 27: Behavioral and Psychiatric Emergencies and Suicide

Match Key Terms

1. (B) Behavior: The manner in which a person acts. (p. 761)

2. (D) Behavioral emergency: When a patient's actions are not typical for the situation; is unacceptable or intolerable to the patient, the patient's family, or the community; or when the patient may harm self or others. (p. 761)

3. (A) Excited delirium: Bizarre and/or aggressive behavior, shouting, paranoia, panic, violence toward others, insensitivity to pain, unexpected physical strength, and hyperthermia. (p. 761)

4. (E) Schizophrenia: A chronic mental disorder that affects how a person thinks, feels, and behaves. People with severe or untreated schizophrenia may seem like they have lost touch with reality. (p. 761)

5. (F) Neurotransmitters: Chemicals within the body that transmit a message in the brain from the distal end of one neuron to the proximal end of the next neuron. (p. 761)

6. (C) Positional asphyxia: Inadequate breathing or respiratory arrest caused by a body position that restricts breathing. (p. 761)

Multiple-Choice Review

1. (D) The physical causes of altered behavior include all of the listed conditions except differing lifestyles. (pp. 748–749)

2. (C) This behavior can be due to any of the listed conditions except for hypoactivity. (pp. 748–749)

3. (C) To calm this patient, you should consider explaining things to the patient honestly in a calm tone. (p. 751)

4. (B) Which one of the following is not usually a common presentation for patient with an acute psychosis event? A calm, neat appearance. (p. 751)

5. (B) He has a handgun and is threatening to kill himself. Your first concern should be your own personal safety. (p. 755)

6. (A) The highest suicide rates occur in the 15- to 25-year-old age group. (p. 754)

7. (C) Which one of the following is not an example of a risk factor for suicide? A patient with suicidal thoughts would not usually deny them when asked. (p. 754)

8. (C) The family member states the patient has actually been exhibiting sudden improvement from depression over the past few days. In this case, you should consider that the patient is still at risk for suicide. (p. 754)

9. (D) When assessing an aggressive patient for a possible threat to you or your crew, take all of the following actions except assessing the patient in the kitchen where knives could be a danger. (pp. 755–756)

10. (A) If your 35-year-old male patient stands in a corner of the room with his fists clenched, screaming obscenities, you should request police backup and keep the doorway in sight. (p. 756)

11. (B) Use of reasonable force to restrain a patient should involve an evaluation of all of the included examples except the family's ability to pay for your services. (p. 756)

12. (A) The use of force by an EMT is generally allowed to defend against an attack by an emotionally disturbed patient. (p. 756)

13. (D) Once the decision has been made to restrain your 22-year-old male patient, which one of the following steps should be avoided? A minimum of four rescuers (one for each limb) should secure the patient. (p. 757)

14. (D) This behavior is best managed by placing a surgical mask on the patient's face. (p. 759)

15. (C) You are treating a 28-year-old male patient who you feel is becoming a danger to himself or the people around him and will need to be transported against his will. You should contact the police for assistance. (p. 757)

16. (B) Which of the following is not considered a cause of altered mental status? Nervousness when speaking to a large group. (pp. 749–750)

17. (B) The patient who has excited delirium is likely to have unexpected physical strength and hyperthermia. (p. 757)

18. (D) The care of the patient with a behavioral or psychiatric emergency should include each activity except going along with their hallucinations. (p. 753)

19. (C) Substance abuse, such as cocaine or amphetamine, can be associated with bizarre and/or aggressive behavior referred to as excited delirium. (p. 757)

20. (B) Catatonia is the exhibiting of an almost complete noninteraction with the environment. (p. 751)

Pathophysiology: Neurotransmitters (p. 748)

1. To transmit messages to and from the brain, from the distal end of one neuron to the proximal end of the next neuron as the impulse travels towards its intended destination.

2. To elevate mood by preventing the reuptake of the neurotransmitter serotonin in the synapse.

Complete the Following

1. List nine factors associated with a risk for suicide. (p. 754)
   A. Depression
   B. High stress level
   C. Recent emotional trauma
   D. Age (highest risk is for people between the ages of 15–25 and over 40)
   E. Alcohol and drug abuse
   F. Threats of suicide
   G. Organized suicide plan
   H. Previous attempts
   I. Sudden improvement from depression

2. When a patient acts as if he or she may hurt him/herself or others, you first concern must be your own safety. List three precautions you should take. Any three of the four below: (p. 754)
   A. Do not argue with the patient.
   B. Make no threats.
   C. Show no indication of using force.
   D. Always have an open route to escape the patient if needed.

3. List behaviors that you may expect to see in an aggressive or hostile patient. (p. 756)
   A. Responding to people inappropriately
   B. Trying to hurt themselves or others
   C. They may have a rapid pulse and breathing
   D. Often display rapid speech and rapid physical movements
   E. They may appear anxious, nervous, or "panicky"

4. List seven common presentations, or signs and symptoms, of patients experiencing a psychiatric emergency. (p. 752)
   A. Panic or anxiety
   B. Unusual appearance, disordered clothing, or poor hygiene
   C. Agitated or unusual activity
   D. Unusual speech patterns
   E. Bizarre behavior or thought patterns
   F. Suicidal or self-destructive behavior
   G. Violent or aggressive behavior or intent to harm others

Case Study: Today Is Not the Day to Die

1. Take Standard Precautions and then, after ensuring that the patient's airway is open and breathing is adequate (the patient is talking to you), control the bleeding with a pressure bandage.

2. Apply direct pressure, and consider elevation and a pressure bandage. If this does not work, it may be necessary to apply a tourniquet or pressure point depending on your Medical Director's policies. Use your best judgment and remember how fast someone can bleed to death if bleeding is left uncontrolled.

3. The oozing is probably coming from a capillary, and the flowing is probably venous. Arteries often spurt, at least till the systolic BP drops.

4. Yes, it is definitely appropriate to ask if the patient was trying to take his own life; document the patient's answer on the PCR in quotation marks.

5. Explain to the patient why it is essential that he be taken to the hospital to deal with the wounds.

6. Restraint should be done with enough help (one person per extremity and, if enough rescuers are available, perhaps one for the head) and with care to avoid hurting the rescuers, and not causing further harm to his self-inflicted injuries. Use your best clinical judgment and follow local protocols. It is good to discuss a case like this with your Medical Director to understand his or her view on restraint and safety.

CHAPTER 28: Hematologic and Renal Emergencies

Match Key Terms

1. (D) Anemia: Deficiency in the number of red blood cells in the circulation. (pp. 779–780)

2. (C) Continuous ambulatory peritoneal dialysis (CAPD): A gravity exchange process for dialysis in which a bag of dialysis fluid is raised above the level of an abdominal catheter to fill the abdominal cavity and then is lowered below the level of the abdominal catheter to drain the fluid out. (pp. 779–780)

3. (B) Continuous cycle assisted peritoneal dialysis (CCPD): A mechanical process for dialysis in which a machine fills and empties the abdominal cavity of dialysis solution. (pp. 779–780)

4. (E) Dialysis: The process by which toxins and excess fluid are removed from the body by a medical system independent of the kidneys. (pp. 779–780)

5. (A) End-stage renal disease (ESRD): Irreversible renal failure to the extent that the kidneys can no longer provide adequate filtration and fluid balance to sustain life. (pp. 779–780)

6. (J) Exchange: One cycle of filling and draining the peritoneal cavity in peritoneal dialysis. (pp. 779–780)

7. (I) Peritonitis: Infection within the peritoneal cavity. (pp. 779–780)

8. (G) Renal failure: Loss of the kidneys' ability to filter the blood and remove toxins and excess fluid from the body. (pp. 779–780)

9. (F) Sickle cell anemia (SCA): An abnormally low number of RBCs in the circulation due to sickle cell disease. (pp. 769)

10. (H) Thrill: A vibration felt on gentle palpation, such as that which typically occurs within an arteriovenous fistula. (pp. 779–780)

11. (K) Coagulopathy: Loss of the normal ability to form a blood clot with internal or external bleeding. (pp. 779–780)

12. (N) Urinary catheter: Drainage tube placed into the urinary system to allow the flow of urine out of the body. (pp. 779–780)

13. (M) Pyelonephritis: An infection that begins in the urinary tract and ascends up the ureter into the kidney. (pp. 779–780)

14. (L) Sickle cell disease (SCD): An inherited disease in which patients have a genetic defect in their hemoglobin that results in an abnormal structure of the red blood cell. (pp. 779–780)

CHAPTER 28: (continued)

Multiple-Choice Review

1. (B) The medical specialty concerned with kidney disorders is nephrology. (p. 765)

2. (A) Blood does not remove oxygen from the cells. It delivers oxygen to the cells. (p. 766)

3. (C) The medical specialty concerned with blood disorders is hematology. (p. 765)

4. (C) White blood cells are a blood component that is critical to the body's response to infection. (p. 766)

5. (B) Platelets are a component of the blood that is designed to aggregate as a response to bleeding. (p. 766)

6. (B) The liquid in which the blood cells and platelets are suspended is called plasma. (p. 766)

7. (B) Chronic anemia is a condition that could be due to a slow GI bleed in thispatient. (p. 768)

8. (C) She called the ambulance today because she has severe pain in her arms, legs, and abdomen. What is a likely cause of this condition? A sickle cell crisis. (p. 770)

9. (D) Complications that may be found in a 35-year-old male, with respiratory distress, who has sickle cell anemia, are: destruction of the spleen, acute chest syndrome, and priapism. (p. 769)

10. (D) During the general management of a patient with sickle cell disease, you should provide: high-flow supplemental oxygen, monitoring for high fever, and treatment for shock. (p. 770)

11. (B) What life-ending disease is highly likely to occur in this patient? Renal failure. (p. 771)

12. (D) Patients who are taking meds such as: Coumadin®, Pradaxa®, Xarelto®, and Eliquis® often have a medical history of: atrial fibrillation, stroke, heart attack. (p. 767)

13. (C) The process by which an external medical system independent of the kidneys is used to remove toxins and excess fluid from the body is called dialysis. (p. 773)

14. (C) Your 56-year-old male patient tells you that he has kidney problems and must go to the clinic three times a week. The reason he goes there is probably to receive hemodialysis. (p. 773)

15. (A) A vibration that can be palpated at the fistula in the arm of the dialysis patient is called a thrill. (pp. 774–775)

16. (D) You are called to the home of a 62-year-old female patient who states that she missed dialysis twice this week because of the storm. What are the symptoms that she may exhibit? Shortness of breath, fluid in the lungs, and swollen ankles, hands, and face. (p. 776)

17. (A) The most commonly transplanted organ(s) are the kidneys. (p. 778)

18. (A) All of the following are complications of dialysis except development of an aortic aneurism. (p. 777)

19. (B) The most common serious complication of ESRD patients on peritoneal dialysis is peritonitis. (p. 777)

20. (C) When encountering an ESRD patient who missed dialysis and is experiencing problems the EMT should do each of the following except check the blood pressure on the arm with the fistula. (p. 777)

Complete the Following

1. List two types of peritoneal dialysis. (p. 776)
   A. Continuous ambulatory peritoneal dialysis (CAPD)
   B. Continuous cycler-assisted peritoneal dialysis (CCPD)

2. What is the difference between the two types of peritoneal dialysis?
   A. CAPD – fluid is left in the peritoneal cavity for 4–6 hours multiple times a day.
   B. CCPD – a machine is used to fill and empty the abdominal cavity 3–5 times as they sleep.

3. List seven steps in the assessment and care of ESRD patient who missed dialysis. (p. 777)
   A. Assess the patient.
   B. When you obtain vital signs, obtain a blood pressure on an arm that does not have a fistula.
   C. Place the patient in a position of comfort.
   D. Administer high-flow oxygen by NRB mask for those in respiratory distress.
   E. Consider the use of noninvasive positive pressure ventilation in cases of severe respiratory distress.
   F. Monitor the patient's vital signs carefully and be prepared to attach the AED if patient becomes unresponsive.
   G. Transport the patient to a hospital with renal dialysis capabilities.

Case Study: Simply No Comfortable Position

1. He is most likely attempting to pass a renal calculus (a kidney stone).

2. It is not uncommon for patients with renal calculi to drink lots of fluids to keep their urinary system flowing.

3. No, you still need to make sure there is nothing else going on (e.g., cardiac or GI problems or shock) that may be masked by the very distracting severe flank pain.

4. No, because his vitals are good and his SpO_2 is fine for now.

5. Do not cancel the medic unit. Take the patient out to your ambulance and get another set of vitals. By the time you have done that, the medic will be there.

Interim Exam 2

1. (A) The key size-up elements are maintained throughout the call, to prevent dangerous surprises later. (p. 290)

2. (D) When multiple patients are confirmed at any scene the EMT should immediately call for additional ambulances. (pp. 307–308)

3. (B) Assessing mental status is the step of the primary assessment that comes after the general impression. (p. 315)

4. (C) The "V" in AVPU stands for "verbal." (p. 321)

5. (B) The "P" in AVPU stands for "painful." (p. 321)

6. (D) When a patient is not breathing adequately the EMT must assist the patient's ventilation with 100% oxygen. (p. 323)

7. (C) If a patient is talking or crying, assume an open airway. This condition may change, however, so you need to monitor the patient. (p. 322)

8. (B) Pale, clammy skin often indicates shock. (p. 327)

9. (B) An infant has an airway that is different from an adult's, so the head should be placed in a neutral position—not tilting it back the way an adult's airway is opened. (p. 332)

©2021 Pearson Education, Inc.
Emergency Care, 14th Ed.

10. (B) Special consideration with a patient with suspected TB includes EMTs wearing N-95 respirators when caring for the patient and providing treatment. (pp. 672–673)

11. (C) The capillary refill test is used to evaluate the circulation of infants and children but is no longer advocated as an effective, reliable test for adults. (p.332)

12. (B) When assessing the pupils, you should look for three things: size, equality, and reactivity. (p. 349)

13. (C) Documenting examination findings that are negative (things that are not true) is called documenting a pertinent negative. (p. 481)

14. (C) Pulse oximeter is an electronic device for determining the amount of oxygen carried in the blood. (p. 359)

15. (B) An important concept of EMS documentation is "If it is not written down, you did not do it." (p. 482)

16. (A) If a patient does not want to go to the hospital, document with a refusal-of-care form. Be sure to consult medical direction whenever there is a patient refusal. (p. 483)

17. (B) Failure to perform an important part of patient assessment or care is an error of omission. Errors of commission are performing actions that are wrong or improper. (p. 486)

18. (C) Making up vitals is falsification and could endanger the patient's care. (p. 486)

19. (A) Stating that "the patient is alert and oriented" is an example of objective information that you are able to observe. (p. 481)

20. (D) Statements from patients, bystanders, or family should be put in quotes on the PCR. (p. 481)

21. (A) After establishing the patient's mental status in the primary assessment, you should proceed to open the airway. (p. 315)

22. (B) The vital signs are pulse; respirations; blood pressure; pupils; and skin condition, color, and temperature. (p. 340)

23. (B) The normal adult pulse rate at rest is between 60 and 100 beats per minute. (p. 341)

24. (D) The initial pulse rate for patients 1 year and older is normally taken at the radial pulse. (p. 344)

25. (D) A weak and thin pulse force is described as thready. (p. 344)

26. (B) Normal adult at-rest respiration rates vary from 12 to 20 breaths per minute. (p. 345)

27. (D) Crowing is a noisy, harsh sound heard during inhalation that indicates a partial airway obstruction. (p. 346)

28. (C) The systolic blood pressure is the arterial pressure that is created when the left ventricle of the heart contracts. (p. 350)

29. (B) Diastolic blood pressure is the arterial pressure that is created by relaxation and refilling of the left ventricle of the heart. (p. 350)

30. (A) Determining blood pressure by palpation is not as accurate as by the auscultation method. This procedure is used when there is a lot of noise around a patient. (p. 352)

31. (A) Information that you see, hear, feel, or smell is a sign and can be measured. Information that the patient tells you is a symptom. (p. 406)

32. (B) When you ask the patient, "Have you recently had any surgery or injuries?" you are inquiring about the patient's pertinent past history. (p. 406)

33. (C) Croup is an upper respiratory infection that includes dyspnea and a bark-like cough. (pp. 672–673)

34. (C) An acronym that is used to remember what questions to ask about the patient's present problem and past history is SAMPLE. AVPU is the level of responsiveness, PEARL is the status of the pupils, and DCAP-BTLS helps to remind the EMT what to look for in a soft-tissue exam. (p. 408)

35. (C) A normal blood glucose level is usually 70–100 mg/dL. (p. 364)

36. (A) When performing CPR, capnography will show an increased reading in end-tidal CO_2 when there is a return of spontaneous circulation. (p. 365)

37. (B) In adults, we normally perform the physical exam in head-to-toe order; on pediatric patients, you might need to modify the examination to start with the extremities first. (p. 378)

38. (D) Orthopnea occurs in several respiratory conditions, including heart failure. (p. 379)

39. (C) In taking a patient's blood pressure, the stethoscope is placed over the brachial artery. (pp. 353–354)

40. (D) Because the patient's signs and symptoms suggest hepatitis B, you should avoid contact with the patient's blood. This would mean full PPE, not just a gown. (pp. 672–673)

41. (B) When there are no apparent hazards at the scene of a collision, the danger zone should extend 50 feet in all directions from the wreckage. (p. 294)

42. (C) Patients on blood thinners are more prone to life-threatening bleeding when they are injured, often they bleed into their brain after even minor head trauma. (p. 767)

43. (C) The purpose of the primary assessment is to discover and treat life-threatening conditions. (p. 314)

44. (B) Deficiency in the normal number of red blood cells (low hemoglobin) in the circulation is called anemia. (p. 768)

45. (C) The "S" in OPQRST stands for severity. (p. 408)

46. (D) Vital signs should be reassessed every 5 minutes because this is an unstable patient. The BP in this patient is low, making him unstable. (p. 415)

47. (B) The rapid assessment evaluates areas of the body where the greatest threats to the patient are likely to be. (p. 406)

48. (A) The secondary (detailed) examination is most often performed on the trauma patient with a significant mechanism of injury. (p. 448)

49. (A) To obtain a history of a patient's present illness, ask the OPQRST questions. These questions focus on the chief complaint and potential causes. (p. 408)

50. (C) The "P" in OPQRST stands for "provocation," which refers to questions such as "Can you think of anything that might have triggered this pain?" (p. 408)

51. (C) For a stable patient, the EMT should perform the reassessment every 15 minutes. For an unstable patient, the EMT should perform the reassessment every 5 minutes. (p. 457)

52. (A) During the reassessment, whenever you believe that there may have been a change in the patient's condition, you should repeat the primary assessment. (p. 454)

CHAPTER 28: (continued)

53. (D) Pale, clammy skin most likely indicates shock. Exposure to cold causes dry, cold skin. Fever results in clammy, warm or hot skin. (p. 327)

54. (D) As an EMT, your overriding concern at all times is your own safety. Your crew's safety has a high priority, but your personal safety must come first. (p. 290)

55. (C) The chief complaint is what the patient tells you is the matter. (p. 420)

56. (C) Infants and young children under the age of 8 years are primarily abdominal breathers. (p. 447)

57. (A) The presence of JVD in a sitting patient means that blood is backing up in the veins because the heart is not pumping effectively. (p. 437)

58. (C) If possible, position yourself facing the patient, at or below the patient's eye level. This position will be less threatening to the patient than standing above him or her. (p. 471)

59. (B) The first item that is given to the hospital in your medical radio report to the receiving facility is your unit identification and level of provider. (p. 468)

60. (B) The neck offers less support because muscles and bone structures are less developed. (p. 444)

61. (C) A medical radio report should paint a picture of the patient's problem in words. (p. 468)

62. (A) In infants, the lateral lung fields are best evaluated from the mid-axillary position to ensure the sounds appreciated are not referred from the opposite lung. (p. 446)

63. (D) Any action of a drug other than the desired action is called a side effect. (p. 504)

64. (D) Administering a drug subcutaneously means injecting the drug under the skin. (p. 506)

65. (D) Aspirin reduces the blood's ability to clot and works to prevent clot formation that causes damage to the heart. (p. 497)

66. (B) The adequate rate of artificial ventilation for a nonbreathing adult patient with a pulse is 10–12 breaths per minute. (p. 600)

67. (C) The adequate rate of artificial ventilation for a nonbreathing infant or child patient with a pulse is 12–20 breaths per minute. (p. 600)

68. (A) An unresponsive adult who makes snoring or gurgling sounds most likely has a serious airway problem requiring immediate intervention. (p. 524)

69. (D) The skin of a patient with inadequate breathing may be blue (or pale) in color and will feel cool and clammy. (p. 524)

70. (C) If a patient is experiencing breathing difficulty but is breathing adequately, it is usually best to place him or her in a position of comfort. This is generally a sitting-up position. (p. 534)

71. (D) The cause of adult chest pain due to a decreased blood supply to the heart is angina pectoris. Dysrhythmia is an irregular heart rhythm. (p. 570)

72. (C) Most heart attacks are caused by narrowing or occlusion of a coronary artery. The coronary arteries supply the heart muscle with blood. (p. 558)

73. (D) Acute myocardial infarction is the condition in which a portion of the heart muscle dies because of oxygen starvation. (p. 572)

74. (B) An irregular or absent heart rhythm is called dysrhythmia. (p. 572)

75. (A) A pulse slower than 60 beats per minute is called bradycardia. (p. 559)

76. (C) An at-rest heart beat faster than 100 beats per minute is referred to as tachycardia. (p. 559)

77. (A) Heart failure is the condition caused by excessive fluid buildup in the lungs and/or other organs and body parts because of inadequate pumping of the heart. (p. 574)

78. (A) A diabetic with a weak, rapid pulse and cold, clammy skin who complains of hunger pangs is probably suffering from hypoglycemia. Hyperglycemic patients often have warm, red, dry skin and an acetone breath. (p. 628, 634)

79. (B) In hyperglycemia, the patient's breath smells like acetone. (p. 634)

80. (A) A conscious, hypoglycemic patient who is able to swallow is frequently administered oral glucose, with permission given by medical direction or standing orders. (p. 626, 632)

81. (C) If you cannot administer glucose to the diabetic patient because she or he is not awake enough to swallow, you should treat the patient like any other patient with altered mental status. Secure the airway, provide artificial ventilations if necessary, and be prepared to perform CPR if needed. (p. 632)

82. (C) The first time a person is exposed to an allergen, the person's immune system forms antibodies. (p. 653)

83. (C) To be considered a severe allergic reaction, a patient must have signs and symptoms of shock or respiratory distress. (p. 655)

84. (D) When patient has no history of allergies and is having his or her first allergic reaction, try to determine what the cause might be. (p. 655)

85. (C) Carbon monoxide, chlorine, and ammonia are examples of inhaled poisons. (p. 698)

86. (A) It is important for the EMT to determine when the ingestion of a poison occurred because different poisons act on the body at different rates. (p. 700)

87. (B) The principal prehospital treatment of a patient who has inhaled poison is administering high-concentration oxygen. (p. 709)

88. (B) Patients who have mixed alcohol and beta blockers can present with depressed vital signs. (p. 716)

89. (C) Most cases of poisoning involve young children. (p. 697)

90. (C) Poisons that are swallowed are ingested poisons. (p. 698)

91. (C) A late sign of respiratory distress is bradycardia. Nasal flaring and stridor are early signs. (pp. 532–534)

92. (B) Swelling or edema in both lower extremities is associated with a history of heart failure. (p. 574)

93. (B) The actions of nitroglycerin will relax blood vessels and decrease the workload of the heart. (p. 569)

94. (A) A heart rate less than 60 beats per minute in an infant should be considered non-perfusing and should indicate chest compressions. (p. 587)

95. (D) Renal failure occurs when the kidneys lose their ability to adequately filter the blood. (p. 771)

96. (B) The organs that are found outside the peritoneum and between the abdomen and the back are in the retroperitoneal space. (p. 728)

97. (C) The spleen is located in the upper left abdominal quadrant. (p. 727)

98. (D) He may have an aortic aneurysm. (pp. 732–733)

99. (B) The patient probably has a bleeding ulcer. (p. 732)

100. (D) Your first step when called to care for any attempted suicide victim is to ensure your own safety. This may mean waiting for police assistance, depending on the circumstances of the suicide attempt. (p. 751, 755)

101. (C) If you are unable to perform normal assessment and care procedures because the patient is aggressive and hostile, you should seek advice from medical direction. (p. 756)

102. (B) Diabetes is a condition brought about by decreased insulin production or the ability of the body cells to use insulin properly. Insulin moves glucose into cells. (pp. 624–625)

103. (C) When a patient presents with more than one condition or a familiar condition but under unusual circumstances, the EMT should assess the patient as usual and then seek guidance if necessary. (p. 634)

104. (A) Because of the retroperitoneal location of the pancreas, behind the stomach, the pain may radiate to the back and/or shoulders. (p. 732)

105. (D) If this area with pain is palpated first and causes additional pain, it will mask or alter the patient's response to palpation of the other quadrants. Thus palpate the quadrant with the pain last. (p. 739)

106. (D) The patient with slurred speech may have had a stroke, an overdose, or a seizure. (p. 634)

107. (B) The kidneys filter the blood and remove wastes and excess fluid from the body. (p. 771)

108. (C) Because of the importance and vulnerability of the fistula obtaining a BP in the same arm should be avoided. (p. 775)

109. (C) Transient ischemic attack (TIA) or mini-stroke presents with symptoms of stroke that resolve within 24 hours. (p. 639)

110. (A) The conclusion that an EMT makes about a patient's condition after assessing the patient is called field diagnosis. (p. 392)

111. (C) Critical thinking is the analytical process that assists the EMT in reaching a field diagnosis. (p. 392)

112. (C) Epinephrine when administered as a medication, will constrict blood vessels (helping to raise the BP and improve perfusion) and dilate the bronchioles (helping to open the airway and improve breathing). (p. 660)

113. (C) The differential diagnosis is a list of conditions that may be the cause of the patient's current condition. (p. 393)

114. (B) Signs and symptoms are similar to adults, but the treatment can differ. The dose of epinephrine for a child is less than for an adult. (p. 662)

115. (D) Signs and symptoms of poisoning from insecticides include slow pulse, excessive salivation, sweating, nausea, vomiting, diarrhea, difficulty breathing and constricted pupils. (p. 698)

116. (A) The traditional approach to diagnosis involves narrowing down a long list of possibilities. (pp. 392–396)

117. (B) Specifically looking for evidence that supports the diagnosis you already have in mind is called a confirmation bias. (p. 398)

118. (D) Availability is the urge to think of things because they are more easily recalled, often because of recent exposure. (p. 397)

119. (B) It is critical that the EMT take protective measures to prevent exposure to these substances. The patient may need to be decontaminated by a HAZMAT team prior to assessing the patient. (p. 712)

120. (A) Stopping the search for a diagnosis too soon can lead to missing out on the secondary diagnosis. (p. 398)

121. (B) With the mental status rapidly diminishing in this patient who is already on CPAP, you should remove the CPAP and ventilate the patient with a BVM device. (p. 537)

122. (C) This was a long flight, and the patient's history of smoking and DVT and the shortness of breath suggest that she may have a pulmonary embolism. (p. 639)

123. (A) They both have numerous stings, but the daughter is experiencing the signs of an anaphylactic reaction, not the simple allergic reaction the father is having. The daughter will most likely have hypotension, which is a critical sign. (p. 652)

124. (B) She may have attempted suicide by mixing chemicals to produce hydrogen sulfide. CO is odorless. CO_2 and cyanide do not smell like rotten eggs. (p. 712)

125. (A) The complications of sickle cell disease can include destruction of the spleen, acute chest syndrome, priapism, and stroke but not destruction of the pancreas. (p. 769)

CHAPTER 29: Bleeding and Shock

Match Key Terms

1. (G) Arterial bleeding: Bleeding, from an artery, which is characterized by bright red blood and is rapid, profuse, and difficult to control. (p. 821)

2. (C) Capillary bleeding: Bleeding from capillaries, which is characterized by a slow, oozing flow of blood. (p. 821)

3. (H) Cardiogenic shock: Shock, or lack of perfusion, brought on not by blood loss but by the heart's inadequate pumping action. It is often the result of heart attack or heart failure. (p. 821)

4. (B) Compensated shock: When the patient is developing shock but the body is still able to maintain perfusion. (p. 821)

5. (E) Decompensated shock: When the body can no longer compensate a shock state which results in hypotension and death. (p. 821)

6. (J) Hemorrhage: Bleeding, especially severe bleeding. (p. 821)

7. (K) Hemorrhagic shock: Shock resulting from blood loss. (p. 821)

8. (I) Hemostatic agents: Substances applied as powders, dressings, gauze, or bandages to open wounds to stop bleeding. (p. 821)

9. (F) Hypoperfusion: The body's inability to adequately circulate blood to the body's cells to supply them with oxygen and nutrients. (p. 821)

10. (D) Hypovolemic shock: Shock resulting from blood or fluid loss. (p. 821)

CHAPTER 29: (continued)

11. (A) Neurogenic shock: Hypoperfusion caused by a spinal cord injury that results in systemic vasodilatation. (p. 821)

12. (N) Perfusion: The supply of oxygen to, and removal of wastes from, the cells and tissues of the body as a result of blood flow through the capillaries. (p. 821)

13. (O) Pressure dressing: A bulky dressing held in position with a tightly wrapped bandage, which applies pressure to help control bleeding. (p. 821)

14. (P) Shock: A general or lay term used to describe the inability to adequately circulate blood to the body's cells in order to supply them with oxygen and nutrients; a life-threatening condition. (p. 821)

15. (M) Tourniquet: A device used for bleeding control that constricts all blood flow to and from an extremity. (p. 821)

16. (L) Venous bleeding: Bleeding from a vein, which is characterized by dark red or maroon blood and a steady, easy-to-control flow. (p. 821)

17. (R) Distributive shock: Hypoperfusion due to lack of blood vessel tone. Blood vessel dilation leads to decreased pressure within the circulatory system. (p. 821)

18. (Q) Obstructive shock: A type of shock in which the heart cannot pump blood due to a blockage of blood flow into or out of the heart. (p. 790)

Multiple-Choice Review

1. (B) Blood that has been depleted of oxygen and loaded with carbon dioxide and other wastes empties into the veins, which carry it back to the heart. (p. 787)

2. (D) Cells and tissues of the brain, spinal cord, kidneys, and heart are the most sensitive to inadequate perfusion. (p. 789, 799)

3. (B) Police are on the scene, and it is now safe for you to begin your assessment and treatment. The use of Standard Precautions is essential whenever bleeding is discovered or simply anticipated. (p. 801)

4. (C) The process of substances such as hormones, water, and enzymes that are carried by the blood and the body's functions is referred to as regulation. (p. 788)

5. (B) Which statement about arterial bleeding is correct? Arterial bleeding is often rapid and profuse. (p. 800)

6. (B) There is a steady flow of dark red or maroon blood, which is most likely a result of venous bleeding. (p. 800)

7. (C) Bleeding described as oozing is usually a result of capillary bleeding. (p. 801)

8. (B) When a patient is losing blood hemorrhagic shock begins to occur. When blood is lost so are the platelets, which affect the blood's ability to clot, and hemoglobin, which affects the blood's oxygen carrying ability. (p. 789)

9. (C) Pediatric patients are excellent compensators when confronted with blood loss from trauma. They can successfully shunt blood to their core; their heart rate can speed up quickly; and they are able to maintain their BP even with up to 40% blood loss; however, they cannot produce very forceful heart contractions. (p. 792)

10. (B) Each of the listed causes of shock are distributive in nature, except obstructive shock. (p. 790)

11. (A) Conditions that obstruct the flow of blood cause obstructive shock. Brain hemorrhage is not a cause of an obstructive. (p. 790)

12. (D) The body's natural responses to bleeding are constriction of the injured blood vessel and clotting. (p. 787)

13. (B) Your assessment of external bleeding includes all the mentioned steps except waiting for signs and symptoms of shock to appear before beginning treatment. (p. 802)

14. (B) The major methods that are used to control massive external extremity bleeding include all those mentioned except for hemolytic dressing. (A major method of controlling such bleeding is hemostatic dressing. The term "hemolytic" refers to the rupture or destruction of red blood cells.) (p. 803)

15. (B) Why is administration of supplemental oxygen an important treatment for the trauma patient? Supplemental oxygen helps provide a higher level of oxygen in the limited amount of blood reaching the tissues. (p. 803)

16. (C) The most common and effective way to control massive external extremity bleeding is by tourniquet. (p. 803, 811)

17. (C) The initial layer of dressing should not be removed from a bleeding wound because it is a necessary part of clot formation. (p. 806)

18. (A) Wound packing can be effective, especially when hemostatic gauze is used, for the following areas: extremities and junctional areas. (p. 808)

19. (C) When you suspect that a patient is in late stages of shock, an additional sign of late shock may be cyanosis around the lips and nail beds. (p. 797)

20. (B) You should be especially careful when evaluating pediatric patients for shock because children may display few signs until a large percentage of blood volume is lost. (p. 792)

21. (B) What method of bleeding control should you use? Direct pressure with a dressing and bandage should work. (p. 806)

22. (D) Use of direct pressure may not be effective if the wound involves a profusely bleeding artery. (pp. 806–808)

23. (A) Which of the following is true about the use of an air splint? It is effective for controlling venous and capillary bleeding. (p. 817)

24. (B) Which of the following is not a guideline for supplementing bleeding control with cold application? Pour ice chips directly into the open skin. (p. 817)

25. (B) The best treatment would be to utilize hemostatic gauze into the wound while beginning to transport the patient by Medevac to the regional trauma center. (pp. 810–811)

26. (C) Bleeding from a clean-edged amputation is usually cared for initially with a tourniquet. (p. 814)

27. (C) When the body has lost the battle to maintain perfusion to the organ systems and the systolic BP begins to drop, the patient is experiencing decompensated shock. (p. 793)

28. (A) Once a tourniquet is in place, it must not be removed or loosened unless ordered by medical direction. (p. 815)

29. (D) Early signs of shock that are actually the body's compensating mechanisms include all of the following except shorter capillary refill time in children. (p. 793)

30. (D) If you note bleeding or leakage of CSF from the patient's ears or nose, you should allow the drainage to flow freely. (p. 817)

31. (B) The medical term for a nosebleed is epistaxis. (p. 817)

32. (D) To stop or control a nosebleed, try each method except applying cold packs to the bridge of the nose and face. (p. 817)

©2021 Pearson Education, Inc.
Emergency Care, 14th Ed.

33. (A) The leading cause of internal injuries and bleeding is blunt trauma. (p. 818)

34. (A) Which of the following is not *typically*.an example of a penetrating trauma? A blast injury. (Blast injuries *can* include penetrating trauma but typically do not.) (p. 819)

35. (B) Signs of internal bleeding include all of the listed findings except bradycardia and a flushed face. (p. 819)

36. (D) Internal bleeding may be signaled by all but bleeding from a laceration in the forearm, which is external bleeding only. (p. 819)

37. (C) Because of internal injury, the patient is developing inadequate tissue perfusion. This condition is referred to as hypoperfusion. (*Shock* and *hypoperfusion* are synonyms.) (p. 819)

38. (D) Which cause is least likely to result in a state of shock or hypoperfusion? A closed head injury. (pp. 789–790)

39. (C) The most common mechanism of shock for a heart attack patient is pump failure. (p. 790)

40. (C) Shock caused by the failure of the nervous system to control the diameter of blood vessels is called neurogenic shock. (p. 790)

41. (A) This is often referred to as compensated shock. (p. 792)

42. (A) What is causing this symptom of feeling nauseated? Blood is diverted from the digestive system. (p. 797)

43. (C) The pulse rate of a female in an early shock state will be increased. (p. 797)

44. (D) The patient in question 42 has a drop in her systolic BP. This is a late sign of shock. (p. 797)

Pathophysiology: Fight-or-Flight (p. 791)

1. The blood vessels constrict, especially in skin, kidneys, and GI tract. Sweat glands empty their contents, causing sweaty skin.

2. When blood vessels in the kidneys constrict, the kidneys produce less urine, thus preventing the loss of fluid.

3. Constriction of blood vessels in the GI tract causes the stomach to try to empty its contents, leading to nausea and vomiting.

Complete the Following

1. List four categories of shock and key interventions. (p. 799)
   A. Hypovolemic shock – control bleeding, provide rapid transport.
   B. Cardiogenic shock – Request ALS and place the patient in an appropriate position to help maintain blood pressure.
   C. Distributive shock (anaphylaxis) – Administer epinephrine to vasoconstrict blood vessels.
   D. Distributive shock (sepsis) – Recognize and notify receiving hospital; contact ALS and position the patient appropriately, provide rapid transport.

2. List five signs of shock. (p. 797)
   A. Altered mental status
   B. Pale, cool, and clammy skin
   C. Nausea and vomiting
   D. Vital sign changes
   E. Late sign (sometimes, cyanosis around the lips and nail beds).

3. List seven principles of care for patient with external hemorrhage. (p. 818)
   A. If possible, begin hemorrhage control with direct pressure.
   B. Consider hemostatic agents to augment direct pressure.
   C. Consider the need for wound packing.
   D. Consider the use of a junctional tourniquet.
   E. If direct pressure fails or is inappropriate, immediately apply a tourniquet.
   F. Initiate rapid transport.
   G. Consider the need for ALS.

Label the Diagram (p. 788)

1. Artery

2. Arteriole

3. Capillary

4. Venule

5. Vein

Case Study: Convenience Store Shooting

1. Ensuring that the shooter is no longer on the scene is critical to the safety of the EMS crew, patient, and bystanders.

2. Safety issues, proper BSI precautions, number of patients, and need for additional resources.

3. Internal and external bleeding are present. She is going into decompensated shock, which is demonstrated by the fast, weak (almost unpalpable) radial pulse. Her blood pressure can be estimated to be less than 90 systolic.

4. The patient is in decompensating hypovolemic or hemorrhagic shock from blood loss.

5. The patient's brain interprets her blood loss (fluid) as low fluid volume. Therefore, she asks for fluids. In this case, it is too late to restore her fluid volume by asking her to drink oral fluids. She needs IV fluids and blood products on arrival at the regional trauma center.

6. Bullet fragments can easily ricochet into the chest. Always listen to the lung sounds of a trauma patient so that you will not miss possible injuries to the lungs (e.g., pneumothorax).

7. Use a nonrebreather mask at 15 liters per minute. It would be helpful to obtain the SpO_2. Monitor the patient's ventilations closely in case you need to switch to a BVM and assist her ventilations.

8. Call for ALS immediately. This is definitely a Gray Zone, depending on your individual EMS system and your Medical Director's point of view as well as your best clinical judgment. If ALS has not arrived when you are ready to transport, you may want to arrange an intercept en route to the hospital. Time is very critical on this call, and it makes no sense to delay the patient on the scene or wait for ALS to arrive. For further discussion on operations in a case like this, consult your Medical Director.

9. As little as possible, the goal is to spend no more than 10 minutes on the scene.

10. Because the patient is likely to need surgery at the regional trauma center to stop her internal bleeding, take as little time as possible and call ahead to the emergency department (ED) to let them know the patient's condition as soon as you can. This will save a lot of time by having all the right providers in the ED when you arrive.

CHAPTER 29: (continued)

11. Insert an oral airway if the patient has no gag reflex. Continue to assist ventilations as required. When the paramedics arrive, they may choose to insert an advanced airway en route to the hospital.

12. The question of spinal immobilization could be controversial and depends on your state or regional protocols. This is a Gray Zone area in which you should use your best clinical judgment. Because the patient is able to move all four extremities, it is probably not worth taking the extra time to immobilize her. You could also ask whether there is paresthesia ("pins and needles") in the legs, which might indicate spinal cord injury and the need for the immobilization. Using the long backboard does act as a "full body splint."

13. Because this patient is being ventilated (at this time), she is considered critical. In fact, she is in decompensated (severe) shock and may die without your quick interventions, possible ALS intercept, and transport to the most appropriate facility.

14. Administer two large-bore IVs of normal saline or lactated Ringer solution, insert an advanced airway, monitor ECG, and administer assisted ventilations.

15. Review your sample radio report with your instructor.

CHAPTER 30: Soft-Tissue Trauma

Match Key Terms

Part A

1. (N) Abrasion: A scratch or scrape. (pp. 864–865)

2. (O) Amputation: The surgical removal or traumatic severing of a body part, usually an extremity. (pp. 864–865)

3. (H) Avulsion: The tearing away or tearing off of a piece or flap or other soft tissue. This term also may be used for an eye pulled from its socket or a tooth dislodged from its socket. (pp. 864–865)

4. (C) Bandage: Any material used to hold a dressing in place. (pp. 864–865)

5. (F) Closed wound: An internal injury with no pathway from the outside. (pp. 864–865)

6. (M) Contusion: A bruise. (pp. 864–865)

7. (J) Crush injury: An injury caused when force it transmitted from the body's exterior to its internal structures, often causing massive internal injuries and bone fractures. (pp. 864–865)

8. (L) Dermis: The inner (second) layer of the skin found beneath the epidermis. It is rich in blood vessels and nerves. (pp. 864–865)

9. (I) Dressing: Any material (preferably sterile) used to cover a wound that will help control bleeding and prevent additional contamination. (pp. 864–865)

10. (B) Epidermis: The outer layer of the skin. (pp. 864–865)

11. (G) Full-thickness burn: A burn in which all the layers of the skin are damaged. There are usually areas that are charred black or areas that are dry and white. (pp. 864–865)

12. (A) Hematoma: A swelling caused by the collection of blood under the skin or in damaged tissues as a result of an injured or broken blood vessel. (pp. 864–865)

13. (D) Laceration: A cut. (pp. 864–865)

14. (K) Occlusive dressing: Any dressing that forms an airtight seal. (pp. 864–865)

15. (E) Open wound: An injury in which the skin is interrupted, exposing the tissue beneath. (pp. 864–865)

Part B

1. (E) Partial-thickness burn: A burn in which the epidermis (first layer of skin) is burned through and the dermis (second layer) is damaged. Burns of this type cause reddening, blistering, and a mottled appearance. This is also called a second-degree burn. (pp. 864–865)

2. (H) Pressure dressing: A dressing applied tightly to control bleeding. (pp. 864)

3. (F) Puncture wound: An open wound that tears through the skin and destroys underlying tissues. This type of wound can be shallow or deep. (pp. 864–865)

4. (B) Rule of nines: A method for estimating the extent of larger burns. (pp. 864–865)

5. (C) Rule of palm: A method for estimating the extent of smaller burns. The palm of the patient's hand, which equals about 1% of the body's surface area, is compared with the patient's burn to estimate the size of the burn. (pp. 864–865)

6. (G) Subcutaneous layers: The layers of fat and soft tissues found below the dermis. (pp. 864–865)

7. (D) Superficial burn: A burn that involves only the epidermis, the outer layer of the skin. It is characterized by reddening of the skin and perhaps some swelling. A common example is sunburn. This is also called a first-degree burn. (pp. 864–865)

8. (A) Universal dressing: A bulky dressing. (pp. 864–865)

Multiple-Choice Review

1. (C) The soft tissues of the body include all of the following except teeth and cartilage. (p. 825)

2. (D) Which of the following is not a function of the skin? White blood cell production. (p. 825)

3. (D) The layers of the skin include all of the following except epithelial. (p. 826)

4. (A) The outermost epidermis is the layer of the skin that is composed of dead cells, which are rubbed or sloughed off and are replaced continuously. (p. 826)

5. (B) Specialized nerve endings in the dermis are involved in the senses of touch, cold, heat, and pain. (p. 827)

6. (C) Shock absorption and insulation are major functions of the subcutaneous layer of the skin. (p. 827)

7. (C) There is no external bleeding. This wound is called a closed injury. (p. 827)

8. (B) A patient has experienced a closed wound involving tissue damage and a collection of blood at the injury site. This is called a hematoma. (p. 828)

9. (C) A patient has experienced a soft-tissue injury from a force that caused a rupture or bleeding of internal organs. This injury is called a closed crush injury. (p. 828)

©2021 Pearson Education, Inc.
Emergency Care, 14th Ed.

10. (B) The oozing of blood from her capillary beds is from an injury called a(n) abrasion. (p. 830)

11. (C) A 28-year-old male sustained a cut on his hand while slicing carrots for a stew. The wound that he sustained is called a laceration. (p. 830)

12. (B) When a sharp or pointed object, such as an ice pick or bullet, passes through the skin or other tissue, a puncture wound has occurred. (p. 831)

13. (A) The tip of his nose was almost completely cut off by the knife. This is an avulsion injury. (p. 832)

14. (D) Various types of guns, when fired at close range, can cause all the described injuries except significant cold injuries. (p. 837)

15. (A) Emergency care in the field for this patient includes stabilizing the object in place. (p. 838)

16. (C) Which of the following is not correct about an injury caused by an impaled object? (p. 839)

17. (A) Which of the following is false about this impaled object? It should never be removed. (p. 841)

18. (C) If a 22-year-old female patient has an impaled object in her right eye, the care that you provide should include use of a combination of 4 x 4s and a paper cup. (p. 842)

19. (D) You should do all of the described treatments except tearing it off and cooling it during transport. (p. 843)

20. (C) The amputated parts torn from her body should be wrapped and placed in a plastic bag on top of a sealed bag of ice. (p. 843)

21. (A) The most effective treatment for an amputation is to apply a tourniquet and cool the lower leg. (p. 836)

22. (A) Your 19-year-old male patient has sustained a very serious injury, and it will be necessary to apply an occlusive dressing to the wound. An occlusive dressing is used to form an airtight seal. (p. 861)

23. (B) The primary injuries that occur from a blast are caused by a pressure wave. (p. 834)

24. (C) Your treatment should include each described intervention except for packing his genitals in ice as soon as possible. (p. 844)

25. (D) The victim of an electrical accident may have the following signs and symptoms: elevated BP or low BP with shock signs and symptoms, seizures, muscle tenderness or twitching. (p. 857)

26. (A) In terms of injuries, you expect to find a mixture of open and closed injuries. (p. 834)

27. (C) This type of injury is called a crush injury. (pp. 828–829)

28. (A) Blast injuries often include all of the described findings except potentially infectious disease. (p. 835)

29. (B) In addition to the physical damage caused by burns, patients often suffer emotional and psychological problems. (p. 845)

30. (A) When caring for a 22-year-old male who was burned do not neglect assessment in order to begin burn care. (p. 845)

31. (D) Examples of agents that can cause burns include all of the following except distilled water. (p. 846)

32. (A) A burn that involves only the epidermis is called a superficial burn. (p. 846)

33. (B) Which of the following types of burns will result in deep, intense pain; blisters; and mottled skin? Partial-thickness. (p. 847)

34. (C) To distinguish between a partial-thickness burn and a full-thickness burn, look for charred or dry and white areas, which indicate a full-thickness burn. (p. 847)

35. (B) Electrical burns are of special concern because they pose a great risk of severe internal injuries. (p. 856)

36. (C) Chemical burns are of special concern because the chemicals may remain on the skin and continue to burn for hours. (p. 853)

37. (D) Burns to the face are of special concern because they may involve airway injury. (p. 848)

38. (B) Using the rule of nines, approximate the size of the burn area. The burn estimate for this patient is 27%. (p. 848)

39. (D) Using the rule of nines, approximate the size of the burn area. The burn estimate for this patient is 54%. (p. 849)

40. (A) This burn would cover approximately 5% of the patient's total body surface area. (p. 849)

41. (B) The age of the patient is an important factor in burns. Patients under 5 and over 55 years of age have the most severe body responses to burns. (p. 849)

42. (D) Burn center criteria include all of the following except partial thickness burns on the wrist. (p. 850)

43. (A) A 22-year-old male patient who has a partial-thickness burn to the entire back should be wrapped in a dry, sterile burn sheet. (p. 852)

44. (B) The primary care for a patient with a chemical burn to the eyes is to wash away the chemical with flowing water. (p. 855)

45. (C) This patient probably suffered an electrical burn. (p. 857)

46. (A) if dry lime is the burn agent, brush it from the patient's skin and then flush the patient's skin with water. (p. 854)

Pathophysiology: Acids and Alkalis (p. 854)

1. The alkali liquefies dead tissue allowing it to penetrate and continue burning much deeper than an acid burn.

2. Hydrofluoric acid is flushed longer because it penetrates deeper into the skin.

Complete the Following

1. List three ways that burns can be classified. (p. 845)
   A. By type of burn
   B. By depth of burn
   C. By severity of burn

2. List eleven parts of the adult body that account for 9% each, using the rule of nines. (p. 849)
   A. The head
   B. Right arm
   C. Left arm
   D. Upper back
   E. Lower back

CHAPTER 30: (continued)

    F. Right front leg
    G. Left front leg
    H. Right back of leg
    I. Left back of the leg
    J. Upper chest
    K. Abdomen

3. List seven criteria for patients who should be treated at a burn center. (p. 850)
    A. Second-degree (partial thickness) burns greater than 10 percent of the total body surface area
    B. Burns involving the face, genitalia, or perineum, hands, feet, or major joints
    C. Third-degree (full thickness) burns
    D. Electrical burns
    E. Inhalation burns
    F. Other medical problems or trauma
    G. Other needs that a typical hospital will not be able to meet

Label the Diagram (p. 846)

1. Superficial
2. Partial thickness
3. Full thickness
4. Red skin
5. Blisters
6. Charring

Case Study: No Patience for Lighter Fluid

1. On the basis of information so far—blistered skin on his right (1%) and left palms (1%), the anterior and posterior surfaces of his right (4.5%) and left (45%) forearms, and his entire chest (9%)—approximately 20% of his body surface was burned.

2. The significance of the singed facial hair is that there could be burns to the face or he might have inhaled superheated gases, which can cause respiratory burns.

3. Lighter fluid burns, but generally the fumes do not explode easily. Gasoline emits fumes that can easily find a heat source and explode.

4. Blisters are the indication of a partial-thickness (second-degree) burn, which is very painful because of the exposed nerve endings.

5. Yes. The patient burned his hands, and the total burns are 20%. Use your best judgment in evaluating this patient and, if needed, consult with your Medical Director in making the decision on where the patient should be transported.

6. In most regions, protocols call for putting out the fire and then using a dry, preferably sterile dressing. The dressing can be accomplished by spreading the burn sheet on the stretcher and then covering the patient once he is on the sheet. Monitor vitals and treat for shock as well as calling for ALS.

7. His watch and rings needed to be removed because his hands and forearms are going to swell, and the rings will act as tourniquets, damaging the tissue in his fingers.

8. This question could have many answers. Use your best clinical judgment to consider allergies (such as an allergy to pain medicine) or medication the patient may have taken (which could speed up shock or affect respirations) or specific past medical history that could make him a higher priority (cardiac or respiratory problems). If the history identifies something that you feel may be relevant to this case, feel free to discuss it with your medical director.

9. During your physical examination, listen to this patient's lung sounds to make sure he is not exhibiting any signs of a respiratory burn, such as wheezing.

10. Either ask the paramedic or place the electrodes on the unburned surfaces of the limbs. Do not place them on burn blisters.

CHAPTER 31: Chest and Abdominal Trauma

Match Key Terms

1. (C) Tension pneumothorax: A type of chest injury in which air that enters the chest cavity is prevented from escaping causing the lung to collapse and the heart to shift. (p. 890)

2. (E) Sucking chest wound: An open chest wound in which air is "sucked" into the chest cavity. (p. 890)

3. (D) Evisceration: An intestine or other internal organ protruding through a wound in the abdomen. (p. 890)

4. (F) Flail chest: Fracture of two or more adjacent ribs in two or more places that allows for free movement of the fractured segment. (p. 890)

5. (B) Pneumothorax: Air in the chest cavity. (p. 890)

6. (A) Paradoxical motion: Movement of ribs in a flail segment that is opposite to the direction of movement of the rest of the chest cavity. (p. 890)

Multiple-Choice Review

1. (D) Of the over 150,000 traumatic injury deaths in 2018, over 75% were associated with chest and abdominal trauma. (p. 869)

2. (C) Three consecutive ribs were fractured in at least two places each. This patient has a flail chest. (p. 874)

3. (B) When the patient with a large flail section takes a breath, the EMT may notice that he is exhibiting paradoxical chest wall motion. (p. 875)

4. (B) When a penetrating injury to the heart causes blood to flow into the pericardial sac and to compress the heart, this injury is called cardiac tamponade. (p. 882)

5. (C) Your patient has sustained an open chest wound. A chest cavity that is open to the atmosphere is referred to as a sucking chest wound. (p. 878)

6. (B) The treatment for a patient with an open chest wound includes all of the following except binding the chest tightly. (pp. 878–879)

7. (D) When air becomes trapped in the chest cavity, it can affect the body in all of the following ways except by increasing the ventilatory volume of the chest. (p. 881)

8. (D) The signs of pneumothorax or tension pneumothorax include all of the following except increased depth of respiration. (p. 881)

9. (B) Which of the following is not a sign of traumatic asphyxia? Wide pulse pressure. (p. 882)

10. (C) When you are taping an occlusive dressing in place, tape the dressing in place quickly because this is a life-threatening situation. (p. 878)

11. (B) An open wound to the abdomen that is so large and deep that organs protrude through the opening is called an evisceration. (p. 885)

12. (D) Potential signs of an abdominal injury include all of the described findings except contusions over the upper ribs. (p. 885)

13. (C) Of the injuries listed, which is most likely the reason why his upper body is blue and he is in cardiac arrest? Traumatic asphyxia. (pp. 881–882)

14. (B) How would you consider positioning a patient who has an abdominal injury? Place the patient supine, with legs flexed at the knees, to reduce pain and relax the abdominal muscles. (p. 888)

15. (C) When covering an exposed abdominal organ, the EMT should apply a sterile saline-moistened dressing and then an occlusive dressing. (p. 889)

16. (D) What is her likely condition? *Commotio cordis*. This patient needs CPR and immediate defibrillation. (p. 883)

17. (C) The treatment of an evisceration should never include replacing or touching the exposed organ. (p. 889)

18. (C) Common signs of abdominal injury include all of the listed findings except headache and photophobia. (p. 887)

19. (D) When a small child (typically younger than 8 years old) is compared to an adult the child would have abdominal organs more exposed to injury, a more pliable chest, and less calcified bones. (p. 872)

20. (C) A punctured lung is an open pneumothorax; the flutter valve would help relieve the excessive pressure from the chest. (p. 879)

Pathophysiology: The Path of the Bullet (p. 888)

1. Yes, especially with bullet tumble or secondary bullet fragments taking different paths.

2. Yes, depending on the position of the lungs in the chest. They take up a lot more room on inspiration, and the liver and spleen, which lie posterior to the lowest left and right ribs, might have been missed with the large, inflated lungs. On the other hand, if the lungs were deflated because of exhalation, the liver and spleen would become more prominent targets.

Complete the Following

1. Explain what the following injuries are: (pp. 881–883)
   A. *Commotio cordis*: An uncommon condition when someone gets hit in the center of the chest at the precise moment in the cardiac cycle that interferes with electrical activity, causing them to go into ventricular fibrillation.
   B. Cardiac tamponade: An injury to the heart causes blood to flow into the surrounding pericardial sac and compress the heart. This will lead to cardiac arrest if not treated promptly.
   C. Traumatic asphyxia: An event associated with sudden compression of the chest. The sternum and ribs exert severe pressure on the heart and lungs, forcing blood back into the jugular veins and neck.
   D. Hemothorax: Filling of the chest cavity with blood.
   E. Pneumothorax: Filling of the chest cavity with air.
   F. Aortic injury: Damage to the largest artery usually from blunt trauma to the chest or penetrating injury directly to the artery.

2. List seven signs of a tension pneumothorax: (pp. 883–884)
   A. Respiratory difficulty
   B. Uneven chest wall movement
   C. Reduction or absence of breath sounds on the affected side of the chest
   D. Increasing respiratory difficulty and signs of hypoxia, including cyanosis
   E. Indications of developing shock
   F. Distended neck veins
   G. Tracheal deviation to the uninjured side

3. For each organ below, list the abdominal quadrant, type or organ (solid or hollow), and primary function. (p. 872)
   A. Gallbladder: RUQ, hollow, digestion
   B. Intestine (large and small): all four quadrants, hollow, digestion
   C. Kidneys: RUQ/LUQ/retroperitoneal, solid, blood filtration, excretion
   D. Liver: RUQ, solid, blood filtration
   E. Pancreas: RUQ/LUQ/retroperitoneal, solid, digestion, endocrine functions
   F. Spleen: LUQ, solid, blood filtration
   G. Stomach: LUQ, hollow, digestion
   H. Urinary bladder: RLQ/LLQ, hollow, stores urine
   I. Uterus and ovaries: RLQ/LLQ, solid (nonpregnant), reproduction

Case Study: Assault with an Ice Pick

1. No, the scene is not safe. You really do not know who is in that crowd. Make sure the police have been dispatched and always be aware of what is going on around you.

2. This is a judgment call. Get some help from people you can trust to hold back the crowd and begin assessment with the idea that you might have to leave right away. You can always load and go and then pull over in a location that is safer for you, your partner, and the patient.

3. After scene safety, your top priority is the primary assessment.

4. This is a judgment call, and you may have local protocols or a Medical Director's advice on how to handle this situation, but if there is no obvious trauma to the head or neck and a witness saw the patient go to his knees before collapsing to the ground, it is probably not necessary to take the time to do a spine motion restriction precautions. This patient is critical and needs a surgeon.

5. The injuries could be pneumothorax, tension pneumothorax, cardiac tamponade, hemothorax, or other internal injuries leading to shock and massive internal injuries.

6. The patient is in shock (decompensating), and his blood pressure is low already, just a few minutes after the stabbing.

7. Because the patient's respirations are shallow and increasing, he is decompensating in shock, and he has no lung sounds on one side. He needs more than a nonrebreather mask to assure adequate oxygenation. It is time to start assisting ventilations with the BVM and get to the appropriate hospital.

8. A 45-year-old male stabbed in area of the heart with ice pick. The patient is critical, and we have a 10-minute arrival at your department. The patient is unconscious, tachycardic, and hypotensive, and we are assisting ventilations.

CHAPTER 32: Musculoskeletal Trauma

Match Key Terms

1. (P) Angulated fracture: A fracture in which the broken bone segments are at an angle to each other. (p. 945)

2. (R) Bones: Hard but flexible living structures that provide support for the body and protection to vital organs. (p. 945)

3. (I) Cartilage: Tough tissue that covers the joint ends and bones and helps to form certain body parts, such as the outer ear. (p. 945)

4. (Q) Closed extremity injury: Any injury to an extremity with no associated opening in the skin. (p. 945)

5. (S) Comminuted fracture: A fracture in which the bone is broken in several places. (p. 945)

6. (T) Compartment syndrome: Injury caused when tissues such as blood vessels and nerves are compressed from swelling or because of a tight dressing or cast. (p. 945)

7. (E) Crepitus: A grating sensation or sound that is made when fractured bone ends rub together. (p. 945)

8. (B) Dislocation: The disruption or "coming apart" of a joint. (p. 945)

9. (H) Extremities: The portions of the skeleton that include the clavicles, scapulae, arms, wrists, and hands and the pelvis, thighs, legs, ankles, and feet. (p. 945)

10. (G) Fracture: Any break in a bone. (p. 945)

11. (O) Greenstick fracture: An incomplete fracture from excessive bending force. (p. 945)

12. (L) Joints: Places where bones articulate, or meet. (p. 945)

13. (N) Ligaments: Connective tissues that connect bone to bone. (p. 945)

14. (K) Manual traction: The process of applying tension to straighten and realign a fractured limb before splinting. (p. 945)

15. (A) Muscles: Tissues or fibers that cause movement of body parts and organs. (p. 945)

16. (C) Open extremity injury: An injury in which the skin has been broken or torn through from the inside or from the outside. (p. 945)

17. (M) Sprain: The stretching and tearing of ligaments. (p. 945)

18. (J) Strain: Muscle injury caused by overstretching or overexertion of the muscle. (p. 945)

19. (F) Tendons: Tissues that bind muscles to bones. (p. 945)

20. (D) Traction splint: A splint that applies constant pull along the length of the lower extremity to help stabilize the fractured bone and to reduce muscle spasms in the limb; used primarily on femoral shaft fractures. (p. 945)

Multiple-Choice Review

1. (B) As we age, our bones because deficient in calcium, resulting in bones that are more brittle and easier to break. (p. 894)

2. (C) The strong white fibrous material that covers the bones is called the periosteum. (p. 894)

3. (B) In children, the majority of long bone growth occurs in the growth plate. (p. 899)

4. (D) Musculoskeletal injuries care caused by direct, indirect, and twisting force. (p. 901)

5. (D) Fractures of the pelvis typically cause a 3 pint blood loss over the first 2 hours. (p. 903)

6. (C) The traction splint reduced the death rate post- WWI. (p. 903)

7. (B) Objective or purpose of realignment is to assist in restoring circulation. (p. 908)

8. (C) You are managing a 32-year-old male patient who is suffering from a stretching or tearing of a ligament. This injury is called a sprain. (p. 904)

9. (B) A break in the continuity of the skin of a fractured extremity is considered an open bone or joint injury. (p. 907)

10. (C) Proper splinting of this closed fracture is designed to prevent closed injuries from becoming open ones. (p. 907)

11. (C) The signs and symptoms of a bone or joint injury include all those described except vomiting. (p. 906)

12. (A) The head of the humerus appears to move in front of the shoulder. This is a sign of a possible anterior dislocation. (p. 916)

13. (C) Which procedure is done at least twice whenever a splint is applied/ Assessment for circulation, sensation, and motor function (CSM) distal to the injury. (p. 911)

14. (B) In what order will you take the following steps? 4, 1,2,3 (p. 913)

15. (C) Multiple fractures, especially of the femur, can cause life-threatening external and internal bleeding. (p. 907)

16. (A) Applying cold packs to fractures helps to reduce swelling. (p. 907)

17. (D) Care should include all of the described steps except splinting each injury individually. Splinting individual injuries would delay getting this unstable patient to the hospital. (p. 907)

18. (D) A splint properly applied to a closed bone injury should help prevent all of the described changes to the extremity except proper circulation to the extremity. (p. 907)

19. (D) Fractures can introduce complications, which may include all those described except increased distal sensation. (p. 907)

20. (D) A properly applied splint should do those things described in the question except prevent the need for surgery. Need for surgery depends on the injury. (p. 907)

21. (A) There is a severe deformity of the right extremity about midway between the knee and the ankle, and the extremity distal to this injury lacks sensation. You should align with manual traction before splinting to allow return of circulation. (pp. 908–909)

22. (A) What are the three basic types of splints? Rigid, formable, and traction. (p. 909)

23. (D) Which of the following is not true about rigid splints? It is not true that they are preferred for immobilizing joint injuries in the position found. Formable splints are preferred for immobilizing joint injuries in the position found. (pp. 909–910)

24. (C) Your patient has a serious fracture to which you will be applying a traction splint. The femur is most likely the bone that was fractured. (p. 910, 914)

25. (D) When applying a traction splint, the EMT should first manually stabilize the leg and then apply manual traction distally. (p. 915)

26. (C) To ensure proper stabilization and increase comfort when applying a rigid splint, you should pad the spaces between the body part and the splint. (p. 910)

27. (B) The method of splinting should be dictated by the severity of the patient's condition and the priority decision. (p. 910)

28. (D) You should do all interventions listed except for applying two traction splints before securing the patient on a long spine board. Speed is important in caring for the unstable patient. (p. 910)

29. (D) Hazards of improper splinting may include aggravation of a bone or joint injury, reduced distal circulation, delay in transport of the patient with a life threatening injury. (p. 910)

30. (C) If his lower leg is cyanotic or lacks a pulse when a knee joint injury is assessed, you should realign the knee joint with gentle traction if no resistance is met. (p. 908)

31. (B) Examples of bipolar traction splints include all of the following except the Sager. (p. 914)

32. (B) The amount of traction that the EMT should pull when applying a Sager traction splint is about 10% of the patient's body weight up to 15 pounds (6.8 kg). (p. 915)

33. (B) The indications for a traction splint are a possible midshaft femur fracture with no joint or lower leg injury. (p. 923)

34. (D) The signs and symptoms of a knee injury may include any of the following except discoloration to the thigh. (p. 924)

35. (A) Elderly patients are more susceptible to hip fractures because of brittle bones or bones weakened by disease. (p. 921)

36. (B) Your suspicion of a fractured hip is based on the injured limb appearing shorter than the other extremity. (p. 921)

37. (C) She may have experienced a pelvic fracture. (p. 917)

38. (D) When stabilizing him, you should do all of the following except raising the lower legs. (p. 918)

Complete the Following

1. List eight signs and symptoms of musculoskeletal injury. (p. 906)
- **A.** Pain and tenderness
- **B.** Deformity or angulation
- **C.** Grating, or crepitus
- **D.** Swelling
- **E.** Bruising
- **F.** Exposed bone ends
- **G.** Joints locked into position
- **H.** Nerve and blood vessel compromise

2. List eight signs and symptoms of a hip fracture (p. 921)
- **A.** Pain is localized, although some patients also complain of pain in the knee.
- **B.** Pain or sensitivity to pressure exerted on the lateral prominence of the hip.
- **C.** Surrounding tissues are discolored.
- **D.** Swelling may be evident.
- **E.** The patient is unable to move the limb.
- **F.** Patient complains about being unable to stand.

G. Foot or injured side usually turns outward; however, it may rotate inward (rarely).

H. Injured limb may appear shorter.

3. List the "six Ps" in assessing compromise to an extremity. (pp. 906–907)
- **A.** Pain
- **B.** Pallor
- **C.** Paresthesia
- **D.** Pulses
- **E.** Paralysis
- **F.** Pressure

Label the Diagram (p. 985)

1. Skull
2. Cervical vertebrae
3. Clavicle
4. Sternum
5. Ribs
6. Thoracic vertebrae
7. Lumbar vertebrae
8. Ilium
9. Pubis
10. Tibia
11. Fibula
12. Tarsals
13. Metatarsals
14. Phalanges
15. Maxilla
16. Mandible
17. Scapula
18. Humerus
19. Ulna
20. Radius
21. Sacrum
22. Coccyx
23. Carpals
24. Metacarpals
25. Phalanges
26. Ischium
27. Femur
28. Patella

Pathophysiology: Fracture or No Fracture?

1. Patients who experience long bone fractures often experience shock in addition to the bone injury because the bones are vascular and bleed a significant amount over the first 2 hours. (p. 894)

2. The EMT should splint on suspicion of a fracture rather than confirming an actual fracture because it often takes an X-ray in the emergency department to confirm that the patient has a fracture. Some types of fractures do not have deformity but could be made worse if the patient is allowed to walk or bear his or her weight on them. (p. 902)

3. Swelling is due to the destruction of blood vessels in the periosteum and bone and loss of blood from adjacent damaged blood vessels. (p. 896)

Case Study: Just a Slip on Ice

1. In addition to mental status assessment, the airway, breathing, and circulation are the essential components of the primary assessment.

2. Yes, once you are sure that there is no need for spinal motion restriction precautions and there are no other injuries that need your immediate attention. It is cold, she is shivering, and you need to get her into the warm ambulance to complete further assessment, examination, medical history, and management. Use your best clinical judgment here. This is a good case to discuss with your medical director.

3. A quick head-to-toe trauma examination to make sure it is appropriate to move her.

CHAPTER 32: (continued)

4. You will document that you assessed pulses, motor function, and sensation before and after applying splints for any musculoskeletal injuries.

5. Shock is very likely. She injured two or possibly four bones (radius and ulnar bones in two arms). Because bones will bleed even with an uncomplicated fracture, she could lose a pint or two of blood in the first two hours. Her vital signs are normal but should be, and it would be smart to use your best clinical judgment, considering that she is probably in the compensated stage of shock.

6. Ask about the SAMPLE history, in particular her medical history and medications. For example, she could be taking a blood thinner (because of previous stroke or cardiac problem), which might cause her to bleed excessively internally from the fractures that she has sustained.

7. She may have neurologic deficits left over from the stroke or be on medication that could affect bleeding. This injury could also have resulted from a new stroke.

8. Splinting helps to reduce pain, as does local application of cold to the fractures.

CHAPTER 33: Trauma to the Head, Neck, and Spine

Match Key Terms

Part A

1. (P) Autonomic nervous system: Controls involuntary functions. (p. 994)

2. (K) Central nervous system: The brain and spinal cord. (p. 994)

3. (I) Cerebrospinal fluid (CSF): The fluid that surrounds the brain and spinal cord. (p. 994)

4. (B) Concussion: Mild closed head injury without detectable damage to the brain. Complete recovery usually expected but effects may linger for weeks, months, even years. (p. 994)

5. (J) Contusion: A bruised brain caused when the force of a blow to the head is great enough to rupture blood vessels. (p. 994)

6. (H) Cranium: The bony structure making up the forehead, top, back, and sides of the skull. (p. 994)

7. (N) Orbits: The bony structures around the eye sockets. (p. 994)

8. (A) Peripheral nervous system: All of the body's nerves except for the brain and spinal cord. (p. 994)

9. (E) Spinous process: The bony bump on a vertebra. (p. 994)

10. (L) Temporal bones: The bones that form part of the sides of the skull. (p. 994)

11. (G) Temporomandibular joint (TMJ): The movable joint formed between the mandible and the temporal bones; also called the TMJ. (p. 994)

12. (R) Laceration: In brain injuries, a cut to the brain. (p. 994)

13. (D) Malar: The cheek bone. Also called the zygomatic bone. (p. 994)

14. (Q) Mandible: The lower jaw bone. (p. 994)

15. (F) Vertebrae: The bones of the spinal column (singular vertebra). (p. 994)

16. (M) Nasal bones: The bones that form the upper third, or bridge, of the nose. (p. 994)

17. (C) Nervous system: provides overall control of thought, sensation, and the voluntary and involuntary motor functions of the body. The components of this system are the brain and the spinal cord as well as the nerves that enter and exit the brain and spinal cord and extend to various parts of the body. (p. 994)

18. (O) Neurogenic shock: A state of shock (hypoperfusion) cause by nerve paralysis that sometimes develops from spinal injuries. (p. 994)

Part B

1. (F) Dermatome: An area of the skin that is innervated by a single spinal nerve. (p. 994)

2. (A) Foramen magnum: The opening at the base of the skull through which the spinal cord passes from the brain. (p. 994)

3. (E) Hematoma: In a head injury, a collection of blood within the skull or brain. (p. 994)

4. (D) Herniation: Pushing of a portion of the brain downward towards the foramen magnum as a result of increased intracranial pressure. (p. 994)

5. (B) Intracranial pressure (ICP): Pressure inside the skull. (p. 994)

6. (C) Maxillae: The two fused bones forming the upper jaw. (p. 994)

7. (I) Spinal motion restriction: Limiting the movement of the spine to prevent additional injury. (p. 994)

8. (K) Cheyne-Stokes breathing: A distinct pattern of breathing characterized by quickening and deepening respirations followed by a period of apnea. (p. 994)

9. (G) Pulmonary air embolism: A blockage in the blood circulation of the lung caused by a air bubble. (p. 994)

10. (H) Air embolism: A bubble of air in the bloodstream. (p. 994)

11. (J) Ataxic respirations: A pattern of irregular and unpredictable breathing commonly caused by brain injury. (p. 994)

12. (L) A pattern of rapid and deep breathing caused by injury to the brain. (p. 994)

Multiple-Choice Review

1. (B) The function of the spinal column is to protect the spinal cord. (pp. 951–952)

2. (C) The spine is made up of 33 vertebrae. (p. 951)

3. (C) When a patient has a scalp injury, the EMT should expect profuse bleeding. (p. 953)

4. (C) You notice that he has a bruise behind the ear. This is called Battle sign. (p. 958)

5. (B) Assessment of a patient with blunt head trauma and discoloration of the soft tissues under both eyes. This finding is called raccoon eyes. (p. 958)

6. (A) Her signs and symptoms may include blood or fluid flowing from the ears and/or nose. (p. 958, 959)

©2021 Pearson Education, Inc.
Emergency Care, 14th Ed.

7. (B) Traumatic brain injury may result in altered mental status and unequal pupils. (p. 958)

8. (A) Which of the following is a late sign of traumatic brain injury? A temperature increase (fever). (p 960)

9. (C) Hypoperfusion is generally not a sign of traumatic brain injury, except in infants. (p. 960)

10. (D) Based on the NEXUS study the current spinal assessment used in the field should incorporate determining if the patient is reliable, determining if there are distracting injuries, and close attention to the MOI in younger children. (p. 975)

11. (D) In some EMS systems, she would be taken to a trauma center if her Glasgow Coma Scale (GCS) score was less than 14. (p. 961)

12. (A) You are treating a construction worker who has a 4-foot steel rod penetrating his skull. You should shorten lengthy objects, using any appropriate tools to minimize vibration. (p. 963)

13. (B) The primary concern for emergency care of a facial fracture or jaw injury is the patient's airway. (p. 963)

14. (D) The cervical and lumbar vertebrae are the vertebrae most susceptible to injury because they are not supported by other bony structures. (p. 970)

15. (C) When the spine is excessively pulled, which commonly occurs during a hanging, this is called a distraction injury. (p. 969)

16. (C) In calling for a backup ambulance you should report that both the driver and the passenger may require spinal motion restriction. (p. 971)

17. (C) Which of the following would be least likely to cause a spine injury? A trauma patient who was shot in the abdomen. (p. 971)

18. (D) All of mechanisms described are cervical-spine injuries that can result from a diving accident except lateral bending. (p. 971)

19. (B) It is important to remember that a lack of spinal pain does not rule out the possibility of spinal-cord injury because other distracting painful injuries may mask it. (p. 975)

20. (A) Damage to the nerves that innervate the intercostal muscles will result in abdominal breathing only as the muscles between the ribs no longer are contracting. (p. 973)

21. (B) When a child who was in a car seat needs to be taken to the hospital after a high-speed motor vehicle collision, the best procedure is to use the rapid extrication from car seat procedure. (pp. 987–988)

22. (A) If the patient who was in a serious high-speed collision is up and walking around at the scene, you should still assess for a potential spinal injury. (p. 971)

23. (A) Do not ask the patient to move just to determine if it will cause pain. (p. 972)

24. (A) After performing the primary assessment on a supine spinal cord injured patient, your next step is to apply an appropriately sized rigid cervical collar. (p. 973)

25. (B) If he complains of pain when you attempt to place his head in a neutral inline position you should steady the head in the position found so you do not create further injury to the area. (p. 978)

26. (B) When treating the patient who you suspect has a spine injury, one EMT on your crew should maintain manual spine motion restriction until the patient is secured. (p. 978)

27. (C) Which of the following statements about the rigid cervical collar is false? The collar completely eliminates neck movement. (p. 978)

28. (B) If a stable male patient is found in a sitting position of a car and is complaining about back pain, the EMT should guide and lower the patient to a long spine board. (p. 973)

29. (B) You would use the long spine board in all of the scenarios except when a stable, low-priority patient must be immobilized. (p. 979)

30. (A) When immobilizing a 6-year-old or younger child on a long backboard provide padding beneath the shoulder blades. (p. 987)

31. (B) You should consider keeping the helmet on the patient if it has a snug fit that allows no head movement. (p. 990)

32. (B) Which is the correct order of steps for applying a vest-type extrication device? 3, 1, 2, 4. (p. 981)

33. (D) Before and after spinal motion restriction with a vest-type extrication device the EMT should assess pulses in all extremities, motor function in all extremities, and sensation in all extremities. (p. 980)

34. (A) The time it takes to develop the symptoms from an increased ICP depend on the location of the bleed and the rate of bleeding into the head (pp. 956)

35. (C) The patient went into sudden cardiac arrest. An air embolism is the most likely cause. (p. 965)

Pathophysiology: Dysfunction from Spine Injury (pp. 973–974)

1. This patient may have an injury to the nerve that controls the movement of the diaphragm, the main muscle of breathing. This nerve is called the phrenic nerve. As such he may have respiratory arrest.

2. Loss of smooth muscle control allows the dilation of the blood vessels, especially in the periphery, which causes distal pooling of the blood and ultimately hypotension.

3. Because the messages from the brain to the adrenal gland, which secretes epinephrine to increase the heartbeat, travel through the spinal cord. In this instance, the spinal cord may be damaged or severed so the message to increase the heart rate never makes it to the body.

Complete the Following

1. List 15 signs of a skull fracture or brain injury. (pp. 958–960)

(Any 15 of the following)
- Visible bone fragments and bits of brain tissue
- Altered mental status
- Deep laceration or severe bruise or hematoma to the scalp of forehead
- Depressions or deformity of the skull, large swellings (goose eggs), or anything unusual about the shape of the cranium
- Severe pain at the site of head injury
- Battle sign
- Pupils are unequal or nonreactive to light

CHAPTER 33: (continued)

- Raccoon eyes
- One eye appears to be sunken
- Bleeding exists from the ears and/or nose
- Clear fluid flowing from the ears and/or nose
- Personality changes ranging from irritable to irrational
- Increased BP and decreased pulse rate (Cushing reflex)
- Irregular breathing patterns
- Blurred or multiple-image vision in one or both eyes
- Impaired hearing or ringing in the ears
- Equilibrium problems
- Forceful or projectile vomiting
- Decorticate or decerebrate posturing
- Paralysis or disability on one side of the body
- Seizures may be present
- Temperature increase (late sign due to inflammation, infection, or damage to temperature regulating centers)
- The patient has deteriorating vital signs

2. List five high-risk mechanisms for spinal injury. (p. 971)
   A. Falls from higher than 3 feet (about 1 meter)or down more than five stairs
   B. Axial loading (compression) injuries such as diving injuries
   C. High-speed, motor-vehicle crashes, especially with rollover or ejection
   D. Motorized recreational vehicle (ATV) crashes
   E. Bicycle collisions

3. Glasgow Coma Scale: (p. 962)
   - Eye opening (Items A to D)

     Spontaneous – 4

     To Voice – 3

     To Pain – 2

     None – 1
   - Verbal Response (Items E to H)

     Oriented – 5

     Confused – 4

     Inappropriate words – 3

     Incomprehensive sounds – 2

     None – 1
   - Motor Response (Items K to P)

     Obeys Commands – 6

     Localizes Pain – 5

     Withdraws (pain) – 4

     Flexion (pain) – 3

     Extension (pain) – 2

     None – 1

4. A patient has a significant epidural hematoma after being struck on the side of the head with a baseball. List seven stages in the progression of this patient. (p. 957)
   A. She appears all right at first or may have a brief LOC.
   B. After about 10 minutes, she develops a slightly altered mental status.
   C. The AMS worsens. Soon the patient responds to loud verbal stimulus only by moaning. Her BP begins to increase.
   D. She has a generalized seizure as ICP rises.
   E. Patient is now totally unresponsive to stimuli. Blood pressure continues to rise and the pulse is dropping. Pupils are unequal or nonreactive.
   F. Respirations become slightly irregular. BP continues to increase. Pulse continues to drop.
   G. The patient may begin to develop decorticate posturing, followed by decerebrate posturing. Death follows if the condition is uncorrected by intervention at a trauma center.

Label the Diagram

1. Cervical spine
2. Thoracic spine
3. Lumbar spine
4. Sacral spine (sacrum)
5. Coccygeal spine (coccyx)

Case Study: Deep Dive in a Shallow Pool

1. You would want to know whether the patient struck his head, where he entered the pool, whether there was any loss of consciousness, exactly how he flipped over, and whether at any point he had any movement or sensation in his arms or legs.

2. As long as the patient is floating with assistance and as long as manual in line motion restriction of his head and neck is being maintained, you can float him to the shallow end of the pool, where it will be easier to apply a long backboard.

3. Equipment needed includes a long backboard that floats, a rigid cervical collar, a head immobilizer, some padding, and straps or cravats.

4. Ask the patient whether he remembers what happened, whether he is having trouble breathing, and whether he has feeling or sensation in his arms and legs. You should ask the OPQRST questions about his chief complaint and begin to get the SAMPLE history.

5. Tell the patient that you are going to do everything you can to immobilize his spine properly and get him to the most appropriate hospital as quickly as possible.

6. Your partner should complete the primary assessment; take baseline vital signs; make sure the patient is securely immobilized; and reassess distal circulation, sensation, and motor function. Use your best clinical judgment in managing this patient, as spinal shock may develop over the next hour or so. Not all patients who are injured in a pool need spinal motion restriction, but in this case, the combination of the witness report that the patient jumped headfirst into the shallow area, and the physical findings make the spinal motion restriction imperative.

7. Many spine injury calls go to court, so make sure the prehospital care report (PCR) is very accurate. Be sure to document the actions of the bystander who was in the pool when you arrived and how the injury was reported to have occurred (MOI). Be very specific that the patient stated that he had no sensation or movement in his arms and legs before your arrival and that distal circulation, sensation, and motor function were checked and rechecked before and after spinal motion restriction. This is a good case on which to discuss the specific documentation and management with your Medical Director in training.

CHAPTER 34: Multisystem Trauma

Match Key Terms

1. (C) Multiple trauma: More than one serious injury. (p. 1010)

2. (A) Multisystem trauma: One or more injuries that affect more than one body system. (p. 1010)

3. (B) Trauma score: A numerical rating system for trauma patients to determine severity. (p. 1010)

Multiple-Choice Review

1. (B) She has sustained a fractured right femur and crushed pelvis. She would be considered a multiple-trauma patient. (p. 998)

2. (C) What is the highest priority for this multiple-trauma patient? Managing his airway takes priority over the other options. (p. 998)

3. (A) The patient, described in question 2, would not be considered stable until he has been treated at the emergency department. (p. 998)

4. (A) The three "Ts" are timing, transport, and teamwork. (p. 999)

5. (B) The guidelines for trauma triage and transport released by the CDC take into consideration all of the listed factors except the patient's sex. (p. 1000)

6. (B) When a trauma patient begins to make gurgling sounds while breathing, you should suction the airway. (p. 1003)

7. (D) Sometimes a long backboard can act as a universal splint when the critical patient must be immobilized quickly. (p. 1005)

8. (D) You should not take the time to apply two traction splints, but you should apply tourniquets to both legs if there is severe bleeding and set up an ALS intercept en route to the hospital. (p. 1103–1004)

9. (C) You will most likely perform any or all the listed interventions at the scene except bandaging all of the lacerations. (p. 1004)

10. (C) Even when you are trying to limit on-scene time for a multiple-trauma patient, the one thing that you do not leave out is ensuring scene safety. (p 1006)

11. (B) An example of a patient who requires triage to a higher level of trauma care would be the geriatric patient who fell and is on anticoagulant medications. (p. 1002)

12. (A) The scoring system for trauma patients also helps to allow the trauma centers to evaluate themselves in comparing outcomes of trauma patients with similar trauma scores. (p. 1008)

13. (C) Physiologic criteria according to the CDC Trauma Triage Guidelines include all the answers except two or more proximal long-bone fractures. (p. 1000)

14. (B) According to the CDC Trauma Triage Guidelines, all of the answers are considered MOI criteria except for a crushed, degloved, mangled, or pulseless extremity. (p. 1001)

15. (D) In the context of multiple trauma, when assessing a pediatric patient you will need to consider MOI considerations for spinal motion restriction, additional emotional support, and the keeping family members together if possible. (p. 1007)

16. (C) Pediatric trauma patients may compensate for blood loss more effectively than adults. In this situation there may be a sudden appearance of decompensation. (p. 1007)

Pathophysiology: Internal Injuries

1. You should suspect that the patient has sustained a pneumothorax. (p. 1002)

2. You should suspect that the patient has a cardiac tamponade. (p. 1002)

Complete the Following

1. List eight examples of treatments that would be appropriate on the scene of a critical trauma patient. (p. 1006)
   A. Providing spine motion restriction of the cervical spine during all interventions
   B. Suctioning the airway
   C. Inserting an oral or nasal airway
   D. Sealing a sucking chest wound
   E. Ventilating with a BVM
   F. Administering high-concentration oxygen
   G. Controlling bleeding
   H. Restricting spinal motion

2. The four principles of multisystem trauma management are the following: (pp. 1006–1007)
   A. Scene safety is paramount.
   B. Ensure an open airway.
   C. Perform urgent or emergency moves as necessary.
   D. Adapt to the situation.

3. Fill in the missing information for the Revised Trauma Score chart below: (p. 1009)

Characteristic	Criterion	RTS Points
Glasgow Coma Scale	13–15	4
	9–12 **(A)**	3
	6–8	2
	4–5	1 **(D)**
	3	0
Systolic BP	>89 mmHg	4
	76–89 mmHg **(B)**	3
	50–75 mmHg	2
	1–49 mmHg	1
	0	0
Respiratory Rate	10–29/min	4 **(E)**
	> 29/min **(C)**	3
	6–9/min	2
	1–5/min	1
	0	0
Revised Trauma Score	TOTAL	

CHAPTER 34: (continued)

4. Using the Revised Trauma Score, chart and compile the appropriate score for each of the following patients and decide if they should be transported to the trauma center:
   A. (3+4+3=10) Yes
   B. (3+2+4=9) Yes
   C. (3+3+2=8) Yes

Case Study: A Fastball to The Head

1. Do the primary assessment, which involves general impression, mental status, airway, bleeding, circulation and priority. Treat only the immediate life-threats found in the primary assessment at this point.

2. Apply painful stimuli and see whether he withdraws or exhibits neurologic posturing (decorticate or decerebrate or is totally unresponsive).

3. Yes, since the patient sustained significant injury above the clavicles and may have both head and neck injuries.

4. If you have the patient on a nonrebreather mask, remove it and quickly roll the long backboard to its side, making sure you do not compromise the spine motion restriction. Then clear out the airway, suction quickly, then return to oxygenation and ventilation as needed. Remember that vagal stimulus is the enemy of a child in distress and that retching and stimulating the back of the throat cause vagal stimuli.

5. He was a high priority before and is still a high priority, and now you also have a likely airway compromise. You need to get going and call ahead so that the trauma center will be ready for his arrival.

6. After the call when you are completing the PCR is the best time to calculate the Trauma Score.

CHAPTER 35: Environmental Emergencies

Match Key Terms

Part A

1. (C) Active rewarming: Application of an external heat source to rewarm the body of a hypothermic patient. (pp. 1047–1048)

2. (H) Central rewarming: Application of heat specifically to the lateral chest, neck, armpits, and groin of a hypothermic patient. (pp. 1047–1048)

3. (J) Conduction: The transfer of heat from one material to another through direct contact. (pp. 1047–1048)

4. (D) Convection: Carrying away of heat by currents of air, water, or other gases or liquids. (pp. 1047–1048)

5. (G) Decompression sickness: A condition resulting from nitrogen trapped in the body's tissues, caused by coming up too quickly from a deep, prolonged dive. (pp. 1047–1048)

6. (I) Drowning: The process of experiencing respiratory impairment from submersion or immersion in liquid, which may result in death. (pp. 1047–1048)

7. (A) Evaporation: The change from liquid to gas. When the body perspires or gets wet, evaporation of the perspiration or other liquid into the air has a cooling effect on the body. (pp. 1047–1048)

8. (B) Hyperthermia: An increase in the body temperature above normal, which is a life-threatening condition in its extreme. (pp. 1047–1048)

9. (E) Hypothermia: Generalized cooling that reduces body temperature below normal, which is a life-threatening condition in its extreme. (pp. 1047–1048)

10. (F) Air embolism: Gas bubble in the blood stream. The more accurate term is arterial gas embolism (AGE). (pp. 1047–1048)

Part B

1. (E) Local cooling: Cooling or freezing of particular parts of the body. (pp. 1047–1048)

2. (B) Passive rewarming: Covering a hypothermic patient and taking other steps to prevent further heat loss and help the body rewarm itself. (pp. 1047–1048)

3. (C) Radiation: Sending out energy, such as heat, in waves. (pp. 1047–1048)

4. (D) Respiration: Breathing. Refers to the loss of body heat through breathing. (pp. 1047–1048)

5. (G) Toxins: Substances produced by animals or plants that are poisonous to humans. (pp. 1047–1048)

6. (F) Venom: A toxin (poison) produced by certain animals such as snakes, spiders, and some marine life forms. (pp. 1047–1048)

7. (H) Water chill: Chilling caused by conduction of heat from the body when the body or clothing is wet. (pp. 1047–1048)

8. (A) Wind chill: Chilling caused by convection of heat from the body in the presence of air currents. (pp. 1047–1048)

Multiple-Choice Review

1. (A) Heat will flow from a warmer material to a cooler one. Water conducts heat away from the body 25 times faster than still air. (p. 1015)

2. (C) When there is more wind, there is greater heat loss. (p. 1015)

3. (C) Most radiant heat loss occurs from a person's head and neck. (p. 1016)

4. (D) The factors that could predispose him include all of the following except headache. (p. 1016)

5. (D) Which of the following is not a reason that infants and children are more prone to hypothermia? They have more body fat than adults do. (p. 1017)

6. (B) Besides the fracture, you should consider hypothermia. (p. 1017)

7. (B) You determine that her body temperature is below 90°F. With a core body temperature in this range, she may no longer be shivering. (p. 1019)

8. (A) All of the listed are signs and symptoms of hypothermia except high BP and low pulse. (p. 1019)

9. (B) This procedure involves removing wet clothing and covering the patient. (p. 1019)

10. (C) Her treatment may include all of the listed interventions except rapidly giving the patient plenty of hot liquids. (p. 1020)

11. (A) you are actively rewarming a patient. If your medical director has authorized this treatment, you should apply heat to the chest, neck, armpits, and groin. (p. 1020)

©2021 Pearson Education, Inc.
Emergency Care, 14th Ed.

12. (A) The reason why you should rewarm the body's core first is to prevent blood from collecting in the extremities due to vasodilation. (p. 1020)

13. (B) EMT care of a patient with moist, pale, and normal or cool skin includes all of the listed interventions except fanning the patient so that he or she begins to shiver. (p. 1027)

14. (C) If a patient with moist, pale, and normal or cool skin is responsive but not yet nauseated, you should have the patient drink small sips of water. (p. 1027)

15. (C) You should provide high-concentration oxygen passed through a warm humidifier. (p. 1021)

16. (B) Because patients with extreme hypothermia might not reach biological death for over 30 minutes, the medical philosophy is they are not dead until they are warm and dead. (p. 1022)

17. (A) A cold injury usually occurring to expose areas of the body that is brought above by direct contact with a cold object or exposure to cold air is called an early or superficial local cold injury. (p. 1022)

18. (B) The skin color of a patient with light skin who has a superficial local cold injury will change from white to red. (p. 1022)

19. (C) You should not re-expose the injury to cold. (p. 1023)

20. (C) If the muscles, bones, deep blood vessels, and organ membranes become frozen in the patient exposed to the outside cold elements for a long period of time, this type of injury is referred to as a deep local cold injury. (p. 1023)

21. (B) In frostbite, the affected area first appears white and waxy. (p. 1023)

22. (C) Do not allow a frostbite patient to smoke or drink alcohol because constriction of blood vessels and decreased circulation to the injured tissues may result. (p. 1024)

23. (A) This procedure is seldom recommended in the field. (p. 1024)

24. (D) When assessing an unconscious adult patient who you suspect is in extreme hypothermia, check the carotid pulse for at least 60 seconds. (p. 1022)

25. (C) The environmental condition(s) associated with hyperthermia include heat and high humidity. (p. 1025)

26. (B) The higher the humidity the less your perspiration evaporates. (p. 1025)

27. (D) When the body loses salts through sweating, the patient may have all of the findings except fluid buildup in the lungs. (p. 1026)

28. (B) You suspect that he may have heat exhaustion, which means that he is likely to have moist, pale, and normal or cool skin. (p. 1026)

29. (B) The signs and symptoms of a heat emergency in patients who have hot, dry, or moist skin include seizures. (p. 1028)

30. (C) When responding to a water-related emergency. You should suspect, in addition to a drowning, all of the listed situations except that profuse perspiration is the likely cause. (p. 1030)

31. (D) The signs and symptoms of an air embolism associated with scuba diving include altered mental status, blurred vision, paresthesia in extremities, and seizures or stroke. (p. 1035)

32. (C) During a drowning submersion incident, water that hits the epiglottis causes a reflex spasm of the larynx. (p. 1030)

33. (B) About 10% of drowning submersion victims die from lack of air. (p. 1030)

34. (A) If you are not an experienced swimmer, you should not attempt to go into the water to do a rescue. (p. 1029)

35. (B) if you suspect that this patient has a possible spine injury, you should maintain inline stabilization until a backboard is used for spinal motion restriction. (p. 1033)

36. (C) Two special medical problems that are seen in scuba diving accidents are decompression sickness and arterial gas embolism. (p. 1035)

37. (A) The risk of decompression sickness is increased by air travel within 18 hours of a dive. (p. 1035)

38. (C) A toxin produced by some animals that is harmful to humans is venom. (p. 1041)

39. (D) Sources of injected toxins in USA include spider bites, scorpion stings, snakebites, and insect stings. (pp. 1039–1041)

40. (B) After getting the history and doing an assessment, you believe it is possible that the patient was bitten by a poisonous spider. (pp. 1042–1043)

41. (D) Apparently, a snake has crawled out into the sunshine, and you suspect that the patient has been bitten by that snake. You should do all of the following except capture the snake and bring it alive in the ambulance to the ED. (pp. 1043–1044)

42. (C) The patient got nervous and ascended much too fast. Blurred vision or convulsions are signs and symptoms that would not likely be found in this patient. (p. 1036)

43. (D) If the patient who ascended too rapidly has convulsions and lapses rapidly into unconsciousness leading to respiratory or cardiac arrest, you should suspect that she may have an air embolism. (p. 1035–1036)

44. (D) If you have not been appropriately water rescue trained methods you can use to assist a patient who has fallen into a body of water include reach, throw and tow, and row. (p.1038)

45. (C) A condition that can occur when an inexperienced hiker (over 8,000 feet) experiences a diffuse headache, fatigue, and dehydration is acute mountain sickness. (p. 1039–1040)

46. (D) Common signs and symptoms of high altitude cerebral edema include loss of balance and coordination, seizures, and headache that worsens over time. (p. 1040)

Complete the Following

1. List six signs and symptoms that are likely in a heat emergency patient with moist, pale, normal or cool skin. (p. 1026)
   A. Muscle cramps, usually legs and abdomen
   B. Weakness or exhaustion, and sometimes dizziness or periods of faintness
   C. Rapid, shallow breathing
   D. Weak pulse
   E. Heavy perspiration
   F. Loss of consciousness is possible but is usually brief if it occurs

2. list seven signs and symptoms that are likely in a heat emergency patient with hot and dry or hot and moist skin. (pp. 1027–1028)
   A. Loss of consciousness or AMS
   B. Rapid, shallow breathing.
   C. Full, and rapid pulse.
   D. Generalized weakness.

CHAPTER 35: (continued)

    E. Little to no perspiration.
    F. Dilated pupils.
    G. Potential seizures: no muscle cramps.

3. List 13 signs and symptoms of injected envenomation. (pp. 1042–1043)

    (Any 13 of these)
- AMS
- Noticeable stings or bites on skin
- Puncture marks
- Blotchy (mottled) skin
- Localized pain or itching
- Numbness in a limb or body part
- Burning sensations at the site
- Pain to the rest of the extremity
- Redness
- Swelling or blistering at the site
- Weakness or collapse
- Difficulty breathing and abnormal pulse rate
- Headache and dizziness
- Chills
- Fever
- Nausea and vomiting
- Muscle cramps, chest tightness, joint pain
- Excessive saliva, formation, profuse sweating
- Anaphylaxis

4. List eight signs and/or symptoms of snake bite. (p. 1044)
    A. Noticeable bite on the skin, which may appear as nothing more than a discoloration
    B. Pain and swelling in the area of the bite
    C. Rapid pulse and labored breathing
    D. Progressive general weakness
    E. Vision problems (dim or blurred)
    F. Nausea and vomiting
    G. Seizures
    H. Drowsiness or unconsciousness

5. List ten signs and/or symptoms of hypothermia. (p. 1019)
    A. Shivering in early stages when the core temp is above 90°F (32°C). In severe cases, shivering decreases or is absent.
    B. Numbness, or reduced or lost sense of touch
    C. Stiff or rigid posture in prolonged cases
    D. Drowsiness and/or unwillingness or inability to do even the simplest activities. In prolonged exposures, the patient may become irrational, drift into a stuporous state, or actually remove clothing.
    E. Rapid breathing and rapid pulse in early stages, and slow or absent breathing and pulse in prolonged cases
    F. Loss of motor coordination, such as poor balance, staggering, or inability to hold things
    G. Joint/muscle stiffness, or muscular rigidity
    H. Decreased LOC or unconsciousness. In extreme cases, the patient has a "glassy stare."
    I. Cool abdominal skin temperature
    J. Skin may appear red in early stages. In prolonged cases, skin is pale or cyanotic. In most extreme cases, some body parts are stiff and hard (frozen)

Case Study: Too Cold for Comfort

1. Mental status, A-B-Cs, and ruling out trauma.

2. No. A parent is on the way, but there is no need to wait for the parent's arrival before you talk to the patient and the other children. The more quickly you gather information the better. Waiting before gathering information and formulating a treatment plan is likely to be detrimental to the child.

3. SAMPLE history and OPQRST of the chief complaint, which is altered mental status in this case.

4. Comfortable, lying supine, wrapped in blankets.

5. Using your best judgment and considering that the patient is still shivering and has no relevant medical history, you suspect a mild case of hypothermia. Consider that because she wandered away from the others, there is always the possibility that she also suffered some type of trauma.

6. Yes, oxygen via nonrebreather mask would be helpful.

7. A slightly decreased temperature but not as low at 90°F, which is considered severe hypothermia.

8. Using your best judgment, consider that the patient is a child, is thin and frail with little fat insulation, and has been playing in cold water and the wind all afternoon.

9. Children love to swim and will do so all day long if given the opportunity. Suggest that the parent mandate frequent breaks for the children to warm up out of the water and wind.

CHAPTER 36: Obstetrics and Gynecologic Emergencies

Match Key Terms

Part A

1. (I) Abortion: Spontaneous (miscarriage) or induced termination of pregnancy. (pp. 1098–1099)

2. (R) Abruptio placentae: A condition in which the placenta separates from the uterine wall. (pp. 1098–1099)

3. (D) Afterbirth: The placenta, membranes of the amniotic sac, part of the umbilical cord, and some tissues from the lining of the uterus that are delivered after the birth of the baby. (pp. 1098–1099)

4. (K) Amniotic sac: The "bag of waters" that surrounds the developing fetus. (pp. 1098–1099)

5. (M) Breech presentation: When the baby's buttocks or legs appear first during birth. (pp. 1098–1099)

6. (A) Cephalic presentation: Normal birth presentation, where the baby appears head first. (pp. 1098–1099)

7. (B) Cervix: The lower neck of the uterus at the entrance to the birth canal. (pp. 1098–1099)

8. (O) Crowning: The point during childbirth when part of the baby is visible through the vaginal opening. (pp. 1098–1099)

9. (Q) Eclampsia: A severe complication of pregnancy that produces seizures and which is very dangerous to the infant and mother. (pp. 1098–1099)

10. (C) Ectopic pregnancy: When implantation of the fertilized egg is not in the body of the uterus, occurring instead in the fallopian tube (oviduct), cervix, or abdominopelvic cavity. (pp. 1098–1099)

11. (E) Fetus: The baby from 8 weeks of development to birth. (pp. 1098–1099)

12. (G) Induced abortion: Expulsion of a fetus as a result of deliberate actions taken to terminate the pregnancy. (pp. 1098–1099)

©2021 Pearson Education, Inc.
Emergency Care, 14th Ed.

13. (J) Labor: The three stages of the delivery of a baby, which begin with the contractions of the uterus and end with the expulsion of the placenta. (pp. 1098–1099)

14. (H) Lightening: The sensation of the fetus moving from high in the abdomen to low in the birth canal. (pp. 1098–1099)

15. (N) Limb presentation: When an infant's arm or leg protrudes from the vagina before the appearance of any other body part. (pp. 1098–1099)

16. (L) Meconium staining: Amniotic fluid that is greenish or brownish-yellow rather than clear as a result of fetal defecation; an indication of possible maternal or fetal distress during labor. (pp. 1098–1099)

17. (F) Miscarriage: Spontaneous abortion. (pp. 1098–1099)

18. (P) Multiple birth: When more than one baby is born during a single delivery. (pp. 1098–1099)

19. (S) Braxton-Hicks contractions: Irregular prelabor contractions of the uterus. (pp. 1098–1099)

Part B

1. (J) Ovary: The female reproductive organ that produces ova. (pp. 1098–1099)

2. (F) Ovulation: The phase of the female reproductive cycle in which an egg is released from the ovary. (pp. 1098–1099)

3. (D) Fallopian tube: The narrow tube that connects the ovary to the uterus. Also called the oviduct. (pp. 1098–1099)

4. (N) Perineum: The surface area between the vagina and the anus. (pp. 1098–1099)

5. (O) Placenta: The organ of pregnancy where exchange of oxygen, foods, and wastes occurs between mother and fetus. (pp. 1098–1099)

6. (I) Placenta previa: A condition in which the placenta is formed in an abnormal location (low in the uterus and close to or over the cervical opening). (pp. 1098–1099)

7. (M) Preeclampsia: A complication of pregnancy in which the woman retains large amounts of fluid and has hypertension, and which may progress to eclampsia. (pp. 1098–1099)

8. (C) Premature infant: Any newborn weighing less than 5 ½ pounds or born before the 37th week of pregnancy. (pp. 1098–1099)

9. (A) Prolapsed umbilical cord: When the umbilical cord presents first at the opening of the vaginal canal during birth. (pp. 1098–1099)

10. (L) Spontaneous abortion: When the fetus and placenta deliver before the 20th week of pregnancy; commonly called in miscarriage. (pp. 1098–1099)

11. (E) Stillborn: Born dead. (pp. 1098–1099)

12. (B) Supine hypotensive syndrome: Dizziness and a drop in blood pressure caused when the mother is in a supine position and the weight of the pregnant uterus compresses the inferior vena cava, reducing return of blood to the heart and cardiac output. (pp. 1098–1099)

13. (G) Umbilical cord: The fetal structure that contains the blood vessels that carry blood to and from the placenta. (pp. 1098–1099)

14. (K) Uterus: The muscular abdominal organ where the fetus develops. (pp. 1098–1099)

15. (H) Vagina: The birth canal. (pp. 1098–1099)

16. (R) Labia: Soft tissues that protect the entrance to the vagina. (pp. 1098–1099)

17. (P) Mons pubis: Soft tissue that covers the pubic symphysis; area where hair grown as a woman reaches puberty. (pp. 1098–1099)

18. (Q) Embryo: The baby from fertilization to 8 weeks of development. (pp. 1098–1099)

19. (S) Neonate: A newly born infant or an infant less than 1 month old. (pp. 1098–1099)

Multiple-Choice Review

1. (C) The nine months of pregnancy are divided into three-month trimesters. During the second trimester, the uterus is often seen reaching up to the epigastrium. (p. 1057)

2. (B) The normal birth position is head first and is called a cephalic birth. (p. 1063)

3. (C) The first stage of labor begins with regular contractions of the uterus. (p. 1059)

4. (A) The third stage of labor begins after the birth of the baby. (p. 1059)

5. (B) The process by which the cervix gradually widens is called dilation. (p. 1059)

6. (C) Greenish or brownish-yellow fluid is being expelled from the amniotic sac. This is called meconium staining and could indicate potential fetal distress. (p. 1061)

7. (C) When your patient, who is in labor, suddenly states, "I need to go to the bathroom right now!" this most likely means that the delivery is nearing. (p. 1061)

8. (B) When you are timing the duration of a contraction, time it from the beginning of the contraction to when the uterus relaxes. (p. 1061)

9. (A) The contraction interval, or frequency, is timed from the start of one contraction to the start of the next. (p. 1061)

10. (B) Delivery is said to be imminent when the contractions last 30 seconds and are 2 to 3 minutes apart. (p. 1061)

11. (B) The EMT's primary roles at a normal childbirth scene are to determine whether the delivery will occur at the scene and, if so, to assist the mother as she delivers the infant. (p. 1061)

12. (C) The sterile OB kit does not contain heavy, flat twine to tie the cord. Clamps are provided to clamp the umbilical cord. (p. 1067)

13. (B) When you are evaluating the mother for a possible home delivery, you should check the frequency and duration of contractions. (p. 1061)

14. (A) It is important to ask the patient whether you can examine for crowning if she is having an urge to push during contractions. (p. 1063)

15. (C) What should you do next in the eight month pregnant patient having labor pains every 15 minutes? Ask whether her water broke and prepare for a quiet ride to the hospital. (p. 1062)

16. (A) If you determine that delivery is imminent because of the presence of crowning and other signs, you should contact medical direction if local protocol requires, as you will likely be delivering this baby at home. (p. 1064)

17. (B) When a full-term pregnant woman lying on her back complains of dizziness and you note a drop in her BP, this could be due to a condition called supine hypotensive syndrome. (p. 1059)

18. (B) To counteract the pressure of the uterus on the inferior vena cava, you should transport the patient on her left side. (p. 1059)

19. (C) Which findings which would not be a possible indication for a neonatal resuscitation? The infant's umbilical cord is looped around the neck. This is a common finding and does not necessarily mean that neonatal resuscitation will be required. (p. 1070)

20. (D) During the delivery, you should encourage the mother to breathe deeply through her mouth. (p. 1068)

21. (A) When supporting the baby's head during the delivery, the EMT should do all the steps except pull on the baby's shoulders when they appear. (pp. 1068–1070)

22. (B) If the amniotic sac has not broken by the time the baby's head is delivered, you should use your finger to puncture the membrane. (p. 1070)

23. (C) If you cannot loosen or unwrap the umbilical cord from around the infant's neck you should clamp the cord in two places and cut between the clamps. (p. 1070)

24. (A) Most babies are born face down and then rotate to either side. (p. 1069)

25. (B) When suctioning a newborn compress the bulb syringe before placing it in the baby's mouth. (p. 1070)

26. (B) Once the baby's feet are delivered lay the baby on his or her side with the head slightly lower than the torso. (p. 1070)

27. (D) To assess the newborn, the EMT should do all of the steps except check the response to a sternal rub. (p. 1071)

28. (B) If assessment of the infant's breathing reveals shallow, slow, or absent respirations, the EMT should provide a gentle but vigorous rubbing of the infant's back. (p. 1075)

29. (B) You just delivered a full-term infant who is not breathing and has a heart rate of 58. You should begin chest compressions. (p. 1076)

30. (D) The first umbilical cord clamp should be placed about 10 inches from the baby. (p. 1073)

31. (C) The second umbilical cord clamp should be placed about 7 inches from the baby. (p. 1073)

32. (D) If the placenta does not deliver within 20 minutes of the baby's birth, transport the mother and baby to a medical facility without delay. (p. 1078)

33. (B) During the delivery of a full-term newborn, the mother sustains a tear in her perineum. The EMT should apply a sanitary napkin and gentle pressure. (p. 1080)

34. (D) Which action is appropriate to take for a breech presentation? Initiate rapid transport upon recognition. (p. 1081)

35. (A) During the exam of a woman in labor, you see the umbilical cord presenting first. You should gently push up on the baby's head or buttocks to take pressure off the cord. (p. 1083)

36. (D) When a baby's limb presents first, you should begin rapid transport of the patient immediately. (p. 1081)

37. (B) When you are assisting with the delivery of twins, clamp the cord of the first baby before the second baby is born. (p. 1085)

38. (B) Newly born infants lose heat rapidly. Heat loss not only affects their comfort but also can affect their ability to carry oxygen in their blood. (p. 1072)

39. (D) If after delivery the mother continues to bleed profusely, what should you do besides rapidly transporting? Massage the uterus, encourage the mother to nurse the infant, and place a sanitary napkin and treat for shock. (p. 1079)

40. (B) If you suspect meconium staining when the infant is born, avoid stimulating the infant before suctioning the oropharynx. (p. 1087)

41. (D) A condition in which the placenta is formed low in the uterus and close to the cervical opening, preventing normal delivery of the fetus is called placenta previa. (p. 1088)

42. (D) Which statement is true of seizures in pregnancy? They are usually associated with extreme swelling of the extremities. (p. 1090)

43. (C) The greatest danger associated with blunt trauma to the woman's abdomen and pelvis is massive bleeding and shock. (p. 1092)

44. (A) Which statement is true about the physiology of a pregnant woman? Her heart rate may be interpreted as suggestive of shock when they are actually normal. (p. 1092)

45. (B) Which statement is true of the treatment necessary for this patient? Assume that the woman is pregnant and transport. (p. 1089)

46. (C) You are preparing for a neonatal resuscitation. If breathing is absent or the neonate is gasping, with a heart rate less than 100, you should begin positive pressure ventilations. (p. 1075)

Complete the Following

1. List seven things you should do when evaluating a woman who is in labor and considering a transport decision. (pp. 1062–1063)
   A. Ask what her expected due date is.
   B. Ask if this is her first pregnancy.
   C. Ask her if she has seen a doctor regarding her pregnancy.
   D. Ask her when the labor pain started.
   E. Ask her if her "water" has broken and if she has any bleeding or bloody show.
   F. Ask her if she feels the urge to push or if she feels as though she needs to move her bowels.
   G. Examine the mother for crowning.

2. List seven steps you should take when providing care for a woman who presents with a prolapsed cord. (p. 1083)
   A. Position the mother with her head down and the pelvis raised with a blanket or pillow, using gravity to lessen pressure on the birth canal.
   B. Provide the mother with high-concentration oxygen by way of a nonrebreather mask to increase the concentration carried over to the infant.
   C. Check the cord for pulses, and wrap the exposed cord, using a sterile towel from the OB kit. The cord must be kept warm.
   D. Insert several fingers of your gloved hand into the mother's vagina so you can gently push up on the baby's head or buttocks to keep pressure off the cord.
   E. Keeping mother, child, and EMT as a unit for transport. Be prepared to stay in this position until you reach the hospital.

©2021 Pearson Education, Inc.
Emergency Care, 14th Ed.

F. Provide rapid transport to the hospital. Have your partner obtain vital signs while en route to the hospital if possible.

G. Notify the receiving facility of the limb presentation so they can prepare the necessary obstetrical and neonatal resources.

3. Complete the chart: (p. 1072)
A. Extremities blue, trunk pink.
B. Greater than 100.
C. No reaction.
D. Only slight activity (flexing extremities).
E. Good breathing, strong cry.

Label the Diagrams (p. 1057)

1. Amniotic sac (or amniotic fluid)
2. Umbilical cord.
3. Placenta
4. Uterus.
5. Cervix.
6. Pubic bone.
7. Vagina

Pathophysiology: Physiologic Changes of Pregnancy (pp. 1057–1058)

1. A pregnant woman who has a more pink coloration to her skin has an increased blood volume on the "inside."

2. A pregnant woman who exhibits nausea, vomiting, and heartburn has hormonal changes and a GI tract that has been displaced by the growing uterus on the "inside."

3. A woman in active labor has a contraction on the "inside." She might tell the EMT that she has regular pain with contraction and the urge to push (or defecate) with each strong contraction.

4. If the fetus is not in the head-first position in the birth canal on the "inside," the EMT may observe a limb presentation on the "outside."

Case Study: More Than a Speeding Ticket

1. Gloves, mask, eye shield, and a gown as needed.

2. The key components are bulb syringe, cord clamps, sanitary napkins, sterile scalpel or scissor, a bag for the placenta, and some drapes.

3. In a short time, you need some important history. Ask about prenatal care; any expected complications this time; what the position of the baby is; when the last contraction was; whether the water broke; is there any recent history of drug abuse and, if so, when; and how many prior pregnancies and deliveries she has had.

4. At this point, oxygen is not necessary. Those vital signs are basically normal for a woman who is pregnant.

5. It is probably best to downgrade the response (no need for light and siren) but not cancel at this point.

6. It is useful to know that she has had no prior complications in giving birth. This being her third delivery, it is likely to go faster than the first two.

7. The fact that she has been getting prenatal care is an excellent indicator that it is not a problem pregnancy, and the patient should have a lot of useful information. It will also confirm that you are headed to the correct hospital.

8. This birth was a cephalic birth. If the baby had presented both feet first, that would have been a breech birth.

9. The third stage is the delivery of the placenta. Books usually say not to wait more than 20 minutes for delivery of the placenta. Common sense should prevail here, as the patient is already in your ambulance and the baby has delivered. Just head to the hospital without all the lights and sirens, and if the placenta delivers, then handle it. Be sure to call the hospital and inform them of what has transpired and when you will be arriving.

10. Stillbirth, prolapsed cord, limb presentation, meconium staining, cord looped around the neck, breech with a large head that does not easily deliver, and multiple births, are some potential complications of childbirth.

CHAPTER 37: Emergencies for patients with Special Challenges

Match Key Terms

1. (O) Autism spectrum disorders (ASD): Developmental disorders that affect, among other things, the ability to communicate, self-regulate behaviors, and interact with others (p. 1137)

2. (D) Automatic implanted cardiac defibrillator (AICD): A device implanted under the skin that can detect life-threatening cardiac dysrhythmias and deliver a shock to the heart. (p. 1137)

3. (P) Bariatrics: The branch of medicine that deals with the causes of obesity as well as its prevention and treatment. (p. 1137)

4. (J) Central IV catheter: A surgically inserted for long-term delivery of medications or fluids into the central circulation. (p. 1137)

5. (L) Continuous positive airway pressure (CPAP): A device worn by a patient that blows oxygen or air under constant low pressure through a tube and mask to keep airway passages from collapsing at the end of a breath. (p. 1137)

6. (I) Dialysis: The artificial process of filtering the blood to remove toxic or unwanted wastes and fluids. (p. 1137)

7. (A) Disability: A physical, emotional, behavioral, or cognitive condition that interferes with a person's ability to carry out everyday tasks such as working or caring for oneself. (p. 1137)

8. (E) Feeding tube: A tube used to provide delivery of nutrients to the stomach. (p. 1137)

9. (C) Ventricular assist device: A battery-powered mechanical pump that is implanted in the body to assist a failing heart in pumping blood to the body. (p. 1137)

10. (M) Obesity: A condition of having too much body fat, defined as a body mass index of 30 or greater. (p. 1137)

11. (K) Ostomy bag: An external pouch that collects fecal matter diverted from the colon or ileum through a surgical opening in the abdominal wall. (p. 1137)

12. (N) Pacemaker: A device that is implanted under the skin with wires implanted into the heart to modify the heart rate as needed to maintain an adequate heart rate. (p. 1137)

13. (G) Stoma: A surgically created opening into the body, as with a tracheostomy, colostomy, or ileostomy. (p. 1137)

CHAPTER 37: (continued)

14. (F) Tracheostomy: A surgical opening in the neck into the trachea. (p. 1137)

15. (H) Urinary catheter: A tube inserted into the bladder through the urethra to drain urine from the bladder. (p. 1137)

16. (B) Ventilator: A device that breathes for a patient. (p. 1137)

17. (Q) Wearable cardioverter defibrillator (WCD): An external vest worn by a patient to detect any life-threatening dysrhythmia and deliver a shock to the heart. (p. 1137)

Multiple-Choice Review

1. (D) To ensure proper care for the patient with special needs, the EMT must be able to recognize, understand, and evaluate the patient's specific health care needs in addition to the chief complaint. (p. 1111)

2. (A) The EMT may find patients with special care needs when responding to calls in any of these locations except the ED. (p. 1112)

3. (C) One of the best resources to help you when you have a special needs patient who is on a specific device would be the family member who is with the patient. (p. 1113)

4. (C) A condition that is present at the birth of the patient is considered congenital. (p. 1116)

5. (B) A device that is used to help them sleep and by EMS providers in certain medical emergencies to keep the air passages from collapsing at the end of a breath and is called a CPAP. (p. 1116)

6. (D) His wife tells you that suctioning is commonly required during times of distress, within a few weeks of tracheostomy tube insertion, and when the patient has an infection. (p. 1118)

7. (C) This device is called a ventilator. (p. 1119)

8. (C) A patient who is attached to an artificial ventilator at home is experiencing an electrical or battery failure, so you need to begin bag-valve-mask ventilation. (p. 1119)

9. (D) This device is most likely an AICD. (p. 1120)

10. (C) A family member tells you that he has a cardiac chamber that pumps blood through the aorta to the body. This is a ventricular assist device. (p. 1121)

11. (B) The tube that is inserted into a patient who has lost the ability to regulate his or her urine is a urinary catheter. (p. 1124)

12. (A) This procedure is done to filter her blood to remove toxic wastes. (p. 1125)

13. (C) Devices that are commercially available under the brand names Groshong®, Hickman®, and Broviac® are central venous lines. (p. 1126)

14. (A) A Huber is a special type of needle that is required to access a device implanted under the patient's skin. (p. 1126)

15. (C) A major health risk that is on the rise in the United States is obesity which will ultimately increase the occurrence of type 2 diabetes. (p. 1106)

16. (A) One of the easiest ways to communicate with a patient who has hearing loss is to write questions on a pad of paper. (p. 1127)

17. (D) A cardiac patient who has an AICD and is suddenly shocked by the device is usually instructed to call EMS for all these reasons except if this was the second shock in a 24-hour period. A third shock in a 24-hour period would warrant a call or visit to the emergency department. (p. 1121)

18. (D) In dealing with a patient who has a history of autism and who is having a meltdown, the best advice for the EMT is to remember that calm creates calm. (p. 1109)

19. (C) This includes all of the actions except providing all treatments as quickly as possible. (p. 1109)

20. (D) Example include all the listed conditions except strokes and TIAs. (p. 1107)

21. (A) Parkinson's disease is not considered a developmental disability. (p. 1104)

22. (B) Appropriate questions to ask a caregiver would not include why did you wait so long to call 911? (p. 1113)

23. (B) Your patient need an AICD installed but is waiting for insurance to authorize the surgery. He is wearing a wearable cardioverter defibrillator designed to detect and shock a life-threatening dysrhythmia. (p. 1121)

24. (A) You note the patient is unresponsive and the wearable cardioverter defibrillator (WCD) alarm says do not touch the patient. What should you do next? Prepare for CPR but wait to see if the WCD shocks the patient. (p. 1121)

25. (D) Evidence of child abuse can include all listed findings except a parent who seems concerned about the child's injuries. (pp. 1130–1131)

26. (C) When you respond to the home of a person who you think may be a child abuser, look for all of the following except torn clothing on the child. (p. 1131)

27. (D) Other signs of intimate partner violence may include delays in seeking treatment, history that does not match injuries or injury patterns, and fear of the victim of talking to EMS. (p. 1134)

28. (B) You might suspect human trafficking due to no identification and an older person taking control and not allowing the patient to speak. (p. 1136)

Complete the Following

1. List four ways in which the concept of "basic" applies to the management of a patient with autism. (pp. 1108–1109)
   A. Keep your instructions basic.
   B. Ask basic questions.
   C. Basic means less stuff.
   D. Keep your treatment basic.

2. List ten medical conditions in which obesity increases the risk for patients. (p. 1106)
   A. Some cancers
   B. Type 2 diabetes
   C. Hypertension
   D. Heart attack
   E. Stroke
   F. Liver disease
   G. Gallbladder disease
   H. Arthritis
   I. Sleep apnea
   J. Respiratory problems

3. List four groups of children with special challenges. (p. 1110)
   A. Premature infants with lung disease
   B. Infants and children with heart disease
   C. Infants and children with neurologic disease
   D. Children with chronic disease or altered function from birth

©2021 Pearson Education, Inc.
Emergency Care, 14th Ed.

4. To address an emergency involving a home ventilator what does the memory aid DOPE stand for? (p. 1119)
   A. D – displacement of the tube?
   B. O – obstruction of the tube?
   C. P – pneumothorax or pneumonia?
   D. E – equipment mechanical failure?

CHAPTER 38: EMS Operations

Match Key Terms

1. (B) Due regard: A legal term that appears in most states' driving laws and refers to the responsibility of the emergency vehicle operator to drive safely and keep the safety of all others in mind at all times. (pp. 1153–1154, 1156)

2. (A) EMD: Emergency Medical Dispatcher. (p. 1151)

3. (D) Landing zone (LZ): A large, flat area without aerial obstruction in which a helicopter can land to pick up a patient. (p. 1172)

4. (C) A call in which the driver of the emergency vehicle is excused from obeying certain traffic laws such as speed limits and stop signs because loss of life or limb is possible. (p. 1156)

Multiple-Choice Review

1. (C) The federal agency that develops specifications for ambulance vehicle designs is the U.S. Department of Transportation. (p. 1144)

2. (A) The purpose for carrying an EPA-registered disinfectant solution on the ambulance is to clean up equipment after calls. (p. 1146)

3. (B) Each of the following are checked with the engine off on the ambulance except dash-mounted gauges. (p. 1150)

4. (B) When inspecting the ambulance, which is checked with the engine running? The brake pedal. (p. 1150)

5. (A) All of the listed are pieces of equipment used for airway and ventilation care except sphygmomanometer. (p. 1145)

6. (B) Of the listed BLS medications, oxygen is not optional to carry on the ambulance, it must be carried on all ambulances. (p. 1147)

7. (B) According to Federal specifications an ambulance that is a "van type" is called a Type II. (p. 1144)

8. (D) If you carry a toy on your ambulance, such as a teddy bear, to calm a frightened child, it should be sanitized, soft or padded, and brightly colored. (p. 1163)

9. (C) Activities while at the hospital after delivering the patient include each of the following except fill the vehicle with fuel. (pp. 1166–1067)

10. (B) Which of the following pieces of equipment carried on an ambulance or EMS vehicle for defibrillation or assisting with cardiopulmonary resuscitation is optional? Mechanical CPR compressor. (p. 1147)

11. (D) Equipment that is carried on an ambulance or EMS vehicle for immobilization includes all those listed except a burn sheet. (p. 1145)

12. (D) Supplies used for wound care should include all of the listed except a Hare® or Sager® traction device. (p. 1146)

13. (D) What is the purpose of carrying sterilized occlusive dressing on the ambulance or EMS vehicle? To seal a hole in the chest or abdomen. (p. 1146)

14. (C) The supplies for childbirth include all of the listed except large safety pins. (p. 1146)

15. (A) Of the following items checked on the ambulance or EMS vehicle, which is checked with the engine on? The side to side motion of the steering wheel. (p. 1150)

16. (D) The responsibilities of the EMD include all of the listed except advising the caller that an ambulance is not needed. (pp. 1151–1152)

17. (C) When an EMD questions a patient or caller, which of the following is not routinely asked? Has the patient been in the hospital recently? (p. 1152)

18. (D) Activities to terminate the call when back at quarters include sanitize your hands, clean and sanitize respiratory equipment as required, and remove and clean patient-care equipment as required. (p. 1169)

19. (D) To be a safe ambulance operator, the EMT should be tolerant of other drivers, always wear glasses or contact lenses if required, and have a positive attitude about his or her ability as a driver. (p. 1153)

20. (D) Under certain circumstances, vehicle operators can do all of the listed except pass a school bus that has its red lights blinking. (p. 1154)

21. (A) Once at the scene, you find just one patient, a 24-year-old female, and determine that she is stable. This situation is no longer a true emergency. (p. 1154)

22. (D) Which guideline for the use of the ambulance siren is inappropriate? Keep the siren on until the call is completed. (p. 1155)

23. (B) Which of the following is true about the use of lights and sirens? The decision about the use of lights and sirens should be based on the patient's medical condition. (p. 1155)

24. (B) Use of escorts or multivehicle responses is a very dangerous means of response. (p. 1156)

25. (D) Factors that can affect ambulance responses include all of the listed except the type of emergency. (p. 1156)

26. (B) You should park your vehicle in front (upstream) of the wreckage until the fire apparatus arrives. (p. 1158)

27. (B) The sequence of operations to ready a patient for transfer is called packaging. (p. 1160)

28. (B) Which of the following is an action that you would not perform en route to the hospital? Forming a general impression of the patient is one of the first actions of the EMT when arriving at the scene. (pp. 1163–1164)

29. (D) When describing the landing zone to the air rescue service tell them: the terrain, major landmarks, and estimated distance to nearest town. (p. 1172)

30. (B) When delivering a patient to the hospital, the EMT should never move a patient onto the hospital stretcher and just leave. (p. 1165)

31. (C) When approaching a helicopter, first wait for the pilot crew personnel to wave you in. Then approach from the front or side of the craft. (p. 1173)

32. (C) Which of the following patients is least likely to be transported in a helicopter? A cardiac arrest patient is the least likely patient to be transported in a helicopter. (p. 1172)

33. (A) The EMT should remember that the benefits of GPS is all of the listed except an excellent substitute for knowledge of the response area. (pp. 1157–1158)

CHAPTER 38: (continued)

Complete the Following

1. List the seven questions an EMD should ask a caller who is reporting a medical emergency. (p. 1152)
   - **A.** What is the exact location of the patient?
   - **B.** What is your call-back number?
   - **C.** What is the problem?
   - **D.** How old is the patient?
   - **E.** What's the patient's sex?
   - **F.** Is the patient conscious?
   - **G.** Is the patient breathing?

2. List seven factors that can affect an ambulance response. (pp. 1156–1157)
   - **A.** Day of the week
   - **B.** Time of day
   - **C.** Weather
   - **D.** Road maintenance and construction
   - **E.** Railroad crossings
   - **F.** Bridges and tunnels
   - **G.** Schools and school buses

3. List the four major ways in which the EMT on the scene of a collision should describe the landing zone (LZ) to the air rescue service. (p. 1172)
   - **A.** Terrain
   - **B.** Major landmarks
   - **C.** Estimated distance to nearest town
   - **D.** Other pertinent information (such as electric wires, fences, etc).

4. List five steps in terminating a call (pp. 1166–1167)
   - **A.** Quickly clean the patient compartment while taking appropriate Standard Precautions.
   - **B.** Prepare respiratory equipment for service.
   - **C.** Replace expendable items.
   - **D.** Exchange equipment according to your local policy.
   - **E.** Make up the ambulance cot.

Case Study: The Ambulance Collision

1. Yes, the ambulance driver should have stopped before proceeding through the intersection.
2. Yes, by wearing a shoulder harness.
3. It would be necessary to assign another ambulance to handle that call.
4. Do no harm.
5. The service may lose business. The EMS personnel may be ridiculed, and some patients may actually be afraid to get into your ambulance.
6. Because he or she is allowed to look into incidents of this nature with close scrutiny. This is especially true in the public sector when injury has occurred through fault of the public servant.
7. Absolutely. Civilian motorists are not required to drive with "due regard for the safety of all others."
8. She does, unless her service is willing to assist her or unless she has some insurance or legal aid.
9. Yes, she could.
10. Proper driver screening and qualification, driver training, driving SOPs (which include always wearing a shoulder harness in the front of the vehicle, how to negotiate an intersection, and proper use of emergency lights and siren), ongoing retraining, keeping the emergency vehicles in good shape, and a good quality improvement program.

CHAPTER 39: Hazardous Materials, Multiple-Casualty Incidents, and Incident Management

Match Key Terms

1. (O) Cold zone: Area where the Incident Command post and support functions are located. (p. 1211)
2. (L) Command: The first on the scene to establish order and initiate the Incident Command System. (p. 1211)
3. (V) Decontamination: A chemical and/or physical process that removes contamination from people or equipment; the removal of hazardous substances from employees and their equipment to the extent necessary to preclude foreseeable health effects. (p. 1211)
4. (U) Disaster plan: A predefined set of instructions for a community's emergency responders. (p. 1211)
5. (M) Hazardous material (HAZMAT): Any substance or material in a form that poses an unreasonable risk to health, safety, and property when transported in commerce or kept in storage. (p. 1211)
6. (N) Hot zone: Area immediately surrounding a HAZMAT incident; extends far enough to prevent adverse effects outside the zone. (p. 1211)
7. (Q) Incident Command: The person or persons who assumes overall direction of a large-scale incident. (p. 1211)
8. (R) Incident Command System (ICS): A subset of the National Incident Management System designed specifically for management of multiple-casualty incidents. (p. 1211)
9. (J) Multiple-casualty incident (MCI): Any medical or trauma incident involving multiple patients. (p. 1211)
10. (K) National Incident Management System (NIMS): The management system used by federal, state, and local governments to manage emergencies in the United States in a consistent manner. (p. 1211)
11. (P) Single incident command: A command organization in which a single agency controls all resources and operations. (p. 1211)
12. (H) Staging area: The area where ambulances are parked and other resources are held until needed. (p. 1211)
13. (I) Staging supervisor: The person who is responsible for overseeing ambulances and ambulance personnel at a multiple-casualty incident. (p. 1211)
14. (G) Transportation supervisor: The person who is responsible for communicating with sector officers and hospitals to manage transportation of patients to hospitals from a multiple-casualty incident. (p. 1211)
15. (E) Treatment area: The area in which patients are treated at a multiple-casualty incident. (p. 1211)
16. (F) Treatment supervisor: The person who is responsible for overseeing treatment of patients who have been triaged at a multiple-casualty incident. (p. 1211)
17. (C) Triage: The process of quickly assessing patients at a multiple-casualty incident and assigning each a priority for receiving treatment. (p. 1211)
18. (B) Triage area: The area in which secondary triage takes place at a multiple-casualty incident. (p. 1211)

©2021 Pearson Education, Inc.
Emergency Care, 14th Ed.

19. (D) Triage supervisor: The person who is responsible for overseeing triage at a multiple-casualty incident. (p. 12110)

20. (A) Triage tag: A colored-coded tag indicating the priority group to which a patient has been assigned. (p. 1211)

21. (T) Unified command: A command organization in which several agencies work independently but cooperatively. (p. 1211)

22. (S) Warm zone: The area where personnel and equipment decontamination and hot zone support take place. (p. 1211)

23. (W) Surge capacity: A measurable representation of ability of a medical facility to manage a sudden influx of patients. (p. 1211)

Multiple-Choice Review

1. (B) Using the Emergency Response Guidebook, you would find that benzene (benzol) is a chemical that has toxic vapors that can be absorbed through the skin. (p. 1179)

2. (D) The regulations that are meant to enhance the knowledge, skills, and safety of emergency response personnel, as well as bring about a more effective response to HAZMAT emergencies, are found in OSHA 29 CFR 1910.120. (p. 1179)

3. (B) What level of training does this statement describe? First Responder Operations. (p. 1180)

4. (A) What level of training does this describe? First Responder Awareness. (p. 1180)

5. (C) The standard that deals with competencies for EMS personnel at a hazardous materials incident is NFPA #473. (p. 1180)

6. (D) Which is least likely to be a potential hazardous material location? A pet store. (p. 1180)

7. (C) Unless EMS personnel are trained to the level of Hazardous Materials Technician, they must remain in the cold zone. (pp. 1180–1181)

8. (C) All victims leaving the hot zone should be considered contaminated until proven otherwise. (p. 1181)

9. (A) The primary concern at the scene of a hazardous materials incident is the safety of the EMT and crew, patients, and the public. (p. 1181)

10. (B) The safe zone of a hazardous materials incident should be established in an upwind/same level location. (p. 1181)

11. (C) The role of Command at a hazardous materials incident is to delegate responsibility for all the listed except for immediately initiating rescue attempts. (p. 1181)

12. (A) When a contaminated victim of a HAZMAT incident comes into contact with people who are not contaminated, this is referred to as secondary contamination. (p. 1182)

13. (C) The designations on the sides of tanker trucks are called hazardous material placards. (p. 1182)

14. (B) The commonly used placard system for fixed facilities is called the NFPA 704 system. (p. 1182)

15. (B) All employers are required to post, in an obvious spot, the information about all the chemicals in the workplace on a form called a safety data sheet (SDS). (p. 1185)

16. (A) Resources that the EMT should use at a hazardous materials incident include all of the described except copies of NFPA rules. (pp. 1185–1186)

17. (A) What is CHEMTREC? A twenty-four-hour service for identifying hazardous materials. (p. 1186)

18. (B) You have been dispatched to an incident involving hazardous chemicals. EMS personnel at the scene of a hazardous materials incident are responsible for taking care of the injured and monitoring and rehabilitating HAZMAT team members. (p. 1186)

19. (A) Which of the following is not a characteristic of the rehabilitation operations at a hazardous materials incident? They are located in the warm zone, rather, they should be located in the cold zone. (p. 1187)

20. (D) As soon as possible after a HAZMAT team member exits the hot zone, the EMT in the rehab operations should reassess the team member's vital signs. (p. 1187)

21. (C) Which of the following actions is not recommended? Flush runoff water down the nearest drain. (p. 1188)

22. (D) Which of the following is not a feature of a good local disaster plan? The plan should be generic and meet national standards. (p. 1192)

23. (D) On arrival of the first EMS unit at the scene of an MCI, the crew leader should do all of the following except begin patient treatment. (p. 1196)

24. (C) Which of the following is not a principle of good communication at an MCI? The majority of communications should be done via radio transmission. (p. 1197)

25. (D) Some services administer oral fluids in their rehab sectors. What fluid would be appropriate to offer the team members? Watered-down sports drink. (p. 1187)

26. (A) You are quickly reviewing the roles of the management personnel at a major incident while en route. The individual at an MCI who is responsible for sorting and prioritizing patients is the triage supervisor. (p. 1201)

27. (A) If any children at an MCI incident are assessed as having decreased mental status, they should be considered Priority 1. (p. 1202)

28. (A) If any children at an MCI incident are assessed as having signs of shock, they will be considered Priority 1. (p. 1202)

29. (B) If any children at an MCI incident are assessed as having multiple-bone or joint injuries but no airway problems, they will be considered Priority 2. (p. 1202)

30. (D) The driver of a vehicle involved in an MCI event was assessed as having died at the MCI scene. The driver should be considered a Priority 4. (p. 1202)

31. (C) The individual at an MCI incident who is responsible for maintaining a supply of vehicles and personnel at a location away from the incident site is the staging supervisor. (p. 1201)

32. (C) The individual at an MCI incident who is responsible for determining patient destinations and notifying the hospitals of the incoming patients is the transportation supervisor. (p. 1209)

33. (D) Patient transport decisions at the MCI described in question 26 will be based on all of the listed parameters except patient's family preferences. (p. 1209)

34. (A) The characteristics of the rehabilitation area must include all of the listed except being located in the warm zone. (p. 1187)

35. (C) What should you do next with this team member? Have the team member sit for 15 minutes and reevaluate. (p. 1187)

CHAPTER 39: (continued)

36. (B) Aside from confirming the incident and calling for additional help what is one of the first steps in beginning triage using the START System? Use the PA system to instruct those who can walk to go to a specific location. (p. 1204)

37. (D) You will be using the START system during an MCI event. This system uses all of the listed parameters except the number of broken bones each patient has. (p. 1204)

38. (B) In the START system, the amount of treatment provided before tagging the patients is limited to opening an airway, applying pressure on a bleeding wound, or elevating an extremity. (p. 1204)

39. (C) In the SALT system, patients who have a survivable severe injury get an Immediate or red tag and should answer "yes" to these questions: Does the patient have a peripheral pulse?, Is the patient not in respiratory distress?, Is hemorrhage controlled?, and Does the patient follow commands or make purposeful movements? (p. 1208)

Complete the Following

1. List eleven pieces of information that you should be prepared to give when you call for assistance from CHEMTREC. (p. 1186)
   A. Give your name, agency, and callback number.
   B. Explain the nature and location of the problem.
   C. Report the identification number(s) of the material(s) involved, if there is a safe way for you to obtain this information.
   D. Give the name of the carrier, shipper, manufacturer, consignee, and point of origin.
   E. Describe the container type and size.
   F. Report if the container is on a rail car, on a truck, in open storage, or in housed storage.
   G. Estimate the quantity of material transported and released.
   H. Report local conditions.
   I. Report injuries and exposures.
   J. Report local emergency services that have been notified.
   K. Keep lines of communication open at all times.

2. List six characteristics of the rehabilitation area at a hazardous materials incident. (p. 1187)
   A. Located in the cold zone
   B. Protected from weather extremes
   C. Large enough to accommodate multiple rescue crews
   D. Easily accessible to EMS units
   E. Free from exhaust fumes
   F. Allows for rapid reentry into the emergency operation

3. List seven common mechanisms for performing decontamination. (p. 1190)
   A. Emulsification
   B. Chemical reaction
   C. Disinfection
   D. Dilution
   E. Absorption and adsorption
   F. Removal
   G. Disposal

Complete the Chart (p. 1201)

1. Staging Officer.
2. Safety Officer.
3. Transportation Officer.
4. Triage Supervisor.
5. Rehab Supervisor.
6. P-2 Tx Leader.

Case Study: School Bus MCI

1. Size up the situation, establish command, make contact with the fire and police command officers.
2. You should don the Command vest.
3. Your responsibilities are the overall management of the medical aspects of the incident; working directly with the chief officers of the police and fire departments; ensuring the safety of all your personnel; and designating triage, treatment, transport, and staging area supervisors.
4. Triage supervisor.
5. Set up the triage area and begin tagging patients and classifying them into priority for removal from the scene to the treatment area.
6. Use your best clinical judgment. Every situation is different, but here is one workable recommendation: Have three ambulances respond to the scene and seven to a staging area about a mile away with easy access to the scene. The ambulances responding to the scene help to fill out the complement of command officers and provide personnel to triage patients.
7. The first crew leader at the staging area should be designated as the staging officer, or supervisor and should be responsible for release of ambulances and personnel to the scene as directed by Command.
8. Yes, but only on direction of Command and/or the staging supervisor.
9. Transportation and treatment area supervisors would be helpful in managing the flow of patients.
10. On long backboards with rigid extrication collars applied.
11. The patients should be taken to the respective section of the treatment area depending on their triage tag priority.
12. Priority 2.
13. Priority 1.
14. Priority 4 (or zero).
15. Priority 1.
16. Allow one parent per child to assist and stay with the child in the treatment area if space permits.
17. Transportation area supervisor.
18. Rapidly contact the hospitals for bed availability and the number of patients of each priority they can handle.
19. Consider the use of a helicopter for priority 1 patients.
20. Priority 3 patients with minor injuries who are medically cleared can ride the bus. Medical personnel are still needed on the bus in case a patient's status changes.
21. Appoint a public information officer, plan for rehabilitation operations and a light meal after the incident, and consider setting up plans for critical incident stress management (CISM) for all personnel who were at the scene and who are interested in talking about what they saw and did.

©2021 Pearson Education, Inc.
Emergency Care, 14th Ed.

CHAPTER 40: Highway Safety and Vehicle Extrication

Multiple-Choice Review

1. (B) One of the greatest hazards that emergency responders face on a daily basis is oncoming traffic at highway incidents. (p. 1214)

2. (B) The phases of extrication include all of the listed except defining patient care. (p. 1219)

3. (A) An important part of a rescue scene size-up is determining the extent of entrapment. (p. 1220)

4. (C) During size-up of a collision, you must be able to "read" a collision and develop an action plan based on your knowledge of rescue operations and your estimate of the patient's condition and priority. (pp. 1219–1220)

5. (B) When developing an action plan for patient extrication, always keep in mind that time is very critical to some patients' trauma management. (p. 1220)

6. (C) If a vehicle has an airbag that deployed, the manufacturer recommends lifting the bag and examining the steering wheel and dash for bodily impact damage. (p. 1225)

7. (A) The unsafe act that contributes most to injuries at collision scenes is crossing over lanes of still flowing traffic on foot. (p. 1220)

8. (D) Factors that may contribute to injuries of rescuers at a collision include all of the listed except limiting the inner circle to rescuers who are in protective gear. (p. 1220)

9. (D) Good protective gear at the scene of a collision includes all of the following except plastic "bump caps." Headgear that offers adequate protection is a rescue helmet that meets NFPA 1951 Standards for USAR PPE. (p. 1220, 1223)

10. (A) To ensure adequate eye protection at the collision scene, the EMT should wear safety goggles with a soft vinyl frame. (p. 1223)

11. (C) During extrication, an aluminized rescue blanket may be used to protect the patient from poor weather. (p. 1223)

12. (A) When using flares, the EMT should watch for spilled fuel or other combustibles before igniting. (p. 1224)

13. (C) When there is an electrical hazard, the safe zone should be far enough away to ensure that an arcing wire does not cause injury. (p. 1226)

14. (C) As of 2009, federal highway standards have required that all emergency responders wear ANSI safety vests when working highway operations. (p. 1222)

15. (C) If a vehicle has been involved in a front-end collision and you notice that the airbag did not deploy, for safety of the crew working around the airbag, you should consider disconnecting the battery and wait 2 – 3 minutes to carefully work near the bag. (p. 1225)

16. (B) In wet weather, a phenomenon known as ground gradient may provide your first clue that a wire is down. (p. 1226)

17. (A) Which action should you take? Turn 180 degrees and shuffle with both feet together to safety. (p. 1226)

18. (D) If there is a fire in the car's engine compartment and people are trapped in the vehicle, you should do all of the listed steps except applying a short spine board to the driver right away. (p. 1229)

19. (C) When a vehicle's hood is closed and there is an engine fire, you should do all of the listed steps except fully opening the hood to extinguish the fire. (p. 1229)

20. (A) When a vehicle rolls off the roadway into a field of dried grass, a fire may be caused by the catalytic converter. (p. 1229)

21. (C) "Try before you pry" is the foundation for the simple access procedure. (p. 1236)

22. (D) Once the vehicle to which you were assigned is stabilized and an entry point has been gained, you should immediately complete the described steps except pulling the patient out of the access hole. (p. 1236)

23. (A) Which is the best approach to disentanglement of this patient? Displace the doors, cut the roof, and then displace the dash. (p. 1237)

24. (D) Which of the following is not a reason for removing the roof to access a patient? It helps to stabilize the vehicle quickly. (p. 1237)

Complete the Following

1. List the ten phases of the extrication or rescue process. (p. 1219)
   A. Preparing for rescue
   B. Sizing up the situation
   C. Recognizing and managing hazards
   D. Stabilizing the vehicle prior to entering
   E. Gaining access to the patient
   F. Providing primary patient assessment and a rapid trauma assessment
   G. Disentangling the patient
   H. Immobilizing and extricating the patient from the vehicle
   I. Providing assessment, care, and transport to the most appropriate hospital
   J. Terminating the rescue

2. List six items that can be used to protect a patient from heat, cold, flying particles, and other hazards. (pp. 1223–1224)
   A. An aluminized rescue blanket
   B. A lightweight, vinyl-coated paper tarpaulin
   C. A wool blanket
   D. Short and long spine boards
   E. Hard hats, safety goggles, industrial hearing protectors, disposable dust masts, and thermal masks
   F. Emotional support for the patient

3. List the PPE that you should wear at a collision site where you will be providing patient care within the inner circle on a patient who is entrapped. (pp. 1222–1223)
   A. Helmet
   B. Eye protection
   C. Body protection
   D. Hand protection

4. List eight examples of alternative fuels in vehicles on the road today. (p. 1230)
   A. Biodiesel
   B. Flex fuel
   C. Natural gas
   D. Propane

CHAPTER 40: (continued)

    E. Hydrogen
    F. Solar
    G. Battery
    H. Hybrid

Case Study: Bad Wreck: Patient Pinned Under the Dash

1. As close to the damaged vehicle as safely possible so that they can have access to their tools for the extrication.

2. Heavy protective turnout style coat with reflective striping or ANSI vest and a helmet, eye protection, gloves, high top steel toe shoes/boots, heavy protective pants.

3. In terms of assessment, your next steps should include completing the primary assessment (general impression, mental status, A-B-Cs, priority), then a rapid trauma examination for a trauma patient with significant MOI.

4. Considering your training and clinical judgment, you should take the information from your primary assessment as well as noting the patient's pulse and skin color, temperature, and condition to determine whether she is in decompensating shock (e.g., a barely felt radial pulse could indicate hypotension already). The injuries to her chest and abdomen most definitely could cause significant internal bleeding.

5. Yes, but given the extent of the potential internal bleeding as well as altered mental status, you should be considering rapid extrication rather than taking the time to apply a more complex extrication device. Consult with medical direction or the paramedic on the scene if you need help making this decision.

6. Cervical collar, oxygen by nonrebreather mask. Once you actually see the patient's legs, determine whether there is life-threatening bleeding that must be controlled right away and get ready to do a rapid extrication. Plan ahead and have plenty of help ready to go. Also have the suction unit nearby because the patient could vomit.

7. Yes, most trauma centers want early notice of the patient condition so that they can be ready.

CHAPTER 41: EMS Response to Terrorism

Match Key Terms

1. (I) Contamination: Contact with or presence of a material that is present where it does not belong and that is somehow harmful to persons, animals, or the environment. (p. 1280)

2. (C) Dissemination: Spreading. (p. 1280)

3. (A) Domestic terrorism: Terrorism directed against one's own government or population. (p. 1280)

4. (D) Exposure: The dose or concentration of an agent multiplied by the time or duration. (p. 1280)

5. (H) International terrorism: Terrorism that is purely foreign-based or directed. (p. 1280)

6. (E) Permeation: The movement of a substance through a surface or, on a molecular level, through intact materials; penetration, or spreading. (p. 1280)

7. (B) Rem: A measure of radiation dosage. (p. 1280)

8. (F) Routes of entry: Pathways into the body, generally by absorption, ingestion, injection, or inhalation. (p. 1280)

9. (G) Multiple devices: Destructive devices, such as bombs, including both those used in the initial attack and those placed to be activated after an initial attack and timed to injure emergency responders and others who rush in to help care for those targeted by an initial attack. (also known as "*secondary devices*".) (p. 1280)

10. (O) Strategies: Broad general plans designed to achieve desired outcomes. (p. 1280)

11. (M) Tactics: Specific operational actions to accomplish assigned tasks. (p. 1280)

12. (K) Terrorism: The unlawful use of force or violence against persons or property to intimidate or coerce a government, the civilian population, or any segment thereof, in furtherance of political or social objectives (FBI definition). (p. 1280)

13. (J) Weaponization: Packaging or producing a material, such as a chemical, biologic, or radiologic agent, so that it can be used as a weapon. (p. 1280)

14. (L) Weapons of mass destruction (WMD): Weapons, devices, or agents that are intended to cause widespread harm and/or fear in a population. (p. 1280)

15. (N) Zoonotic: Able to move through the animal-human barrier: Transmissible from animals to humans. (p. 1280)

Multiple-Choice Review

1. (B) In addition to armed attacks, the types of terrorism incidents may be remembered by using the mnemonic CBRNE. (p. 1248)

2. (C) Environmental terrorists, antigovernment militias, and racial-hate groups are examples of domestic terrorists. (p. 1246)

3. (B) The EMT should be alert to clues when on the scene of a suspicious incident. An acronym that was designed to help with this process is TRACEM-P. (p. 1251)

4. (D) Potential high-risk targets of terrorists typically include controversial businesses, infrastructure systems, and public buildings. (p. 1250)

5. (B) Why is April 19 a day when the U.S. government stands at heightened security awareness for government facilities? It is the anniversary of the bombing of the Murrah building in Oklahoma City. (p. 1251)

6. (A) Examples of unexplained patterns of illness or deaths may include all of the following except car crashes involving more than two patients with serious traumatic injuries. (p. 1251)

7. (C) The acronym TRACEM-P is designed to help rescuers understand the types of harm to which they can be exposed. The letter E stands for "etiologic." (pp. 1251–1252)

8. (B) Danger from alpha particles, beta particles, or gamma rays is caused by radiologic harm. (p. 1257)

9. (C) The major routes through which WMD agents can enter the body include all of the listed routes except osmosis. (p. 1255)

10. (D) The types of harm from radiologic or nuclear incidents include radiological, chemical, and psychological, mechanical, and thermal harm. (p. 1257)

11. (B) The primary harm from a nuclear explosion involves thermal harm. (p. 1257)

12. (B) The mainstays of self-protection at a radiologic incident include all of the listed except Standard Precautions. (p. 1257)

13. (C) You are on the scene where there is a suspicion that someone may have been exposed to anthrax. Inhalation is the most lethal route of exposure to anthrax. (p. 1266)

14. (D) The "OTTO" clues that should arouse suspicion of terrorist involvement include on-scene clues, type of event, and timing of the incident. The OTTO acronym stands for occupancy or location; type of event; timing; on-scene clues. (p. 1276)

15. (D) Features that influence the potential for a biologic agent's use of a weapon include infectivity and virulence, toxicity and incubation period, transmissibility and lethality. (pp. 1263–1264)

16. (B) When a terrorist incident is suspected at an explosion you should do each step listed except quickly moving in and evacuating patients from the scene due to risk of personal harm. (p. 1276)

17. (C) The relative ease with which an agent causes death in a susceptible population is referred to as the lethality of the agent. (p. 1264)

18. (D) The WHO declared smallpox eradicated worldwide in 1980 through immunization efforts. (p. 1268)

19. (C) During an explosion a direct consequence of the high energy over pressurization and most common cause of death is blast lung. (p. 1271)

20. (B) A virus with high human-to-human transmission would be smallpox. (p. 1264)

21. (C) In addition to mechanical harm, all of the listed types of harm can occur from an explosive incident except water damage. (p. 1258)

22. (B) What is the danger to this patient? There are often toxic particles, such as asbestos, in the dust. (p. 1258)

23. (C) In recent years, investigations in the U.S. have uncovered groups manufacturing a chemical called ricin, which is designed to interrupt the body's protein-manufacturing process at the cellular level by altering the RNA needed for proper proteins. (p. 1267)

24. (D) What could be the cause of this sickness? A viral hemorrhagic fever. (p. 1269)

Complete the Following

1. List four major routes of entry of poisons into the body. (p. 1255)
   A. Absorption
   B. Ingestion
   C. Injection
   D. Inhalation

2. List four chemical agent properties. (p. 1260)
   A. Physical considerations
   B. Volatility considerations
   C. Chemical considerations
   D. Toxicologic considerations

3. What are the five classifications of chemical agents used as a weapons? (pp. 1260–1261)
   A. Choking agents
   B. Vesicating agents

C. Cyanides
D. Nerve agents
E. Riot control agents

4. What do the letters in the mnemonic SLUDGEM stand for as a means of recalling the signs and symptoms of nerve agents? (p. 1260)
   A. Salivation
   B. Lacrimation
   C. Urination
   D. Defecation
   E. GI upsets
   F. Emesis
   G. Miosis

5. Understand what kind of harm can result from a terrorist incident and plan self-protection measures the TRACEM-P harms are: (p. 1276)
   A. Thermal
   B. Radiologic
   C. Asphyxiation
   D. Chemical
   E. Etiologic
   F. Mechanical
   G. Psychological

Interim Exam 3

1. (B) When a trauma patient is making gurgling sounds as she or he breathes, you should suction the patient's airway. (p. 1003)

2. (D) Sometimes a scoop stretcher can act as a full body splint when a critical patient must be immobilized quickly. (p. 979)

3. (A) Compared to an adult the pediatric patient in shock relies more on the heart rate to compensate for shock. (p. 792)

4. (A) Because internal bleeding is not visible, the EMT must base severity of blood loss on signs and symptoms exhibited. MOI may also be a good clue to internal injury. What the patient tells you does not reveal how much blood has been lost. (pp. 818–819)

5. (B) In a contusion, the epidermis remains intact, but cells and blood vessels in the dermis are damaged. Crush injuries may have intact skin, but often the bones and organs within the body are severely injured. (p. 827)

6. (B) Blood that oozes and is dark red is most likely from a capillary. Venous bleeding will be a steady flow of dark red or maroon blood. Arteries spurt, and their blood is usually bright red. (p. 801)

7. (C) After trying direct pressure and elevation to control the bleeding, the next step would be to apply a tourniquet to the lower arm. (p. 814)

8. (C) The care of an amputated finger or toe includes sealing the digit in a plastic bag and cooling it. (p. 843)

9. (D) You are caring for a patient that was struck by lightning. This type of injury is classified as an electrical burn. (p. 850)

10. (A) In caring for a patient with an open chest wound the EMT should rapidly prevent air from entering the chest wall injury. (p. 878)

11. (A) The signs and symptoms of internal bleeding are the same as those of shock. Patients with these signs are difficult to stabilize in the field. (p. 819)

CHAPTER 41: (continued)

12. (B) Hydrophobia is another name for a fear of water. Obstructive, cardiogenic, and neurogenic are all types of shock. (pp. 789–790)

13. (C) When the body can no longer compensate for the low blood volume, decompensated shock begins. (p. 793)

14. (C) The brain and spinal cord are the major components of the central nervous system. The peripheral nervous system includes the cranial nerves and the nerves that branch out from the spinal cord. (p. 950)

15. (D) Voluntary is a type of skeletal muscle that allows movement. The nervous system is divided into the central, peripheral, and autonomic nervous systems. (p. 950)

16. (D) The cranium consists of the temporal, occipital, frontal, and parietal bones. The maxilla is the upper jaw, and the mandible is the lower jaw. (p. 950)

17. (A) The bones that form the face include the zygomatic bones, mandible, and maxillae. Vertebrae are bones of the spine. (p. 950)

18. (A) The brain and spinal cord are bathed in cerebrospinal fluid. Lymphatic fluid is responsible for maintaining our immune system. Synovial fluid lubricates the joints. (p. 951)

19. (B) When a traumatic injury to the chest causes blood to flow into the sac surrounding the heart the condition is called cardiac tamponade. (p. 882)

20. (C) A patella dislocation is associated with which joint? Knee. (p. 895)

21. (D) The method used most often to immobilize a dislocated shoulder is the sling and swathe. (p. 928)

22. (B) Memory loss after a head injury is referred to as amnesia. (p. 954)

23. (A) She could not find a pediatric cervical collar that was the right size. What should she do? Use a rolled towel to support the neck. (p. 980)

24. (D) A collection of blood within the skull or the brain after a blunt head injury is called a subdural, epidural, or intracerebral hematoma, depending on the specific location, such as epidural (outside the dura), subdural (below the dura), or intracerebral (within the brain). (p. 955)

25. (C) The state of shock associated with a significant spinal cord injury is neurogenic. (p. 993)

26. (B) An assessment strategy that is used to check an extremity for injury or paralysis in the conscious patient is assessing equality of strength by checking hand grip or pushing against the patient's hands and feet. (p. 975)

27. (B) Which MOI is often associated with multi-system trauma? Fall > 20 feet. (p. 1001)

28. (D) In a patient who has a significant brain injury with skull fracture, the pupils tend to be unequal. (p. 957)

29. (D) A patient with a TBI has increased blood pressure and decreased pulse. (p. 957)

30. (B) The spinal column is made up of 33 irregularly shaped bones. (p. 951)

31. (B) Any blunt trauma above the clavicles may damage the cervical vertebrae. (p. 952)

32. (A) Priapism is a persistent erection of the penis. (p. 974)

33. (B) The EMT should consider that any fall injury to an older adult could be an indicator of possible abuse or neglect. (p. 951)

34. (C) Obesity is defined as a condition of having a body mass index or BMI of 30 or more. (p. 1106)

35. (D) As a normal process of aging, geriatric patients lose skin elasticity and sweat glands shrink. This results in thin, dry, wrinkled skin. (p. 1016)

36. (D) When caring for a child with autism the EMT should remember that communication can be challenging so consider using a picture card system to help the patient express their needs. (p. 1108)

37. (D) The EMT may be called to care for an infant with a congenital disease. This means that the patient was born with an abnormal condition. (p. 1116)

38. (C) An unstable foreign object impaled through the cheek wall should be pulled out if both ends of the object can be seen and this can be easily done. This minimizes the potential for bleeding into the airway. (p. 841)

39. (D) The femoral artery is most likely bleeding, and a tourniquet will be needed to control the bleeding. (p. 816)

40. (A) A tracheostomy is a surgical opening in the neck that provides an opening into the trachea. (p. 1117)

41. (B) The best method for control of nasal bleeding is pinching the nostrils together. (p. 817)

42. (C) The first step in caring for possible internal bleeding is treating for shock. Do not place the patient in a sitting position if you suspect shock. (p. 820)

43. (D) The condition in which a flap of skin is torn loose completely is called an avulsion. (p. 832)

44. (C) After controlling profuse bleeding in a patient who has an object impaled in the forearm, you should stabilize the object. Do not remove the object. (p. 840)

45. (D) Pale, cool, clammy skin is a sign of shock. (p. 796)

46. (A) An object impaled in the eye should be stabilized with gauze and protected with a disposable cup. It is also important to cover the other eye to limit movement of the eyes. (p. 842)

47. (B) The EMT may be called to care for a patient with a stoma in the neck because it has become blocked, thereby obstructing the patient's airway. (p. 1118)

48. (C) Before moving a supine patient with possible spinal injuries onto your stretcher, you should always apply a cervical collar. (p. 978)

49. (A) The initial effort to control bleeding from a severed neck artery should be direct pressure or pinching. Then apply the occlusive dressing. Remember Standard Precautions. (p. 965)

50. (B) The most reliable sign of spinal-cord injury in conscious patients is paralysis of extremities. Tenderness along the spine may indicate injury to the bones or muscles. (p. 972)

51. (D) When caring for an open abdominal wound with evisceration, do not replace the organ but cover it with a moistened dressing. (p. 889)

52. (C) A patient in acute abdominal distress without vomiting should be transported in the supine position (face up) with the knees bent to relieve the pressure on the abdominal muscles. (p. 888)

53. (D) There is a power outage in your area of response and you are called to the home of a patient with a home ventilator. What should you be prepared to do when you arrive? Assist ventilations with a bag-valve-mask. (p. 1119)

54. (D) A fracture to the proximal end of the humerus is best cared for by immobilizing with a sling and swathe. (p. 916)

55. (B) The best way to immobilize a fractured elbow when the arm is found in the bent position and there is a distal pulse is to keep the arm in its found position and apply a short, paddled splint. Do not straighten fractured joints that have pulses. (p. 931)

56. (B) When splinting, if a severe deformity exists or distal circulation is compromised, you should align to the anatomical position with gentle traction. (p. 908)

57. (D) A patient with a fractured pelvis should be immobilized on a long spine board with a pelvic wrap. (pp. 918–919)

58. (D) A fractured femur is best immobilized with a traction splint. (p. 914)

59. (A) Before immobilizing a fractured knee, assess for distal circulation and sensory and motor function. If there is no pulse, you may need to manipulate the extremity. (p. 925)

60. (B) A sprain is an injury in which ligaments are torn. (p. 904)

61. (C) Definitive care for open extremity injuries is not provided in the prehospital setting. (p. 904)

62. (D) Muscle is attached to bone by tendons. (p. 902)

63. (A) The entire back of an adult patient's right upper extremity is 4.5% (the entire arm is 9%, so half is 4.5%), and the entire chest is 9%; therefore 9 + 4.5 = 13.5%. (p. 849)

64. (A) Partial-thickness burns cause swelling and blistering. (p. 847)

65. (D) A patient who suffers chemical burns to the skin caused by dry lime should be treated by first brushing away the lime. Dry lime should not be mixed with water or phenol. (p. 854)

66. (D) Acid burns to the eyes should be flooded with water for at least 20 minutes. (p. 855)

67. (A) A method for estimating the extent of a burn is the rule of nines. (p. 848)

68. (D) If a woman is having her first baby, the first stage of labor will usually last an average of 16 hours. (p. 1062)

69. (B) During the most active stage of labor, the uterus usually contracts every 2 to 3 minutes (with contractions commonly lasting 30 seconds to 1 minute). (p. 1061)

70. (C) If the amniotic sac does not break during delivery, the EMT should puncture it with a finger, then remove the membranes from the baby's nose and mouth. (p. 1070)

71. (B) To assist the mother in delivering the baby's shoulders, gently support the baby's head. Do not pull on the infant. (p. 1070)

72. (C) If spontaneous respiration does not begin after the baby's mouth and nose have been suctioned, the EMT should vigorously rub the baby's back, then consider mechanical ventilatory assistance. (p. 1075)

73. (D) An implanted pacemaker helps the patient by delivering an electrical shock to restore a normal rhythm. (p. 1120)

74. (D) The AICD is permanently placed under the patient's skin. (p. 1121)

75. (C) The steps in order should be sizing up the situation, stabilizing the vehicle, gaining the access, and disentangling the patient. (p. 1219)

76. (B) A battery powered mechanical pump that is implanted in the body to assist the heart in pumping blood is the ventricular assist device. (p. 1121)

77. (C) To minimize injuries at a collision, EMTs should wear highly visible clothing to minimize the risk of getting hit by another vehicle while attending to the patient. (p. 1217)

78. (A) Opening the trunk and disconnecting the battery cable are not priority tasks. The three-step process of disentanglement described in the text includes creating exit ways by displacing doors and roof posts, disentangling occupants by displacing the front end, and gaining access by disposing of the roof. (pp. 1237–1238)

79. (B) If a vehicle's electrical system must be disrupted, disconnect the negative (ground) cable from the battery. (p. 1230)

80. (D) When positioning flares, use a formula that includes the stopping distance for the posted speed plus the margin of safety. (p. 1218)

81. (C) Once the vehicle has been stabilized, the next part of an extrication procedure for patient rescue is to displace doors and roof posts. (p. 1237)

82. (D) A nasogastric tube is used to: administer medications, suction out the stomach contents, and deliver nutrients. (p. 1123)

83. (C) The EMD does not need to ask the person's name in order to initiate EMS response. All other questions are pertinent. (p. 1152)

84. (A) The continuous sound of a siren could worsen a patient's condition. The noise from the siren can also damage your ears over a period of time. Not all motorists will hear and honor the siren. If you use the siren continuously, there should be a valid reason for doing so. (p. 1154)

85. (A) A common problem that the EMT will find associated with urinary catheters is infection. (p. 1125)

86. (C) When transferring a nonemergency patient to ED personnel, you should check to see what should be done with the patient. (p. 1164)

87. (C) At the hospital, as soon as you are free from patient-care activities, you should prepare the prehospital care report. (p. 1164)

88. (C) The patient that requires dialysis has renal failure. (p. 1125)

89. (B) A patient that is receiving dialysis will have a fistula that is most commonly located on the arm. (p. 1125)

90. (C) The first clamp placed on the umbilical cord should be about 10 inches from the baby. (p. 1073)

91. (A) The maximum amount of time to wait for the placenta to be delivered before transporting is 20 minutes. (p. 1078)

92. (A) Delivery of the placenta is usually accompanied by the loss of no more than 500 cc of blood. (p. 1079)

93. (B) Along with physical and mental fitness, ambulance operators should be able to perform under stress. (p. 1153)

94. (B) A child with special health needs may have a ventriculoperitoneal (VP) shunt which drains fluid from the brain. (p. 1127)

95. (B) If upon viewing the vaginal area, you see the umbilical cord presenting first (a prolapsed cord delivery), you should gently push up on the baby's head or buttocks to keep pressure off the cord. Do not cut the cord because it is the infant's blood supply. Never attempt to push the cord back into the vagina. (p. 1083)

96. (C) If you note an arm presentation without a prolapsed cord, transport immediately, providing high-concentration oxygen. (p. 1082)

97. (C) A baby is considered premature if the baby weighs less than 5 pounds or is born before the thirty-seventh week. (p. 1085)

98. (C) The three primary ways in which elders can be abused or neglected are physically, psychologically, and financially. (p. 1133)

99. (A) The most effective technique to slow the spread of venom after a snakebite may be to immobilize the affected extremity. (p. 1045)

100. (A) When a patient who was working in a hot environment complains of severe muscle cramps in the legs and feeling faint, you should move the patient to a cool place and begin care by administering oxygen. (p. 1027)

101. (A) An emergency vehicle operator must drive with due regard for other drivers on the road. (p. 1153)

102. (C) Injuries to the back, legs, and upper arms might lead you to consider child abuse. Multiple skinned knees and sprained ankles are common in children. (p. 1129)

103. (D) With early frostbite, the patient may complain of burning or tingling at the site. (p. 1023)

104. (A) The initial sign of hypothermia is shivering. (p. 1019)

105. (A) Extreme hypothermia is characterized by unconsciousness and absence of discernible vital signs. If there is shivering, numbness, and drowsiness, the patient is not yet in severe hypothermia. (p. 1022)

106. (D) Having a police car escort an ambulance to the hospital creates additional hazards for the ambulance. (p. 1156)

107. (D) What agency has a system for identifying hazardous materials via placards that indicate the nature of the hazardous contents? National Highway and Traffic Safety Association. (p. 1182)

108. (B) The best way to stabilize a vehicle involved in a collision before gaining access to a patient is to use three step chocks. (p. 1232)

109. (C) Considering blast injury patterns, the parts of the body that are especially vulnerable to injuries are the lungs, ears, brain, and abdomen. (p. 1271)

110. (B) Terrorists have a history of setting traps for emergency responders that arrive on the scene of an initial attack. The term related to harming the responders in this way is secondary devices. (p. 1249)

111. (D) The strong, white, fibrous material covering the bones is the periosteum. (p. 894)

112. (C) The coming apart of a joint is referred to as a dislocation. (p. 904)

113. (A) Overstretching or overexertion of a muscle is called a strain. (p. 904)

114. (B) A patient with hot and dry or hot and moist skin is experiencing a true emergency that requires rapid cooling and immediate transport. (p. 1028)

115. (B) The primary type of harm from biologic incidents is etiologic. (p. 1256)

116. (C) To treat a patient with deep frostbite, cover the frostbitten area, handle it as gently as possible, and transport the patient. Do not rub the area or apply cold. Do not rewarm the area unless you can ensure that it will not refreeze. (p. 1024)

117. (C) The indications for a traction splint are painful, swollen, and deformed mid-thigh with no joint or lower leg injury. (p. 915)

118. (C) The Hazardous Materials Technician actually plugs, patches, or stops the release of a hazardous material. (p. 1181)

119. (C) The safe zone should be established on the same level as and upwind from the hazardous materials accident site. This positioning prevents flowing liquids or burning gases from spreading into the safe zone. (p. 1181)

120. (B) A resource that must be maintained at the work site by the employer and that must be available to all employees working with hazardous materials is the safety data sheets. This SDS generally names the substance, its physical properties, fire and explosion hazard information, health hazard information, and emergency first-aid treatment. (p. 1185)

121. (B) EMS personnel at a hazmat incident are responsible for caring for the injured and monitoring and rehabilitating the hazmat team members. (p. 1186)

122. (D) Categorizing a patient as Priority 1 at an MCI means the patient has treatable life-threatening illness or injuries. (p. 1202)

123. (B) The MCI officer who is responsible for communicating with each treatment area to determine the number and priority of the patients in that sector is the triage supervisor. (p. 1209)

124. (C) A Priority 2 patient at an MCI would be color-coded yellow. Priority 1 patients would be coded red, Priority 3 would be coded green, and Priority 4 would be coded black or gray. (p. 1202)

125. (C) Patients at an MCI who are assessed to have minor injuries are categorized as Priority 3. (p. 1202)

APPENDIX A: Basic Cardiac Life Support Review

Multiple-Choice Review

1. (D) Once clinical death occurs, brain cells begin to die within 4 to 6 minutes. However, it usually takes 10 minutes for biological death to occur. (p. 1283)

2. (C) In the CAB sequence of cardiopulmonary resuscitation, the A stands for "airway." (p. 1283)

©2021 Pearson Education, Inc.
Emergency Care, 14th Ed.

3. (C) In the CAB sequence of cardiopulmonary resuscitation, the C stands for "circulation" (or "compressions" since the circulation portion of the CAB procedure starts with chest compressions). (p. 1283)

4. (D) To determine whether an adult or child is pulseless, the EMT should check for a pulse at the carotid artery. (p. 1283)

5. (A) To determine pulselessness in an infant, the EMT should use the brachial artery because the carotid pulse is difficult to determine in an infant. (p. 1283)

6. (B) If you are alone and have determined unresponsiveness in an adult, the next thing you should do before starting CPR is to activate EMS. (p. 1283)

7. (C) When an unconscious patient's head flexes forward, the tongue could cause an airway obstruction. (pp. 1284–1285)

8. (C) The head-tilt, chin-lift maneuver should not be used on a diving accident victim because of the potential for cervical-spine injury. (p. 1285)

9. (A) The recommended maneuver for opening the airway of a patient with possible cervical-spine injury is the jaw-thrust maneuver. (p. 1285)

10. (B) In an adult patient who requires rescue breathing, the EMT should watch for chest rise while ventilating 10 to 12 times a minute. (p. 1286)

11. (C) Initial ventilations did not result in chest rise. Your next step is to perform the steps of CPR. (p. 1293)

12. (B) A problem in the resuscitation of infants and children caused by improper head position or too quick ventilations is gastric distention. (p. 1286)

13. (C) In child rescue breathing, the EMT provides 12–20 breaths every minute. (p. 1287)

14. (A) Infants should be ventilated at the rate of 12 to 20 breaths per minute, which is one breath every 3 to 5 seconds. (p. 1286)

15. (C) When a patient has a distended abdomen due to air being forced into the stomach, the EMT should be prepared to suction if the patient vomits (and if trained and prepared to do so). Do not decrease the oxygen concentration. Pressing on the abdomen would produce vomiting. (p. 1288)

16. (A) The recovery protects the airway and allows for drainage from the mouth. It also prevents the tongue rolling back to block the airway. (p. 1288)

17. (D) The adult CPR compression point is located on the middle of the sternum, centered between the nipples. (p. 1289)

18. (A) Before beginning CPR, the health care provider should assess the patient's pulse for a maximum of 10 seconds. (p. 1290)

19. (D) For an adult, the one-rescuer compression-to-ventilations ratio is 30:2. (p. 1290)

20. (C) The adult CPR compression rate in one-rescuer CPR is 100 to 120 times a minute. (p. 1292)

21. (C) The child CPR compression rate in two-rescuer CPR is 100 to 120 times a minute. (p. 1292)

22. (B) The compression depth for an adult should be at least 2 inches.(p. 1292)

23. (C) The compression depth for an infant should be one-third the depth of the chest (approximately 1½ inches). (p. 1292)

24. (B) The compression-to-ventilation ratio for a young child or infant when there are two rescuers should be 15:2. (p. 1292)

25. (C) The compression-to-ventilation ratio for a young child or infant when there is only one rescuer doing the CPR is 30:2. (p. 1292)

26. (C) When opening the airway of an infant, use a slight head- tilt. Full hyperextension of the neck can cause the airway to occlude. (p. 1290)

27. (B) With effective CPR, the patient's pupils may constrict. Dilation occurs when the patient is hypoxic. (p. 1290)

28. (C) CPR compressions are delivered to children with the heel of one hand. The fingertips are used to deliver compressions for infants. (p. 1291)

29. (B) Except when defibrillation and advanced cardiac life support measures are being initiated, CPR should not be interrupted for more than 10 seconds. (p. 1291)

30. (B) If you are treating a patient with a partial airway obstruction, poor air exchange, and gray skin, you should treat the patient for a complete airway obstruction. (p. 1293)

31. (B) Complete airway obstruction in a conscious patient is indicated by an inability to speak. Crowing, gurgling, and snoring are all sounds of partial airway obstruction. (p. 1293)

32. (C) When you recognize complete airway obstruction in a conscious adult patient, you should deliver manual abdominal thrusts until the obstruction is relieved. Only unconscious patients are placed in a supine position when ventilations are attempted. (p. 1293)

33. (D) You should continue with chest thrusts, look in the mouth to remove visible objects, and provide ventilations, in that order. (pp. 1293–1294)

34. (C) When treating a woman who is eight months pregnant and has a complete airway obstruction, use chest thrusts. (p. 1293)

35. (B) If a patient has a partial airway obstruction and is able to speak and cough forcefully, you should carefully watch the patient. Do not interfere with the patient's attempts to expel the foreign body. However, be prepared to provide help if the partial airway obstruction becomes a complete obstruction. (p. 1293)

36. (C) Which of the following is not correct procedure for clearing an obstructed airway? Do not use blind finger sweeps with infants or adults. Only remove objects you can see. Blind sweeps may push an object deeper into the airway (p. 1293)

37. (A) If opening the airway, looking in the mouth, and attempting to ventilate fail, begin CPR compressions. (p. 1293)

38. (B) Your next step is to perform back blows and chest thrusts. (p. 1293)

39. (D) Signs of choking in an infant are lack of a strong cry, ineffective cough, agitation, wheezing, blue color, and breathing difficulty. (pp. 1293–1294)

40. (B) In health care provider CPR training, infants are up to 1 year of age, children are from 1 year to puberty, and adults are from puberty to death. Remember that citizen CPR courses do not teach this distinction and still define a child as age 1 to 8 years. (p. 1292)

APPENDIX A: (continued)

Complete the Following

1. List six special circumstances in which CPR should *not* be initiated by the EMT even though the patient has no pulse. (pp. 1291–1292)
   A. A line of lividity is present
   B. Obvious decomposition
   C. Obvious mortal wounds
   D. Rigor mortis
   E. Stillbirth
   F. Valid DNR

2. Once the EMT has started CPR, list six situations in which CPR and be stopped. (p. 1292)
   A. Spontaneous circulation occurs (then provide rescue breathing as needed).
   B. Spontaneous circulation and breathing occur.
   C. Another trained rescuer can take over for you.
   D. You turn care of the patient over to a person with a higher level of training.
   E. You receive a "no CPR" order from a physician or other authority per local protocols.
   F. You are too exhausted to continue.

3. The information missing from the chart is as follows: (p. 1292)
   • **(A):** at least 2 inches
   • **(B):** 100 to 120/minute
   • **(C):** 1 second
   • **(D):** Carotid artery (throat)
   • **(E):** 30:2
   • **(F):** 30:2 15:2 (2 rescuers)

Comprehensive Final Exam

1. A	2. B	3. D	4. D	5. A	6. A
7. C	8. A	9. B	10. C	11. A	12. C
13. A	14. A	15. C	16. D	17. C	18. D
19. C	20. B	21. A	22. B	23. B	24. A
25. C	26. C	27. C	28. A	29. A	30. D
31. D	32. B	33. A	34. D	35. D	36. C
37. B	38. C	39. A	40. D	41. A	42. B
43. D	44. C	45. D	46. C	47. C	48. B
49. D	50. C	51. B	52. C	53. B	54. D
55. B	56. A	57. D	58. B	59. C	60. A
61. C	62. C	63. A	64. B	65. D	66. C
67. A	68. D	69. C	70. B	71. A	72. C
73. C	74. D	75. D	76. A	77. B	78. C
79. A	80. B	81. B	82. D	83. A	84. C
85. C	86. B	87. D	88. B	89. C	90. B
91. B	92. C	93. D	94. C	95. C	96. A
97. D	98. B	99. D	100. C		